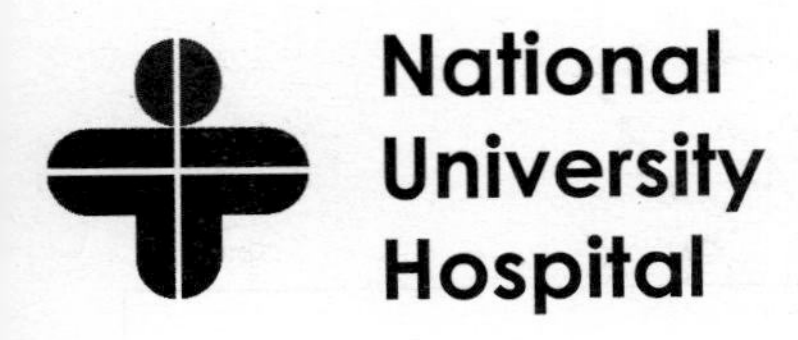

W9-BFL-961

GUIDE TO THE ESSENTIALS IN Emergency Medicine

edited by
Shirley Ooi
Peter Manning

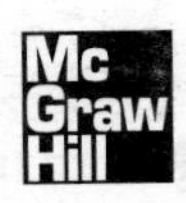

Singapore • Boston • Burr Ridge, IL • Dubuque, IA • Madison, WI • New York • San Francisco
St. Louis • Bangkok • Bogotá • Caracas • Kuala Lumpur • Lisbon • London • Madrid
Mexico City • Milan • Montreal • New Delhi • Santiago • Seoul • Sydney • Taipei • Toronto

The McGraw·Hill Companies

Notice

Medicine is an ever-changing science. As new research and clinical experience broaden our knowledge, changes in treatment and drug therapy are required. The authors and publisher of this work have checked with sources believed to be reliable in their efforts to provide information that is complete and generally in accord with the standards accepted at the time of publication. However, in view of the possibility of human error or changes in medical sciences, neither the authors nor the publisher nor any other party who has been involved in the preparation or publication of this work warrants that the information contained herein is in every respect accurate or complete, and they disclaim all responsibility for any errors or omissions or for the results obtained from use of the information contained in this work. Readers are encouraged to confirm the information contained herein with other sources. For example and in particular, readers are advised to check the product information sheet included in the package of each drug they plan to administer to be certain that the information contained in this work is accurate and that changes have not been made in the recommended dose or in the contraindications for administration. This recommendation is of particular importance in connection with new or infrequently used drugs.

Guide to the Essentials in Emergency Medicine

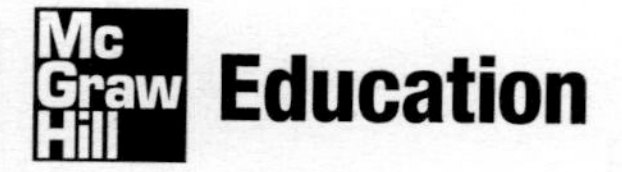

Copyright © 2004 by McGraw-Hill Education (Asia). All rights reserved. No part of this publication may be reproduced or distributed in any form or by any means, or stored in a data base or retrieval system, without the prior written permission of the publisher.

2 3 4 5 6 7 8 9 10 LG SLP 08 07 06 05 04

When ordering this title, use ISBN 007-122631-1

Printed in Singapore

To

God, the source of all my inspiration, perseverance and strength

my family for their love, sacrifice and support

Shirley Ooi

the teaching of Emergency Medicine in Singapore

Peter Manning

all past and present staff of NUH EMD

Shirley Ooi and Peter Manning

… this long-needed local guide to the practice of Emergency Medicine … is eminently readable, current, succinct and systematically presented.

Clinical Assoc. Prof. V Anantharaman, President, Society for Emergency Medicine in Singapore and Senior Consultant Emergency Physician, Singapore General Hospital

… *Guide to the Essentials in Emergency Medicine* represents an outstanding effort … is clearly written and … [a] most useful reference for any individual working or training in an Emergency Department.

Prof. W. Brian Gibler, Chairman, Department of Emergency Medicine, University of Cincinnati College of Medicine

… there is accumulated experience and wisdom in its pages … This book should be in the lab coat pocket or on the desk of all doctors who have to deal with emergencies and urgent medical problems in one way or another.

Assoc. Prof. Goh Lee Gan, Dept. of Community, Occupational and Family Medicine, Medical Faculty, National University of Singapore, and Regional President, World Organisation of Family Doctors (WONCA), Asia Pacific Region

Emergency departments see an enormous range of illnesses, injuries and problems. ... This book ... is an excellent source of practical guidelines and should be widely used.

Dr. Robin Illingworth, Consultant in Accident and Emergency Medicine, St James's University Hospital, Leeds, UK, and Senior Clinical Lecturer in Accident and Emergency Medicine, University of Leeds.

A handy and practical guide for the management of common emergencies … clearly presented in point form for quick reference: a good book for medical students and postgraduate trainees.

Prof. Lee Eng Hin, Director of Graduate Medical Studies, National University of Singapore

Pocket-sized and highly practical, readers will find this book evidence-based and representing the best practices of … Emergency Medicine.

Prof. John Wong Eu-Li, Dean, Faculty of Medicine, National University of Singapore

Contents

Foreword

Most doctors have only limited exposure to the Emergency Department during their undergraduate training. Except for a few short weeks, students deal mainly with stable patients, and are taught medicine in a compartmentalized manner. Most of the time, the patients they come into contact with are already labelled with a diagnosis, and classified by disease or organ system according to the posting they are doing. It is not surprising that when they are posted to the Emergency Department during the early years of postgraduate training, most feel inadequate to deal with the myriad of medical and surgical emergencies in patients of all age groups. Apart from seniors' guidance, most would welcome a readable handbook for quick reference.

The *Guide to the Essentials in Emergency Medicine* is written almost exclusively by staff at the Emergency Medicine Department, National University Hospital, Singapore. Despite their busy clinical and teaching duties, the authors managed to produce this concise but informative book which addresses the many situations and emergencies commonly encountered in a busy emergency department. The book is written in an easy to read style, and its content is evidence-based. The format allows for rapid access to information on assessment, diagnosis, investigation and management of emergency patients.

I congratulate Drs Manning and Ooi, and their colleagues, for writing this book, which will benefit medical/dental students, and doctors doing their emergency posting. I believe even nursing and other ancillary staffs who work in the environment will find this book handy and useful.

Associate Professor Lim Yean Teng
Chairman Medical Board/Senior Consultant Cardiologist
National University Hospital, Singapore

Preface

The contents of this handbook have been developed from the National University Hospital's Emergency Medicine Department (NUH EMD) Clinical Guidelines. First established by the department's senior physicians in 1998, the purpose of the guidelines was to ensure a minimum standard of medical care for the hospital's patients. Through the years, resident doctors serving their Emergency Medicine (EM) postings with the hospital have found these guidelines to be very helpful in their daily practice, leading to its publication in the form of a handbook.

This handy pocket guide aims to be a comprehensive and updated resource for all levels of practitioners who encounter emergency situations, from medical students to medical officers to practising Emergency Physicians. Its contributors are mainly current and former department staff, with some invited 'guest contributions'. To ensure that representative views are reflected, peer review was sought from colleagues from medical departments of various hospitals.

As this is not meant to be a textbook on EM, we have not included detailed pathophysiology, and clinical descriptions are kept concise. The emphasis of this handbook is on the practical management of 90–95% of common emergency conditions.

This book is divided into 3 main sections:

Section 1: Common Presentations

- This section is essential reading for junior doctors, general practitioners and medical students, and it presents a *symptom-based approach* to problems before a clear-cut diagnosis is made.
- Presented from the balanced viewpoint of an Emergency Physician, long and impractical lists of diagnoses are excluded and emphasis is on the most life-threatening and common conditions. For example, when an approach to chest pain is given by a cardiologist, the cardiac causes of chest pain are given more emphasis than the non-cardiac causes. This is not so when it is written by an Emergency Physician who sees the cases presented in an *undifferentiated form.*
- A unique feature of this book is the section on *Caveats*, where we share the pitfalls likely to be encountered in medical practice. This will be particularly useful to those involved in this area.
- *Special Tips for GPs* is a section written specially for general practitioners and those who provide prehospital care for patients such as paramedics.

It highlights what can be done before a patient arrives at a hospital's Emergency Department (ED).

Section 2: Specific Conditions

- This section covers both adult and paediatric conditions.
- Chapters in this section are a practical guide to managing the various conditions that commonly occur after a diagnosis has been made. Medical conditions mentioned in Section 1 are referred to Section 2 for more details.

Section 3: Other Useful Information

- This section covers miscellaneous topics such as useful formulae, tetanus immunization schedules, conscious sedation, pain management, views of X-rays to order, list of drugs to avoid in pregnancy, G6PD deficiency as well as simple statistics.

This book is meant for:

- *Medical Officers (Residents)* serving their *EM rotations* and *Emergency Nurses*. This will be a quick reference for at least 90–95% of the most commonly encountered conditions in their daily practice.
- *Basic and Advanced Emergency Medicine Trainees preparing for their postgraduate exams*. The information in this book provides a good foundation for most of the common conditions encountered in the practice of EM.
- *Medical Students serving their rotations at the ED*. This is the first locally written book detailing virtually all the common conditions that they may encounter during their EM posting. Section 1 is practical, focused and concise, and students should be able to finish reading it within their 3-week posting.
- *House Officers* and *Medical Officers serving their rotations other than EM*. This book will assist them in treating multidisciplinary emergencies as these can arise unexpectedly in the course of their work. It will help them to manage the patient in that first half-hour while awaiting additional help.
- *General Practitioners*. This book will guide them on how to treat multidisciplinary emergencies within the first half-hour while arrangements are made to send their patients to a hospital's ED. Of particular interest will be the *Special Tips for GPs* sections.
- *Paramedics* and *Prehospital Care Personnel*. Section 1 and *Special Tips for GPs* will be very useful in guiding them on the symptom-based approach to emergency conditions.

This book would not have been possible without the invaluable help of the numerous contributors and reviewers. We wish to specially acknowledge the tireless and dedicated efforts of our department executive, Joyce Loke, who has assisted us in countless ways from start to finish. Without her, this book would not have been possible. Our Registrar, Dr. Lee Kuan Wee and our former Medical Officer, Dr. Loh Chi Yuan, deserve special mention for putting in countless hours to proofread the manuscript. We also wish to thank our former staff nurse, David Koo, for his help in formatting a few chapters. We are also grateful to our former and present Medical Officers who have given us useful feedback on our department's clinical guidelines. Eunice Toh, former Director of the NUH Endowment Fund and Corporate Affairs, also deserves special mention for her advice and general support. We would like to acknowledge the NUH Endowment Fund for its support towards medical education. We are also grateful to Associate Professor Lim Yean Teng, Chairman, Medical Board of NUH for penning the Foreword, Professor John Wong, Dean of the Faculty of Medicine National University of Singapore (NUS), Professor Lee Eng Hin, Director of Graduate Medical Studies NUS, Clinical Associate Professor V Anantharaman, President of the Society of Emergency Medicine in Singapore, and Associate Professor Goh Lee Gan, Censor-in-Chief from College of Family Physicians, Dr. Robin Illingworth, Consultant in Accident and Emergency Medicine, St. James's University Hospital, Leeds, UK, and Professor Brian Gibler, Chairman of the Department of Medicine, University of Cincinnati College of Medicine for endorsing the book. Finally, we would like to thank Ms. Cheong Yun Wan, former Senior Editor of McGraw-Hill Education (Asia), for her help in publishing this book.

We hope that you will find this guide useful and welcome your feedback about the book. You can email your feedback to lokepc@nuh.com.sg.

Dr Shirley Ooi Beng Suat
Clinical Associate Professor Peter George Manning

Contributors

Emergency Medicine Department, National University Hospital, Singapore

Chong Chew Lan
MBBS (S'pore), MRCSEd (A&E)
Registrar

Ibrahim, Irwani
MBBS (S'pore), FRCSEd (A&E)
Registrar

Lee Kuan Wee
MBBS (S'pore), MRCSEd (A&E), MMed (Emergency Med)
Registrar

Lee Sock Koon
MBBS (S'pore), MRCSEd (A&E), MMed (Emergency Med)
Registrar

Leong Sieu-Hon, Benjamin
MBBS (S'pore), MRCSEd (A&E), MMed (Emergency Med)
Registrar

Mahadevan, Malcolm
MBBS (S'pore), MRCP (UK), FRCSEd (A&E), FAMS
Consultant

Manning, Peter George
MBBS (London), FACEP
Chief and Senior Consultant

Ooi Beng Suat, Shirley
MBBS (S'pore), FRCSEd (A&E), FAMS
Senior Consultant

Peng Li Lee
MBBS (S'pore), FRCSEd (A&E)
Associate Consultant

Pillai, Suresh
MBBS (S'pore), FRCSEd (A&E)
Consultant

Quek Lit Sin
MBBS (S'pore), FRCSEd (A&E), MMed (Emergency Med)
Registrar

Seet Chong Meng
MBBS (S'pore), MRCP (UK), FRCSEd (A&E)
Consultant

Guest Contributors

The late Alexandre Chao
Consultant
Department of Surgery
Tan Tock Seng Hospital, Singapore

Khor Sek Hoon, Elizabeth
MBBS (S'pore), MMed (Paeds) FAMS
Senior Consultant
Department of Paediatrics
National University Hospital, Singapore

Lee Chun Yue, Francis
MBBS (S'pore), FRCSEd (A&E), FAMS
Chief and Consultant
Department of Emergency Medicine
Alexandra Hospital, Singapore

Lee Yin Mei
MB ChB, MRCP (UK)
Consultant
Department of Medicine
National University Hospital, Singapore

Lim Seng Gee
MBBS, MD, FRACP, CertImm (Monash), FAMS
Senior Consultant and Associate Professor
Department of Medicine
National University Hospital, Singapore

Mak Seck Wai, Kenneth
MBBS, FRCS (Edin)
Consultant
Department of Surgery
National University Hospital, Singapore

Nalachandran, Sanjay
MB BCh BAO (Ireland), MRCS (Surgery) (Edin), AFRCS (Ire) 2001
Registrar
Department of Surgery
Tan Tock Seng Hospital, Singapore

Rajnakova, Andrea
MD (Slovakia), MMed (Int Med) (Slovakia), MRCP (UK), MMed (Int Med) PhD
Registrar
Department of Medicine
National University Hospital, Singapore

Travers, James Peregrine
BSc (Hons), MBChB, FRCS (England), PhD
Senior Consultant
Department of Emergency Medicine
Alexandra Hospital, Singapore

Tsang Bih Shiou, Charles
MBBS (S'pore), MMed (Surg), MS (Exp. Surg), FRCS (Edin), FRCS (Glasg), FICS, FAMS
Consultant
Department of Surgery
National University Hospital, Singapore

Wong Chin Khoon
MBBS (S'pore), MMed (Paediatrics), FAMS
Consultant
Children's Emergency
National University Hospital, Singapore

Yam Pei Yuan, John
MBBS (S'pore), MRCOG (London), MMed O&G (S'pore), HRANZCOG (Australia & New Zealand
Associate Consultant
Department of General Obstetrics and Gynaecology
KK Women's and Children's Hospital

Reviewers

Alexandra Hospital, Singapore
Dr. Pang Weng Sun
Senior Consultant
Department of Geriatrics
Geriatric emergencies

Changi General Hospital, Singapore
Dr. Goh Siang Hiong
Chief and Senior Consultant
Department of Emergency Medicine
Alcohol intoxication, Assault, Diving emergencies, Electrical & lightning injuries, Hyperthermia, Near drowning, Useful formulae, Violent/suicidal patient, Tetanus immunization schedule, Tetanus

KK Women's and Children's Hospital, Singapore
Dr. Ang, Angelina
Associate Consultant
Department of Emergency Medicine
Child with breathlessness, Febrile fit, Child, fitting

Dr. Ng Kee Chong
Consultant
Department of Emergency Medicine
Child/baby, crying, Child with diarrhoea, Child with vomiting, Fluid replacement in paediatrics, Paediatric drugs and equipment, Child with abdominal pain, Conscious sedation

Dr. Tham Lai Peng
Consultant
Department of Emergency Medicine
Child with fever

Ministry of Health, Singpore
Dr. Chan Yiong Huak
Head of Statistics
Clinical Trials & Epidemiology Research Unit
Simple statistics

National University Hospital, Singapore

Dr. Ang Kian Chuan
Consultant
Department of Orthopaedic Surgery
Crush syndrome

A/Prof. Biswas, Arijit
Senior Consultant
Department of Obstetrics & Gynaecology
Bleeding, vaginal, abnormal, Pelvic inflammatory disease

Dr. Chan Poon Lap, Bernard
Consultant
Department of Medicine
Stroke

A/Prof. Chew Tec Kuan, Paul
Chief and Senior Consultant
Department of Ophthalmology
Blurring of vision, acute, Red and painful eye

Prof. Chia Boon Lock
Senior Consultant
Cardiac Department
Palpitations

Dr. Chionh Siok Bee
Consultant
Department of Medicine
Adrenal insufficiency, acute, Diabetic ketoacidosis (DKA), Hyperosmolar hyperglycaemic state (HHS), Hypoglycaemia, Thyrotoxic crisis

Dr. Consigliere, David Terrence
Ag. Chief and Senior Consultant
Department of Urology
Urinary retention, acute, Pain, scrotal and penile, Urolithiasis

Dr. Goh Boon Cher
Consultant
Department of Haematology – Oncology
Oncology emergencies

Dr. Goh Poh Sun
Consultant
Department of Diagnostic Imaging
Views of x-rays to order

A/Prof. Goh Yam Thiam, Daniel
Consultant
Department of Paediatrics
Bronchiolitis, Asthma, paediatric

Dr. Habib, Abdulrazaq G
Associate Consultant
Department of Medicine
Dengue fever, Malaria

Asst. Prof. Hui Hoi Po, James
Consultant
Department of Orthopaedic Surgery
Trauma, upper limb, Trauma, lower limb

Dr. Khor Sek Hoon, Elizabeth
Senior Consultant
Department of Paediatrics
Non-accidental injury in paediatrics

A/Prof. Koh Kwong Fah
Former Senior Consultant
Department of Anaesthesia
Airway management / Rapid sequence intubation

A/Prof. Kum Cheng Kiong
Former Consultant
Department of Surgery
Appendicitis, acute

A/Prof. Lee Kam Yiu, Timothy
Former Senior Consultant
Department of Surgery
Trauma, head, Subarachnoid haemorrhage (SAH)

A/Prof. Lee Kang Hoe
Senior Consultant
Department of Medicine
Haemoptysis

A/Prof. Lim Beng Hai
Chief and Senior Consultant
Department of Hand & Reconstructive Microsurgery
Trauma and infections, hand

A/Prof. Lim Seng Gee
Senior Consultant
Department of Medicine
Hepatic encephalopathy, acute

A/Prof. Lim Thiam Chye
Senior Consultant
Department of Surgery
Burns, major, Burns, minor, Wound care, Trauma, maxillofacial

A/Prof. Lim Tow Keang
Senior Consultant
Department of Medicine
Asthma, Respiratory failure, acute, Chronic obstructive lung disease, Pnemonia, community acquired (CAP), Pneumothorax, Pulmonary embolism

Dr. Mak Seck Wai, Kenneth
Consultant
Department of Surgery
Pain, abdominal, Bleeding, GIT, Intestinal obstruction, Ischaemic bowel

A/Prof Mongelli, Joe M
Former Consultant
Department of Obstetrics & Gynaecology
Eclampsia, Ectopic pregnancy

A/Prof. Oakley, Reida
Former Consultant
Department of Cardiac, Thoracic and Vascular Surgery
Aortic dissection, Trauma, chest

Prof. Oh Min Sen, Vernon
Senior Consultant
Department of Medicine
Poisoning, paracetamol, Poisoning, salicylate, Poisoning, organophosphate

Dr. Ong, Adrian
Former Associate Consultant
Department of Surgery
Trauma, abdominal, Trauma, paediatric, Trauma, multiple, Trauma, pregnancy

Dr. Pang Yoke Teen
Senior Consultant
Department of Otolaryngology (ENT) – Head & Neck Surgery
ENT emergencies

A/Prof. Tambyah, Paul
Consultant
Department of Medicine
Dermatology in emergency care, Needle-stick injury protocol, Bites, mammalian and human

Dr. Tan Hock Soon, Kenneth
Consultant
Department of Anaesthesia
Shock/Hypoperfusion states, Sepsis/Septic shock

Dr. Tan Huay Cheem
Chief and Senior Consultant
Cardiac Department
Coronary syndromes, acute, Myocardial infarction, acute, Pulmonary oedema, cardiogenic

A/Prof. Tan Kim Siang, Luke
Chief and Senior Consultant
Department of Otolaryngology (ENT) – Head & Neck Surgery
Stridor

Dr. Thambiah, Joseph
Senior Consultant
Department of Orthopaedic Surgery
Trauma, pelvic

Dr. Sivaraman, Pary
Consultant
Department of Medicine
Renal emergencies

A/Prof. Wilder-Smith, Einar
Consultant
Department of Medicine
Meningitis, Seizure, Temporal arteritis

A/Prof. Wong Hee Kit
Chief and Senior Consultant
Department of Orthopaedic Surgery
Cervical spine clearance, Spinal cord injury

National University Of Singapore
Dr. Saw Seang Mei
Assistant Professor
Department of Community, Occupational and Family Medicine
Simple statistics

Raffles Hospital, Singapore
Dr. Ng Wai Lin
Consultant Cardiologist
Heart failure, Hypertensive crisis

Singapore General Hospital
Dr. Lateef, Fatimah
Consultant
Department of Emergency Medicine
Allergic reactions/anaphylaxis, Diarrhoea and vomiting, Pain, low back, Lower limb swelling

Dr. Leong Kwok Fai, Mark
Senior Consultant
Department of Emergency Medicine
Commonly used scoring systems, Administration of blood products in the ED, Pain management

Dr. Lim Swee Han
Head and Senior Consultant
Department of Emergency Medicine
Pain, chest, acute

Dr. Ponapalam, R
Consultant
Department of Emergency Medicine
Poisoning, benzodiazepine, Poisoning, carbon monoxide, Poisoning, cyclic antidepressant, Poisoning, general principles, Bites, snake

Tan Tock Seng Hospital, Singapore
Dr. Seow, Eillyne
Head and Senior Consultant
Department of Emergency Medicine
Breathlessness, acute, Hyperventilation

Dr. Tham Kum Ying
Consultant
Department of Emergency Medicine
Altered mental state, Fever, Giddiness, Headache, Syncope

Abbreviations

AAA	abdominal aortic aneurysm
ABC	airway, breathing, circulation
ABG	arterial blood gas
AIS	Abbreviated Injury Scale
ALP	alkaline phosphatase
ALT	alanine transaminase
AMI	acute myocardial infarction
ANOVA	analysis of variance
AP	anteroposterior
ARDS	Adult Respiratory Distress Syndrome
AST	aspartate transaminase
AXR	abdominal x-ray
BBB	bundle branch block
BCI	blunt cardiac injury
BCU	body cooling unit
bd	twice daily
BIPAP	biphasic positive airway pressure
BP	blood pressure
BVM	bag-valve-mask
BW	body weight
BZD	benzodiazepine
C&S	culture and sensitivity
Ca	calcium
CAGE	cerebral arterial gas embolism
CAP	community acquired pneumonia
CAPD	continuous abdominal peritoneal dialysis
CCF	congestive cardiac failure
CCU	Coronary Care Unit
CK	creatine kinase
CNS	central nervous system
CO	carbon monoxide
CO_2	carbon dioxide
COHB	carboxyhaemoglobin
COLD	chronic obstructive lung disease
CONSB	carbon monoxide neuropsychiatric screening battery
CRAO	central retinal artery occlusion
CRVO	central retinal vein occlusion
CSF	cerebrospinal fluid
CSM	carotid sinus massage
CT	computed tomography

CVA	cerebrovascular accident
CVS	cardiovascular system
CXR	chest x-ray
D_5W	5% dextrose-water
DBP	diastolic blood pressure
DCI	decompression illness
DIPJ	distal interphalangeal joint
DIVC	disseminated intravascular coagulation
DKA	diabetic ketoacidosis
DL	direct laryngoscopy
DM	diabetes mellitus
DPL	diagnostic peritoneal lavage
DVT	deep vein thrombosis
ECG	electrocardiogram
ECM	external cardiac massage
ESRF	end stage renal failure
ETT	endotracheal tubes
FAST	focused assessment using sonography in trauma
FB	foreign body
FBC	full blood count
FDP	flexor digitorum profundus
FDS	flexor digitorum superficialis
FFP	fresh frozen plasma
FRC	functional residual capacity
g	gram
GA	general anaesthesia
GCS	Glasgow coma scale
GE	gastroenteritis
GGT	gamma glutaryl transaminase
GI	gastrointestinal
GOLD	global initiative for chronic obstructive lung disease
GTN	glyceryl trinitrate
GXM	group and cross match
HA	hyperventilation attack
Hb	haemoglobin
HCG	human chorionic gonadotrophin
HCW	health care worker
HD	high dependency
H,E,E,N,T	head, eyes, ear, nose and throat
HHNK	hyperosmolar hyperglycaemic non-ketotic state
HHS	hyperosmolar hyperglycaemic state
I&D	incision and drainage
IV	intravenous
ICH	intracerebral haemorrhage
ICU	intensive care unit
IDL	indirect laryngoscopy

IHD	ischaemic heart disease
IPPV	intermittent positive pressure ventilation
IS	ischaemic stroke
ISDN	isosorbide dinitrate
ISS	Injury Severity Score
IVC	inferior vena cava
K^+	potassium
KUB	kidney, ureter and bladder x-ray
l	litre
LBBB	left bundle branch block
LBP	low back pain
LDH	lactate dehydrogenase
LFT	liver function test
LOC	loss of consciousness
LOV	loss of vision
M&R	manipulation and reduction
MAP	mean arterial pressure
MCPJ	metacarpophalangeal joint
mg	milligram
Mg	magnesium
ml	millilitre
MMR	measles, mumps, rubella
MRI	magnetic resonance imaging
MRI-A	magnetic resonance imaging with angiogram
MSP	Munchausen Syndrome by Proxy
Na^+	sodium
NAI	non-accidental injury
NBM	nil by mouth
NG	nasogastric
NIV	non-invasive ventilation
NS	normal saline
NSAIDs	non-steroidal antiinflammatory drugs
NWB	non-weight-bearing
O_2	oxygen
OM	occipitomental
ORIF	open reduction and internal fixation
PA	posteroanterior
PCP	phencyclidine
PEEP	peak end-expiratory pressure
PID	pelvic inflammatory disease
PIPJ	proximal interphalangeal joint
PO_4	phosphate
PPV	positive pressure ventilation
PR	pulse rate
PSA	procedural sedation and analgesia
PT	prothrombin time

PT/PTT	coagulation profile
PUD	peptic ulcer disease
PUO	pyrexia of unknown origin
qds	four times daily
RBBB	right bundle branch block
RBCs	red blood cells
RHC	right hypochondrial pain
RICE	rest, ice, compression and elevation
RLQ	right lower quadrant
RSI	rapid sequence intubation
RTA	road traffic accidents
rtPA	recombinant tissue plasminogen activator
RTS	Revised Trauma Score
SAH	subarachnoid haemorrhage
SBI	serious bacterial infection
SBP	systolic blood pressure
SC	subcutaneous
SIRS	systemic inflammatory response syndrome
SK	streptokinase
SL	sublingual
SLE	systemic lupus erythematosus
SOB	shortness of breath
SOC	specialist outpatient clinic
SP	special precautions
SVT	supraventricular tachycardia
SXR	skull x-ray
SYNC	synchronization
T&S	toilet and suture
TCA	tricyclic antidepressant
TCM	traditional Chinese medicine
tds	three times daily
TEE	transoesophageal echocardiography
TIA	transient ischaemic attack
TWC	total white count
u	units
UC9	urine dipstick
URTI	upper respiratory tract infection
UTI	urinary tract infection
V/Q	ventilation-perfusion
VBI	vertebrobasilar insufficiency
VF	ventricular fibrillation
VT	ventricular tachycardia
VZV	varicella zoster virus
WBCs	leukocytes

Common presentations

1 Altered mental state

Peter Manning • Peng Li Lee • Lee Kuan Wee

CAVEATS

The primary focus of the ED evaluation of a patient with altered mental state (AMS) is:

- To address easily reversible causes, eg hypoxaemia, hypercarbia, hypoglycaemia.
- To differentiate structural from toxic-metabolic causes since the former require emergent CNS imaging, whereas the latter are usually more readily identified by laboratory studies.
- Refer to *Commonly Used Scoring System* under Glasgow Coma Scale for definition of coma.

> ☛ **Special Tips for GPs**
>
> - Always consider reversible causes of AMS that you can initiate treatment for in your office: hypoglycaemia (oral sugar or IV dextrose 50%), hypoxaemia (supplemental oxygen), heat stroke (cooling measures and IV normal saline) before sending the patient to the ED by ambulance.

MANAGEMENT

Initial priorities

- See Figure 1 for approach to differential diagnosis of altered mental state.
- Patient should be managed initially in the critical care area.
- If a promptly reversible cause of AMS is found, then the patient can be downgraded to the intermediate acuity area.
- **Positive airway control/C spine immobilization**.
  1. Open the airway and search for foreign bodies.
  2. Insert oral or nasopharyngeal airway.
  3. Apply stiff collar or manual immobilization if history does not exclude trauma.
  4. Definitive airway if patient comatose: intubation with/without rapid sequence intubation **or** perform surgical airway such as emergency cricothyrotomy.

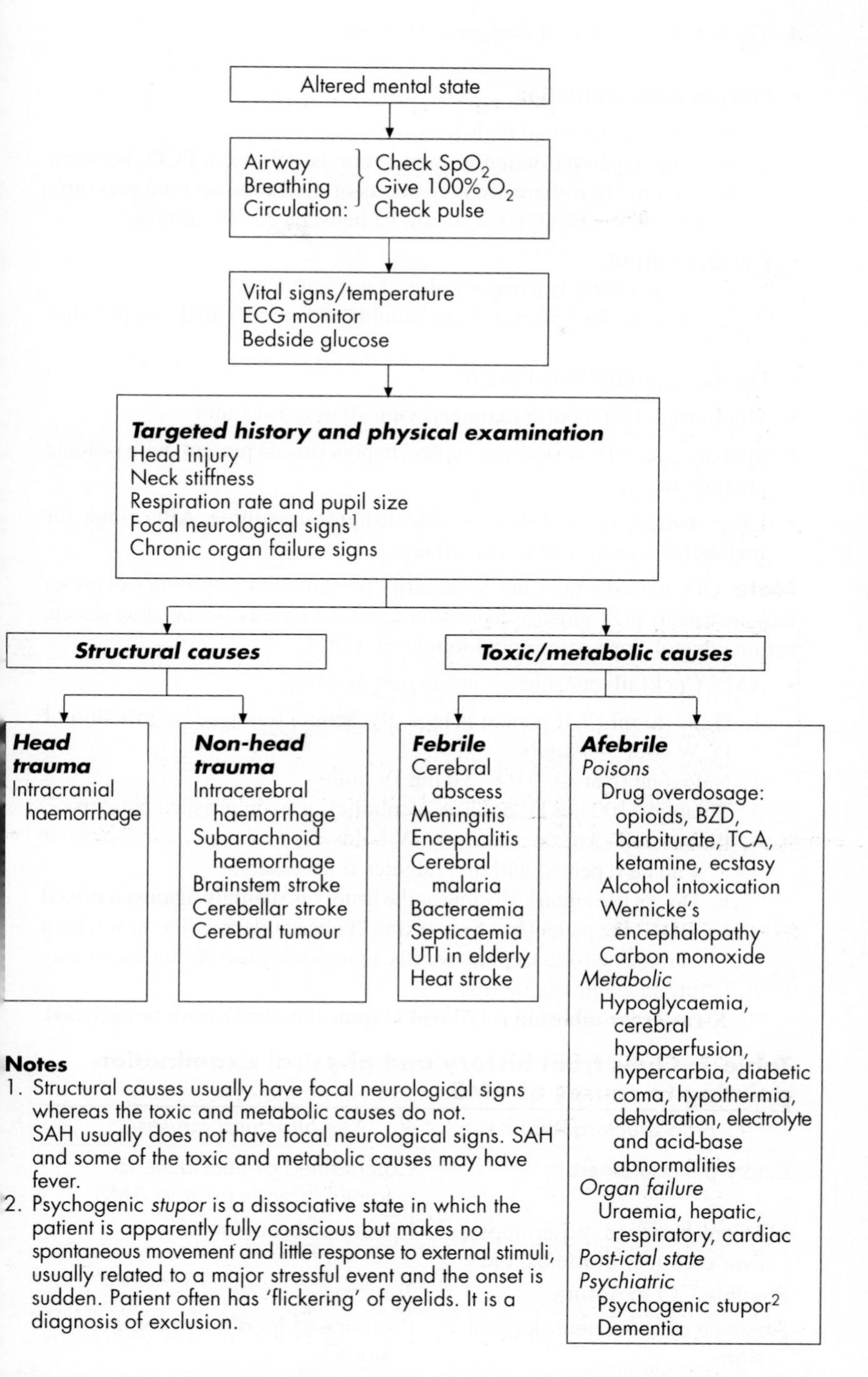

Figure 1: Approach to differential diagnosis of altered mental state

- **Oxygenation/ventilation**.
  1. Provide supplemental high-flow oxygen.
  2. Institute hyperventilation in moderation to achieve a PCO_2 between 30–35 mm Hg if there are indications of raised intracranial pressure. In general, the PCO_2 level should be between 35–40 mm Hg.
- **Cardiac output**.
  1. Check that there is a major pulse; if not start CPR!
  2. Obvious external haemorrhage should be stopped with direct pressure only.
- **Do stat capillary blood sugar**.
- Monitoring: ECG, pulse oximetry, vital signs q 5–15 min.
- Start peripheral IV at slow rate (unless hypoperfusion present) with isotonic crystalloid.
- Labs: mandatory for FBC, urea/electrolytes/creatinine, ABG (look for metabolic acidosis and hypercarbia).

Note: CO_2 narcosis does not necessarily present with respiratory distress; they are usually in respiratory depression. Consider serum calcium, drug screen, serum ethanol, carboxyhaemoglobin level, GXM.

- **AMS Cocktail**: consider its use in part or whole.
  1. $D_{50}W$ 40 ml IV if patient is hypoglycaemic, followed by **infusion of** $D_{10}W$ over 3–4 hours
  2. Naloxone (Narcan®) 0.8–2.0 mg IV bolus
  3. Thiamine 100 mg IV bolus in alcoholics or malnourished patients
  4. Flumazenil (Anexate®) 0.5 mg IV bolus
     a. Can be repeated within 5 minutes if necessary.
     b. Do not use empirically unless the history is **strongly against a mixed OD**. If the patient has been taking cyclic antidepressants or is taking chronic benzodiazepines for fits, unnecessary use of flumazenil may produce intractable fits.
  5. **X-ray cross-table lateral film of C spine** if trauma cannot be excluded.

Table 1: Clues from history and physical examination pointing to causes of AMS

Non-structural causes	Structural causes
Empty pill containers	Complained of headache to family/friends prior to AMS
Medical diseases, eg epilepsy, liver disease, diabetes, etc	History of brain tumour
Possible CO exposure	Trauma
Absence of focal neurological signs	Presence of focal neurological signs
Signs of metabolic acidosis	Head trauma
Anticholinergic signs	

- **Clinical evaluation**: the focus is on differentiating structural from toxic-metabolic causes of AMS (Table 1).
- **History**: rarely clear-cut; look for clues from patient's family, friends, belongings and information at scene from paramedic/ambulance officer.
- **Examination**: brief external assessment of patient searching for stigmata of numerous disease processes. While a head-to-toe examination is important, in AMS pay most attention to a **focused neurological examination**.

AMS due to suspected structural causes

- Give supplemental oxygen to maintain SpO_2 of at least 95%.
- Start IV at slow rate.
- Perform head CT scan.
- **Lower intracranial pressure** if indicated.
  1. Controlled ventilation: works fastest. See p. 4 for details.
  2. **IV Mannitol** useful in conjunction with neurosurgical consult. Dose is 1 g/kg body weight (BW), ie BW × 5 mls/kg BW of 20% Mannitol solution.
  3. Steroids are debatable.

AMS due to suspected toxic–metabolic causes

- Do gastric lavage; to be performed with airway protection if required.
- Use activated charcoal in suspected drug overdoses. Refer to *Poisoning, General Principles*.
- Check rectal temperature and consider heat stroke if temp >40°C and taking anticholinergics.
- If meningitis is suspected, consider early lumbar puncture (after CT head scan). **Start empiric antibiotics before either of the tests** together with a neurological consult. Refer to *Meningitis*.

Disposition

- Admit all cases of AMS. Admit to ICU those who are intubated or with haemodynamic instability.

References/further reading

1. Hamilton GC. Altered mental status: Depressed level of consciousness. In: Hamilton GC, ed. *Presenting Signs and Symptoms in the Emergency Department: Evaluation and Treatment*. Baltimore: William and Wilkins; 1993:528–536.
2. Peterson J. Coma. In: Rosen R, Barkin RM, Braen CR, et al, eds. *Emergency Medicine: Concepts and Clinical Practice*. 3rd ed. St. Louis: Mosby Year Book; 1992:1747–1750.

2 Bleeding, GIT

JP Travers • Peter Manning

CAVEATS

- The **management** of GIT bleeding is **essentially** to:
  1. Identify shock and resuscitate.
  2. Identify potential causes of the bleeding and reverse where possible (eg reverse over-anticoagulation).
  3. Identify physiologic compromise resulting from shock (cardiac ischaemia, renal compromise or symptomatic anaemia requiring blood transfusion).
- Always be aware that **aortic aneurysm** may present as GIT bleeding.
- Always do a **rectal examination** to establish whether frank melaena is present or there is local bleeding from the anal canal/perianal area.
- Black stools due to iron treatment are green/black in colour.
- **Common causes** of GI bleeding are:
  1. Peptic ulcer
  2. Gastric erosions
  3. Varices from the upper GI tract
  4. Haemorrhoids from the lower part
  5. Malignancy

☛ Special Tips for GPs

- Assess if shock is present (tachycardia and/or hypotension). If it is, call for ambulance and transfer to the nearest ED. Set up IV line(s) and infuse NS stat in the first instance.
- If vomiting blood and conscious, place in recovery position and establish IV lines.
- Examine abdomen for tenderness and do rectal examination to confirm melaena.
- Establish if any history of alcohol abuse or anticoagulation treatment.
- Always bear in mind abdominal pulsation and aortic aneurysm.
- Ask patient regarding use of NSAIDs and traditional Chinese medicine (TCM).
- Advise patient to stay NBM.

MANAGEMENT

Supportive measures

A. Haemodynamically unstable patient

- Patient must be managed in critical care area.
- Maintain airway. Consider intubation if haematemesis is copious and patient is unable to protect own airway, eg depressed mental state from previous CVA.
- Provide supplemental high flow oxygen to maintain SpO_2 >94%.
- Monitoring: ECG, vital signs every 5 min, pulse oximetry.
- Perform 12-lead ECG to exclude cardiac dysrhythmia.
- Establish 2, or more, large-bore peripheral IV lines (14/16G).
- **Labs**:
  1. GXM for at least 4 units.
  2. FBC, urea/electrolytes/creatinine, coagulation profile.
  3. Order liver function tests if patient is jaundiced.
  4. Order cardiac enzymes if there is ECG evidence of myocardial ischaemia/injury.
- Infuse 1 litre normal saline rapidly and reassess parameters. Arrange for blood transfusion if there is no significant improvement after the initial fluid challenge.
- Insert nasogastric tube to free drainage for diagnostic purposes (and to prevent aspiration if patient vomits). **Do not** insert nasogastric tube if oesophageal varices are suspected.
- Insert urinary catheter to monitor urine output.

Note: Role of omeprazole (proton pump inhibitor). Current evidence suggests there may be some benefit in reducing haemorrhage in the short term (increases stomach pH, allowing optimal conditions for clot formation) but further trials are needed for effects on mortality and morbidity. Administer IV omeprazole 40 mg.

B. Haemodynamically normal patient

- Patient can be managed in intermediate care area though it must be remembered that the patient may decompensate after his first evaluation due to continued blood loss.
- Provide supplemental oxygen to maintain SpO_2 >94%.
- Monitor vital signs every 10–15 min, pulse oximetry. Establish at least one peripheral IV (14/16G).
- Perform 12-lead ECG.
- **Labs**:
  1. GXM 2 units.

2. FBC, urea/electrolytes/creatinine, coagulation profile.
3. Liver function tests if patient is jaundiced or shows signs of chronic liver disease.
4. Cardiac enzymes if ECG shows signs of myocardial ischaemia/injury.

- Start normal saline infusion 500 ml over 1–2 hours.
- Insert nasogastric tube to free drainage for diagnostic purposes (and to prevent aspiration if patient vomits).
- Give IV **omeprazole** 40 mg.
- Upgrade to critical care area if instability develops.

Specific Measures

- Look for scar of previous abdominal aortic aneurysm surgery: this episode of GIT bleeding may represent an **aortoenteric fistula**. If this is suspected, consult General Surgical registrar and Cardiothoracic registrar.
- If **oesophageal varices** are suggested by the clinical picture, consider the use of IV **somatostatin** 250 μg bolus, followed by an IV infusion of 250 μg/h (successful in up to 85–90% of cases). If somatostatin is unsuccessful in stopping the bleeding, and there is the risk of patient exanguinating before endoscopy can be arranged, then the insertion of a **Sengstaken–Blakemore tube** should be considered. This should be inserted only by an experienced operator.

Disposition

- Consultations for admission to either General Surgery or Gastroenterology depending on institutional practice.

References/further reading

1. Gilbert G, Chan CH, Thomas E. Peptic ulcer disease: How to treat it now. *Postgraduate Medicine*. 1991;89(4):91–98.
2. Larson DE, editor-in-chief. *Mayo Clinic Family Health Book*. New York: William Morrow and Company, Inc. 1990.
3. Masoodi JGI, Zargar SA, Khan BA, et al. Omeprazole as adjuvant therapy to endoscopic combination injection sclerotherapy for treating bleeding peptic ulcer. *Am J Med*. 2001;111(4):280–284.
4. Gisbert JP, Gonzalez L, Calvet X, et al. Proton pump inhibitors versus H_2-receptor antagonists: A meta-analysis of their efficacy in treating bleeding peptic ulcer. *Aliment. Pharmacol. Ther.* 2001;15(7):917–926.
5. Geus WP. Are there indications for intravenous acid-inhibition in the prevention of upper GI bleeding? *Scand J Gastroenterol*. Suppl 2000;232:10–20.
6. Bustamante M, Stollman N. The efficacy of proton-pump inhibitors in acute ulcer bleeding: a qualitative review. *J Clin Gastroenterol*. 2000;30(1):7–13.
7. Li Y, Sha W, Nie Y, et al. Effect of intragastric pH on control of peptic ulcer bleeding. *J Gastroenterol Hepatol*. 2000;15(2):148–154.

3 Bleeding, vaginal, abnormal

John Yam Pei Yuan

CAVEATS

- A careful history is important in the assessment of abnormal vaginal bleeding. This should include a complete menstrual history (including date of last menstrual period), medical and drug history, obstetric history and sexual history (including use of birth control). The presence of pain, its location, duration, onset and severity should also be assessed.
- Pregnancy should be excluded in all patients who are pregnancy-capable.
- It is also important to exclude, from the outset, bleeding from the urinary tract and bowel.
- See Table 1 for **emergency causes of abnormal vaginal bleeding**.
- See Table 2 for other **important but not immediately life-threatening causes** of abnormal vaginal bleeding.

Table 1: Emergency causes of abnormal vaginal bleeding

1. Ectopic pregnancy
2. Incomplete abortion (may be *septic*) and inevitable abortion
3. Placenta praevia
4. Abruptio placentae
5. Postpartum haemorrhage (1–5 are all *complications of pregnancy*)
6. Vaginal trauma
7. Menorrhagia in a non-pregnant woman
8. Bleeding from any lower genital tract tumours (eg *cervical or endometrial carcinomas*)

☛ Special Tips for GPs

- Pregnancy should be excluded in all patients who are pregnancy-capable.
- Refer all patients with bleeding in pregnancy to the ED. An exception to this is patients who have a threatened miscarriage but experience no pain and in whom foetal viability can be demonstrated.

Table 2: Important but not immediately life-threatening causes of abnormal vaginal bleeding

1. Pregnancy-related	• Threatened miscarriage • Missed abortion • Gestational trophoblastic disease (*rare*) • Show (*may occur in normal pregnancies prior to delivery*) • Lochia (*occurs normally after delivery*)
2. Non-pregnancy-related	• Bleeding in a pre-pubertal girl • Irregular vaginal bleeding • Prolonged vaginal bleeding • Postcoital bleeding • Intermenstrual bleeding • Postmenopausal bleeding

MANAGEMENT

- Ensure vital signs are stable. Intravenous infusion for volume replacement should be started immediately if the patient is unstable. Specimens for FBC, GXM and a pregnancy test should be obtained.
- If there is heavy bleeding, administer supplemental oxygen, pulse oximetry and BP monitoring.
- The amount of bleeding can be assessed from the history and by examining the clothing and pads.
- The general resuscitative measures outlined above should be instituted while awaiting specialist review.
- Patients with bleeding in early pregnancy should have an ultrasound examination to assess foetal viability and localization. However, if there are signs of intraabdominal bleeding (eg in ruptured ectopic pregnancy), prompt resuscitation, followed by emergency surgery, is indicated. Refer to *Ectopic Pregnancy* for further details.
- In pregnant patients in whom the uterus is palpable per abdomen, a Doptone should be used to assess foetal viability.
- Patients with antepartum haemorrhage should be sent urgently to the labour ward. Coagulation studies should be done. It may sometimes be difficult to differentiate show from antepartum haemorrhage. When in doubt, the patient should be sent to the labour ward.
- See Figure 1 for management plans.

References/further reading

1. Ratnam SS, Rao KB, Arulkumaran S, eds. *Obstetrics & Gynaecology for Postgraduates*. Vols. 1 & 2. Madras: Orient Longman; 1993.

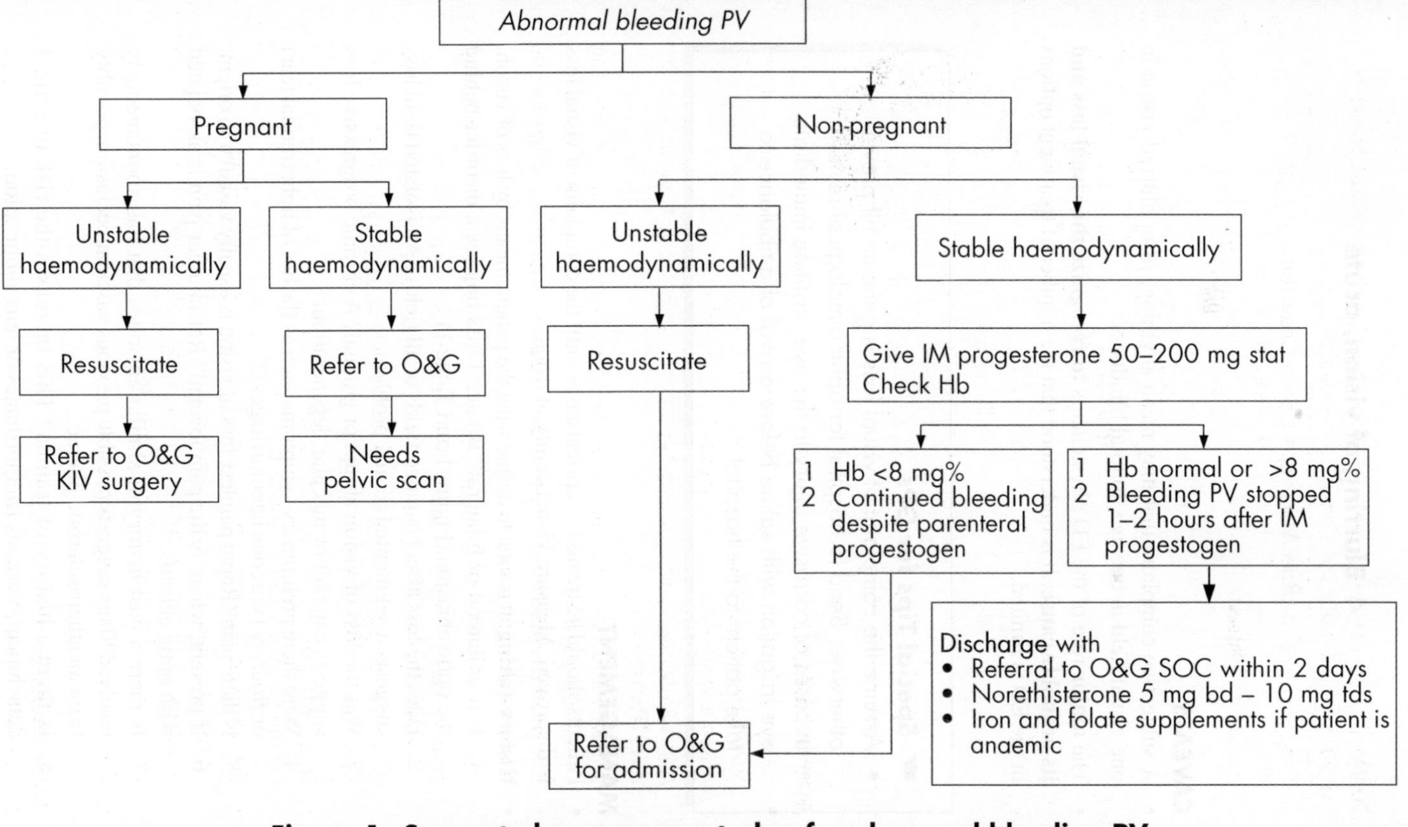

Figure 1: Suggested management plan for abnormal bleeding PV

4 Blurring of vision, acute

Peter Manning • Chong Chew Lan

CAVEATS

- A subjective complaint that may mean anything, from blurred vision in one visual field in one eye, to total blindness.
- The **major** role of the ED physician is **to recognize the visual loss and its probable cause**. It is understood that the number of treatment options in the ED is limited.

> **☛ Special Tips for GPs**
> - Assume the complaint of visual loss is genuine till proven otherwise. Send to hospital for ophthalmological review.
> - In cases of corrosive injury to the eye, institute immediate eye irrigation with saline before arrival of ambulance to take patient to the hospital.

MANAGEMENT

- Patients should be treated as critical cases until the complaint of visual loss is disproved. Measure visual acuity at triage.
- **History-taking**: it is vital to define what the patient means by loss of vision.
  1. Is it unilateral or bilateral? Bilateral loss implies a disorder behind the optic chiasma (Figure 1 and Table 1).
  2. Does the loss affect isolated fields or all fields? An isolated field loss suggests a segmented retinal problem.
  3. Was the loss of vision abrupt or gradual? A chronic progressive loss suggests cataract or macular degeneration.
  4. Were there preliminary symptoms such as flashes of light (retinal tear) or *floaters* (vitreous haemorrhages)?
  5. Is there pain? Rapid painless loss of vision is usually vascular in origin.
  6. If present, where is the pain located? Retrobulbar pain is associated with optic neuritis.
  7. Is there a past history of similar episodes that had spontaneously resolved? This suggests possible previous vascular occlusion, possibly from an atherosclerotic plaque.
  8. Is there a history of trauma? This increases the risk of retinal detachment, vitreous haemorrhages or lens subluxation.

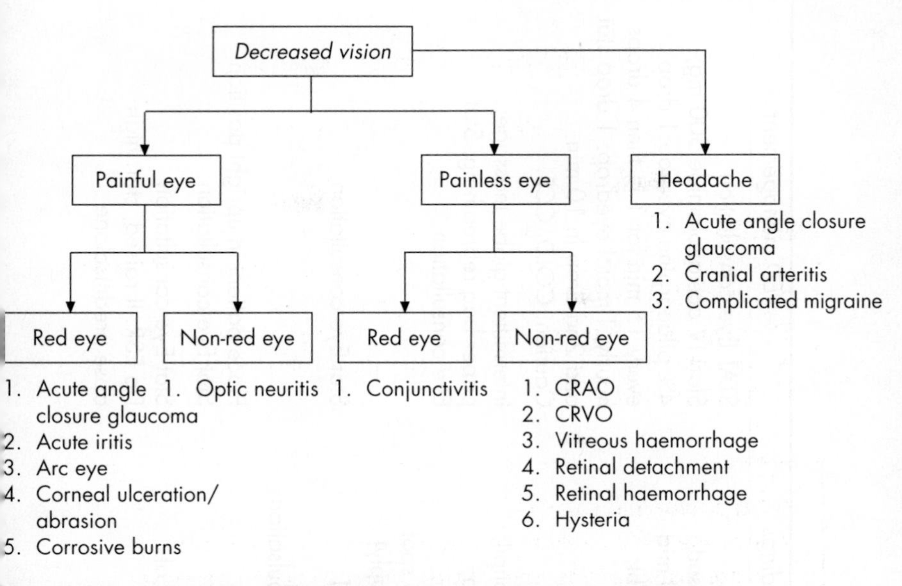

Figure 1: Suggested flow chart for patients presenting with loss of vision

9. Is there a history of potential toxin ingestion? Methanol, salicylates and quinine can affect vision.
10. Is there a history of corrosive injury to the eye? This can cause significant damage to the globe. Acids cause coagulative necrosis that is usually superficial, whereas alkalis cause a liquefaction necrosis that tends to be deep, leaving corneal ulcerations.

EXAMINATION (SPECIFIC)

- **Visual acuity**: check with and without corrective lenses.
  1. A Snellen or hand-held chart is used: the patient must read 50% of letters on a line to be said to have that acuity.
  2. If the patient cannot use a Snellen chart, then assess the ability to count fingers, detect hand motion or perceive light.
  3. A pinhole cover will correct refractive error to help you discern if this is the cause of decreased visual acuity.
- **Inspection**: important points that indicate significant pathology include:
  1. Corneal opacities from infectious or infiltrative processes.
  2. Iridodonesis (a shimmering movement of the iris) may represent traumatic subluxation of the lens.
  3. Difficulty in visualizing the retina: may be due to cataract, blood in the vitreous or retinal detachment.
  4. Pupillary reaction: check response to light and accommodation.

Table 1: Specific entities presenting as loss of vision (LOV)

	History	*Examination findings*	*ED management*
Acute angle closure glaucoma	Unilateral dull aching ocular pain; nausea and vomiting; decreased vision; haloes around light	Diffusely reddened congested eye; decreased VA; hazy cornea; pupil mid-dilated and fixed to light; increased intraocular pressure	STAT Eye consultation Start IV acetazolamide 500 mg; 4% pilocarpine eyedrop: 1 drop every 15 min for 1 h, then 4 drops hourly, Timolol eyedrop: 1 drop stat and 2nd drop in 10 min Caution: COLD, CCF
CRAO (central retinal artery occlusion)	Unilateral, painless LOV; ±previous amaurosis fugax	Reduced VA; afferent pupil; pale oedematous retina; markedly reduced vasculature; cherry red spot (intact fuveal blood supply)	Intermittent globe massage; paper bag rebreathing; Stat Eye consultation
CRVO (central retinal vein occlusion)	Unilateral LOV	Reduced VA; engorged tortuous retinal veins without physiological pulsations	Stat Eye consultation
Vitreous haemorrhage	Varies from a few floaters to profound, painless LOV	Reduced VA; vitreous floaters on fundoscopy	Place patient in upright position Stat Eye consultation
Cranial arteritis	Elderly patient; unilateral headache; jaw claudication and muscle aches	Tender temporal artery of decreased pulse	Stat Eye consultation Do ESR. If raised, start high dose prednisolone

Optic neuritis	Unilateral LOV over hours to days; pain increased by eye movements; a/w multiple sclerosis	Reduced VA and painful Note: Papillitis (looks like papilloedema but is unilateral and has greater loss of VA)	Stat Eye consultation
Retinal detachment	Acute LOV; usually total with preceding streaks or flashes of light common	Fundoscopy shows grey, billowed or folded area of retina with overlying vessels having an undulating course	Stat Eye consultation
Retinal haemorrhage	Painless, acute focal or generalized LOV	Focal or generalized reduction in VA; fundoscopy shows retinal haemorrhages	Stat Eye consultation
Migraine	Headache consistent with migraine; scintillating scotoma	Fundus usually normal; EOM paralysis; pupillary dilatation	Stat Eye/Neurology consultation
Hysteria	Often total bilateral LOV	Normal optokinetic nystagmus; variable responses to different techniques of testing VA	Stat Eye/Psychiatry consultation
Corrosive burn	Sudden pain with LOV; tearing	Ulcerations of cornea esp with alkali burns; pain++; photophobia with tearing	Stat Ophth consultation. Immediate irrigation with NS to pH neutral using pink/blue litmus paper. (Normal pH of tears is 6.5–7.0)

5. Check for Marcus Gunn pupil: indicates an afferent or prechiasmal defect such as retinal or optic nerve dysfunction. See Figure 2 for the swinging flashlight test.

- **Ophthalmoscopy**: you rarely need to dilate the pupil with a short-acting mydriatic (tropicamide 1%). Contraindications include known closed-angle glaucoma or a need to monitor pupillary changes as in head-injured patients.
  1. Check for retinal defects: noted by their position on a clock face.
  2. Check for central retinal artery or vein occlusion, retinal detachment, hypertensive or diabetic retinopathy, papilloedema or papillitis.
- **Check visual fields and extraocular movements**.

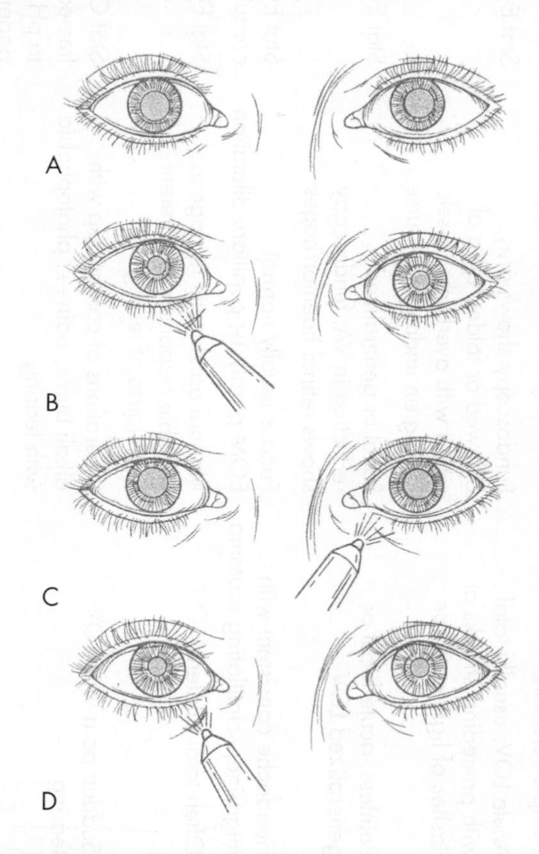

Figure 2: "Swinging flashlight test" revealing an afferent papillary defect (Marcus-Gunn pupil) of the left eye. B. The test is positive when the affected pupil dilates in response to light. Reproduced with permission of the McGraw-Hill Companies, from Tintinalli JE, Kelen GD, Stapczynski JS, et al, eds. *Emergency Medicine: A Comprehensive Study Guide*. New York: McGraw-Hill; 2000:1502, Fig. 230–3.

EXAMINATION (ADJUNCTS)

- **Slit lamp examination**: check for flare and cells, posterior keratitic precipitates, and/or hyphema in the anterior chamber.
- **Tonometry** is performed after topical anaesthesia, to measure intraocular pressure. An abnormal pressure is >20 mm Hg.
- **Disposition**: refer for immediate ophthalmology consults if there is a documented visual loss or a high index of suspicion of visual loss.

References/further reading

1. Markoff D and Chacko D. Common ophthalmologic emergencies: examination, differential diagnosis, and target management. *Emerg Med Report.* 1999;20(1):1–12.
2. Rosen R, Barkin RM, Braen CR, et al, eds. *Emergency Medicine: Concepts and Clinical Practice*. 3rd ed. St. Louis: Mosby Year Book; 1992:2453–2456.

5 Breathlessness, acute

Chong Chew Lan

CAVEATS

- When approaching a patient suffering acute breathlessness, always consider those **causes** that can be **dealt with immediately** (ie within seconds or minutes).
  1. Acute upper airway obstruction: Heimlich manoeuvre or Magill's forceps
  2. Acute tension pneumothorax: needle thoracostomy, followed by insertion of chest tube
  3. Acute respiratory failure: endotracheal intubation
- The **common causes** of acute breathlessness are shown in Table 1.
- Note that psychogenic hyperventilation is a diagnosis of exclusion.
- In general, it is useful to clinically elucidate the causes by dividing the patients into those without lung findings (refer to *Hyperventilation*) and those with lung findings.
- Remember that not all who wheeze have asthma or COLD.
- Consider the diagnosis of other conditions, such as cardiac asthma, anaphylaxis and aspiration.
- Look out for signs and symptoms of heart failure, eg orthopnoea, pedal oedema and raised jugular venous pressure, to differentiate cardiac asthma from respiratory asthma.
- Not all severely tachypnoeic patients with generalized crepitations are due to pulmonary oedema. They may have pneumonia or bronchiectasis, for example.

☛ Special Tips for GPs

- Give oxygen and obtain intravenous access for breathless patients who need referral to the ED.
- Send the patient by ambulance if a serious pathology is suspected.

Table 1: Common causes of acute breathlessness

Cardiac	Acute pulmonary oedema	Refer to *Pulmonary Oedema, Cardiogenic*
	Heart failure	Refer to *Heart Failure*
	Cardiac tamponade	
Respiratory	Severe asthma or chronic obstructive airway disease	Refer to *Asthma* and *Chronic Obstructive Lung Disease*
	Chest infection	Refer to *Pneumonia*
	Pulmonary embolism	Refer to *Pulmonary Embolism*
	Pneumothorax both tension and simple	Refer to *Pneumothorax*
	Pleural effusion	
	Chest trauma, eg tension pneumothorax, haemothorax, pulmonary contusion, flail chest	Refer to *Trauma, Chest*
	Aspiration, including acute foreign body upper airway obstruction	
	Near drowning	Refer to *Near Drowning*
Others	Respiratory compensation for metabolic acidosis, eg DKA, uraemia	
	Poisoning, eg salicylate poisoning	Refer to *Poisoning, Salicylates*
	Adult respiratory distress syndrome	
	Fever	Refer to *Fever*
	Anaphylaxis	Refer to *Allergic Reactions/Anaphylaxis*
	Hyperventilation syndrome	Refer to *Hyperventilation*

MANAGEMENT

- Use ABC approach and resuscitate as necessary: most dyspnoeic patients will need to be evaluated in the intermediate or high acuity areas.
- The **history** will help to point to the diagnosis. In particular, exacerbating and relieving factors, as well as the associated symptoms, will be helpful. There may not be a history of exposure to allergens or poisons but do entertain the possibility of anaphylaxis or poisoning.
- Always apply a pulse oximeter and monitor the respiratory rate.
- **Investigations** will be guided by history and may include ECG, FBC, ABG, bedside glucose level and CXR.
- **Disposition** of the patients will depend on the diagnosis and the clinical state of the patient.
  1. Patients in mild heart failure not due to myocardial infarction and clinically comfortable without tachycardia or evidence of pulmonary oedema on chest x-ray may be treated and referred to cardiologist as an outpatient. Interim review by the GP or polyclinic can be arranged until the patient is seen by the cardiologist. Refer to *Heart Failure*.
  2. Patients with hyperventilation syndrome may need a medical social worker or psychiatric referral, especially if recurrent. Refer to *Hyperventilation*.
- Start **treatment** of the identified cause of the acute breathlessness.

References/further reading

1. Wyatt JP, Illingworth RN, Clancy MJ, et al, eds. *Oxford Handbook of Accident and Emergency Medicine*. Oxford: Oxford University Press; 1999:96.
2. Stapczynski JS. Respiratory Distress. In Tintinalli JE, Kelen GD, Stapczynski JS, et al, eds. *Emergency Medicine: A Comprehensive Study Guide*. 5th ed. New York: McGraw-Hill; 2000:443–452.

6 Child with abdominal pain

Peter Manning

CAVEATS

- The duration of pain is useful since a surgical diagnosis is less likely in a child with chronic abdominal pain.
- The presence of fever suggests an infective course or peritonitis.
- Children under 5 years old usually have an organic cause for their pain.
- The possibility of functional abdominal pain should be considered in older children.
- The age of the child is useful since the diagnosis is narrowed accordingly.
- Bilious vomiting or persistent vomiting in the presence of abdominal pain is always an ominous sign and should be considered due to a mechanical obstruction till proven otherwise.

> ☛ **Special Tips for GPs**
>
> - The physical examination is especially important given that the history may be inconclusive and up to one-third of children display atypical presentations of specific diseases.
> - Palpation should be left till last in the examination so as not to lose the trust of the child.
> - Do not forget to examine the genital area and perform a rectal examination.

THE MOST COMMON LIFE-THREATENING CAUSES OF ABDOMINAL PAIN

Table 1 lists the most common life-threatening causes of abdominal pain for four age groups.

MANAGEMENT

- Most children with abdominal pain can be managed in the ambulatory area.
- Assess the child's ABCs and transfer to the intermediate or critical care area if necessary to implement supplemental oxygen therapy, monitoring of vital signs and oximetry, and administration of crystalloids via peripheral IV lines.

Table 1: Common life-threatening causes of abdominal pain

Neonatal	*Infancy (<2 years)*	*Childhood (2–10)*	*Adolescence*
Severe gastroenteritis	Severe gastroenteritis	Appendicitis	Toxic overdose
Sepsis	Toxic overdose	Trauma	Trauma
Incarcerated hernia	Sepsis	Intussusception	Appendicitis
Malrotation/volvulus	Intussusception	Toxic overdose	Ectopic pregnancy
Pyloric stenosis	Appendicitis	Sepsis	Peptic ulcer disease
Hirschsprung's disease	Incarcerated hernia	Diabetic ketoacidosis	Pancreatitis
Trauma	Meckel's diverticulum	Megacolon	Diabetic ketoacidosis
	Trauma		Aortic dissection/aneurysm
	Diabetic ketoacidosis		Megacolon

HISTORY

- However thorough this may be inconclusive.
- Characteristics of the pain are useful for differentiating disease processes.

Onset

- Sudden onset is more likely associated with perforation, intussusception, torsion and ectopic pregnancy.
- Slow or insidious onset occurs in appendicitis, pancreatitis and cholecystitis.
- Colicky pain characterizes hollow viscus irritation or obstruction.
- Chronic severe pain is more likely associated with inflammatory bowel disease.

Location of pain at the onset

- Periumbilical pain suggests pathology in the small bowel or proximal colon.
- Epigastric pain suggests proximal GI tract disease including pancreas.
- Hypogastric pain correlates with disease of the distal colon, pelvic pathology, including incarcerated hernia.
- Referred pain to the shoulder suggests diaphragmatic irritation.

Associated symptoms

- Vomiting preceding or coincidental with the onset of pain suggests intussusception, gastroenteritis or ureteric colic.
- Vomiting following well after the onset of pain is more suggestive of peritoneal irritation as in appendicitis, bowel obstruction or cholecystitis.
- Bilious vomiting is always significant and indicates mechanical obstruction.
- **Diarrhoea** suggests gastroenteritis **but can be seen in surgical conditions too**.
- Fever and vomiting are non-specific in children, occurring in both intraabdominal and extraabdominal causes of abdominal pain as well as various viral infections.

Past medical history

- Episodes of previous abdominal pain and outcome should be noted as should recent illnesses in the household or day care. Chronic medical illnesses such as diabetes mellitus, nephrotic syndrome, and sickle cell disease in Afro-Americans are important to note and document.

PHYSICAL EXAMINATION

- Importance is underlined by the fact that the history may be inconclusive and up to one-third of children display atypical presentations of specific diseases. It also requires a great deal of patience starting with observation from a distance while the parents are giving the history.

- Note the child's:
  1. Activity level
  2. Interaction with parents
  3. Apparent degree of discomfort
- Generally:
  1. A writhing, rocking or moaning child has a colicky pain.
  2. An ill-appearing and lethargic child suggests dehydration or sepsis.
  3. A motionless child lying with knees drawn up suggests peritoneal irritation.
- A complete set of vital signs should be reviewed and documented.
- Perform abdominal examination last following complete physical examination:
  1. **Inspection**: Is abdomen scaphoid or distended? Look for scars, abdominal wall defects and peristaltic waves.
  2. **Auscultation**: In all four quadrants:
     a. Hypoactive bowel sounds suggest peritonitis or bowel obstruction (ileus).
     b. Hyperactive bowel sounds suggest gastroenteritis or early bowel obstruction (mechanical).
  3. **Percussion**: Avoid most tender area; an alternative is to shake couch/trolley to assess for peritoneal irritation.
  4. **Palpation**: The most informative part of the examination but should be left till last due to the pain likely to be induced. Distraction techniques or palpating the abdomen over the child's own hand may be useful.
     a. Involuntary guarding or rebound tenderness suggests peritoneal irritation.
     b. Rigidity usually indicates perforation.
     c. Do not forget to examine the genital area and perform a rectal examination.

INVESTIGATIONS

- Investigations are useful in patients with an unclear diagnosis, a history suggestive of a surgical aetiology, and signs of peritoneal irritation.
  1. **FBC**: useful to identify an infectious process or blood loss. Note that the total white cell count may be elevated in any intraabdominal condition or febrile condition and so the interpretation may be difficult.
  2. **Urea/electrolytes/creatinine and blood sugar**: useful in patients requiring IV fluid resuscitation as in bowel obstruction, peritonitis or gastroenteritis.
  3. **Others**: liver function tests and amylase should be obtained if indicated clinically.
  4. **Urinalysis** is indicated in any age patient with abdominal pain looking

Table 2: Common causes of abdominal pain

Neonatal	*Infancy (<2 years)*	*Childhood (2–10)*	*Adolescence*
Non-surgical			
Colic	Gastroenteritis	Gastroenteritis	Gastroenteritis
Milk allergy	Viral syndrome	Constipation	Viral syndrome
Gastroenteritis	Constipation	Functional pain	Functional pain
Gastroesophageal reflux	Urinary tract infection	Viral syndrome	Pneumonia
	Sepsis	Urinary tract infection	
		Pneumonia	
Surgical			
Volvulus/malrotation	Intussusception	Appendicitis	Appendicitis
Incarcerated hernia	Incarcerated hernia	Trauma	Trauma
Pyloric stenosis	Trauma	Meckel's diverticulum	Ectopic pregnancy
Intestinal anomalies	Meckel's diverticulum	Intussusception	Testicular torsion
Hirschsprung's disease	Appendicitis	Tumour	Tumour
Intestinal perforation	Tumour (Wilm's)		
Trauma			

for pyuria, haematuria and ketonuria ± glycosuria.

5. **Urine pregnancy test** is indicated in any teenage girl who is pregnancy capable regardless of her menstrual or sexual history.
6. **Plain abdominal x-rays** are most likely to be significant in cases of:
   a. prior abdominal surgery
   b. foreign body ingestion
   c. abnormal bowel sounds
   d. abdominal distention
   e. signs of peritoneal irritation

   Abnormalities to be sought include:
   a. air fluid levels
   b. decreased intestinal gas
   c. sentinel loops
   d. faecaliths
   e. free air
   f. foreign bodies
   g. masses
   h. constipation
7. **Abdominal ultrasonography**: a sensitive method to detect intraabdominal pathology including intussusception, appendicitis, pyloric stenosis, masses and abscesses. It is particularly useful in the adolescent female with lower abdominal pain to differentiate appendicitis from other pelvic pathology.

SPECIFIC ENTITIES ACCORDING TO AGE OF CHILD

The most common causes of abdominal pain, both surgical and non-surgical are presented in Table 2.

NON-ABDOMINAL CAUSES OF ABDOMINAL PAIN

Table 3 presents non-abdominal causes of abdominal pain.

Table 3: Extraabdominal causes of abdominal pain

Inflammatory	*Toxicologic*
Viral illness	Heavy metal poisoning
Strep pharyngitis	Ingestions of alcohol, aspirin, insecticides
Henoch-Schönlein purpura	
Sepsis	*Referred from extraabdominal sources*
Acute rheumatic fever	Pneumonia
Collagen-vascular disease	Pyelonephritis
	Urolithiasis
Metabolic/haematologic	Testicular torsion
Diabetic ketoacidosis	Epididymitis
Leukaemia	Abdominal migraine
Sickle cell crisis	Myocarditis and pericarditis
	Functional abdominal pain

DISPOSITION

- Any child with a probable surgical abdomen requires an immediate surgical consultation.
- A liberal policy regarding admission is suggested for children with equivocal signs and symptoms. If parents insist on taking the child home, full documentation of advice given must be recorded.

References/further reading

1. Singer J. Acute abdominal conditions that may require surgical intervention In: *Pediatric Emergency Medicine: A Comprehensive Study Guide.* American College of Emergency Physicians. New York: McGraw-Hill; 1995:311–319.

7 Child with breathlessness

Elizabeth Khor • Peter Manning

CAVEATS

- Remember the ABCs: **do not** delay transfer of an acutely dyspnoeic child to the critical care area of ED by asking the parents to give the history.
- A **breathless child with no audible cry** is in imminent danger of respiratory arrest: transfer to critical care area of ED.
- A child with good cry and screaming volubly is demonstrating good lung function.
- A breathless child could be in severe pain from eg biliary colic (choledochal cyst), acute abdomen (peritonitis, intussusception). Anyone in pain can be breathless!
- A breathless child with normal chest examination and a normal chest x-ray could have DKA (findings: typical air hunger, raised stat capillary blood sugar, ketones on breath and in urine).
- When attempting to auscultate the chest of a child you may need to distract the child first since it is very easy to miss physical findings in a screaming child.
- In auscultating the chest of a child, **pay attention to air entry**, not only the crackles and wheezing: diminished air entry over one lobe or one lung may be the only clue to the diagnosis of lobar consolidation **before** the development of localized crackles or bronchial breath sounds, the presence of a pleural effusion or pneumothorax.
- Aspirin or other drug overdose may present with breathlessness as a reflection of metabolic acidosis.
- Always consider cardiac causes of breathlessness such as heart failure due to congenital heart disease, myocarditis or supraventricular tachycardia (SVT).

☛ Special Tips for GPs

- Place a breathless child in a position of comfort for that child: **do not force** him/her to lie flat.
- If the child is frightened by the application of an oxygen mask, then administer 'blow by' oxygen by having the mother hold the mask a short distance from the child's face, directing the flow on to the face.

QUESTIONS TO ASK PARENTS OR CAREGIVER

- **Onset of breathlessness**.
  1. Is breathlessness abrupt while playing with a toy or while eating?
  2. Child becomes breathless while vomiting: vomiting and cyanosis suggest aspiration.
  3. Vomiting, chest pain and dyspnoea may suggest lower lobe pneumonia.
  4. Vomiting, dyspnoea and wheeze may indicate sticky phlegm, eg bronchitis.
- **Exposure of family members to PTB, recent pneumonia or chest infections, or viral illnesses**.
- **History of asthma or previous wheeze**.

EXAMINATION

Note:

1. A breathless child could be in **cardiac failure**, yet presents like bronchiolitis with wheezing; the heart sounds may be difficult to hear.
2. The breathless child with **head retractions** may have signs of **meningeal irritation**: remember to look for signs of increased intracranial pressure in a drowsy, breathless or apnoeic child.
3. A breathless child with **failure to thrive** could have gastroesophageal reflux, tracheoesophageal fistula, cystic fibrosis, or be immunocompromised.

- The **most important sign** to recognize is the mental state: this is an early indicator of hypoxaemia or hypercarbia. Beware irritability, drowsiness, inability to recognize parents and inappropriate social responses.
- Look for presence of **central cyanosis**: if noted, transfer the child immediately to the critical care area of ED and administer 100% supplemental oxygen by face mask.
- Look for **signs of respiratory distress**: cyanosis, head retractions, use of accessory muscles, tracheal tug, retractions, grunting or flaring of the nostrils, or stridor. If noted, transfer immediately to the critical care area of ED: place child in position of comfort and administer 100% supplemental oxygen by face mask.
- Count the **respiratory rate** of the child.
- Do the signs suggest upper or lower respiratory tract disease?
  1. **Upper respiratory tract obstruction** is suggested by snoring and stridor (presence of the latter demands transfer to the critical care area).
  2. **Grunting** suggests alveolar pathology requiring PEEP to clear the alveoli as in consolidation of pneumonia, or pulmonary oedema, or sepsis.
- **Observe chest** for signs of unequal expansion; palpate position of trachea; palpate for subcutaneous emphysema: vocal resonance is best evaluated by asking the child to repeat the names of favourite cartoon characters.
- Complete the examination by evaluating the **ENT system**.

MANAGEMENT

- **X-ray considerations**
  1. A clinical diagnosis should be made before ordering a chest x-ray for any breathless child.
  2. Chest x-ray is useful in dyspnoeic infants since you can ascertain pulmonary findings as well as cardiac size.
  3. Not all asthmatic patients need chest x-rays but it is useful to exclude FB aspiration, or presence of pneumonia or atelectasis.
  4. Chest x-ray is indicated in all first wheezes and the clinical triad of fever, cough and dyspnoea.
  5. It may be dangerous to send a child to x-ray rather than having the child x-rayed in the critical care area, eg croup and epiglottitis.

- **Severely dyspnoeic child**
  1. Manage the child in the critical care area.
  2. Evaluate and support the airway.
  3. Administer 100% supplemental oxygen by mask.
  4. Monitoring: ECG, vital signs q 5–15 min, pulse oximetry.
  5. Perform careful examination of the chest.
  6. Chest x-ray as needed (see above).
  7. Nebulized salbutamol therapy for the wheezing child.
     Dosage: **0.5 ml: 1.5 ml saline for age <1 year**
     1 ml: 3 ml saline for age >1 year – can be repeated q 20 min
     Obtain paediatric consultation and transfer to Paeds ICU.
  8. Set heparin plug in a peripheral vein: obtain venous blood gas since this is useful in assessing the pH and PCO_2.

- **Mildly or moderately dyspnoeic child**
  1. Can be managed in the intermediate care area of ED.
  2. Monitoring: pulse oximetry.
  3. Administer supplemental oxygen if SpO_2 <96%.
  4. In asthmatics
     a. PEFRs if child can perform the technique adequately (generally age 6–7 years and above).
     b. Nebulized salbutamol therapy as needed q 20 min.
     c. Start oral prednisolone 1–2 mg/kg **early** if discharge from ED is likely.

DISPOSITION

- **Admit**
  1. Children who are intubated, following appropriate paediatric consultation.
  2. Children who do not improve with therapy.
  3. Children whose SpO_2 on room air is <96%.
  4. Children whose parents/caregivers do not seem competent to follow instructions.

- **Discharge to outpatient care**
  1. Children who respond appropriately to therapy.
  2. Children with competent parents/caregivers who will/can follow instructions.

References/further reading

1. Strange GR, Ahrens WR, Lelyveld S, et al, eds. *Pediatric Emergency Medicine: A Comprehensive Study Guide*. New York: McGraw-Hill; 1996.

8 Child/baby, crying

Elizabeth Khor • Peter Manning

CAVEATS

- Refers to the child who cries continually and refuses to be pacified.
- Be cognizant that this is a situation that is fraught with anxiety, since the caregivers cannot tolerate the crying and have brought the child to the ED out of sheer desperation.
- **Avoid** prescribing sedating agents: **do not** accede to parents' request for such treatment. The crying is a symptom of a problem and sedating the child will simply mask the underlying cause.

> ☛ **Special Tips for GPs**
> - Remember to undress the child totally to expose abdomen, perineum and extremities fully.

MANAGEMENT

Is the child in pain?

- **Abdominal conditions**
  1. Acute **intussusception**: non-stop screaming, vomits and refuses to feed.

Note: Do rectal exam looking for blood or redcurrant jelly stools.

  2. **Volvulus**: abdominal distension.
  3. **Obstructed inguinal herniae** (baby boys and girls): remember to look at the groin and feel the testes in boys for acute **torsion**.
  4. **Ureteric colic**, **biliary colic** or acute **UTI**: Urine dipstick leukocytes for blood, nitrites.
- **H, E, E, N, T conditions**
  1. Acute **otitis media**: beware the 'normal' injected tympanic membrane of the crying infant.
  2. Check oropharynx for scalds or burns, and herpangina or gingivostomatitis with oral ulcers.
  3. Look for **corneal abrasions**.
  4. Examine head for **bulging fontanelles** (for those <15 to 18 months old).
- **Extremity conditions**
  1. **Circumferential ligature** ('pseudoainhum'): the infant's toes, fingers or even penis can be strangulated by a loose thread from a mitten, blanket or maternal hair.
  2. **Long bone injury**: think of non-accidental injury.

3. **Osteomyelitis**: examine extremities for local tenderness, swelling and redness.

- **Chest pain** (rare, but possible)
  1. Cardiac **ischaemia**: Kawasaki's disease or pericarditis.
  2. **SVT** may present with crying and poor perfusion: **remember** to count the pulse rate.
- Consider **meningeal irritation**
  1. A crying child with a high-pitched cry.
  2. May show head retraction, bulging fontanelle, drowsiness or stiff neck.
- Consider **shaken baby syndrome**: suspect this if the child is pale, drowsy with unexplained physical injuries and/or retinal haemorrhages.

Disposition

- Admit child to hospital: This is prudent since the caregivers are probably sleep-deprived and too weary to cope with the incessant crying. This allows caregivers to sleep. This also permits further investigation of cause, eg possible non-accidental injury (NAI).

References/further reading

1. Barkin, RM, Caputo GL, Jaffe DM, et al, eds. *Pediatric Emergency Medicine Concepts and Clinical Practice*. 2nd ed. St. Louis, MI: Mosby; 1997.
2. Reisdorff EJ, Roberts MR, Wiegenstein JG. *Pediatric Emergency Medicine*. Philadelphia, PA: WB Saunders; 1993.
3. Green M, Haggerty RJ, Weitzman M, eds. *Ambulatory Pediatrics*. 5th ed. Philadelphia, PA: WB Saunders; 1999.

9 Child with diarrhoea

Elizabeth Khor • Peter Manning

CAVEATS

- Refers to child with diarrhoea only, without vomiting.
- Consider the possibility that the **diarrhoea** is 'spurious' and caused by:
  1. Constipation: can palpate faecal masses in the abdomen
  2. Laxatives, antacids or antibiotics
  3. Too much sorbitol-containing fruit juice (eg apple juice)
- Most cases are due to **acute GI infections**:
  1. **Viral** eg rotavirus: URTI symptoms followed by non-bilious vomiting, then profuse and watery diarrhoea.
  2. **Invasive** – *Salmonella*, *Shigella*, *Campylobacter jejuni* or *E. coli* – blood-stained mucoid stools, high fever, tenesmus, 'sick' appearance.
  3. **Toddler's diarrhoea**: often begins after a bout of acute GE but child looks well without fever, weight loss or tenesmus; parents are concerned about frequent passage of soft, pasty stools with undigested vegetables in the stool.
- **Do not** prescribe Lomotil® or Imodium®-type products in children <6 years of age as these medications may cause paralytic ileus.
- Teach parents that **even with treatment, some diarrhoea should be expected**: the aim of therapy is to prevent dehydration in the child.

> ☛ **Special Tips for GPs**
> - Remember to perform a focused hydration history and examination (see below).

QUESTIONS TO ASK PARENTS OR CAREGIVER

- **What has been the recent bowel habit?** eg constipation
- **What is in your child's diet?** eg fibre, sorbitol-containing juices
- **Has your child recently been prescribed laxatives, antacids or antibiotics?**

EXAMINATION ESSENTIALS

- **Quick hydration check**:
  1. Is diaper dry or wet? If dry, ask when the child last passed urine; no urine for more than 8 hours is a symptom of dehydration.
  2. Beware crying child who sheds no tears.

- **Focused hydration check** (Table 1):
  1. Look for sunken eyes, dry mouth, poor peripheral perfusion, reduced skin turgor.
  2. If patient is severely dehydrated, there is danger of hypovolaemic shock: start IV resuscitation in ED prior to admission.
- **Tachypnoea** may indicate hyperpyrexia or the air hunger of metabolic acidosis.
- **H, E, E, N, T conditions**:
  1. Examine ears for acute otitis media.
  2. Auscultate lung bases for basilar pneumonia.
  3. Check throat for signs of pharyngitis or tonsillitis: absence of these signs makes diagnosis less likely.
- **Examine abdomen for**:
  1. Tenderness (appendicitis or peritonitis)
  2. Hepatomegaly (may have sepsis)
  3. Masses (intussuception)
  4. Distension (intestinal obstruction or paralytic ileus)
- **Perform rectal examination** (you may be able to disimpact faecal masses): any blood should already be obvious on the diaper.

MANAGEMENT

- **Stool cultures** have no place in emergency medicine.
- **Urinalysis** for **ketonuria**: useful, particularly in the obese child in whom signs of dehydration are difficult to assess.
- **Urinalysis** for nitrites/white blood cells: for presumptive diagnosis of UTI.
- **X-rays**: KUB if child has abdominal distension or is passing bloody diarrhoea.
- **Stat capillary blood sugar** if altered mental state exists.
- **Rehydration of the severely dehydrated child (10% dehydration)**: Refer to *Fluid Replacement in Paediatrics*
  1. Establish peripheral IV line.
  2. Administer crystalloid (normal saline or Hartman's solution) at 20 ml/kg body weight as bolus over 20–30 min.
  3. Labs: FBC, urea/electrolytes/creatinine, stat capillary blood sugar.
  4. Obtain paediatric consultation and transfer child to Paeds ICU.

DISPOSITION

1. **Admit** for IV fluid therapy:
   a. A neonate or young infant with profuse diarrhoea.
   b. Children with signs of moderate/severe diarrhoea and who refuse oral fluids.

Table 1: Clinical assessment of severity of dehydration

Signs and symptoms	*Mild dehydration (5%)*	*Moderate dehydration (7%)*	*Severe dehydration (10%)*
General appearance and condition			
Infants and young children	Thirsty, alert, restless	Thirsty, restless, lethargic but irritable or drowsy	Drowsy, limp, cold, sweaty, cyanotic extremities, may be comatose
Older children and adults	Thirsty, alert, restless	Thirsty, alert, postural hypotension	Cold, sweaty, muscle cramps, cyanotic extremities, conscious
Radial pulse	Normal rate and strength	Rapid and weak	Rapid, sometimes impalpable
Respiration	Normal	Deep ± rapid	Deep and rapid
Anterior fontanelle	Normal	Sunken	Very sunken
Systolic BP	Normal	Normal or low	<90 mmHg; may be unrecordable
Skin elasticity	Pinch retracts immediately	Pinch retracts slowly	Pinch retracts slowly (>2 s)
Eyes	Normal	Sunken (detectable)	Grossly sunken
Tears	Present	Absent	Absent
Mucous membranes	Moist	Dry	Very dry
Urine flow	Normal	Reduced amount, dark	None for several hours
Body weight loss (%)	4–5	6–9	10 or more
Estimated fluid deficit (mL/kg)	40–50	60–90	100–110

Source: Adapted with permission of the McGraw-Hill Companies, from Powell EC, Reynolds S. Gastroenteritis. In: Strange GR, Ahrens W, Lelyreld S. et al., eds. *Paediatric Emergency Medicine: A Comprehensive Study Guide*. New York: McGraw-Hill; 1995:291.

   c. Children with pathological chronic diarrhoea with failure to thrive, or signs of colitis and possible electrolyte and water deficiencies.
2. **Discharge to outpatient care** children who are not toxic-looking and whose urinalysis shows absent or trace ketones only.
   a. Oral rehydration solutions (ORS), eg Servidrat or diluted rice cereal.
   b. Continue breast feeding when possible.
   c. If duration of diarrhoea >24 hours, children may be offered lactose-free milk, eg O-Lac or any soy-based milk formula or HNMilupa 25 for 48–72 hours.
   d. Allow child to eat solid food as soon as tolerated and appetite has returned: most solids are acceptable.
   e. Kaolin products are not useful: instead Smecta will reduce, but not eliminate totally, the number of stools by 30–40%.
   f. Toddler's diarrhoea: avoid lactose and sorbitol-containing products, and reduce dietary fibre for one week.

References/further reading

1. Barkin, RM, Caputo GL, Jaffe DM, et al, eds. *Pediatric Emergency Medicine Concepts and Clinical Practice*. 2nd ed. St. Louis, MI: Mosby; 1997.
2. Reisdorff EJ, Roberts MR, Wiegenstein JG. *Pediatric Emergency Medicine*. Philadelphia, PA: WB Saunders; 1993.
3. Green M, Haggerty RJ, Weitzman M, eds. *Ambulatory Pediatrics*. 5th ed. Philadelphia, PA: WB Saunders; 1999.

10 Child with fever

Wong Chin Khoon

CAVEATS

- Fever is a normal response.
- Fever is a symptom, not a disease.
- Fever persists until the disease process resolves.
- Fever determination need not always be exact.
- Fever is often a useful body defence.
- Fever, especially low grade, need not always be treated.
- Clinical appearance is usually more important than the height of the fever.

PHYSIOLOGICAL EFFECTS OF FEVER

- Fever appears to increase:
  1. The phagocytic and bactericidal activity of neutrophils
  2. The cytotoxic effects of lymphocytes
- For each 1°C elevation of body temperature there is:
  1. 13% increase in O_2 consumption
  2. Tachycardia (10 beats per min/°C)
  3. Tachypnoea (2.5 breath per min/°C)
- The increased metabolic demand may stress foetuses as well as patients with marginal cardiac or cerebral vascular supply.

POTENTIAL COMPLICATIONS OF FEVER

- Dehydration
- Fits
- Delirium (especially in younger ones)
- Hyperpyrexia (>41.1°C): must consider serious bacterial infection (SBI)

Note: **SBI** are meningitis, pneumonia, sepsis, osteomyelitis, UTI, *Salmonella enteritis, Listeria, E. coli, Staph/Strep* infection. **Symptoms and signs** are irritability, decreased activity, weak cry, poor feeding, diarrhoea and vomiting, abdominal distension, drowsiness, respiratory distress, hypothermia or hyperthermia, poor peripheral perfusion. Rate of SBI = 9.5% (<40°C) vs. 36% (>40°C).

MANAGEMENT: POINTS TO BE CONSIDERED

Consider whether there is a fever

- **Definition of fever**: body temperature of 1°C or greater above the mean standard deviation at the site of recording.

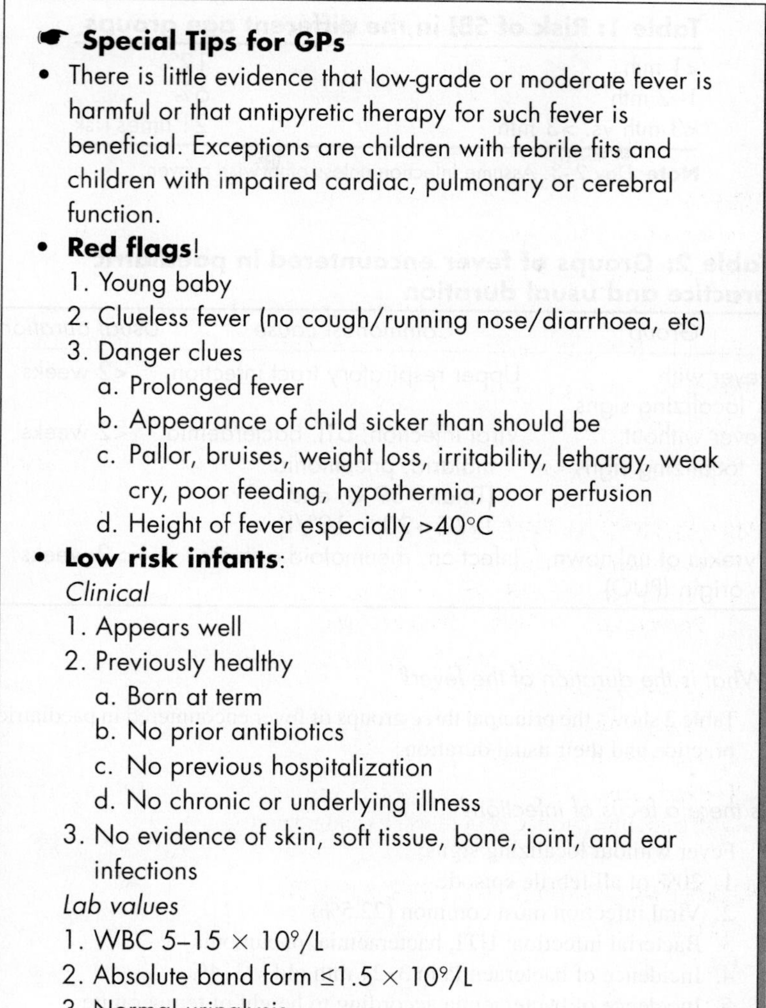

☛ Special Tips for GPs

- There is little evidence that low-grade or moderate fever is harmful or that antipyretic therapy for such fever is beneficial. Exceptions are children with febrile fits and children with impaired cardiac, pulmonary or cerebral function.
- **Red flags**!
  1. Young baby
  2. Clueless fever (no cough/running nose/diarrhoea, etc)
  3. Danger clues
     a. Prolonged fever
     b. Appearance of child sicker than should be
     c. Pallor, bruises, weight loss, irritability, lethargy, weak cry, poor feeding, hypothermia, poor perfusion
     d. Height of fever especially >40°C
- **Low risk infants**:

  Clinical
  1. Appears well
  2. Previously healthy
     a. Born at term
     b. No prior antibiotics
     c. No previous hospitalization
     d. No chronic or underlying illness
  3. No evidence of skin, soft tissue, bone, joint, and ear infections

  Lab values
  1. WBC 5–15 × 10^9/L
  2. Absolute band form ≤1.5 × 10^9/L
  3. Normal urinalysis

- Normal baby temperature according to site of recording:
  1. Rectal route: ≤38.0°C
  2. Oral route: ≤37.5°C
  3. Axillary route: ≤37.5°C
  4. Tympanic route: ≤38.0°C

What is the age of the child?

- The age of the child correlates with the risk of SBI. See Table 1.

Table 1: Risk of SBI in the different age groups

<1 mth	12%
1–2 mth	6%
<3 mth vs. >3 mth	21 times risk

Note: Day 2–3: Assume infection unless otherwise proven.

Table 2: Groups of fever encountered in paediatric practice and usual duration

Group	*Commonest cause*	*Usual duration*
Fever with localizing signs	Upper respiratory tract infection	<2 weeks
Fever without localizing signs	Viral infection, UTI, bacteraemia, malaria, pneumonia (Tmax >39°C, and TWC >20 × 10^9/L)	<2 weeks
Pyrexia of unknown origin (PUO)	Infection, rheumatoid arthritis	>2 weeks

What is the duration of the fever?

- Table 2 shows the principal three groups of fever encountered in paediatric practice and their usual duration.

Is there a focus of infection?

- Fever without localizing signs:
  1. 20% of all febrile episodes
  2. Viral infection most common (22.5%)
  3. Bacterial infection: UTI, bacteraemia, pneumonia
  4. Incidence of bacteraemia in 3–24 mth old = 3–4%
  5. Incidence of bacteraemia according to height of temperature
     40°C–40.4°C = 1.7%
     40.5°C–40.9°C = 2.4%
     >40.9°C = 2.8%
  6. Septicaemia: meningitis, pneumonia, otitis media due to Group B *Strep, E. coli, Listeria* (neonate), *Strep pneumoniae, H. influenzae*
- Pyrexia of unknown origin (PUO):
  1. 38.3°C on several occasions
  2. >1 week after investigations and diagnosis still uncertain
  3. Infection 50–60% (viral 15%)
  4. Collagen disease 20%
  5. Malignancy 5%

6. Miscellaneous 5–10%
7. Undiagnosed 5%

Are there any red flags?

See *Special Tips for GPs*.

MANAGEMENT: TO TREAT OR NOT TO TREAT?

- Antipyretics **do not** shorten the duration of the febrile episode or interfere directly with pyrogen formation or heat loss.
- **Indications for antipyretics**:
  1. Fever >38.5°C associated with painful or unpleasant symptoms, eg otitis media, myalgia, discomfort.
  2. Fever >39°C without obvious symptoms.
  3. Poor nutrition, cardiovascular diseases, burns or postoperative state.
  4. History of fits or delirium secondary to fever.

Note: In the Singaporean context, it may be difficult to convince parents to give antipyretics only if fever >38.5°C, so 37.5°C is a practical threshold.

- **Antipyretics**:
  1. **Paracetamol**
     a. Dosage: 10–15 mg/kg dose 4–6 h oral or rectal routes.
     b. Maximum daily dosage: 65 mg/kg/day.
     c. Onset of action at 30 min, nadir of fever 3 h later, duration 3–6 h.
     d. Improves activity and alertness but not mood or appetite.
     e. Side effects are rare (GIT upset, rash, thrombocytopenia, hypoglycaemia, bronchospasm).

Note: Use with caution in patients with liver disease or jaundice.

  2. **Ibuprofen (Brufen®)**
     a. The *only* NSAID approved as antipyretic in USA (1984) and UK (1990).
     b. Dosage: 5–10 mg/kg/ dose q 6 h.
     c. Onset of action earlier, more potent, and lasts longer than paracetamol.

Note: There is no documented evidence that alternating paracetamol with NSAIDs provides better control of fever, but NSAIDs can be used together with paracetamol at different intervals because the mechanism of action is different. It is recommended that it be given at least 1 hour after the last dose of paracetamol (to allow paracetamol time to work).

     d. Side effects are few (platelet inhibition and reduced renal blood flow are both extremely rare).

Note: Use with caution in patients with bleeding diathesis and asthma as NSAIDs have antiplatelet effects and may cause bronchospasm.

  3. **Diclofenac (Voltaren®)**: though commonly used as an antipyretic it is not indicated as such, but can be useful for the myalgias sometimes associated with fever.

Note: Prescribing information provided by the manufacturer (Novartis) states *Fever alone is not an indication.*

- **Adjunctive measures for fever**:
  1. Tepid sponging (water temperature 27°C–34°C)
     a. Useful if temp >41°C or 40°C with discomfort
     b. Start after giving antipyretic
  2. Bed rest has no significant effect on temperature control
  3. Total body cooling, ice packs and air-conditioner are indicated only for hyperthermia
  4. Alcohol sponging is contraindicated in children

DISPOSITION

- Age <3 months: Admit for full septic work-up
- Age 3–36 months:
  1. Clear-cut focus: treat focus as appropriate; if discharged, to follow up within 24–48 hours
  2. No clear-cut focus:
     a. Non-toxic and low risk: discharge with follow up within 24 hours
     b. Toxic or high risk: admit for full septic work-up and antibiotics

Note: Urinalysis for all and FBC if fever >3 days.

Other admission criteria

- Life-threatening infections, eg meningitis.
- Severe soft tissue infections, eg septic arthritis, buccal or orbital cellulitis.
- Hypoxia due to lower respiratory tract infection.
- Electrolyte imbalance due to gastroenteritis.
- Impression of parental competence:
  1. Can parents provide adequate care?
  2. Will antibiotics, if indicated, be given as recommended?
  3. Can parents be trusted to return to hospital if needed?
  4. Can follow-up be ensured?

References/further reading

1. Fauci AS, et al, eds. *Harrison's Principles of Internal Medicine*. 14th ed. New York: McGraw-Hill; 1998.
2. Baraff LJ, Bass JW, Fleisher GR, et al. Practice guidelines for the management of infants and children 0 to 36 months of age with fever without source. Agency for Health Care Policy and Research. *Pediatrics*. 1993;22(7):1198–1210.
3. Bachur R, Perry H, Harper M. Occult pneumonias empiric chest radiographs in febrile children with leukocytosis. *Ann Emerg Med*. 1999;33(2):166–173.
4. Lee GM. Risk of bacteraemia in the post Hib era. *Arch Pediatr Adolesc Med*. 1998;152:624–628.

11 Child, fitting

Wong Chin Khoon

CAVEATS

- The **objectives** for the ED **management** are:
  1. Maintenance of adequate airway, breathing and circulation.
  2. Termination of convulsive activity and prevention of recurrence.
  3. Diagnosis and initial therapy of life-threatening causes, which includes the reversal of physiological changes that may have taken place.
  4. Arrangement for the appropriate disposition of the child (eg investigations, admission or referral).
- For purpose of **subsequent management**, there is a need to differentiate between febrile seizure (simple or complex) and non-febrile seizure, both of which can present as status epilepticus.
- When the exact onset of seizure is unknown, any fitting patient arriving at the ED should be managed as though he/she is having status epilepticus.
- Always consider the important **differential diagnosis** in Table 1.

☛ Special Tips for GPs

- Neck stiffness may be absent in children <18 months old or difficult to elicit information from uncooperative children.
- Opisthotonic posturing in a drowsy child suggests increased intracranial pressure.
- An irritable child who is difficult to examine may have meningeal irritation.
- Bradycardia, hypotension and poor perfusion in a fitting child are ominous signs and imply severe hypoxia and an immediate need to establish the airway and ventilate the child.
- Before giving any medication, always get a brief history on seizure disorder, medication usage, chronic disease or drug allergies.
- Do **bedside blood sugar** level in all fitting children.
- Metoclopramide-induced oculogyric crisis may mimic a febrile seizure and has a totally different management, ie IM or IV diphenhydramine (<3 years old) or benztropine (>3 years old).
- A recognized source of infection (eg otitis media) does not exclude the presence of meningitis.

Table 1: Differential diagnosis of seizure

1. Rigors
2. Hypoglycaemic seizure
3. Meningitis/Meningoencephalitis
4. Reye's syndrome
5. Drug intoxication, eg oculogyric crisis
6. Breath-holding attacks
7. Gastroesophageal reflux
8. Syncope
9. Pseudoseizure

MANAGEMENT OF A FITTING CHILD

- Most seizures are brief and do not require any specific treatment.
  1. Position the child semiprone to minimize the chance of aspiration.
  2. Secure airway: if necessary clear the airway with gentle suction.

Note: Put a padded gag between teeth to prevent the biting of tongue **only if** jaw is relaxed; otherwise more damage is done with the use of force. Administer supplemental oxygen by face mask and keep oxygen saturation >95%.

- **If seizure continues**
  1. Give **rectal diazepam** 0.5 mg/kg (max. 10 mg, good guide: infant 2.5 mg, >1 year old 5 mg, may repeat twice) only if unable to insert intravenous (IV) plug. Otherwise give **IV diazepam** 0.1–0.25 mg/kg at rate no faster than 2 mg/min, you may repeat twice every 5 minutes if seizure is not controlled.
  2. Monitor carefully for respiratory depression.
  3. Establish peripheral intravenous line.
  4. Take blood for bedside blood glucose and electrolytes.
  5. Measure and record vital signs and temperature.
  6. If seizure continues, treat as for status epilepticus (see below).
- **After seizure stops**
  1. Continue to monitor respiratory and neurological status.
  2. If child is febrile, bring temperature down with **tepid sponging** and **antipyretics**.
  3. Measure vital signs, temperature and oxygen saturation.
  4. Continue to give supplemental oxygen if oxygen saturation <95%.
  5. Consider investigations: anticonvulsant level, FBC, urea/electrolytes/creatinine, liver function test, ionised calcium, magnesium, lumbar puncture, chest x-ray, urinalysis (depending on clinical suspicion).
- Admit all patients with a first non-febrile seizure. In a child with a **first non-febrile seizure**
  1. Lumbar puncture is of limited value and is used primarily when there is concern about possible meningitis or encephalitis.

2. EEG is recommended as part of the neurodiagnostic evaluation.
3. If a neuroimaging study is obtained, MRI is the preferred modality.

STATUS EPILEPTICUS

Definition

Continuous seizure activity or intermittent seizure activity with failure to regain consciousness between seizures for a duration of longer than 30 minutes.

MANAGEMENT

- Initial management of a fitting child is as mentioned above.
- When setting IV line, take blood for:
    1. Stat capillary blood sugar. Consider FBC, urea/electrolytes/creatinine, liver function tests, ionized calcium, magnesium, phosphate and blood gases in selected cases.
    2. Include anticonvulsant level(s) on all patients on long-term therapy.
- If patient is hypoglycaemic, give IV glucose bolus: 25% dextrose 1–2 ml/kg and 10% dextrose 2–3 ml/kg. Maintain with IV 10% dextrose infusion at 5–10 ml/kg/min to maintain normoglycaemia.
- Prepare intubation equipment in case you are unable to maintain airway and adequate oxygenation.
- **If seizure continues**:
    1. Administer **IV phenytoin** 20 mg/kg diluted in **normal saline** at a rate of 1 mg/kg/min (max. 50 mg/min). Additional 5 mg/kg increments of phenytoin may be given up to a maximum dose of 30 mg/kg (max. 1000 mg) if seizure continues (monitor ECG and BP as it may cause cardiac arrhythmias).

Note: The use of dilution with saline is dependent on institutional policy. Phenytoin can be administered without dilution though the precautions regarding rate of administration still apply.

2. **IV phenobarbitone** 20 mg/kg may be given at a rate of 2 mg/kg/min (max. 30 mg/min) after the loading dose of phenytoin if seizure continues. Additional 5 mg/kg increments may be given up to a maximum total dose of 30 mg/kg (max. 600 mg) if seizure continues (may cause respiratory depression, hypotension and sedation in high doses).

- If seizure continues despite the above measures taken, consider Rapid Sequence Intubation: paralysis and intubation by an individual skilled in airway management.
- **Disposition**:
    1. Admit to the Paeds ICU and obtain an immediate paediatric neurological consult.

2. All children with status epilepticus should have a **CT scan of the head** done. CT scan may be undertaken after the convulsion has terminated and airway, breathing and circulation are stabilized.
3. Start **maintenance therapy of anticonvulsant** (phenytoin or phenobarbitone or both, depending on what has been used in the initial therapy).

Isolated fit in an epileptic

- Take **blood level of anticonvulsants**:
  1. If *low*, administer a double dose of medication.
  2. If the patient is *non-compliant*, strongly encourage compliance.
  3. If the patient is *already compliant* with their medication, increase the dose if the maximum dose has not been reached.
  4. If the *maximum dose* has already been reached, consult the paediatric neurologist for further anticonvulsants.
- **Disposition**: Observe in the ED for 2–3 hours, discharge if no further seizures and refer to the paediatric neurologist in the Specialist Clinic.

References/further reading

1. Practice Parameter: Evaluating a first non-febrile seizure in children. Report of the Quality Standards Subcommittee of the American Academy of Neurology, the Child Neurology Society, and the American Epilepsy Society. *Neurology* 2000;55:616–629. Also available at: www.aan.com/professionals/practice/pdfs/g10081.pdf.
2. The Neurodiagnostic Evaluation of the Child with a First Simple Febrile Seizure. American Academy of Pediatrics Practice Guideline. May 1996. Volume 97, Number 5. Available at: www.aap.org/policy/neuro.htm. Accessed 13 August 2002.
3. Singapore Ministry of Health. A Guide on Paediatrics. 1997:27–28.
4. Management of the Paediatric Patient with Generalised Convulsive Status Epilepticus in the Emergency Department. Position Statement from the Emergency Paediatrics Section, Canadian Paediatric Society, January 2002. Available at: www.cps.ca/english/statements/EP/ep95–01.htm. Accessed 13 August 2002.
5. Tay S. Protocol for Refractory Status Epilepticus. Paediatric Neurology Division, Children's Medical Institute, National University Hospital. Singapore: 2001. Available at: courses.nus.edu.sg/course/paev34/notes/cmi-protocols/index.htm.

12 Child with vomiting

Elizabeth Khor • Peter Manning

CAVEATS

- Not every child who vomits has an acute gastrointestinal problem: be aware of meningitis, increased intracranial pressure, otitis media, acute asthma, lower lobe pneumonia or UTI, which also present with vomiting.
- Beware the infant or neonate who vomits: the diagnosis of 'overfeeding' or 'mild reflux' is made only after medical or surgical conditions have been excluded. Be aware that **vomiting** is **often** the **presenting symptom** of a **septic** neonate, a neonate with inborn error of metabolism, an infant with acute **appendicitis,** or **meningitis,** or **pyloric stenosis**.
- **Avoid** prescribing metoclopramide and prochlorperazine to children under 12 years old since oculogyric crises are a distressing and undesirable side effect.
- Oral promethazine syrup is a safe and mild antiemetic.
- Avoid prescribing Prepulsid in young children since one must be absolutely certain that there are no signs of an acute surgical abdomen.

> ☛ **Special Tips for GPs**
> - Remember to perform a focused hydration history and examination (see below).

QUESTIONS TO ASK PARENTS OR CAREGIVER

- **What is the colour of the vomitus?**
  1. **Bile** (malrotation of the gut) or **blood** points towards an acute surgical condition that warrants admission for further investigation.
  2. Examine the vomitus itself or vomit-stained clothing.

Note: Bile often resembles sugar cane juice and blood may look like Milo.

- **What medication has been prescribed? or How many doctors have you consulted?** Be aware that certain prescribed medications may cause gastric irritation and vomiting, eg macrolide antibiotics, oral theophylline, oral NSAIDs, and oral prednisolone.
- **When did you last note a wet diaper or when did your child last urinate?** No urine for more than 8 hours is a symptom of dehydration.
- **Did your child sustain a recent head injury?**
- **Is there a history of family members/siblings suffering from similar symptoms?** Eg: Rotavirus GE usually starts with URTI symptoms

followed by vomiting and profuse diarrhoea; there is a high risk of dehydration in children <3 years of age.

EXAMINATION ESSENTIALS

- **Quick hydration check:**
  1. Is diaper dry or wet? If dry, ask question above
  2. Beware crying child who sheds no tears
- **Focused hydration check**: refer to *Child with Diarrhoea* Table 1 for clinical assessment of severity of dehydration.
  1. Look for sunken eyes, dry mouth, poor peripheral perfusion, reduced skin turgor
  2. If patient is severely dehydrated, there is danger of hypovolaemic shock: start IV resuscitation in ED prior to admission
- **Tachypnoea** may indicate hyperpyrexia or the air hunger of metabolic acidosis.
- **Tachycardia** may indicate impending shock in the young.
- **H, E, E, N, T conditions**:
  1. Examine ears for acute otitis media
  2. Auscultate lung bases for basilar pneumonia
  3. Check throat for signs of pharyngitis or tonsillitis: absence of these signs makes diagnosis less likely
  4. Check for bulging fontanelles (for those less than 15 to 18 months old)
- **Examine abdomen** for:
  1. Tenderness (appendicitis or peritonitis)
  2. Hepatomegaly (may have sepsis)
  3. Masses, eg pyloric stenosis or intussusception
  4. Distension, eg intestinal obstruction or paralytic ileus
  5. Perform rectal examination to check for blood or redcurrant jelly stools of intussusception
- If there is a history of **head injury**, examine for:
  1. Any boggy scalp swelling
  2. Pupillary response
  3. Fundus
  4. Gait and symmetry of neurological parameters

MANAGEMENT

- **Urine dipstick** for **ketonuria**: useful, particularly in the obese child in whom signs of dehydration are difficult to assess.
- **Urine dipstick** for **nitrites/leukocytes** for presumptive diagnosis of UTI.
- **X-rays**:
  1. **CXR** for vomiting children with respiratory symptoms or abdominal pain/epigastric tenderness.

2. **KUB** if child is vomiting bile or blood.
3. **X-ray** of **skull** is still medically and culturally the norm in Singapore, particularly in younger children in whom the calvarium is very thin.

- **Stat capillary blood sugar** if altered mental state exists:
  1. Drowsy child with low blood sugar and hepatomegaly could have acute sepsis or Reye's syndrome.
  2. Drowsy child with hyperglycaemia and 'air hunger' could have acute DKA.
- **Rehydration of the severely dehydrated child (10% dehydration)**: refer to *Fluid Replacement in Paediatrics*
  1. Establish peripheral IV line.
  2. Administer crystalloid (normal saline or Hartmann's solution) at 20 ml/kg body weight as bolus over 20–30 minutes.
  3. Labs: FBC, urea/eletrolytes/creatinine.
  4. Obtain paediatric consultation and transfer child to Paeds ICU.
- **Disposition**:
  1. **Admit**:
     a. Children who are still vomiting or have diarrhoea, show anorexia or dehydration in spite of outpatient care with antiemetics or antispasmodics, ie failure of outpatient treatment.
     b. Children who have signs of epigastric tenderness with even mild dehydration, since this child is less likely to be able to drink and retain oral rehydration solutions (ORS).
     c. Children with history of head injury with several episodes of vomiting (after skull x-rays: see *Trauma, Head* criteria): admit to Paeds Surgery.
  2. **Discharge to outpatient care**:
     a. Children in whom you are certain of the diagnosis with no or very mild dehydration.
     b. Parents to administer clear fluids like porridge water or ORS (Servidrat, Gastrolyte or Pedialyte) in small, frequent volumes for the next 6–8 hours.
     c. Oral promethazine syrup is a safe and mild antiemetic.
     d. In viral GE, symptoms subside after 24–48 hours: advise parents to return child for review if no improvement noted after 8–12 hours of oral rehydration therapy at home.

References/further reading

1. Barkin RM, Caputo GL, Jaffe DM, et al, eds. *Pediatric Emergency Medicine Concepts and Clinical Practice*. 2nd ed. St. Louis, MI: Mosby; 1997.
2. Reisdorff EJ, Roberts MR, Wiegenstein JG. *Pediatric Emergency Medicine*. Philadelphia, PA: WB Saunders; 1993.
3. Green M, Haggerty RJ, Weitzman M, eds. *Ambulatory Pediatrics*. 5th ed. Philadelphia, PA: WB Saunders; 1999.

13 Diarrhoea and vomiting

Peng Li Lee

CAVEATS

- Diarrhoea and vomiting are common complaints seen in the ED and for the majority of cases, it is due to food-borne toxigenic diarrhoea, which is self-limiting and requires only symptomatic treatment and rehydration therapy.
- The **most disastrous misdiagnosis** in the differential diagnosis of acute diarrhoeal illness is that of a **missed surgical abdomen**, eg appendicitis, intestinal obstruction, ectopic pregnancy, etc.
- In the **paediatric** population, vomiting and diarrhoea may be a non-specific presentation for **varied illnesses** including otitis media, urinary tract infection, metabolic acidosis, raised intracranial pressure, toxins/drugs, intussusception and malrotation.
- In the **elderly**, be wary of the possibility of **ischaemic colitis**, which is associated with high mortality.
- When vomiting occurs without diarrhoea, a search should be made for a non-infective cause.
- In the clinical assessment, the general state of hydration and nutrition should be noted. Having excluded a surgical abdomen and an extraintestinal cause for the diarrhoea/vomiting, the patient can then be treated symptomatically.

☛ Special Tips for GPs

- For travellers going to endemic areas where they may be prone to **traveller's diarrhoea**, the suggested empiric regime is a fluoroquinolone (ciprofloxacin 500 mg or norfloxacin 400 mg or orfloxacin 300 mg) bd for 3 days + loperamide when diarrhoea develops.
- In children do not forget to perform a focused hydration history and physical examination. Refer to *Child with Vomiting* and *Child with Diarrhoea*.

MANAGEMENT

Symptomatic treatment

- See Table 1 for symptomatic treatment of diarrhoea and vomiting.
- **Rehydration therapy**
  1. **IV rehydration**
     a. Indicated in: severe, intractable vomiting; severe dehydration; altered mental state and ileus.
     b. Should be considered in patients with mild dehydration but are unable to tolerate orally. They will usually feel symptomatically better after IV hydration of 1–1.5l of Hartman's solution over a period of 2–4 hours. In children, see *Fluid Replacement in Paediatrics*.
     c. Clinical assessment to guide therapy: other than clinical signs, the presence of ketonuria on urine dipstick may be used as a useful indicator of dehydration.
  2. **Oral rehydration**
     a. It is as effective as IV rehydration in patients who can tolerate orally.
     b. Administer in small amounts repeatedly.
     c. Principle: water and sodium enter the intestinal cell via the linking (coupling) of one organic molecule, eg glucose. Hence the oral fluids should contain glucose to stimulate the absorption of water and electrolytes across the small intestines. This sodium glucose coupled with active absorption mechanism is largely unaffected by enteric toxins. Servidrat, Pedialyte, Gastrolyte are examples of useful oral rehydration agents.

Investigation at ED

- Generally not required unless clinical dehydration and a prolonged course of illness warrants a check for urea/electrolytes.

Use of antibiotics

- Most food toxigenic diarrhoea does not require antibiotics.
- Duration of traveller's diarrhoea (*E.coli*, *Shigella*) can be shortened by half with the use of ciprofloxacin or bactrim.
- **Indications**: invasive diarrhoea characterized by fever and toxicity ± bloody diarrhoea, ie presumed bacterial diarrhoea.
- **Choice**:
  1. **Ciprofloxacin** is the drug of choice when used empirically. Dosage: 500 mg bd. Duration: 3 days (single doses have been used effectively). Contraindicated in paediatrics (<18 years). Use bactrim as an alternative.
  2. **Metronidazole (Flagyl®)**
     Dosage: 800 mg tds. Duration: 5 days. Indicated when protozoa infection (giardiasis or amoebiasis) is suspected.

Table 1: Drugs used in symptomatic treatment of diarrhoea and vomiting

Medication	*Route*	*Dosage*	*Remarks*
Anti-emetic			
Maxolon® (metoclopromide)	IM Tab	10 mg 10 mg 8H	Useful in the symptomatic relief of nausea and vomiting
Stemetil® (prochlorperazine)	IM Tab	12.5 mg 5–10 mg 8H	Caution in paediatric population as it is associated with increased incidence of extra-pyramidal side effects
Phenergan® (promethazine)	IM IM/PO	25 mg (adult) 0.25–1.0 mg/kg (>2 yrs)	
Anti-diarrhoeal			
Lomotil® (diphenoxylate)	PO	2 tabs tds	Used to decrease frequency of diarrhoeal stools
Imodium® (loperamide)	PO	2 mg tds	Not recommended in children <9 years of age
Activated charcoal	PO	1–2 Tab tds/prn	**Note:** The use of antidiarrhoeal agents is generally not recommended for invasive enteritis as they may increase the risk of bowel invasion by the organism. Avoid also in patients with aspirin sensitivity.
Bismuth subsalicylate	 PO PO	*Adults* 2 or 30 ml q 1 h prn *Children* [9–12 y o] 1 tab or 15 ml q 1 h prn up to 8 doses in 24 h [6–9 y o] 2/3 tab or 10 ml q 1 h prn up to 8 doses in 24 h [3–6 y o] 1/3 tab or 5 ml q 1 h prn up to 8 doses in 24 h	
Anti-spasmodic/motility			
Buscopan® (hyoscine-N-butylbromide)	IM PO	20–40 mg 10 mg tds	For symptomatic relief of abdominal colic associated with diarrhoea Generally contraindicated in invasive enteritis

Indications for Admission

- Invasive diarrhoea requiring stool investigations
- Inability to retain oral fluids
- Uncertain diagnosis requiring further evaluation
- Management of complications: severe dehydration, electrolyte abnormality

References/further reading

1. Hogan DE. The emergency department approach to diarrhoea. In: Munter DW, ed. *Emergency Medicine Clinics of North America: Gastrointestinal Emergencies Part II.* Philadelphia: WB Saunders Company; 1996;14(4):673–694.
2. Gilbert DN, Moellering RC, Sunde MA. *The Sanford Guide to Antimicrobial therapy 2000.* 13th ed. USA: Jeb C. Sanford; 2000:14.
3. Ooi SBS, Koh-Tai BC, Aw TC, et al. Assessment of dehydration in adults using haematomlogic and biochemical tests. *Acad Emerg Med* 1997;4(8):840–844.

14 Fever

Suresh Pillai

CAVEATS

- Fever can be caused by a myriad of illnesses ranging from benign, self-limited viral fevers to severe systemic septicaemia.
- It is important to identify and promptly treat febrile patients with potential sources of infection, especially in the paediatric and geriatric age groups, where fever may be the only sign of severe sepsis.
- The treatment of **unstable febrile patients** with overwhelming sepsis includes the maintenance of adequate oxygenation and organ perfusion, obtaining clinical culture specimens and initiation of empiric antibiotic therapy.
- Consider the possibility of **meningococcaemia** in a **febrile** patient with a **purpuric rash**.

> ☛ **Special Tips for GPs**
>
> - It is important to identify febrile septic patients with or without an obvious localizing source of sepsis and refer them to hospital immediately.
> - Indiscriminate antibiotics should not be prescribed for non-specific viral fevers or upper respiratory tract infection.
> - Administer IV crystalline penicillin 4 mega units stat to all patients with suspected **meningococcaemia**, before sending them to hospital by ambulance.
> - The presentation in **geriatric patients** is usually non-specific, eg generalized weakness, confusion and lethargy. Fever is found in approximately 50% of septic elderly.

ASSESSMENT

- The **history** should include details on the magnitude and duration of fever, localizing signs or symptoms, concurrent medical illnesses, any travel history, immunization history, contact history, medication history, allergies, drug or alcohol abuse.

Note: If travel history is positive, the destination is important because specific illnesses are destination-specific, eg in Thailand, falciparum malaria is resistant to many drugs.

- The **physical examination** should include a careful evaluation of the following:
  1. AMS: drowsiness and lethargy may be the only indicators of severe sepsis in the paediatric and geriatric age groups.
  2. Neck stiffness.
  3. Rash: ranging from maculopapular rash caused by viral exanthems, measles or rubella to petechiae caused by dengue haemorrhagic fever, to purpura caused by disseminated meningococcaemia.
  4. Conjunctivitis, jaundice and signs of otitis externa or media.
  5. Pharyngitis, tonsilitis and sinusitis.
  6. Crepitations in the lungs that may indicate pneumonia or a pericardial rub or cardiac murmur to suggest myopericarditis or bacterial endocarditis respectively.
  7. Abdominal tenderness that may suggest peritonitis, appendicitis, cholecystitis, hepatitis or diverticulitis.
  8. Dysuria, frequency or urgency that may suggest urinary tract infection.
  9. Cellulitis, deep venous thrombosis in the lower extremity or pelvic veins or infected decubitus ulcers.

MANAGEMENT

- The management of febrile patients depends on whether the patient is stable with a minor self-limited illness or whether he is unstable with a potentially life-threatening cause.

The stable febrile patient

- Is haemodynamically stable, alert and clinically non-toxic.
- Is tolerating the fever well without decompensation.
- Has no serious underlying medical illness.
- Has a normal physical examination.
- Has probable viral upper respiratory tract infection or non-specific viral fever if the fever is less than one week's duration.
- Includes patients with fever and a rash that may indicate measles, varicella, rubella or infectious mononucleosis.

The unstable febrile patient

- Is hypotensive, with AMS, is in septicaemic shock or clinically toxic.
- Has prolonged fever of more than one week with no response to treatment.
- Has fever with a serious localizing source like meningitis or appendicitis.
- Has a serious underlying medical illness like diabetes or is immunocompromised from cancer chemotherapy or long term steroid therapy.
- Includes patients with a rash that may indicate dengue haemorrhagic fever or disseminated meningococcaemia or malaria (with no rash).

Investigations (usually not necessary for the stable febrile patient)

- FBC: including the total white count, differential count, absolute neutrophil count, platelets.
- Stat capillary blood sugar estimation to look out for associated hyperglycaemic complications like diabetic ketoacidosis, especially in all toxic-appearing febrile patients and **even in the absence of a prior history of diabetes mellitus**.
- Urine dipstick and culture.
- Blood film for malarial parasites.
- Blood culture.
- Chest x-ray.

Treatment

- If the patient is in septic shock, refer to *Sepsis/Septic Shock*.
- Treat symptomatically with antipyretics like paracetamol 1 g every 6 hourly or non-steroidal antiinflammatory drugs such as diclofenac (Voltaren®) or ibuprofen.

Note: Diclofenac (Voltaren®), though commonly used as an antipyretic, is not indicated as such. Prescribing information provided by the manufacturer (Novartis) states 'Fever alone is not an indication'.

- **Empirical antibiotics** (IV ceftriaxone 1 g stat) should be commenced for septic patients after acquisition of first blood culture.
- For patients with neutropenic sepsis IV ceftazidime 1 g with 1–1.5 mg/kg of gentamicin should be commenced. Refer to *Oncology Emergencies*.
- For intraabdominal sepsis, IV ampicillin 500 mg together with IV gentamicin 80 mg and IV metronidazole 500 mg or IV ceftriaxone 1 g and IV metronidazole 500 mg should be commenced.

Disposition

- Admit the unstable febrile patient to the Medical Department (High Dependency Unit or Intensive Care Unit).
- If there is neutropenic sepsis, admit to the High Dependency Oncology Ward.
- If there is a potential surgical source of intraabdominal sepsis, the patient should be admitted to the Surgical Department.
- Refer those suspected of having dengue fever to the Medical SOC for repeat of FBC. Refer to *Dengue Fever.*

References/further reading

1. Zeccardi JA. Bacteraemia, sepsis and meningitis. In: Tintinalli J, Krome RL, Ruiz E, eds. *Emergency Medicine: A Comprehensive Study Guide.* 3rd ed. New York: McGraw-Hill; 1992:454–456.
2. Carter DW. Fever. In: Hamilton GC, ed. *Presenting Signs and Symptoms in the Emergency Department, Evaluation and Treatment*. Baltimore: Williams and Wilkins; 1993:222–228.

15 Giddiness

Francis Lee • Shirley Ooi

CAVEATS

- Although a clear distinction between vertigo and non-specific giddiness or lightheadedness is useful in pinpointing diagnosis, many patients are unable to accurately describe the sensation that they are feeling.
- **Vertigo** tends to point to an **otological** or **brainstem problem** while non-specific giddiness has many other causes (Table 1).
- **Lightheadedness** as a symptom is often **more sinister** and the approach should be that of syncope/presyncope.
- It is important, on first encounter, to ensure that the patient does not have a significant **life-threatening disease**:
  1. Ischaemic heart disease, eg acute coronary syndrome
  2. Cardiac failure
  3. Cardiac dysrhythmias
  4. Stroke
  5. Sources of hypovolaemia, eg GIT bleeding
  6. Gynaecological problems: ectopic pregnancy/vaginal bleeding
  7. Hypoglycaemia
- The evaluation in the elderly is even more complex as chronic problems such as failure of eyesight and gait instability could be interpreted as giddiness.

Table 1: Types of giddiness

Vertigo	An illusion of motion, which is frequently rotatory, but may be rocking, swaying, or a sense of linear propulsion and can be of varying degrees of intensity and persistence. It is indicative of vestibular dysfunction, whether peripheral or central.
Presyncope	Sensation that a faint is about to occur. During episode, the patient often senses vision growing dark or dim. There may be nausea, vomiting, weakness, dyspnoea and anxiety. Transient in nature.
Non-specific giddiness	Vague giddiness symptoms that do not fit into the above.

☛ **Special Tips for GPs**

- **Cardiac syncope** should be considered in **every elderly patient** presenting with giddiness.
- Take **postural vital signs**. If postural hypotension is present do a rectal examination to exclude GIT bleeding.
- Do **stat capillary glucose level** and **ECG** for all patients with non-vertiginous giddiness.

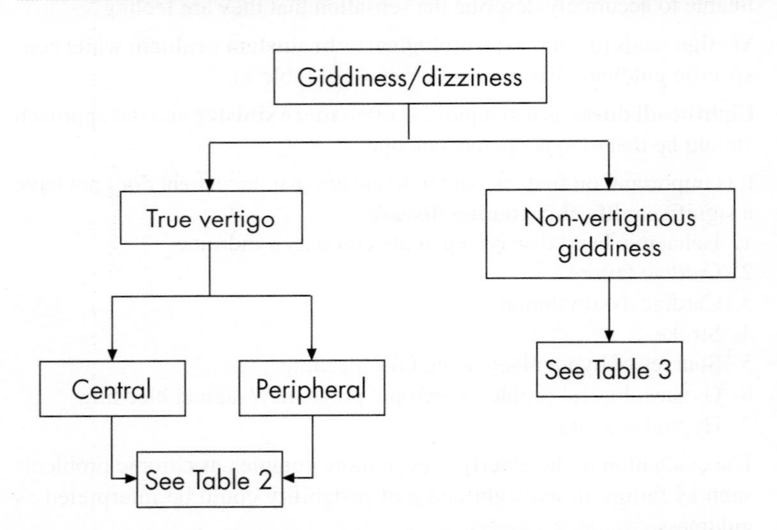

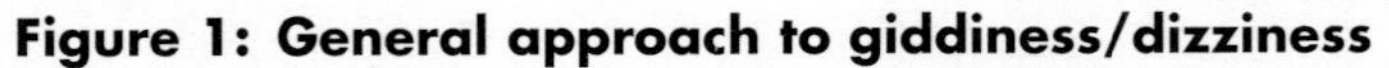

Figure 1: General approach to giddiness/dizziness

MANAGEMENT

Initial management

- Patients with significant giddiness and unsteadiness should be managed in the intermediate care area.
- ABCs of patient should be addressed.
- Low flow supplemental oxygen should be administered.
- Patient should be placed on cardiac monitoring.
- Vitals should be taken and patient should be upgraded to critical care area status if found abnormal.
- Postural parameters should be taken. **Definition of postural hypotension**: decrease in SBP >20 mm Hg on standing and an increase in PR >20/min upon standing may indicate significant volume loss.

Table 2: Characteristics of peripheral and central vertigo

Characteristics	*Peripheral*	*Central*
Onset	Abrupt	Gradual
Intensity	Moderate to intense	Mild to moderate
Temporal pattern	Brief, episodic	Chronic, continuous
Nystagmus	Rotatory/unidirectional/horizontal Suppressed by visual fixation	Any kind/multidirectional including bizarre/vertical Not suppressed by visual fixation
Head motion	Aggravation of symptoms	Little aggravation of symptoms
Tinnitus	Characteristic	Uncommon
Hearing loss	Characteristic	Uncommon
Nausea/vomiting	Common	Uncommon
Differential diagnosis	Vestibular neuronitis Benign positional vertigo Ménière's disease Middle ear infection Cholesteatoma	Vertebrobasilar insufficiency Brainstem infarct Tumour (acoustic neuroma) Haemorrhage (cerebellar) Multiple sclerosis

Table 3: Common important causes of non-vertiginous giddiness

System	*Examples*
Cardiac	Acute myocardial infarction or any condition that causes decreased cardiac output Dysrhythmias Valvular heart disease Congestive heart failure
Orthostatic hypotension	Blood loss, eg GIT bleeding, ruptured ectopic pregnancy Dehydration Drugs: see Table 4
Metabolic	Hypoxia Hypoglycaemia Hyperventilation Drugs Uraemia Hepatic failure
Haematologic	Anaemia Hyperviscosity syndromes

Table 4: Medications associated with giddiness

Alcohol	Antiinflammatory agents, eg salicylates
Antibiotics, eg aminoglycosides	Antiparkinson agents
Antidysrhythmics	Diuretics, eg frusemide
Anticonvulsants, eg phenytoin	Hypoglycaemics
Antidepressants	Phenothiazines
Antihistamines	Sedatives
Antihypertensives	

Investigations

- **Stat capillary glucose** should be considered (mandatory for all diabetics).
- Stat **ECG** for the following patients:
  1. Risk factors
     a. Age >40 years
     b. History of coronary artery disease
     c. History of diabetes mellitus
     d. History of hypertension
     e. History of hypercholesterolaemia
     f. Smoker
  2. Unstable vital signs

- The doctor should pay **special attention** to the following:
  1. Evidence of anaemia.
  2. Evidence of hypovolaemia: blood loss or dehydration.
  3. Cardiovascular system.
  4. Neurological system: nystagmus, focal neurological deficit, cerebellar signs.
  5. Abdomen: sepsis or bleeding. Do rectal examination if there is postural hypotension.
- After excluding the above, the doctor could use the general approach shown in Figure 1 to evaluate the cause of giddiness.

SPECIFIC MANAGEMENT

Vertigo

- Symptomatic treatment:
  1. IV/IM prochlorperazine (Stemetil®) 12.5 mg or
  2. IM promethazine (Phenergan®) 12.5–25 mg
- IV hydration if vomiting is severe.
- Distinguish between peripheral and central vertigo (Table 2).
- **Disposition**: patient can be **discharged** if:
  1. He has true peripheral vertigo.
  2. He has no neurological deficit.
  3. He has no symptoms to suggest an episode of vertebrobasilar insufficiency (VBI), ie no diplopia or visual blurring, dysarthria, dysphagia, drop attacks, focal neurological deficits (weakness).
  4. He is well after observation.
  5. He has no significant medical history.
  6. He has good home support (for elderly).

Presyncope

Refer to *Syncope*.

Non-specific giddiness

- Exclude, if possible, obvious neurological problems such as VBI, multiple sclerosis, brain stem or cerebello-pontine infarction or trauma, or Parkinson's disease.
- Bed rest.
- Symptomatic treatment if giddiness is severe:
  1. IM prochlorperazine
  2. Admit if no improvement
- **Disposition**: **discharge** patient if:
  1. Cerebrovascular disease or VBI has been excluded.
  2. Significant diseases have been excluded.

   a. Ischaemic heart disease
   b. Dysrhythmias
   c. Pneumonia/infection
   d. Bleeding or dehydration
3. Patient has no significant risk factors.
   a. Ischaemic heart disease
   b. Diabetes mellitus
   c. Hypertension
4. Well after observation.
   a. Alert and attentive
   b. No significant giddiness
   c. Able to retain
5. Good home care is available (for elderly patients).
6. General discharge advice should include the following. **Do not**:
   a. drive a motor vehicle
   b. ride a bicycle or motorcycle
   c. climb to heights
   d. operate heavy machinery
   e. drink alcoholic beverages
   f. swim

Ischaemic heart disease

- Giddiness can be the presenting complaint in ACS, acute heart failure and dysrhythmias.
- Diagnosis is based on cardiac risk factors, symptomatology and ECG changes.
- Patients should be managed as for acute coronary syndrome, with the view to early myocardial salvage, eg thrombolysis or PTCA.
- Such patients should be admitted to CCU for evaluation.

Cardiac failure

- Chronic heart failure can present with giddiness if cardiac output is insufficient to meet the demands of daily activities.
- Refer to *Heart Failure*.

Cardiac dysrhythmias

- Both fast or slow heart rhythms can cause giddiness.
- This is detectable on the cardiac monitor and 12-lead ECG.
- The management depends on the cause.
- **Significant rhythms** that should receive immediate management and subsequent CCU placement include:
  1. Significant or unexplained bradycardias
  2. 2nd and 3rd degree heart blocks

3. Ventricular tachydysrhythmias
4. Supraventricular tachycardias with haemodynamic instability
5. Atrial fibrillation with rapid ventricular response and haemodynamic instability

Stroke

- Giddiness, either non-specific giddiness or vertiginous forms, could be a sign of a TIA or impending stroke.
- Patients tend to be middle aged and above and many of them will have hypertension.
- Patient should be examined for evidence of brainstem signs and neurological deficit.
- Refer to *Stroke*.

Hypovolaemia

- Any sources of bleeding or fluid loss producing hypovolaemia can cause symptoms of giddiness. In mild cases, persistent or recurrent non-specific giddiness may be felt. In severe cases, there may be a sensation of *blacking-out* or frank syncope.
- All patients should be screened for common sources of **bleeding**, eg GIT bleeding or in the case of a female, vaginal bleeding.
- Patients should be asked whether **severe vomiting** or **diarrhoea** has occurred.
- Take blood for FBC and electrolyte assessment.

Gynaecological conditions

- Women in the childbearing age should be screened for evidence of vaginal bleeding or lower abdominal pain that may suggest **ectopic pregnancy**.

Hypoglycaemia

- Hypoglycaemia may be an important cause of giddiness in both healthy patients as well as diabetics.

References/further reading

1. Fauci AS, et al, eds. *Harrison's Principles of Internal Medicine.* 14th ed. New York: McGraw-Hill, 1998.
2. Sanders AB. Dizziness. In: Hamilton GC, Sanders AB, Strange GR, et al, eds. *Emergency Medicine: An Approach to Clinical Problem-Solving.* Philadelphia: WB Saunders; 1991:924–936.

16 Haemoptysis

Irwani Ibrahim

DEFINITION

- Haemoptysis is **defined** as the expectoration of blood or blood-stained sputum that originates from below the vocal cords or that has been aspirated into the tracheobronchial tree.
- Haemoptysis can be **classified** as:
  1. **Mild**: less than 5 ml of blood in 24 hours
  2. **Massive**: 50 ml in a single expectoration or more than 600 ml of blood in 24 hours. This accounts for 5% of all haemoptysis

CAVEATS

- Haemoptysis can be confused with haematemesis (Table 1).
- Physical examination is useful in determining the severity of haemoptysis, but is **unreliable** in localizing the site of bleeding.
- A search for **deep vein thrombosis** of the lower extremities is indicated to rule out pulmonary embolism as a cause of haemoptysis (Table 2).
- Massive haemoptysis is life threatening because **asphyxiation**, rather than exsanguination, is the leading cause of death. As little as 150 ml of blood can result in suffocation.
- Bleeding that results in respiratory distress and altered gas exchange is life threatening, regardless of the amount of blood.
- The commonest cause for mild haemoptysis is URTI.

Table 1: Differential points between haemoptysis and haemetemesis

Differential points	*Haemoptysis*	*Haemetemesis*
History	Coughing	GI symptoms
Sputum colour	Bright red	Dark red
pH	Alkaline	Acidic
Character	Frothy	Smooth non-frothy

Table 2: Common causes of haemoptysis

Respiratory	Bronchitis Tuberculosis Carcinoma of the lung Bronchiectasis Aspirated blood from epistaxis Sinusitis
Cardiovascular	Pulmonary oedema Pulmonary embolism Mitral stenosis Aorto-bronchial fistula
Coagulation disorder	Bleeding dyscrasias (congenital or acquired)
Others	Foreign body aspiration Protracted coughing

☛ Special Tips for GPs

- It is advisable to refer all cases of haemoptysis unless CXR can be done in the clinic.
- Insert 2 large bore intravenous cannula before transferring patient with massive haemoptysis.

MANAGEMENT OF MASSIVE HAEMOPTYSIS

- Transfer patient to the resuscitation area.
- Protect airway and administer oxygen. Patients who have **depressed conscious level or who are in imminent danger of asphyxiation** should be intubated.
- Set up 2 large bore IV lines and fluid resuscitate.
- Labs:
  1. FBC
  2. Urea/electrolytes/creatinine
  3. Coagulation profile
  4. GXM 4–6 units blood
  5. ABG
- Chest x-ray is **mandatory** in all patients with haemoptysis.
- Patients with ongoing haemoptysis from one lung (if this is known) should be positioned with the bleeding lung dependent to minimize soiling of the contralateral lung.

- **Disposition**:
  1. Patients with **mild haemoptysis** can usually be sent home with rest and cough suppressant.
  2. Refer to the Respiratory Medicine specialist outpatient clinics for early follow-up unless the cause is due to sinusitis or epistaxis in which case, patients should be in the ENT specialist clinics.
  3. Consider admission in all other patients. Those with massive haemoptysis require admission to the intensive care unit.

References/further reading

1. Young Jr. WF, Stava MW. Hemoptysis. In: Tintinalli JE, Kelen GD, Stapczynski JS, et al, eds. *Emergency Medicine: A Comprehensive Study Guide*. 5th ed. New York: McGraw-Hill; 2000:474–476.
2. Janz TG. Hemoptysis. In: Hamilton GC, et al, eds. *Presenting Signs and Symptoms in the Emergency Department Evaluation and Treatment.* Baltimore: Williams and Wilkins; 1993:627–631.

17 Headache

Seet Chong Meng • Peter Manning • Shirley Ooi

CAVEATS

- Potentially life- and vision-threatening causes of headache are:
  1. **Subarachnoid haemorrhage (SAH)**: patients usually present with **sudden onset** of headache, often with associated nausea, vomiting, diminished consciousness (which may be transient) and neck stiffness. Refer to *Subarachnoid Haemorrhage*.
  2. **Meningoencephalitis**: patients are usually febrile and drowsy with evidence of meningism.
  3. **Space-occupying or mass lesions (brain abscess, tumour)**: the headache is sometimes worse in the morning and aggravated by the Valsalva manoeuvre and coughing. Patients often have focal neurological deficits or fits (seizures).
  4. **Temporal arteritis**: patients are typically females, over 50 years old and often present with severe throbbing, burning and unilateral headache. The ipsilateral temporal artery is tender. Refer to *Temporal Arteritis*.
  5. **Glaucoma**: the headache is usually in and around the eye. The eye is usually injected, the cornea oedematous and the pupil mid-dilated. Refer to *Blurring of Vision, Acute*.
- Pay particular attention to the patient who presents with a first severe headache or with a change in the quality and intensity or character of a prior evaluated headache.
- Hypertension is an over-stated cause of headaches. **Do not** attribute a headache to elevated blood pressure unless the diastolic pressure exceeds 130 mm Hg.
- All patients with a worrisome history require work-up with a head CT scan, and if negative a lumbar puncture to rule out SAH.

☛ Special Tips for GPs

- Do not diagnose migraine if the **first** episode of severe headache occurs after the age of 50 years old.
- Do not give parenteral opioids to a patient with headache as the drowsiness post-injection makes monitoring of the neurological status difficult.

ESSENTIAL FEATURES OF A FOCUSED EXAMINATION

- Review of vital signs (especially temperature and blood pressure)
- Fundi
- Pupils, visual fields, face and extremities for focal abnormalities
- Gait

MANAGEMENT

- Patient with grossly abnormal vital signs and conscious level should be managed in the critical care area.
- Patients with normal vital signs can be managed in the intermediate area.
- Monitoring: ECG, vital signs q 10–15 minutes, pulse oximetry.
- Establish peripheral IV line at 'keep open' rate.
- Refer to *Pain Management* for symptomatic relief of headache.
- Labs: FBC, urea/electrolytes/creatinine, coagulation profile, GXM 2 units, ESR (if temporal arteritis is suspected).
- ECG, CXR.

Indications for ordering head CT scan

- Acute onset of the 'first or worst' headache.
- Increased frequency and increased severity of headache.
- New-onset headache after 50 years old.
- New-onset headache with a history of cancer or immunodeficiency.
- Headache with mental state changes.
- Headache with fever, neck stiffness and meningeal signs.
- Headache with focal neurological deficits if not previously documented as a migraine with aura.

Disposition

Admit the following:

- All life- and vision-threatening causes of headache
- 'Migraine headaches' not responding to non-opioid analgesics
- Complicated migraine headaches of new onset
- Headaches needing head CT scans

Discharge the rest of the headaches with analgesics and referral to the Neurology SOC for a follow-up unless it is a headache due to a fever or a tension headache.

References/further reading

1. Diamond ML. Emergency department management of the acute headache. *Clin Cornerstone*. Review 1999;1(6):45–54.
2. Field AG, Wang E. Evaluation of the patient with nontraumatic headache: An evidence based approach. *Emerg Med Clin North Am.* 1999;17(1):127–152.

18 Hyperventilation

Seet Chong Meng • Peter Manning • Shirley Ooi

CAVEATS

- Although common and benign, hyperventilation attack (HA)/panic attack is a **diagnosis of exclusion** which can be achieved principally on historical and physical findings without extensive investigations.
- A typical episode involves a precipitating stressful event with a past history of similar occurrences.
- Common associated symptoms include numbness and/or cramps of hands and feet, perioral tingling, non-specific dizziness, chest tightness, a sensation of suffocation and near-syncope.
- Do not diagnose a patient with HA if the SpO_2 on room air is below 97%.
- Table 1 shows differential diagnosis of hyperventilation.

Table 1: Differential diagnosis of hyperventilation

1. Respiratory System	• Severe asthma (with silent chest) • Pulmonary embolism • Tension pneumothorax • Primary pulmonary hypertension
2. Cardiovascular System	• Cardiac tamponade
3. Metabolic causes	• DKA • Chronic renal failure • Lactic acidosis from severe sepsis or shock of any cause • Poisoning especially by salicylates
4. Neurological System	• Central neurogenic hyperventilation
5. Gastrointestinal System	• Abdominal distension from whatever causes with splinting of diaphragm
6. Hyperventilation attack/ panic attack	

☛ Special Tips for GPs

- It is important to exclude more serious medical conditions such as metabolic acidosis, eg diabetic ketoacidosis, before diagnosing HA.

MANAGEMENT

- Patient should be managed in the intermediate acuity area. However, if significant altered mental state exists or there is haemodynamic instability, then this patient probably does not have HA but some other significant disease process requiring management in the critical care area.
- Do a stat SpO_2 measurement for every patient before diagnosing HA.
- Provide reassurance.
- Advise on breathing technique.

Note: Rebreathing into a bag has been found to be potentially harmful by causing significant hypoxaemia. It has also been shown to be ineffective in bringing up the PCO_2 level to a significant level.

- Monitoring: most cases require a pulse oximeter only.

Note: A patient with true HA is likely to have a normal SpO_2.

- Labs:
  1. Mandatory: **capillary blood glucose** estimation to exclude a hyperglycaemic state
  2. Optional: **ABG** will show respiratory alkalosis in HA. Alternatively, this test may reveal underlying metabolic acidosis
- **Chest x-ray**: to investigate such entities as pneumothorax, pneumonia or pulmonary embolism.
- **ECG** (especially age >40): to investigate possible pulmonary embolism, pericarditis or ischaemia.
- **Drug therapy** (for those patients who do not respond to rest and reassurance):
  1. **Valium® (diazepam)**. Dosage: 5 mg PO
  2. **Dormicum® (midazolam)**. Dosage: 2.5 mg IV (rarely required)
- **Disposition**: Most cases can be discharged. If this is a recurrent problem in this patient, then he/she should be referred to Psychiatry for outpatient therapy. The occasional patient may benefit from being given a prescription for 1–2 doses of oral alprazolam (Xanax®).

References/further reading

1. Saisch SG, Wessely S, Gardner WN. Patients with acute hyperventilation presenting to an inner-city emergency department. *Chest*. 1996;110(4):952–957.
2. Callaham M. Hypoxic hazards of traditional paper bag rebreathing in hyperventilating patients. *Ann Emerg Med*. 1989;18(6):622–628.

19 Lower limb swelling

Quek Lit Sin • Shirley Ooi

CAVEATS

- Lower limb swelling is a common complaint among patients and will present frequently with associated non-specific signs and symptoms. Table 1 shows the important causes of lower limb swelling.
- As with all consultations, a good history will be able to reduce the number of differentials.

PREGNANCY WITH PREECLAMPSIA

- All pregnant women will have lower limb swelling. As lower limb swelling is an early sign of preeclampsia, a high index of suspicion is necessary.
- The diagnosis of preeclampsia is an emergency and the patient must be treated in the hospital: refer to *Eclampsia*.

Table 1: Important causes of lower limb swelling

System	*Examples*	*Unilateral/Bilateral*
Cardiac	• Heart failure. Refer to *Heart Failure*	Bilateral
Renal	• Acute/chronic renal failure with fluid overload. Refer to *Renal Emergencies* • Nephrotic/nephritic syndrome	Bilateral
Pregnancy	• Preeclampsia. Refer to *Eclampsia*	Bilateral
Hepatobiliary	• Liver failure. Refer to *Hepatic Encephalopathy*	Bilateral
Veins/lymphatics	• Deep vein thrombosis (DVT) • Varicose veins • Lymphoedema	Unilateral Unilateral/bilateral Unilateral/bilateral
Infection	• Lymphangitis • Cellulitis	Unilateral
Orthopaedic causes	• Trauma • Compartment syndrome • Arthritis/gout • Ruptured Baker's cyst • Tumour: bone or soft tissue	Unilateral

> ☛ **Special Tips for GPs**
> - High index of suspicion is necessary to avoid missing important causes of lower limb swelling.
> - The three most likely causes of bilateral lower limb swelling are **congestive cardiac failure**, **renal failure** with fluid overload and **hypoalbuminaemia** (from liver failure or diabetic nephropathy).

VEINS AND LYMPHATICS

- The clinical features of **deep vein thrombosis**:
  1. Fullness of lower limb that increases with standing or walking.
  2. Pain in the lower extremities on coughing or sneezing, which is different from the electric-type pain with cough or sneeze associated with sciatica.
  3. The affected limb is often warmer than the normal side. Palpate for 'cords' which are very specific, although insensitive for thrombosis.
  4. Look for **risk factors** for thromboembolic disease (refer to *Pulmonary Embolism*) to diagnose DVT.
- DVT is usually unilateral unless vena cava occludes, a rare and catastrophic event.
- DVT usually occurs over several days. Hence, a sudden, severe pain is more likely to be due to muscle rupture or injury.
- Look for risk factors for thromboembolic disease (refer to *Pulmonary Embolism*) to diagnose DVT.
- A combination of clinical signs and symptoms that includes tenderness, swelling, redness and the assessment of Homan's sign (pain in the posterior calf or knee on forced dorsiflexion of foot) cannot adequately differentiate patients with or without DVT.
- DVT is unlikely to be the cause if fever is >39°C.
- Lack of discrepancy in calf size does not rule out DVT. However, asymmetric calf swelling of >3 cm is almost always a significant finding in DVT.
- **Varicose veins** are accompanied by skin pigmentation in chronic cases. Superficial thrombophlebitis of the varicose veins results in lower limb swelling. Unilateral varicose veins and swelling requires more careful thought as it may indicate a sinister pathology in the pelviabdominal area.
- Lymphatic obstruction will result in oedema of the lower extremities. Secondary **lymphoedema** follows damage and obstruction to the lymphatic pathways by malignant disease involving the lymph nodes, by filariasis and may be iatrogenic from surgical block dissection.

INFECTIONS: LYMPHANGITIS/CELLULITIS

- The infection spreads along the lymphatics causing **lymphangitis** and they become visible as thin, red, tender streaks on the skin, often with slight oedema of the overlying skin. When the infection gets into the oedema, **cellulitis** ensues.
- **Indications of admission**:
  1. Recurrent fever and chills
  2. Increasing local pain
  3. Spreading erythema
  4. Elderly patients as they become septicaemic easily

ORTHOPAEDIC CAUSES: COMPARTMENT SYNDROME

- Orthopaedic causes have a definite history and a good physical examination will usually clinch the diagnosis. It is important to exclude **compartment syndrome**, which is an orthopaedic emergency, in all traumatic injuries to the lower limbs!

Clinical features

- Severe pain in the limb, pain on passive stretch of muscle, pallor, paresthesia, pulselessness and paralysis are the six classic signs of muscle ischaemia.
- The presence of **pain** with **passive range of motion of the muscle** is the **earliest clinical sign**. Others include delayed capillary refill and loss of 2-point discrimination.
- Palpation of the affected muscles of that compartment will be tense and tenderness will be produced.

Common causes

- Lower limb: fracture of tibia or fibula.
- Upper limb: supracondylar fracture of humerus.
- High voltage electrical burn injuries involving muscles.

Complications

- Severe myoglobinuria, renal failure, hyperkalaemia and death.
- Volkmann's ischaemic contracture and loss of limb function.

GENERAL MANAGEMENT

- Ensure vital signs are stable and that there is no acute coronary event that led to the lower limb swelling. Unstable patients must be managed in the critical care area.
- Labs:
  1. **Mandatory**
     a. Urine dipstick for proteinuria

b. ECG for myocardial injury
c. CXR for heart failure/fluid overload

2. **Optional**: if no obvious cause is found after the mandatory investigations or if specific diagnoses are suspected, do:
   a. Liver function test (to rule out hypoalbuminaemia)
   b. Urea/electrolytes/creatinine (if renal failure suspected)
   c. Cardiac enzymes/troponin T (if cardiac cause suspected)
   d. If DVT is suspected, do D-dimer, INR (to guide treatment), colour-flow duplex scanning (regardless of the pretest probability) and GXM.

Note: A normal D-dimer in a patient with no risk factors for thrombosis makes proximal DVT extremely unlikely. FBC is not useful as the leukocyte count cannot distinguish between DVT and cellulitis and is neither sensitive nor specific for either condition.

   e. Blood C&S for **infection** causes before starting antibiotics

- For **compartment syndrome**: call Orthopaedic surgeon early for fasciotomy.

Note: If elevated pressure is not relieved after approximately 8 hours, irreversible injury to entrapped muscle and nerves will occur.

- Treatment of lower limb swelling depends on the primary cause and this is discussed in the relevant chapters.
- **Disposition**: admit the following causes:
  1. Cardiac causes
  2. Renal failure
  3. DVT (although some critical pathways now emphasize outpatient management when appropriate)
  4. Pregnancy with preeclampsia
  5. Infection
  6. Liver failure
  7. Compartment syndrome
  8. Suspected bone tumours

  The first 7 causes should have treatment started in the ED. Refer the other cause to the relevant outpatient clinic for further investigations and follow-up.

References/further reading

1. Nandi PL, Li WS, Leung R, et al. Deep vein thrombosis and pulmonary embolism in the Chinese population. *HKMJ*. 1998;4(3):305–310
2. Lumley JSP. *Hamilton Bailey's Demonstration of Physical Signs in Clinical Surgery.* 18th ed. Oxford: Butterworth Heinemann; 1997.
3. Braunwald E, et al, eds. *Harrison's Principles of Internal Medicine*. 15th ed. New York: McGraw-Hill; 2001:850–981.
4. Skinner DV, Swain A, Peyton R, et al, eds. *Cambridge Textbook of Accident and Emergency Medicine*. Cambridge: Cambridge University Press; 1997:866–897,1003–1014.

20 Pain, abdominal

JP Travers • Peter Manning • Irwani Ibrahim

CAVEATS

- The role of the emergency physician is to identify the patient with the 'acute abdomen', not to make a specific diagnosis. It is a bonus if you are able to!
- Identify those patients with significant posturing: eg lying perfectly still (perforations/peritonitis), and rolling around in agony (bowel/ureteric colic).
- Always consider the **potentially life-threatening aetiologies** presented in Table 1.
- Always consider the possibility of ectopic gestation in pregnancy-capable females.
- A male patient with pain in the right iliac fossa has appendicitis until proven otherwise.
- There are 3 reasons for doing an **abdominal x-ray** in emergency medicine:
  1. To identify **'free' air** (perforated viscus)
  2. To identify **air/fluid interfaces** (intestinal obstruction)
  3. To identify **ectopic calcification** (urolithiasis, hepatobiliary calculi, pancreatitis, AAA)

Table 1: Potentially life-threatening causes of abdominal pain

1. *Intraabdominal*
   - a. Perforated peptic ulcer
   - b. Intestinal obstruction
   - c. Abdominal aortic aneurysm (AAA)
   - d. Appendicitis
   - e. Pancreatitis
   - f. Ectopic pregnancy
   - g. Ischaemic bowel
   - h. Spontaneous bacterial peritonitis in liver cirrhosis
   - i. SLE peritonitis
   - j. Peritonitis in CAPD renal patients
2. *Extraabdominal*
   - a. Acute myocardial infarction
   - b. Lower lobe pneumonia
   - c. Basal pulmonary embolism
   - d. Diabetic ketoacidosis

- The **chest x-ray** is utilized to identify:
  1. Subdiaphragmatic air
  2. Basal consolidation
  3. Pulmonary embolism

Note: If a perforated peptic ulcer is suspected and the CXR shows no obvious subdiaphragmatic air, the instillation of 200 ml air into the stomach via a nasogastric tube may show 'free' air on x-ray. This practice should be considered in light of local custom/preference since it is controversial: in the presence of signs of perforation, instilling air does nothing to change the management (ie to operate), and can worsen spillage of bowel contents into the peritoneal cavity.

> ☛ **Special Tips for GPs**
> - The site and nature of the abdominal pain will give the best clue as to what is causing it.
> - Always suspect ectopic pregnancy in women of child-bearing age.
> - Always suspect appendicitis in any man with lower abdominal pain.
> - Do not forget to feel for epigastric pulsation.
> - Myocardial infarction may give upper abdominal pain. Perform an ECG.

MANAGEMENT

Haemodynamically unstable patient

- Patient must be managed in the critical care area.
- Maintain airway and give supplemental high-flow oxygen.
- Monitoring: ECG, vital signs q 5 min, pulse oximetry.
- Establish 2 large-bore peripheral IVs (14–16G); fluid challenge of 1 litre crystalloid (if AMI not suspected). Reassess parameters.
- **Labs**:
  1. Mandatory: capillary blood sugar; GXM 2–4 units; FBC; urea/electrolytes/creatinine; serum amylase; urine pregnancy test (where relevant); first blood and urine cultures (if sepsis is suspected)
  2. Optional: urinalysis, cardiac enzymes, liver function tests, coagulation profile
- IV antibiotics in cases of intraabdominal sepsis, eg ceftriaxone 1 g and metronidazole 500 mg. Depending on local practice, other antibiotics to cover gram negative and anaerobic organisms can be used.

Note: Aminoglycosides are best avoided if the patient has, or is at risk of, renal impairment.

- X-rays: CXR, KUB.
- ECG to identify AMI or as preparation for anticipated surgery in suitable age group.
- Insert urinary catheter.
- Keep patient nil by mouth.
- Early consultations with, eg:
  1. General Surgery registrar
  2. Obstetrics and Gynaecology registrar for suspected ectopic pregnancy
  3. Cardiothoracic registrar for suspected abdominal aortic aneurysm
  4. Medical or Cardiology registrar for suspected basilar pneumonia or myocardial infarction.

Haemodynamically stable patient (see next section for specific diagnostic entities)

- This patient can be managed in the intermediate acuity area.
- Keep patient NBM till disposition has been decided.
- Consider precautionary intravenous plug.
- Labs should be based on clinical suspicion of the possible causes of abdominal pain in a particular patient.
- Consider KUB, CXR, ECG.
- Evaluate for signs of acute abdomen with frequent abdominal examinations.

DIFFERENTIAL DIAGNOSIS OF RHC PAIN

If patient is febrile

- Consider:
  1. Cholecystitis
  2. Cholangitis
  3. Liver abscess
  4. Subdiaphragmatic abscess
  5. Hepatitis
  6. Pyelonephritis
  7. Right-sided basilar pneumonia
  8. Diverticulitis
- Evaluate for acute abdomen.
- Establish peripheral intravenous line.
- Administer crystalloids at maintenance rate.
- Labs: FBC; urea/electrolytes/creatinine; serum amylase; urinalysis; liver panel and hepatitis markers (optional); first blood and urine cultures if patient is septic.

- KUB: consider CXR, ECG.
- Analgesia: NSAIDs or antispasmodics.
- Keep patient nil by mouth.
- **Disposition**: admit to General Surgery. Inform the GS medical officer or registrar if any delay is anticipated in the admission process.

If patient is afebrile

- Bear in mind that the elderly patient with a surgical abdomen may not be able to mount a febrile response.
- Consider:
  1. Biliary colic: refer to *Hepatobiliary Emergencies*
  2. Referred pain from chest conditions
  3. Hepatitis
- Evaluate for acute abdomen.
- Labs: FBC; urea/electrolytes/creatinine; serum amylase; urinalysis; liver panel and hepatitis markers (optional)
- KUB: consider CXR, ECG.
- Analgesia: NSAIDs or antispasmodics IM.
- **Disposition**: can be discharged to follow-up in General Surgery Clinic if pain settles, abdomen remains benign; otherwise admit to General Surgery. If hepatitis is suspected, patient can be referred to Gastroenterology Clinic.

DIFFERENTIAL DIAGNOSIS OF FLANK PAIN

- Consider:
  1. Pyelonephritis
  2. Ureteric calculi with or without obstruction: refer to *Urolithiasis*
- Consider **abdominal aortic aneurysm (AAA)** if patient is older than 50 years, or aortic dissection in patients with risk factors (refer to *Aortic Dissection*).

Note: Classically, an AAA presents with central abdominal pain penetrating to the back. However, if the aneurysm involves the renal pedicle, then the pain can simulate ureteric colic.

If patient is febrile

- Labs: FBC; urea/electrolytes/creatinine; blood cultures (at least 7.5 ml blood per bottle); urine cultures if urosepsis is suspected.
- KUB: consider CXR, ECG.
- Intravenous antibiotics: coverage for gram-negative organisms and for anaerobic organisms if a hepatobiliary or enteric source is suspected.
- Analgesics: NSAIDs or narcotics.

- **Disposition**:
  1. Admit to Urology for all complicated urolithiasis
  2. Admit to General Medicine for acute pyelonephritis

If patient is afebrile

- Labs: urinalysis, looking for blood and/or WBCs and positive nitrites.
- KUB to locate the ectopic calcification of a calculus and to assess kidney size.
- Analgesics: NSAIDs or narcotics.
- **Disposition**:
  1. Admit if there is inadequate pain relief in ED **or** any hint of ureteric obstruction with infection. Inform Urology in-house team if any delay is anticipated in the admission process.
  2. Can be discharged to follow-up in Urology Clinic if patient becomes painfree and remains afebrile in ED. Advise to return if:
     a. Fever develops
     b. Gross haematuria appears
     c. Urine output drops

DIFFERENTIAL DIAGNOSIS OF LOWER ABDOMINAL PAIN

- Always consider appendicitis (refer to *Appendicitis*) and ectopic pregnancy (refer to *Ectopic Pregnancy*) as possibilities.
- Rectal examination is useful in both men and women since, in the latter, the cervix and adnexae can be palpated without the stress of a vaginal examination.
- Labs:
  1. Mandatory: urine HCG in pregnancy-capable female
  2. Optional: FBC, urea/electrolytes/creatinine, urine dipstick testing

DIFFERENTIAL DIAGNOSIS OF EPIGASTRIC PAIN

- Consider both abdominal and extraabdominal causes. Suspect abdominal aortic aneurysm in patients more than 50 years old especially if the pain radiates to lower back or one flank:
  1. Other intraabdominal causes include:
     a. Acute exacerbation of peptic ulcer disease: refer to *Peptic Ulcer Disease*
     b. Reflux oesophagitis
     c. Penetrating posterior peptic ulcer
     d. Pancreatitis: refer to *Pancreatitis*
     e. Aortic dissection/ruptured AAA

     The latter three conditions are associated with radiation of pain to the lower back.

2. Extraabdominal causes include
   a. Acute myocardial infarction: refer to *Myocardial Infarction, Acute*
   b. Pneumonia: refer to *Pneumonia, Community Acquired*
   c. Pulmonary embolism: refer to *Pulmonary Embolism*
   d. Diabetic ketoacidosis: refer to *Diabetic Ketoacidosis*

- Establish peripheral intravenous access.
- Administer crystalloids at maintenance rate.
- Labs: bedside blood sugar; FBC; serum amylase; urea/electrolytes/creatinine; cardiac enzymes if suspicious.
- Do ECG.
- Do erect CXR and KUB.
- Give adequate analgesia.
- Keep patient nil by mouth.
- **Disposition**: can be discharged to follow-up in General Surgery Clinic if pain settles, abdomen remains benign and investigations normal; otherwise admit to General Surgery.

DIFFERENTIAL DIAGNOSIS OF COLICKY CENTRAL ABDOMINAL PAIN

- The colicky nature of a pain generally indicates obstruction or irritation of a hollow viscus. Consider:
  1. Acute gastroenteritis: refer to *Diarrhoea and Vomiting.*
  2. Intestinal obstruction in large or small bowel: refer to *Intestinal Obstruction.*
  3. Ischaemic bowel, especially if the pain seems out of proportion to the physical findings: refer to *Ischaemic Bowel.*

Note: Adhesion colic as a diagnosis probably does not exist since uncomplicated adhesions are not thought to cause pain. However, in the setting of a post-operative patient, an incomplete or subacute bowel obstruction due to adhesions can produce a typical colicky pain.

References/further reading

1. Davis MA. Abdominal pain. *J Emerg Med Acute Pri Care*. 2001;5325(20):5991–6247.

21 Pain, chest, acute

Shirley Ooi

CAVEATS

- A **good history** remains the **cornerstone** in the **diagnosis** of the life-threatening causes of chest pain (Table 1).
- After excluding the 6 life-threatening causes, the important but not life-threatening causes shown in Table 2 should then be excluded.

Table 1: Life-threatening causes of chest pain

	Key clinical features
1. Acute myocardial infarction (AMI)	Refer to *Myocardial Infarction, Acute*
2. Unstable angina (as it carries similar short-term prognosis as AMI)	Refer to *Coronary Syndromes, Acute*
3. Aortic dissection	Refer to *Aortic Dissection*
4. Pulmonary embolism (PE)	Refer to *Pulmonary Embolism*
5. Tension pneumothorax	Refer to *Trauma, Chest*
6. Oesophageal rupture	Chest pain following violent vomiting and CXR showing pneumomediastinum

Note: AMI and unstable angina are also known as **acute coronary syndromes**.

Table 2: Important but not life-threatening causes of chest pain

1. Cardiac	Stable angina Prinzmetal angina Pericarditis/myocarditis
2. Respiratory	Simple pneumothorax Pneumonia with pleurisy
3. Gastrointestinal	Reflux oesophagitis Oesophageal spasm (this is often a diagnosis by exclusion as it mimics ischaemic chest pain very closely)
4. Referred pain	Gastritis/peptic ulcer disease Biliary disease Subphrenic abscess/inflammation

- Note that **benign causes**, eg musculoskeletal pain, costochondritis, psychogenic chest pain and early herpes zoster neuralgia, should be **diagnoses by exclusion**.
- In the Multicentre Chest Pain Study (MCPS), chest discomfort that is similar to a prior MI or worse than the patient's usual angina remains the strongest independent risk factors for MI and the likelihood of acute coronary ischaemia.
- In the MCPS the factors identifying patients at **higher risk for AMI and ischaemia** are:
  1. Time since onset of pain ⩽4 hours
  2. Longest episode of pain ⩾30 min
  3. Pain described as 'pressure'
  4. Radiation of pain to the left arm, shoulder, neck or jaw
  5. History of angina or MI
  6. ED ECG changes of ischaemia or infarction
- The single best historical predictor of ACS is a known history of AMI or known CAD. The risk of a coronary event is 5 times more likely in persons with established CAD.
- **Traditional risk factors** from the Framingham study (eg age, male gender, smoking, hypertension, DM, hypercholesterolaemia, family history) have been shown to be predictive of patients who will develop CAD over a 14-year period in an outpatient setting but were never developed or intended to identify which chest pain patient in the ED suffered acute cardiac ischaemia. They have been shown to **perform poorly** in this setting. In fact, **no single specific risk factor** has the power to **predict AMI or acute coronary ischaemia** independently. Thus, the risk factor profile cannot be depended on in isolation to risk stratify or to predict the presence of IHD in the ED.
- Chest pain is **pleuritic** or **exacerbated by movement** in 5–8% of patients with AMI.
- 5% of known AMI have **concomitant chest wall tenderness**.
- The following **3 features together** make chest pain very **unlikely** to be due to **cardiac ischaemia**:
  1. Chest pain sharp or stabbing.
  2. No history of angina or MI.
  3. Pain reproducible by palpating chest wall or has a positional or pleuritic component.
- Chest discomfort associated with nausea should be assumed cardiac until proven otherwise. Similarly for any patient with heartburn or indigestion unless patient has been worked up before and proven non-cardiac.
- Think of **aortic dissection** in any patient with chest pain suggestive of **AMI** but with **neurological** symptoms as well.

- The following **associated symptoms**, ie **diaphoresis**, **dyspnoea** and **syncope**, are seen in AMI, PE and aortic dissection and may not help differentiate among these diagnoses but they are important clues that a **serious illness** is present.
- In chest pain, a normal electrocardiogram (ECG) does not rule out ACS, but it places the patient at less risk of subsequent adverse events. Only 65–78% of ECGs of patients admitted are definite or probable in presenting MI. The key is to repeat serial ECGs.
- People **over the age of 65** are more likely to have atypical presentations with delayed or missed diagnoses.

☛ **Special Tips for GPs**

- **Refer** all the following patients to the **ED**:
1. Typical history of AMI but a normal ECG
2. Atypical history but with risk factors for CAD
- The **major risk factors for CAD** are:
1. Diabetes mellitus
2. Systemic hypertension
3. Hyperlipidaemia
4. Smoking

   Note: A patient who has stopped smoking for <2 years is considered to have smoking as a risk factor for CAD.
- Give aspirin 300 mg stat for all patients with acute coronary syndromes before sending them to the hospital.
- All cases of AMI should be sent by ambulance to the hospital.

MANAGEMENT

- Ensure vital signs are stable. If unstable, patient in distress and diaphoretic, bring patient to resuscitation area immediately. Attend to patients with obvious acute coronary syndrome immediately.
- Put patient on oxygen supplementation, pulse oximetry, continuous ECG monitoring, blood pressure monitoring.
- Do an immediate 12-lead ECG. **Role of ECG** in chest pain includes diagnosis of AMI, ischaemia and PE.
- If ECG is normal or suspicious but non-confirmatory of acute coronary syndrome, repeat serial ECGs at close intervals.
- Set up IV plug and take blood tests for cardiac enzymes and other biomarkers, eg myoglobin and troponin T.

  Remember: do **not** get a false sense of security in excluding ischaemic chest pain from a normal troponin T/cardiac enzymes upon presentation at the ED. See Table 3 for proper interpretation of the various cardiac markers.

Table 3: Cardiac markers

Cardiac markers	Release kinetics: Detected within	Peak levels	Normalized by	Advantages
Myoglobin	1–2 h	6–9 h	24–36 h	1. Earliest marker to rise in AMI. 2. Useful in ruling out AMI early as myoglobin is raised in nearly all AMI at 6 hours.
Creatine kinase (CK)–MB	4–6 h	18–24 h	48–72 h	1. Serologic *gold standard of AMI.* Used in the World Health Organisation criteria of diagnosis of AMI.
Troponin T	4–6 h	12–120 h	10–14 days	1. Useful for late presenting AMI. 2. Useful as prognostic indicator in unstable angina. UA patients with troponin T +ve have poorer prognosis than those with troponin T –ve. 3. The most well-studied prognostic indicator in UA among the troponins.
Troponin I	4–6 h	12–36 h	7–9 days	1. The most cardiac-specific marker. 2. No false positive values in renal failure patients. 3. Can be used as a prognostic indicator in UA as in troponin T.

T_0 = Time of presentation T_s = Serial biomarkers

- Give pain relief depending on provisional diagnosis.
- Do chest x-ray. **Role of CXR** in chest pain includes diagnosis of:
  1. Complications of AMI, eg heart failure and pulmonary oedema
  2. Aortic dissection
  3. Respiratory causes, eg pneumothorax, pneumonia, lung malignancy, rib fractures
  4. Peripheral PE

Disadvantages	*Sensitivity (%) for diagnosis of AMI (95% CI)*	*Specificity (%) for diagnosis of AMI (95% CI)*
1. Not specific for cardiac muscle. Other conditions associated with raised myoglobin include: a. Skeletal muscle or neuromuscular disorders b. Renal failure c. Intramuscular injections d. Strenuous exercise e. Postcoronary bypass surgery f. Heavy use of ethanol Hence myoglobin should not be used alone but with another more cardiac-specific marker.	T_0 49 (43–55) T_s 89 (80–94)	T_0 91 (87–94) T_s 87 (80–92)
1. Not specific for cardiac muscle. 2. May be falsely elevated in renal failure patients. 3. Narrow diagnostic window. 4. Failure of total CK to rise to abnormal values in all AMI. To improve the sensitivity and specificity, **relative % index** defined as $\frac{\textbf{CK-MB (ng/ml)} \times \textbf{100\%}}{\textbf{CK (U/L)}}$ is used. ≥5% is suggestive of AMI.	T_0 42 (36–48) T_s 79 (71–86)	T_0 97 (95–98) T_s 96 (95–97)
1. Some false positive values in chronic renal failure and dialysis patients, especially in First Generation troponin T assays.	T_0 39 (26–53) T_s 93 (85–97)	T_0 93 (90–96) T_s 85 (76–91)
1. Currently not very widely available.	T_0 39 (10–78) T_s 90–100	T_0 93 (88–97) T_s 83–96

5. Pneumomediastinum, eg spontaneous rupture of lung bullae, oesophageal rupture

- Some guidelines about the **disposition** of patients with chest pain:
  1. Admit **acute coronary syndromes with ECG changes** or **continuing pain** to **CCU**.
  2. Admit **unstable angina with no ECG changes**, or if the pain has subsided, to the **Cardiology general ward**.

3. Admit patients with diagnosis of **atypical chest pain syndrome** with **risk factors** for CAD to the **Cardiology general ward** unless your ED has a Chest Pain Observation Unit for further workup of the patient.
4. **Stable angina can be discharged with medications** started (aspirin 300 mg stat and then cardiprin 100 mg OM, isosorbide dinitrate 5–10 mg tds, propranolol 20 mg bd) provided there are no contraindications and referred to the Cardiology specialist clinics. (However, this group of patients is probably not common as patients with CAD would not have presented to the ED if the history is that of their usual **stable angina**. Hence, it is advisable to **admit all chest pain patients** with a **known history of CAD**.)
5. Admit patients with **aortic dissection** to the CT ICU.

Note: Recent onset angina that appears to be **stable** from history is considered as **unstable angina** (UA). Hence **all new onset angina** should be **admitted** to the hospital, even if the ECG is normal.

- For treatment of the first 5 life-threatening causes, please refer to the individual chapters in Section 2.

References/further reading

1. Evaluation of chest pain. *Questions and Answers.* Laser Learning Systems. April 1995:3–9.
2. Wu AHB, ed. *Cardiac Markers*. Totowa, NJ: Humana Press; 1998:104–107,120–121,205–209,231–233,237–239.
3. Balk EM, Joannidis JP , Salem D, et al. Accuracy of biomarkers to diagnose acute cardiac ischaemia in the emergency department: a meta-analysis. *Ann Emerg Med.* 2001;37(5):478–494.
4. Wilkinson K, Severance H. Identification of chest pain patients appropriate for an emergency department observation unit. In: Ross MA, Graff LG, eds. Emergency Observation Medicine. *Emerg Med Clinics N America* 2001;19(1):37–40.
5. Lee TH, Juarez G, Cook EF, et al. Ruling out acute myocardial infarction: A prospective multicentre validation of a 12-hour strategy for patients at low risk. *N Engl J Med.* 1991;324:1239–1246.

22 Pain, low back

JP Travers • Peter Manning

CAVEATS

- Patients with acute low back pain (LBP) who require immediate care on arrival are those with:
  1. haemodynamic instability (the most critical group)
  2. significant trauma
  3. incapacitating musculoskeletal pain
- Patients with concomitant back and abdominal pain are at risk for serious intraabdominal or retroperitoneal bleeding and require prompt evaluation and close monitoring.
- Patients in severe distress from musculoskeletal back pain with stable vital signs can be safely and appropriately given potent analgesics after preliminary evaluation.
- Patients with progressive neurologic deficits or with bladder or bowel dysfunction require prompt surgical decompression.
- The **indications for plain lumbosacral spine x-rays** in the ED are few:
  1. Presentation suggests malignancy with possible metastasis to the lumbar spine.
  2. There is a history of significant trauma to the spine.
  3. Fever and localized tenderness suggest osteomyelitis.
  4. There is acute, unexplained neurologic deficit.
- **Conservative treatment** is the **mainstay** of back pain **management** and consists of muscle relaxation facilitated by bed rest, heat or ice, muscle-relaxing medications, and adequate analgesia. 90% of patients respond to such treatment.
- Outpatient management is the norm, with admission usually reserved for patients with neurologic deficits or intractable pain.

CATASTROPHIC ILLNESSES

These can present as LBP.

- **Ruptured abdominal aortic aneurysm (AAA)**: Usually a middle-aged or elderly male patient with a history of hypertension and cardiovascular disease, who presents with LBP and abdominal pain combined with a rapid pulse, syncope and borderline or actual hypotension.
- **Ruptured ectopic pregnancy**: A pregnancy-capable female with a history of risk factors for ectopic pregnancy, presenting with acute onset of LBP, associated vaginal bleeding, syncope, and unilateral abdominal pain.

- **Cauda equina syndrome**: An uncommon but very serious complication of lumbar disc disease. The patient typically presents with LBP, unilateral or bilateral radiation, perineal anaesthesia, motor weakness of the lower extremities, and sphincter dysfunction (usually urinary retention). Classically, surgical intervention within 6 hours of onset of the symptoms is considered essential to prevent permanent paralysis and bladder dysfunction.
- **Acute spinal cord compression**: Due to an expanding tumour mass, this can present as LBP with lower extremity, bowel, or bladder deficits; it requires immediate intervention to prevent permanent neurologic deficit.

> ☛ **Special Tips for GPs**
> - Patients presenting with musculoskeletal pain and stable vital signs may be treated with analgesics in the first instance. Severe pain with no response to medication should be referred to the ED or Orthopaedic specialist as soon as possible.
> - Back pain with focal neurological signs or bowel/bladder dysfunction is a surgical emergency and must be referred to hospital immediately.
> - Always do an abdominal examination and look for aortic aneurysm.

MANAGEMENT

Patients with haemodynamic instability and/or history of significant trauma

- Patient must be managed in the critical care area.
- Intubation and resuscitation equipment must be immediately available.
- Provide supplemental high-flow oxygen via reservoir mask.
- Establish at least two large-bore IV lines.
- Administer IV Hartmann's solution 1 litre stat and reassess parameters.
- Administer type specific blood if necessary.
- Labs: GXM 4–6 units, FBC, urea/electrolytes/creatinine, urine HCG where relevant.
- Monitoring: ECG, vital signs q 5–10 min, pulse oximetry.
- **Disposition**
  1. Early consultation with Cardiothoracic Surgery (for suspected AAA), or

2. General Surgery and Orthopaedics (in cases of trauma), or
3. O&G (in case of ruptured ectopic pregnancy)

Patients with severe, incapacitating musculoskeletal pain

- Must be managed in at least the intermediate care area and evaluated promptly.
- Reassure patient and move him/her carefully.
- Monitor vital signs q 30–60 min.
- Analgesia
  1. Pethidine® (meperidine). Dosage: 50–100 mg IM or IV
  2. Tramal® (tramadone). Dosage: 50–75 mg IM or IV
  3. Voltaren® (diclofenac). Dosage: 50–75 mg IM
- Muscle relaxation: Valium (diazepam) dosage: 5–10 mg PO or 2–5 mg IV (must be in a monitored area if given via IV route).
- Reassess after 1 hour and attempt thorough examination with patient in four positions: standing, supine, prone and sitting.
- Perform rectal examination and assess anal tone.
- Assess for perianal sensory loss.
- Consider plain x-ray of lumbosacral spine.
- **Disposition**
  1. Uncomplicated cases: discharge to home for bed rest on a firm surface with adequate analgesics and muscle relaxants.
  2. Complicated and in severe pain ± mild neurological changes and no symptoms of sphincter dysfunction: admit to Orthopaedics for traction and pain management.
  3. If evidence exists of spinal cord compression or cauda equina syndrome, then consult Neurosurgery stat.
  4. Other patients to be admitted include:
     a. those with infections who may require IV antibiotic therapy, eg pyelonephritis and prostatitis
     b. those with lumbar spine compression fractures for pain management
     c. those with transverse process fractures for evaluation of associated injuries
     d. those with intractable pain who are unable to walk or care for themselves
     e. those with suspected metastases to the spine as they may require IV dexamethasone to be started early: refer to *Oncology Emergencies*

References/further reading

1. Johnson MT. Low back pain. *J Emerg Med Acute Pri Care*. 2001; 5325(20):5991–6247.
2. La Ban MM. Thoracic and lumbar pain syndromes. In: Tintinalli JE, Ruiz E, Krome RL, eds. *Emergency Medicine: A Comprehensive Study Guide*. 3rd ed. New York: McGraw-Hill; 1992:896–900.

23 Pain, scrotal and penile

JP Travers • Peter Manning

CAVEATS

- The aetiology of an acute scrotum can usually be ascertained by history, physical examination and urinalysis.
- Never diagnose epididymitis in a prepubertal boy with scrotal pain. It is testicular torsion until proven otherwise.
- Colour Doppler ultrasound is additionally helpful if available.
- When in doubt it is always most prudent to surgically explore the patient's scrotum.

> ☛ **Special Tips for GPs**
>
> - Always consider torsion of the spermatic cord as a possible diagnosis in every patient who presents with scrotal pain, whether continuous or intermittent. Remember that the testis can have torsion yet detort spontaneously.

NEWBORNS (2 CAUSES)

Torsion

- The likeliest cause is torsion due to breech delivery.
- Involves twist of the **whole** spermatic cord (unfixed newly descended testis).
- Presents late: almost all are necrotic.
- Pain and tenderness **are not** prominent features.
- Scrotum is usually red and swollen with a hard testicular mass.
- Surgery is almost always required to excise damaged testis.

Trauma

- Usually affects both sides.
- Prominent cutaneous bruising.
- Most resolve but should be followed up.
- Spontaneous idiopathic scrotal haemorrhage: look for separate bruise over superficial inguinal ring.

TODDLERS

- The least commonly affected age group.
- Acute epididymo-orchitis is the commonest cause:
  1. Some cases are viral but most caused by *E. coli*.
  2. Do urinalysis by stick reagent test looking for pyuria.
  3. Admit for:
     a. **exclusion of torsion**, and
     b. **full investigation** of urinary tract for congenital abnormalities
- Idiopathic scrotal oedema.
  1. Sudden bilateral scrotal swelling with redness. It is painless.
  2. Associated with *haemolytic Streptococcus*, Henoch-Schönlein purpura, and rarely acute leukaemia.

ADOLESCENTS/ADULTS

- This age group has the highest prevalence of acute scrotal pathology.

Testicular torsion

- Sudden onset of severe testicular pain which may radiate to the groin.
- May have associated nausea and vomiting.
- Usually has a previous episode of self-limiting pain.
- **There are no specific clinical signs to differentiate torsion from epididymitis** (both may present with enlarged, tender testes), though history of dysuria and urethral discharge suggests epididymitis.
- Examination reveals a high-riding or horizontal testis.
- **Immediate** Urology consultation.
- Doppler ultrasound useful if available immediately, but **must not** delay definitive care.
- Surgical exploration mandatory if diagnosis in doubt.
- Testicular salvage depends on time between start of symptoms and surgery (**6 hours** is generally the accepted interval).

Torsion of the Hydatids

- Occurs principally in prepubertal boys (10–12 years) due to surge of gonadotrophins which cause remnants to enlarge.
- Pain is less acute and may appear over 2–3 days.
- Tenderness is localized to upper part of scrotum.
- Patient often has a reactive hydrocoele and examination reveals a strangulated hydatid (‘blue dot sign’).
- When diagnosis is certain, the majority respond to analgesics/NSAIDs. Inform the patient that pain and swelling may worsen in the next 48–72 hours.

- Surgical exploration and excision of strangulated appendix is required in all questionable cases.

Epididymo-orchitis

- Due to sexually transmitted infection, especially Chlamydia trachomatis.
- In ED, treat with analgesics and Urogesic® (phenazopyridine) 1 tab tds (a urinary tract analgesic for the accompanying dysuria) and refer to centre for treatment of sexually transmitted diseases. Admit if there is doubt in the diagnosis.
- Antibiotic of choice is doxycycline.
- A preceding history of mumps parotitis suggests a viral orchitis.

Testicular tumours

- May present as acutely painful scrotum due to intratumoural bleeding and capsular extension with associated inflammation.
- May mimic epididymo-orchitis.
- Refer to *Urology* for further evaluation.

Fournier's gangrene (idiopathic scrotal gangrene)

- This is a potentially life-threatening disease.
- Aetiology: usually due to infection or trauma of the perineal area.
- Predominant organisms are *Bacteroides fragilis (anaerobe)* and *E. coli (aerobe)*. Other agents are *haemolytic Strep*, *Staph* and *Clostridia* species.
- Clinical picture: an older and immunocompromised patient presents with the acute onset of a painful, erythematous and markedly oedematous scrotum ± crepitance and gangrene. He is febrile and appears toxic.
- **Management**:
  1. General supportive measures
  2. Cultures
  3. IV ceftriaxone 1–2 g plus IV metronidazole 500 mg plus IV gentamicin 60–80 mg
  4. Prompt Urology consultation for surgical debridement and suprapubic urinary diversion
  5. Hyperbaric oxygen

PENILE PROBLEMS

Balanoposthitis

- An inflammation of the glans penis (balanitis) and the foreskin (posthitis). If recurrent, suggests diabetes as the underlying disorder.
- On examination, retraction of the foreskin reveals foul, purulent material and the glans is tender to palpation.

- **Management**:
  1. Good hygiene
  2. Topical antifungal cream (as *Candida* infections are quite common)
  3. Consider referral for circumcision
  4. If secondary infection is present, give broad-spectrum antibiotics, eg ciprofloxacin 500 mg bd PO × 7 days. If sexually transmitted disease is suspected, doxycycline 100 mg bd PO × 14 days can be added.
  5. Work-up for diabetes (if problem recurrent)
  6. Be aware of the possibility of child abuse
  7. If there is phimosis, patients should be referred for circumcision.

Phimosis

- The inability to retract the foreskin behind the glans. It is usually secondary to chronic infection of the foreskin associated with progressive scarring.
- **Management**:
  1. Emergency treatment, ie dilatation with an artery forcep or dorsal slit of the foreskin, is not required unless the patient has difficulty voiding.
  2. Definitive therapy is circumcision.

Paraphimosis

- The inability to pull retracted foreskin forward back over the glans.
- **Management**: emergency treatment is indicated since vascular compromise can occur:
  1. Apply continuous, firm pressure to the glans penis for 5–10 minutes to reduce the oedema and then pull the foreskin over the glans. Pain may be reduced either by use of lignocaine gel or dorsal penile nerve block using 5 ml of 1% plain lignocaine.
  2. If manual reduction is unsuccessful, infiltrate the constricting ring with a local anaesthetic (without adrenaline) and make a superficial vertical incision dorsally in the midline (dorsal slit procedure).
  3. Definitive treatment is circumcision.

Priapism

- A painful sustained erection that may also be associated with urinary retention. **This is a medical emergency** (Table 1).

Table 1: Causes of priapism

Reversible (may respond to medical therapy)	*Irreversible (generally unresponsive to medical therapy)*
Corporal injections for impotence	High spinal cord lesions
Leukaemic infiltration	Medications (phenothiazines, some cyclic antidepressants)
Complication of Viagra use	
Sickle cell disease	Idiopathic

- On examination, both of the corpora cavernosa are engorged and rigid while the corpus spongiosum and glans are soft.
- **Management**:
  1. Obtain immediate urological consultation.
  2. Administer SQ terbutaline 0.25–0.5 mg q 4–6 h. This is the initial treatment for both reversible and irreversible causes of priapism, but do not waste time by delaying Urology consultation, since the response to this therapy may not be 100%.
  3. Application of ice packs, sedation and analgesics can be attempted but are usually ineffective.
  4. Subsequent therapy is determined by the underlying aetiology of the priapism.
  5. If the arrival of the urologist is going to be delayed, you might consider aspirating 50 ml of blood from the corpora cavernosa with 18G or larger needle. If that fails, procedure can be repeated, followed by irrigation of the corpora with warm heparinized saline. Some cases will require corporal injection of 200 μg phenylephrine (monitor vital signs q 5 min).
  6. If all this fails, a surgical drainage procedure will be required.

Torn frenulum

- Generally occurs during overvigorous masturbation.
- On examination, oozing (rarely spurting) is noted from the frenulum area.
- **Management**:
  1. Direct pressure for 5–10 minutes.
  2. If direct pressure is unsuccessful, infiltrate frenulum area with 1% plain lignocaine (without adrenaline) and place 1 or 2 5–0 absorbable sutures.

Fractured penis

- Generally occurs due to poor coordination of couples' movements with women in the 'on top' position.
- On examination the penis is flaccid but distorted and ecchymotic; there is a variable amount of pain.
- **Management**:
  1. Analgesia, which often requires parenteral opioid agonists.
  2. Ice packs.
  3. Immediate Urology consultation.

References/further reading

1. Davenport M. ABC of general surgery: Acute problem in the scrotum. *BMJ*. 1996;312:435–437.
2. Schneider RE. Male genital problems. In: Tintinalli JE, Ruiz E, Krome RL, eds. *Emergency Medicine: A Comprehensive Study Guide*. 4th ed. New York: McGraw-Hill; 1996:631–640.

24 Palpitations

Peter Manning • Shirley Ooi

CAVEATS

- The abnormal heart beat is almost always due to a disturbance of cardiac rhythm, or dysrhythmia, and what the patient is sensing is a secondary change in the cardiac output (remember: cardiac output is directly related to stroke volume and heart rate).
- Tachydysrhythmias cause increased heart rates and reduced stroke volumes whereas premature ventricular contractions (PVCs) produce an increased stroke volume in the beat following the PVC as a result of the increased filling time during the compensatory pause.
- Do not waste time trying to identify the precise nature of the dysrhythmia; rather, the priority is to:
  1. Assess the **haemodynamic status** of the patient.
  2. Decide whether this is a **narrow** or **wide complex dysrhythmia** (Table 1).
- If the patient is **unstable**, with **serious signs** of (1) heart failure or dyspnoea; (2) shock; (3) altered mental state; (4) chest pain, perform ***immediate*** synchronized electrical cardioversion (for both narrow and wide complex types).
- Evidence does not support the use of **lignocaine** to discriminate between perfusing ventricular tachycardia (VT) and wide complex tachycardia of uncertain origin.
- Evidence does not support the use of **adenosine** to discriminate between perfusing VT and supraventricular (SVT) with aberrant ventricular contraction (SVT which is conducted to only 1 ventricle because of transient bundle branch block).
- **Amiodarone** is now the drug of choice in the management of stable tachydysrhythmias due to a broad antidysrhythmic spectrum and less negative inotropic effect compared with most other agents.

Table 1: ECG classification of tachydysrhythmias

Narrow complex		Wide complex	
Regular	*Irregular*	*Regular*	*Irregular*
Sinus tachycardia	Atrial fibrillation	Monomorphic VT (Figures 3, 4 and 5 and Table 2)	Polymorphic VT
Supraventricular tachycardia (SVT) (Figure 1)	Atrial flutter with varying blocks	SVT with aberrancy (Figure 6 and Table 2)	Any irregular, narrow complex tachycardia with BBB or WPW syndrome (Figure 7)
Atrial flutter with 1:1 or 2:1 conduction (Figure 2)	Multifocal atrial tachycardia	Any regular, narrow complex tachycardia with bundle branch block (BBB) or Wolff-Parkinson-White (WPW) syndrome	

☛ Special Tips for GPs

- Patients presenting to your office with palpitations will probably have intermittent symptoms of a fairly minimal nature in the form of either isolated PVCs or short bursts of a tachydysrhythmia.
- Do not waste time deciphering the ECG; your **first priority** is to assess the **clinical status** of the patient.
- Perform a 12-lead ECG. The dysrhythmia may be self-limiting and it is very helpful for the hospital doctor to have a tracing taken during the dysrhythmia.
- Administer supplemental oxygen by nasal cannulae at a rate of 2–6 l/min, adjusted to comfort level.
- Measure blood pressure frequently.
- Insert peripheral IV line with normal saline at slow rate.
- Provide reassurance: these patients are often very anxious and fearful of dying.
- Transfer patient to hospital, preferably by an ambulance equipped to perform continual ECG monitoring.
- Do take note of PVCs with '**R on T phenomenon**' as there is a high risk of VF (Figure 8).

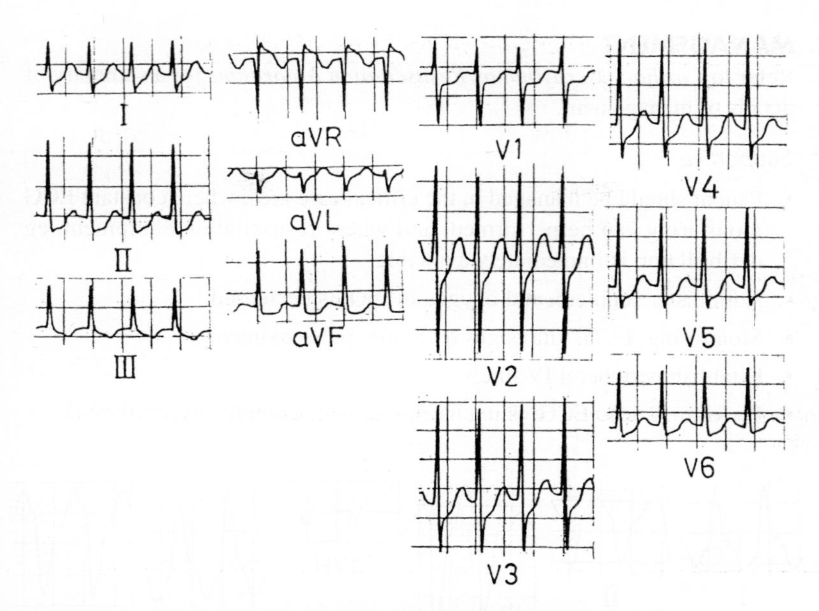

Figure 1: Supraventricular AV nodal reentrant tachycardia in a 35-year-old woman who presented with palpitations

Note: (1) Regular, narrow QRS tachycardia of around 200/min. (2) No P waves are visible. Subsequent electrophysiological study confirmed that the patient was suffering from supraventricular AV nodal reentrant tachycardia. Figure reproduced with permission from Fig. 5.15 Pg 77 (ref. 5).

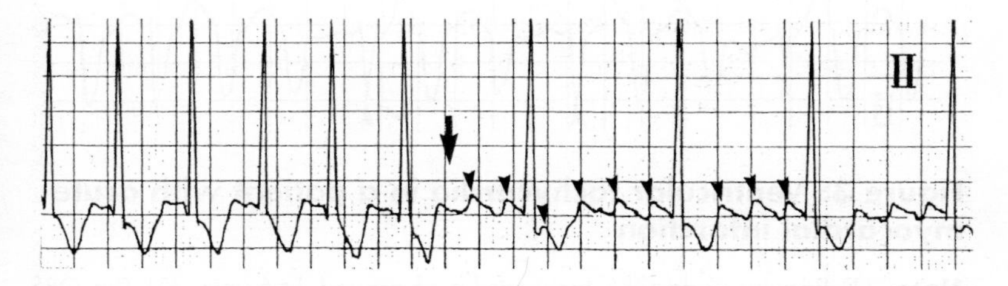

Figure 2: Atrial flutter with 2:1 AV conduction

Note: During 2:1 AV conduction, the flutter ('F') waves are hidden as they are buried within the QRS complexes and the ST/T wave segments. They are evident only when the AV conductions ratio is increased resulting in a slower ventricular rate (arrow). Arrowheads indicate flutter ('F') waves. Figure reproduced with permission from Fig. 5.27 Pg. 88 (ref. 5).

MANAGEMENT

Refer to *Cardiac Dysrhythmias/Resuscitation Algorithms* for a summary of details of management.

Supportive

- Patient should be managed in the critical care area, where constant ECG monitoring can be performed, and where resuscitation equipment, eg defibrillator, is immediately available.
- Administer supplemental oxygen if SpO_2 is decreased.
- Monitoring: ECG, vital signs q 15 min, pulse oximetry.
- Establish peripheral IV line.
- Perform 12-lead ECG: is it a narrow or wide complex dysrhythmia?

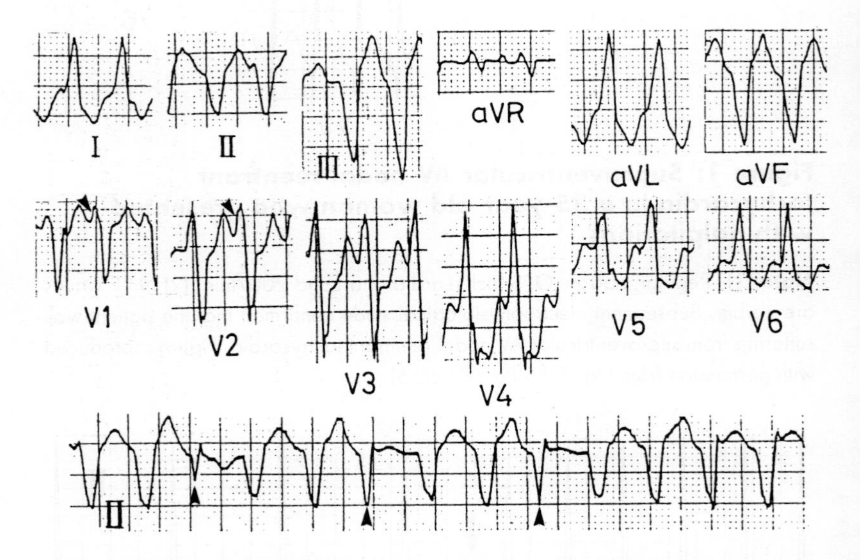

Figure 3: Ventricular tachycardia in a patient with acute myocardial infarction

Note: (1) Regular wide QRS tachycardia of around 166/min. (2) The QRS morphology superficially resembles a left bundle branch pattern, except that the **r waves in V1 and V2** (arrowheads) are broad, thus favouring ventricular ectopy. (3) The rhythm strip in the lower part of the ECG shows **fusion beats** (arrowheads) which are of different morphologies. There is also a suggestion of **AV dissociation**, because some corresponding parts of the ST/T wave segments of consecutive ventricular complexes have slightly different morphologies and appeared deformed, most likely due to the superimposition of P waves occurring at a rate which is different from that of the QRS complexes. Figure reproduced with permission from Fig. 6.11 Pg. 98 (ref. 5).

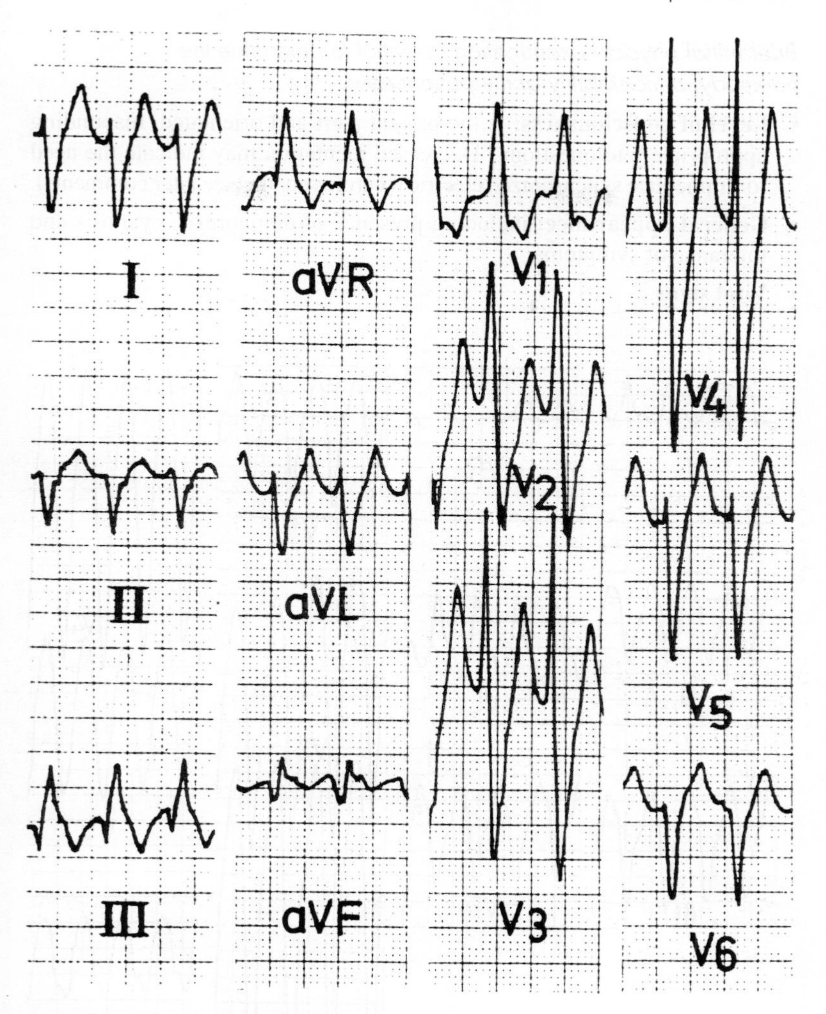

Figure 4: Ventricular tachycardia

Note: (1) Rapid ventricular rate of 158/min. (2) Regular and wide (0.16 sec) QRS complexes. (3) Monophasic R wave in V1. (4) rS complex in V_5 and V_6. (5) Indeterminate axis of appropriately –170°. Figure reproduced with permission from Fig. 6.12 Pg. 99 (ref. 5).

Brief initial physical examination essential to determine the haemodynamic stability of the patient now

- **Level of consciousness:** is the patient alert and orientated, responding appropriately to questions? Decreased mentation may indicate the need for immediate synchronized electrical cardioversion (see later comments).
- **General appearance:** including presence of diaphoresis, cyanosis and tolerance of symptoms.
- **Vital signs.**

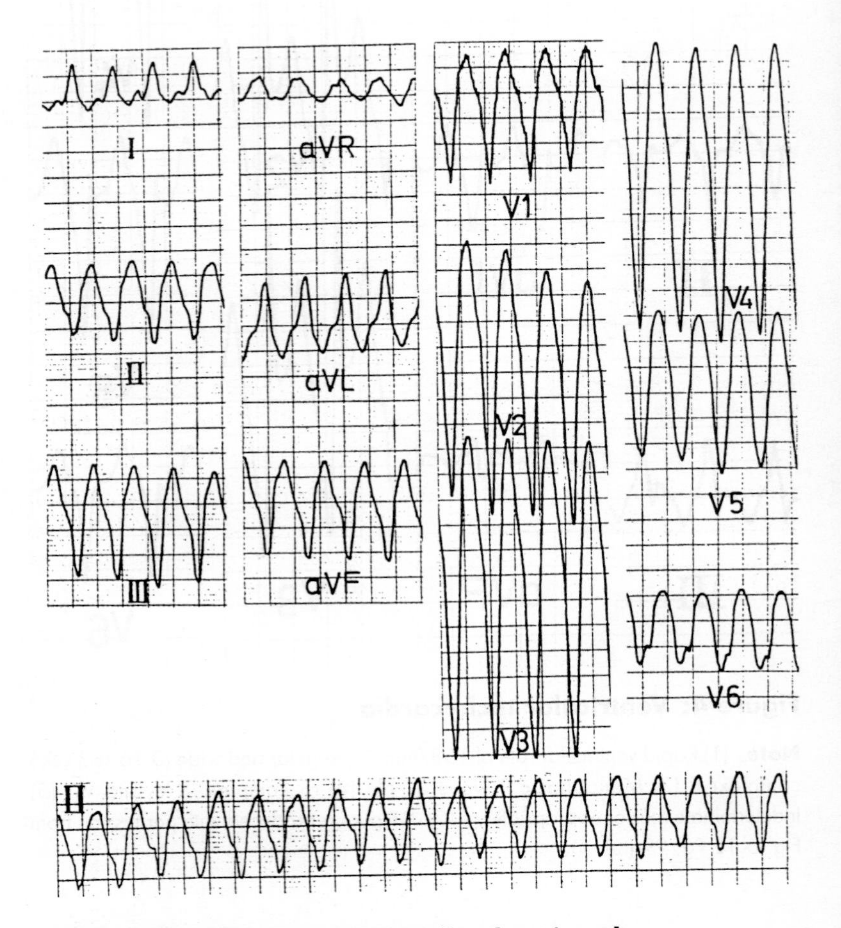

Figure 5: Ventricular tachycardia showing the concordance pattern

Note: (1) Regular, wide QRS tachycardia (190/min). (2) All the QRS complexes in the precordial leads from V_1 to V_6 are negative in polarity. Figure reproduced with permission from Fig. 6.13 Pg. 100 (ref. 5).

- **Technique of cardioversion**:
    1. Place chest patches at the right infraclavicular and apical locations (as in defibrillation).
    2. Administer IV diazepam or midazolam for sedation (if available).
    3. Depress the SYNC (synchronization) button (unlike defibrillation).
    4. Select energy level starting with 100 J for adults with subsequent levels of 200 J, 300 J and 360 J if necessary.

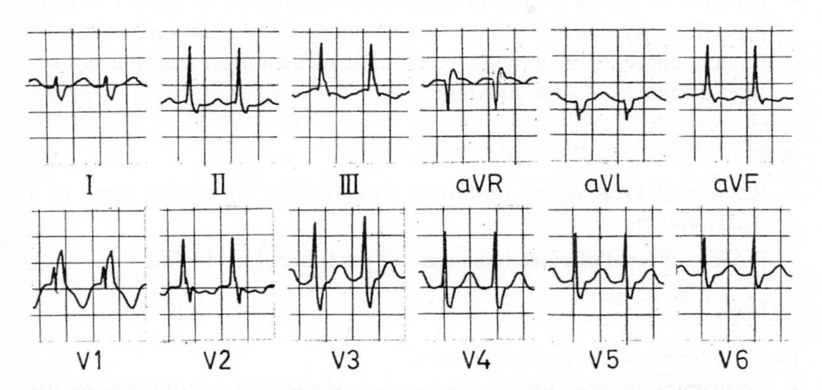

Figure 6: Supraventricular tachycardia with aberrant ventricular conduction induced in the electrophysiological laboratory in a 25-year presenting with palpitation

Note: (1) Rapid heart rate of 160/min. (2) Regular and wide QRS complexes (0.12 sec) with a typical right bundle branch block configuration (triphasic rSR′ pattern in V1). (3) No clearly visible P waves. Figure reproduced with permission from Fig 6.14 Pg. 101 (ref. 5).

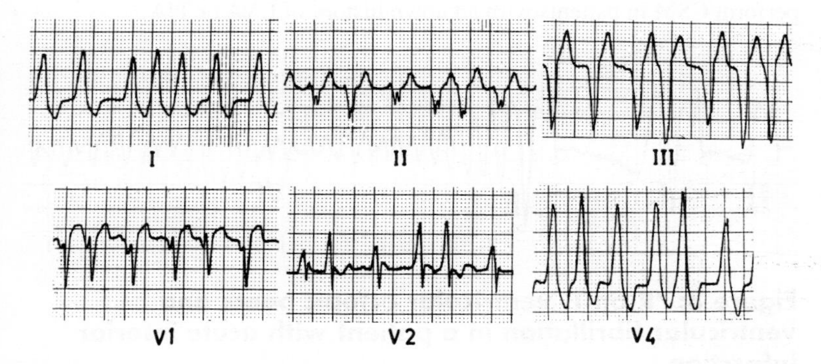

Figure 7: Atrial fibrillation in a 22-year-old man with WPW syndrome

Note: (1) Irregular rhythm and very rapid ventricular rate. (2) The QRS complexes are variably widen. Figure reproduced with permission from Fig. 5.19 Pg. 81 (ref. 5).

Focused history (this is valuable if time permits)

- A previous history of palpitations: if positive, how were they treated: by physical manoeuvres, medications or electrical treatment?
- What has the patient done for the palpitations? Has he/she been taught the Valsalva manoeuvre for home use? If performed, what was the result?
- Associated symptoms of chest pain, dyspnoea, lightheadedness or confusion: indicative of end-organ hypoperfusion and decompensation.
- Personal or family history of cardiovascular disease or history of drug ingestions, eg cold preparations containing sympathomimetic agents, bronchodilator or theophylline-containing medications, or amphetamine-like substances in slimming pills.

Secondary focused physical examination

- Review of **vital signs**: important to detect an improving trend or a deterioration.
- Review of **level of consciousness** and **peripheral perfusion**.

Therapy

Narrow Complex Tachydysrhythmias

- **Treatment depends on the diagnosis**, eg **sinus tachycardia** requires the cause to be addressed (pain, haemorrhage, anxiety, anticholinergic effects, etc)
- **Non-pharmacological**: important as up to 25% of patients with SVT can be converted by Valsalva manoeuvres or carotid sinus massage.

Note: The carotid sinus is located at the level of the angle of the mandible and listen for bruits before performing **carotid sinus massage** (**CSM**). Some clinicians avoid CSM totally in patients over the age of 50 in the anticipation of plaque existence, regardless of the presence or absence of a bruit. Do not perform CSM in patients with a known history of CVA or TIA.

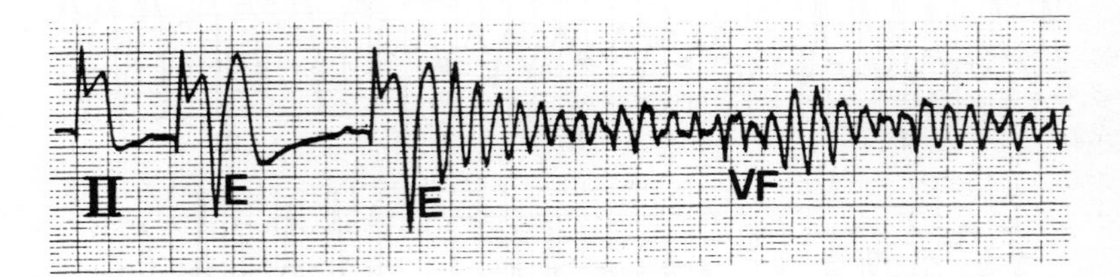

Figure 8: 'R on T' ventricular ectopic beats and ventricular fibrillation in a patient with acute inferior infarction

Note: (1) 'Hyperacute' changes of transmural inferior infarction as reflected by raised ST segment in II. (2) 'R on T' ventricular ectopic beats (E) initiating ventricular fibrillation (VF).

- **Pharmacological**: choices include **adenosine**, **verapamil** or **amiodarone**: all have been found to be equally effective and can be used if another fails to convert the narrow complex tachycardia. Choice of drug depends on availability and experience of clinician.
  1. **Adenosine** is an ultra-short-acting AV nodal blocker (Table 2).
     Dosage: 6 mg IV by **fast** bolus in a **proximal** vein (not hand or wrist), with immediate 20 ml saline flush and elevation of the arm. Can be repeated twice at a dose of 12 mg IV to a total of 30 mg.
  2. **Verapamil** (a calcium channel blocker) is as effective as adenosine. Its disadvantages are: (1) its slower onset of action; and (2) significant side effects of decreased myocardial contractility and peripheral vasodilatation.

Note: Pretreatment with a fluid bolus and calcium chloride (0.5–1.0 gm IV over 5 min) are useful in preventing verapamil-induced hypotension.

     Caution: verapamil should not be used concomitantly with IV beta-blockers and should be avoided in patients with wide complex tachycardias.
     Dosage: 2.5–10 mg IV; can be repeated 15 to 20 min later; maximum total dose of 20 mg.
  3. **Amiodarone** is particularly useful if adenosine has failed and there are signs of congestive heart failure.
     Dosage: 150 mg IV over 10 min; can be repeated once.
  4. **Diltiazem** (another calcium channel blocker) is as effective as verapamil in the management of narrow complex SVT. Its advantage over verapamil is that diltiazem produces less myocardial depression.
     Dosage: 10–20 mg IV over 2 min. If ineffective, can be followed in 15 min by a second bolus of 0.35 mg/kg IV. If needed, an infusion of 5–15 mg/h × 24 h may be initiated.

Table 2: Advantages and disadvantages of giving adenosine over verapamil

Advantages	*Disadvantages*
Short half-life of <10 seconds	Side effects of flushing, dyspnoea and chest pain
Lack of hypotensive and myocardial depressant effects	Recurrence of SVT common (in up to 50–60% of patients)
	Significant drug interactions: antagonized by theophylline and caffeine, and potentiation by dipyridamole and carbamazepine
	Note: Adenosine usually does not convert the dysrhythmia in paroxysmal atrial tachycardia, atrial flutter or atrial fibrillation, but will slow the ventricular rate due to a decrease in atrio-ventricular conduction.

5. **Beta-blockers** such as esmolol and propranolol are also effective:
   Esmolol has a very short half-life and is cardioselective.
   Dosage: 0.5 mg/kg bolus over 1 min followed by an infusion of 0.05 mg/kg/min. The loading dose can be repeated and the infusion rate increased by 0.05 mg/kg/min every 5 min prn to a maximum of 0.2 mg/kg/min.
   Propranolol is the drug of choice for SVT in thyrotoxicosis since it partially blocks the conversion of T3 and T4.
   Caution: avoid in patients with COLD, CCF or asthma, and in patients who are being treated with calcium channel blockers.
   Dosage: 1 mg IV over 1 min; can be repeated q 5 min to a total of 0.1–0.5 mg/kg.
6. **Digoxin**: a vagotonic drug. Its disadvantages are a much slower onset of action compared with the drugs above (may take several hours to work).
   Dosage: 0.5 mg IV bolus initially, with repeated doses of 0.25 mg q 30–60 min prn. Total dose should not exceed 0.02 mg/kg.

Atrial fibrillation (AF) with rapid ventricular response

The presentation of a patient with **atrial fibrillation** and **rapid ventricular response** is a special problem. If the patient is stable haemodynamically, the role of the emergency physician is to slow the ventricular response and **not** to convert the patient to sinus rhythm unless he/she is very sure that the AF is <48 hours' duration. Conversion to sinus rhythm without adequate anticoagulation may result in embolization of a clot attached to the wall of the right atrium. Studies suggest the use of calcium channel blockers (**diltiazem** or **verapamil**) and beta blockers (**esmolol** and **metoprolol**) to be the most effective **rate-controlling medications** in the stable AF patient.

Dosage: **IV diltiazem** 10–20 mg over 2 min.

Note: **Digoxin** has not been shown to be effective for acute rate control. However, if patient is in cardiac failure, the choices would be digoxin or amiodarone.

Overall, **chemical cardioversion** is successful only about 50% of the time. The literature is replete with studies touting the efficacy of one or the other drugs for conversion of AF to sinus rhythm but many are contradictory and not methodologically sound. The choices of drugs include:

- **Class 1A agents (quinidine and procainamide)**: most traditional medications used for cardioversion, with success rates of approximately 40–80%.
- **Amiodarone**: 93% success at restoring sinus rhythm within 24 hours but not as quick as the calcium channel blockers or beta blockers in slowing the rate.
- **Propafenone**: successful in the IV and oral routes.

- **Flecainide**: Successful at cardioversion within 2–3 hours when used as an IV or oral bolus but fear of prodysrhythmic effects limits its use.
- **Ibutilide**: Rapid termination of AF with rates of conversion greater than procainamide but reported incidence of 4.3% of torsades de pointes.

If the patient with rapid atrial fibrillation is unstable haemodynamically, the difficult decision of performing **electrical cardioversion after the administration of heparin 5000 units IV must be made**. The risk of thromboembolism posed by atrial fibrillation seems to persist for a few weeks after cardioversion. Hence anticoagulation should be continued for 3 months unless there is a contraindication.

Note: **Direct cardioversion** is safe and effective **(90% conversion rate)** in conversion of AF to sinus rhythm.

Hospitalization is not required for all patients with atrial fibrillation and can be limited to those:

- with haemodynamic compromise
- with severely symptomatic arrhythmia (eg chest pain, signs of coronary ischaemia, CCF)
- with high risk for embolism (eg heart failure, CCF, mitral stenosis, previous CVA, age >65 years)
- with AF >48 hours' or uncertain duration for rate control and initiation of anticoagulation
- who fail cardioversion in the ED

AF can be considered for **discharge** if:

- <48 hours' duration, who undergo successful cardioversion in the ED, without signs of heart failure or ischaemia.
- Recent-onset AF who have a well-controlled ventricular rate, are well appearing, and have therapeutic anticoagulation arranged. Arrange for follow-up with the cardiologist.

Wide complex tachydysrhythmias

Note: **All regular wide complex tachycardias** should be treated as **ventricular tachycardia**, especially if the patient has a history of **coronary artery disease**.

Exceptions are when the patient has:

- A definite history of SVT and aberrancy is suspected: administer adenosine/verapamil.
- WPW syndrome with preexcitation tachycardias: administer adenosine/amiodarone.

Note: Do not treat irregular wide complex tachycardia (Figure 7) with calcium channel blockers (verapamil or diltiazem), beta-blockers or digoxin because blocking of the AV node may cause the impulses from AF to go down the accessory pathway and cause a VF.

Table 3: How to differentiate VT from SVT with aberrant conduction or prior bundle branch block

	VT	*SVT*
History		
IHD; CCF; Age >35 years	90% specific for VT	However, absence does not establish a diagnosis of SVT
Physical Examination		
1. Irregular cannon 'a' waves in the jugular venous pulse	May be present	Absent
2. Variable intensity of first heart sound	May be present	Absent
ECG		
1. *QRS width*	>140 ms generally	<140 ms
2. *AV relationship*	AV dissociation (<50% VT) (Figure 3) Fusion beats (combination of sinus and tachycardia QRS) (Figure 3) Capture beats (total depolarization of the ventricles by conduction of a sinus beat)	
3. *QRS axis*	Left of –30 degrees or in IV quadrant (Figure 4)	

4. *'Concordance' pattern* (presence of either +ve or –ve QRS complexes in **all** the precordial leads)	Virtually diagnostic of VT (Figure 5)	
5. *QRS morphology* Wide complex tachycardia with *RBBB pattern* (defined as a predominantly +ve QRS in lead V_1)	In V_1: Monophasic R wave .... qR complex .... 'Left rabbit ear' bigger than 'right ear'	In V_1: Triphasic QRS .... 'Right rabbit ear' taller than 'left ear' ....
	In V_6: QS pattern .... r/s ratio <1	
Wide complex tachycardia with *LBBB pattern* (defined as a predominantly –ve deflection in lead V_1)	In V_{1-2}: High and wide initial R wave >0.04 sec with slurring of initial QRS portion .... In V_6: QS or predominantly –ve deflection	

Prior to administering any drugs, assess the patient's haemodynamic status: **any instability mandates immediate sedation followed by synchronized electrical cardioversion**.

- **Amiodarone**: this is the agent of choice as it is effective against VT, SVT with aberrancy and SVT. If it fails, then synchronized cardioversion is indicated.
  Dosage: amiodarone 150 mg IV over 10 min; can be repeated once.
- **Procainamide** is a second choice drug.
  Dosage: 100 mg over 5 min; can be repeated up to a total of 1g, followed by infusion of 1–4 mg/min.
  Precautions: terminate bolus if:
  1. Dysrhythmia is terminated
  2. QRS complex widens by 50%
  3. Hypotension develops
  4. Total of 1 g administered
- **Lignocaine**: still a popular choice due to its long history of usage, relatively low toxicity and ease of administration. However, evidence does not support its use except as a second- or third-line choice.
  Dosage: 1.0–1.5 mg/kg IV push; repeat in 3–5 min to a maximum dose of 3 mg/kg

References/further reading

1. The American Heart Association in Collaboration with the International Liaison Committee on Resuscitation (ILCOR) Guidelines 2000 for Cardiopulmonary Resuscitation and Emergency Cardiovascular Care: An international consensus on science. *Circulation.* 2000;102:11–384.
2. Hood MA, et al. Adenosine versus verapamil in the treatment of supraventricular tachycardia: A randomized double-crossover trial. *Am Heart J.* 1992.
3. Falk RH. Atrial fibrillation. *NEJM.* 2001;334(14):1067–1077.
4. Cooper JS. Atrial fibrillation. In: Frank LF, Jobe KA, eds. *Admission and discharge decisions in Emergency Medicine*, Philadelphia: Hanley & Belfus, Inc; 2002:1–6.
5. Chia BL. *Clinical Electrocardiography*, 3rd ed. Singapore: World Scientific; 1998:77,81, 88,94,98–101.

25 Poisoning

General principles

Shirley Ooi • Peter Manning • Suresh Pillai

CAVEATS

- The history in drug overdose (DO) is often unreliable. Hence one should have a **high index of suspicion** and assume the possibility of a **mixed overdose including alcohol intake**. See Annex for common sources of poisoning in Singapore.
- Pay special attention to the **physical examination** to get clues about the types of DOs.
- A patient with **altered mental state** with a suspicion of DO should have an **ECG** done to exclude the possibility of cyclic antidepressant poisoning and a **stat capillary glucose** done to exclude hypoglycaemia. Consider also the other various differentials of altered mental state. Refer to *Altered Mental State*.
- Remember that prudent management of DO includes paying attention to the emotional/psychiatric state of the patient besides managing the clinical effects of the DO.
- **Gastric lavage** should not be performed routinely for every case of DO. Refer to section on *Gastric decontamination* for details.

☛ **Special Tips for GPs**

- Do **NOT induce emesis** in a patient with DO using syrup Ipecac. This is because Ipecac may delay the administration or reduce the effectiveness of activated charcoal, oral antidotes, and whole bowel irritation.
- It is generally safer to **refer all** patients with DOs to the ED by ambulance. An obvious **exception** is the child who has swallowed **oral contraceptive pills** by mistake. Reassurance can be given and the child can be discharged.
- Consider the possibility of **non-accidental injury** in a paediatric patient with a history of poisoning.
- Attend to the ABCs of the DO patient first before sending the patient to the ED.

Table 1: Differential diagnosis of various vital signs in drug

Temperature	*Pulse rate/rhythm*
HYPOTHERMIA ('COOLS')	BRADYCARDIA ('PACED')
C Carbon monoxide	**P** Propranolol (beta blockers)
O Opiates	**A** Anticholinesterase drugs
O Oral hypoglycaemics, insulin	**C** Clonidine, calcium channel
L Liquor	**E** Ethanol/alcohols
S Sedative hypnotics	**D** Digoxin
HYPERTHERMIA ('NASA')	TACHYCARDIA ('FAST')
N Neuroleptic malignant syndrome, nicotine	**F** Free base (cocaine)
A Antihistamines	**A** Anticholinergics, antihistamines, amphetamines
S Salicylates, sympathomimetics	**S** Sympathomimetics (cocaine, PC
A Anticholinergics, antidepressants	**T** Theophylline
	DYSRHYTHMIAS
	Digoxin
	Cyclic antidepressants
	Sympathomimetics
	Phenothiazines
	Chloral hydrate
	Anticonvulsants

HISTORY

- Definite DO or questionable DO?
- What, when, how much, how, where, why? Any symptoms from exposure?
- Any suicidal risk? If high, psychiatric consult in ED.
- Psychiatric and past medical history (including medications).
- Any previous suicide attempts?

PHYSICAL EXAMINATION

Vital Signs

See Table 1 for details.

Odours

- Obvious odours: kerosene/bleaching agents/insecticides
- Other odours are listed in Table 2.

overdose

Blood pressure	*Respiratory*
HYPOTENSION ('CRASH')	HYPOVENTILATION
C Clonidine (or any antihypertensive)	Opioids
R Reserpine	
A Antidepressants	
S Sedative hypnotics	
H Heroin (opiates)	
HYPERTENSION ('CT SCAN')	HYPERVENTILATION
C Cocaine	Salicylates
T Theophylline	CNS stimulant drugs
S Sympathomimetics	Cyanide
C Caffeine	
A Anticholinergics, amphetamines	
N Nicotine	

Table 2: Odours of poisons

Odours	*Probable poisons*
Fruity	Ethanol
Mothballs	Camphor/naphthalene
Bitter almonds	Cyanide
Silver polish	Cyanide
Stove gas	Carbon monoxide
Rotten eggs	Hydrogen sulphide
Garlic	Arsenic/parathion
Wintergreen	Methylsalicylate

Note: Carbon monoxide is odourless. Stove gas smells because of a stenching agent called mercaptans.

Neurologic Examination

- **Level of consciousness**: see below the selected drugs and toxins that cause coma or stupor.

General CNS depressants
- Anticholinergics
- Antihistamines
- Barbiturates
- Cyclic antidepressants
- Ethanol and other alcohols
- Phenothiazines
- Sedative-hypnotic agents

Cellular hypoxia
- Carbon monoxide
- Cyanide
- Hydrogen sulfide
- Methaemoglobinaemia

Sympatholytic agents
- Clonidine
- Methyldopa
- Opiates

Other or unknown mechanisms
- Bromide
- Hypoglycaemic agents
- Lithium
- Phencyclidine
- Salicyclates

- **Pupils**: selected drugs and toxins and their effects on the pupils are listed below.

MIOSIS ('COPS')
- **C** Cholinergics, clonidine
- **O** Opiates, organophosphates
- **P** Phenothiazines, pilocarpine, pontine bleed
- **S** Sedative-hypnotics

MYDRIASIS ('AAAS')
- **A** Antihistamines
- **A** Antidepressants
- **A** Anticholinergics, atropine
- **S** Sympathomimetics (cocaine, amphetamines)

- **Fits** are caused by the substances listed below ('**OTIS CAMPBELL**')
  - **O** Organophosphates
  - **T** Cyclic antidepressants
  - **I** Insulin, isoniazid
  - **S** Sympathomimetics
  - **C** Camphor, cocaine
  - **A** Amphetamines
  - **M** Methylxanthines
  - **P** PCP (phencyclidine)
  - **B** Beta-blockers
  - **E** Ethanol
  - **L** Lithium
  - **L** Lead
- **Focal signs**: look for other aetiologies, especially trauma.

Skin

- **Diaphoretic skin ('SOAP') and hypoglycaemia**:
  - **S** Sympathomimetics
  - **O** Organophosphates
  - **A** ASA (salicylates)
  - **P** PCP and hypoglycaemia
- **Dry**: anticholinergic

- **Blistering**:
  1. Carbon monoxide
  2. Barbiturates
  3. Poison ivy
  4. Sulphur mustard
  5. Lewisite
- **Colour**:
  Red: Anticholinergic
  Cyanide
  Carbon monoxide
  Blue: Methaemoglobinaemia
- **Needle tracks**: opioids

Toxidromes

- **Opioids**
  1. Coma
  2. Respiratory depression
  3. Pinpoint pupils
  4. Hypotension
  5. Bradycardia
- **Cholinergics ('SLUDGE')**: eg organophosphate/carbamate
  S Salivation
  L Lacrimation
  U Urination
  D Defaecation
  G Gastric emptying
  E Emesis
  1. 'Drowning in their own secretions'
     a. bronchorrhoea
     b. bronchospasm
     c. pulmonary oedema
  2. Altered mental state
  3. Muscle weakness and paralysis
  4. Odour of garlic
- **Anticholinergics**: eg antihistamines, cyclic antidepressants, homatropine, scopolamine
  1. 'hot as a hare' (hyperthermia)
  2. 'red as a beet' (cutaneous vasodilatation)
  3. 'dry as a bone' (decreased salivation)
  4. 'blind as a bat' (cycloplegia and mydriasis)
  5. 'mad as a hatter' (delirium and hallucinations)
  6. Other signs
     a. tachycardia
     b. urinary retention
     c. decreased GIT motility/absent bowel sounds

- **Salicylates**
  1. Fever
  2. Tachypnoea
  3. Vomiting
  4. Lethargy (rarely coma)
  5. Tinnitus
- **Sympathomimetics**: eg cocaine, amphetamines
  1. Hypertension
  2. Tachycardia
  3. Hyperpyrexia
  4. Mydriasis
  5. Anxiety or delirium
- **Sedative-hypnotics**: eg barbiturates, benzodiazepines
  1. Unpredictable pupillary changes
  2. Confusion or coma
  3. Respiratory depression
  4. Hypothermia
  5. Vesicle or bullae ('barb burns')
- **Extrapyramidal**: a 'Parkinsonian' picture (**'TROD'**)
  1. **T**remor
  2. **R**igidity
  3. **O**pisthotonus, oculogyric crisis
  4. **D**ysphonia, dysphagia

  This category of drugs includes the '**zines**'
  1. Chlorpromazine (Largactil®/Thorazine®)
  2. Prochlorperazine (Stemetil®/Compazine®)
  3. Haloperidol (Haldol®)
  4. Metochlopramide (Maxolon®/Reglan®)
- **Haemoglobinopathies**
  1. Carboxyhaemoglobinaemia
     a. Headache
     b. Nausea and vomiting, flu-like illness
     c. Syncope, tachypnoea, tachycardia
     d. Coma, convulsions
     e. Cardiovascular collapse, respiratory failure
  2. Methaemoglobinaemia
     a. Prominent clinical feature is cyanosis ('chocolate blood')
     b. Asymptomatic (<30% methaemoglobin level)
     c. Fatigue, weakness, dizziness, headache (30–50% methaemoglobin level)
     d. Lethargy, stupor, respiratory depression (>55% methaemoglobin level)

DIAGNOSTIC AIDS

Laboratory

- **FBC**: elevated TWC = infection/iron/theophylline/hydrocarbons
- **Serum electrolytes**
  1. Anion gap = $[Na^+] - [HCO_3^-] - [Cl^-]$
  2. Normal anion gap = 8 to 16 mEq/*l*
- **Metabolic acidosis/elevated anion gap**

  C Carbon monoxide, cyanide
  A Alcoholic ketoacidosis
  T Toluene

  M Methanol, methaemoglobin
  U Uraemia
  D Diabetic ketoacidosis
  P Paraldehyde
  I INH/Iron
  L Lactic acidosis
  E Ethylene glycol
  S Salicylates, solvent

- **Serum urea and creatinine**: to identify any preexisting renal dysfunction
- **Toxicology screens**: drug levels are useful in
  1. Paracetamol
  2. Salicylates
  3. Cholinesterases
  4. Iron
  5. Lithium
  6. Theophylline
  7. Carbon monoxide

X-rays

- **Chest**
  1. Pulmonary toxic agents, eg hydrocarbons/toxic gases/paraquat
  2. Non-cardiogenic pulmonary oedema, eg opiates/phenobarbitone/salicylates/carbon monoxide
- **Abdominal**: **toxins radioopaque on x-rays ('CHIPES')**

  C Chloral hydrate
  H Heavy metals
  I Iron
  P Phenothiazines
  E Enteric-coated preps (salicylates)
  S Sustained-release products (theophylline)

ECG

- Cyclic antidepressants affecting cardiac conducting system, eg prolonged PR and QRS intervals.

MANAGEMENT

Patients with altered mental state or haemodynamic instability must be managed in the critical care area. Otherwise most DO cases can be managed in the intermediate care area.

Critical care area cases

- Airway management equipment must be immediately available.

Note: A patient with adequate oxygenation who has an impaired gag reflex and who needs gastric lavage will require prophylactic orotracheal intubation.

- Resuscitation drugs must be immediately available.
- Supplemental oxygen to maintain SpO_2 of at least 95%.
- Monitoring: ECG, vital signs q 5–15 min, pulse oximetry.
- Establish a peripheral IV line.
- Labs (refer to section on *Diagnostic Aids: Laboratory*).
- Place urinary catheter (case dependent).
- Control fits or dysrhythmias: standard approach acceptable except in cases of toxicity by cyclic antidepressants, where cardiac and CNS complications can be prevented by alkalinization of the blood to pH of 7.5. This can be accomplished by either hyperventilation or administration of IV sodium bicarbonate, or both.

'Coma cocktail'

- **Dextrose 50%**: give only for confirmed hypoglycaemia as it may actually worsen neurologic recovery.
- **Naloxone (Narcan®)**:
  Mechanism of action Reverses the effects of opioids including respiratory depression, sedation and hypotension.
  Clinical effect Onset is within 2 minutes.
  Dosage Not a function of age or size (except in neonates); rather it depends on CNS receptor number. 2 mg for both adults and children (can repeat up to 10–20 mg).
  Route of administration IV/endotracheal/intralingual.
  Indications Safe but may add little to patient's diagnostic evaluations as clinical parameters are found to be 92% sensitive in predicting responders to naloxone.
  Caution Potential precipitation of withdrawal symptoms when given to opioid addicts. The half-life of naloxone is sometimes shorter than some opiates. Hence, there is a need for continued monitoring and repeat doses of naloxone.
- **Predicting opioid overdose**: see Table 3.
- **Predicting response to naloxone**: see Table 4.

Table 3: Predicting opioid overdose

Clinical parameter	*Sensitivity (%)*	*Specificity (%)*
Respiratory rate <12/min	79	94
Pinpoint pupils	75	85
Circumstantial evidence	67	95
Any of the above	92	76

Table 4: Predicting response to naloxone

Clinical parameter	*N*	*Sensitivity (%)*
Respiratory rate <12/min	20	80
Pinpoint pupils	22	88
Circumstantial evidence	15	60
Any of the above	24	96

- **Flumazenil (Anexate)**:
  Mechanism of action A benzodiazepine (BZD) structurally related to midazolam. Flumazenil competes with other benzodiazepines at omega 1 receptor sites in the CNS.
  Clinical effect Onset in 1–2 minutes with peak effect in 3–5 minutes.
  Duration of effect 1–4 hours.
  Low dose reverses hypnosis, sedation of BZDs.
  High dose reverses anticonvulsant effect of BZDs.
  Indications Reverses accidental overdose of BZDs in conscious sedation improving ventilatory status.
  Improves level of consciousness in known or suspected BZD overdose to avoid intubation or invasive procedures.
  Dosage Initial 0.2 mg IV; wait 30 seconds, then repeat at 0.3 mg IV; if needed, can give another 0.5 mg/min to a total dose of 3–5 mg.
  Adverse effects BZD withdrawal.
  Fits, especially in cyclic antidepressant or BZD-dependent patients.
  Flush.
  Nausea and/or vomiting.
  Anxiety, palpitations, fear.
  Contraindications Patients taking BDZs for long-term control of fits.
  Anticipated use of BDZs in the near future, eg sedation, muscle relaxation, anticonvulsant.
  Concomitant cyclic antidepressant toxicity.
  Severe head trauma.
- **Thiamine**: Generally safe; indicated in all known alcoholics or the elderly, dishevelled, malnourished patient. Dosage: 100 mg IV bolus over 1–2 minutes.

Decontamination

- Depending on the agent involved, proper protective gear must be worn. At the minimum level, staff should undertake full universal precautions.
- **Decontamination procedure**:
  1. Remove from contaminated area.
  2. Remove all clothing.
  3. Brush off all powder contaminants from the skin to avoid an exothermic reaction when contacting water used for decontamination.
  4. Wash all areas with water and/or soap solution (and shampoo for the hair). Use soft scrubs if available.
  5. Areas to concentrate are the head, axillae, groin and back.
  6. Brush under nails.
  7. Irrigate the eyes if specifically contaminated.
  8. All open wounds must be additionally decontaminated with water.
- **End point of decontamination**:
  1. Till there is pain reduction, if primary dermal exposure is present.
  2. For contamination in the eyes, till pain symptoms abate and/or there is a change in the colour of litmus pH paper according to the nature of the agent involved.
  3. Uncomplicated full decontamination should take 5 to 8 minutes.

Gastric decontamination

- **Dilution**: water/milk.
- **Gastric lavage should not be employed routinely** in the management of poisoned patients. In experimental studies, the amount of marker removed by gastric lavage was highly variable and diminished with time. There is no certain evidence that its use improves clinical outcome and it may cause significant morbidity.

  Indications Should not be considered unless a patient has ingested a potentially life-threatening amount of poison **within 1 hour of ingestion**. Even then, the clinical benefit has not been confirmed in controlled studies.

  Contraindications Ingestion of corrosives.
  Ingestion of petroleum distillates.
  Existence of ongoing fits.
  Non-toxic ingestion.
  Ingestion of sharp materials.
  Significant haemorrhagic diathesis.

  Procedure **Use largest bore tube possible.**
  Protect the airway.
  Place patient in left lateral and mild Trendelenburg position.
  Check correct placement of the tube.
  Aspirate stomach contents and retain specimen to be sent to the ward with the patient.

Instil lavage fluid.
Agitate stomach.
Withdraw fluid.
Repeat until return is clear.

- **Activated charcoal**:
  1. **Single dose**: should not be administered routinely in the management of poisoned patients. Based on volunteer studies, the effectiveness of activated charcoal decreases with time; the greatest benefit is **within 1 hour of ingestion**.
  2. **Indications**: may be considered if a patient has ingested a potentially toxic amount of poison (which is known to be adsorbed by charcoal) within 1 hour; there are insufficient data to support or exclude its use after 1 hour of ingestion. There is no evidence that the administration of activated charcoal improves clinical outcome.
  3. **Multiple dose**: repeated administration (>2 doses) of oral activated charcoal with the intent of enhancing drug elimination. Multiple-dose activated charcoal is thought to produce its beneficial effect by:
     a. Binding any drug which diffuses from the circulation into the gut lumen. After adsorption, a drug will reenter the gut by passive diffusion provided that the concentration there is lower than in the blood. The rate of passive diffusion depends on the concentration gradient and blood flow. Under these 'sink' conditions, a concentration gradient is maintained and the drug passes continuously into the gut lumen where it is adsorbed by charcoal. This process has been termed '**gastrointestinal dialysis**'.
     b. Interrupting the enterohepatic and enterogastric circulation of drugs.
  4. **Indications**: multiple-dose activated charcoal should be considered only if a patient has ingested a life-threatening amount of carbamazepine, dapsone, phenobarbitone, quinine or theophylline.
  5. **Drugs adsorbed by charcoal**:

Acetaminophen	Digoxin	Meprobamate	Phenylpropanolamin
Amphetamines	Ethchlorvynol	Mercuric chloride	Phenytoin
Arsenic	Glutethamide	Methylsalicylate	Propoxyphene
Aspirin	Imipramine	Morphine	Quinidine
Chlorpheniramine	Iodine	Nortryptiline	Quinine
Chlorpromazine	Ipecac	Paraquat	Salicylates
Cocaine	Isoniazid	Phenobarbitone	Secobarbitone

  6. **Substances not adsorbed by activated charcoal**:
     a. Simple ions: iron, lithium, cyanide
     b. Strong acids or bases
     c. Simple alcohols: methanol, ethanol

- **Cathartics**: the administration of a cathartic alone has no role in the management of the poisoned patient and is **not recommended** as a method of gut decontamination. Based on available data, the routine use of cathartic

Table 5: Specific antidotes for toxins

Toxin	*Antidote*	*Dosage*
Acetaminophen, Paracetamol	N-acetylcysteine (Parvolex®)(each ml contains 200 mg Parvolex®)	IV 150 mg/kg in 200 ml $D_5W \times 15$ min, then IV 50 mg/kg in 500 ml $D_5W \times 4$ h, then IV 100 mg/kg in 1000 ml $D_5W \times 16$ h
Arsenic, mercury, lead	BAL (dimercaprol)	5 mg/kg body weight IM
Atropine	Physostigmine	0.5–2 mg IV
Benzodiazepines	Flumazenil (Anexate®)	See section on '*coma cocktail*'
Carbon monoxide	Oxygen	100% O_2 (hyperbaric for moderate-severe exposures and exposure in pregnant women) Refer to *Poisoning, Carbon Monoxide*
Cyanide	Amyl nitrite pearls	Inhalation of contents of 1–2 pearls
	Sodium nitrite (3% sol)	Adults: IV 300 mg (10 ml) over 2–5 min; Children: IV 0.2–0.33 ml/kg (6–10 mg)
	Sodium thiosulphate (25% sol)	Adults: 50 ml IV (12.5 g) over 10 min; can repeat half dose × 1 prn; children: 1.65 ml/kg IV over 10 min
Ethylene glycol, methanol	Ethanol (10%) mixed in D_5W	Loading dose: 800 mg/kg Maintenance: 1–1.5 ml/kg/h
Iron	Desferoxamine	15 mg/kg/h IV

Lead	EDTA: calcium disodium edetate	1000–1500 mg /m^2/day IV continuous infusion
Nitrites	Methylene blue (1% solution)	1–2 mg/kg IV × 5 min
Organophosphates	Atropine	2–4 mg IV q 5–10 min prn (adult); 0.5 mg/kg IV q 5 min prn (child)
	Pralidoxime (2–PAM)	25–50 mg/kg IV (up to 1 g)
Opioids	Naloxone	See section on *'Coma cocktail'*
Phenothiazines	Benztropine (Cogentin®) Diphenhydramine	2 mg IV/IM 50 mg IV/IM/PO
Isoniazid (INH)	Pyridoxine	5 g IV (can repeat if fits persist)
Digoxin, digitoxin, oleander	Digitalis Fab fragments (Digibind®)	Digoxin level unknown: 5–10 vials IV (40 μg Fab/vial): can repeat Digoxin level known: # vials Digibind = $\dfrac{\frac{(\text{serum digoxin}) \times 5.6l/\text{kg} \times \text{wt in kg}}{1000}}{0.6}$

in combination with activated charcoal is not endorsed. If a cathartic is used, it should be limited to a single dose in order to minimize adverse effects.

Mechanism of action Decreases gastrointestinal transit time (controversial).
Neutralizes constipating effect of activated charcoal.
Also useful for whole bowel irrigation.

Contraindications Preexisting diarrhoea.
Bowel obstruction/ileus.
Volume depleted states.
Infants.
Renal failure contraindicates use of magnesium containing cathartics.
Abdominal trauma.

Enhancement of elimination

- **Forced alkaline diuresis**:
  Alkalinization Alkalinizing of the urine to enhance elimination of weak acids has a limited role for salicylates, phenobarbitone, and herbicide 2, 4 (dichlorophenoxyacetic acid [2, 4-D]).
  Regimen A cycle of 1.5*l* fluid/3 hours:
  500 ml 5% Dextrose + 8.4% $NaHCO_3$ at 1–2 ml/kg body weight
  500 ml 5% Dextrose + 30 ml of 7.45% potassium chloride
  500 ml normal saline
  IV frusemide 20 mg at end of each cycle
  Monitor serum pH and electrolytes: urinary pH should be maintained at pH $\leqslant$8.
  Caution Elderly.
  Cardiac patients.
  Renal disease patients.
  Ingestion of poisons which are cardio- and nephro-toxic.
- **Haemoperfusion**: indications are severe intoxications with theophylline and barbiturates.
- **Haemodialysis**: indications are
  1. Ethylene glycol
  2. Methanol
  3. Lithium (with significant CNS alterations)
  4. Salicylates (with fits, altered mental state, severe metabolic acidosis and serum level >100 mg/dl)
- **Specific antidotes**: see Table 5 for details.
- **Disposition**: admission must be to General Medicine in anticipation of later transfer to Psychiatry. Non-life-threatening DOs without convincing suicidal intent may be discharged **after** psychiatry consultation.

Annex

Common sources of poisoning in Singapore

Paracetamol
Benzodiazepines
Bleaching agents
Household detergents
Antidepressants
Salicylates
Organophosphates

References/further reading

1. Hoffman JR. The empire use of naloxone in patients with altered mental status: A reappraisal. *Ann Emerg Med.* 1991;20:246–252.
2. Chyka PA, Seger D. Position statement: Single-dose activated charcoal. The American Academy of Clinical Toxicology, European Association of Poison Centres and Clinical Toxicologists. *J Toxicol Clin Toxicol.* 1997;35(7):721–741.
3. Vale JA. Position statement: Gastric lavage. The American Academy of Clinical Toxicology, European Association of Poison Centres and Clinical Toxicologists. *J Toxicol Clin Toxicol.* 1997;35(7):669–709.
4. Barceloux D, McGuigan M, Hartigan-Go K. Position statement: Cathartics. The American Academy of Clinical Toxicology, European Association of Poison Centres and Clinical Toxicologists. *J Toxicol Clin Toxicol.* 1997;35(7):743–752.
5. Krenzelok EP, McGuigan M, Lheur P. Position statement: Ipecac syrup. The American Academy of Clinical Toxicology, European Association of Poison Centres and Clinical Toxicologists. *J Toxicol Clin Toxicol.* 1997;35(7):669–709.

26 Red and painful eye

Peter Manning

CAVEATS

- The major role of the ED physician is to perform an appropriate examination and recognize potential vision-threatening disorders.
- Always perform a visual acuity on any patient with an eye problem. It defines in a simple way whether the function of this critical organ is impaired.
- Beware the combination of red eye, vomiting, frontal headache and visual loss: This is typical of **acute angle-closure glaucoma** and demands immediate attention as a potential vision-threatening case.
- Infections and penetrating eye injuries should not be patched (photophobia can be minimized by the use of sunglasses or eye shield).
- Steroid-containing drops or ointment should not be prescribed without eye consultation.

☛ **Special Tips for GPs**

Refer for **immediate** Ophthalmology consultation if the patient exhibits any of the following:

- Decreased visual acuity.
- Deep, rather than superficial, pain.
- Pain unrelieved by topical anaesthetics.
- Corneal oedema.
- Flare or cells in the anterior chamber.
- Ciliary flush.
- Pain in the contralateral eye on direct exposure of the unaffected eye.
- Corneal or conjunctival foreign body which cannot be removed after one attempt in the office.
- In the case of a corrosive burn, implement saline irrigation. immediately prior to patient being transported to hospital. Irrigate until the effluent is pH neutral or mildly acidic as shown by the use of blue and pink litmus paper.

MANAGEMENT

Patients are to be triaged as intermediate acuity cases or as critical care cases if there is any hint of visual impairment, eg acute glaucoma (red eye, vomiting, frontal headache and visual loss). They should be managed in a well-equipped Eye examination room in the ED.

Examination (Specific)

- **Check visual acuity** with and without corrective lenses:
  1. Topical anaesthesia may overcome reflex blepharospasm and facilitate examination. Check corneal sensation before giving topical anaesthetics.
  2. A pinhole cover will correct refractive error to help you discern if this is the cause of decreased visual acuity.
- **Inspection** includes the following important points that indicate significant pathology:
  1. Proptosis, which may indicate retroorbital pathology such as abscess.
  2. Irregular corneal light reflex, which indicates corneal oedema (glaucoma) or altered corneal surface (keratitis or corneal abrasion).
  3. Ciliary flush, which indicates anterior chamber pathology (iritis, glaucoma, keratitis).
  4. Evert the lids to search for a foreign body.
  5. Corneal opacities, which are seen with keratitis or corneal ulcer.
- **Check pupillary reaction** in response to light and accommodation:
  1. Pain in contralateral eye on direct light exposure is an early sign of iritis.
  2. An irregular pupil is seen with synechiae in iritis.
  3. A midpoint-fixed pupil is often found in glaucoma or iritis.
- **Ophthalmoscopy**: check for cloudy vitreous humor and yellowish-white patches on the choroid and retina, indicative of chorioretinitis.
- **Check visual fields and extraocular movements**.

Examination adjuncts

- **Slit lamp examination**, optimally, is used on all patients. Examine for flare and cells, posterior keratitic precipitates, and/or hyphema in the anterior chamber, indicative of inflammatory process.
- **Tonometry** is performed after topical anaesthesia to measure intraocular pressure. An abnormal pressure is >20 mm Hg. Avoid this procedure if the eye is infected or if there is the possibility of global rupture.
  1. **Fluorescein staining** is used to elucidate corneal pathology. The stain is taken up by the hydrophilic deep layers of the cornea when the hydrophobic superficial layers are gone, as in abrasion or infection.
  2. **Imaging**: a plain film of globe soft tissue may identify a radioopaque foreign body.
  3. **Topical anaesthesia** is often useful to differentiate keratitis from iritis.

   a. Pain from conjunctivitis, a superficial foreign body, or corneal abrasion and keratitis, is relieved by a topical anaesthetic.
   b. Pain from deeper inflammation, eg iritis, is unrelieved by this therapy.
4. **Homatropine**: use of this agent, a mydriatic/cycloplegic drug, should decrease deep eye pain in deep inflammation of the anterior pole structures, eg iritis by reduction of ciliary and iris muscle spasm.

Disposition

- Refer for **immediate** ophthalmology consult if the patient exhibits any of the points listed in Special Tips for GPs.
- **Most patients** can be discharged to home with follow-up in Eye SOC in 24–48 hours.

DOCUMENTATION

- Visual acuity on all charts.
- Brief history of present illness, medications, allergies, past medical and surgical history.
- Document complete examination, even if results are normal, including adjunctive tests.
- Document telephone advice if given by staff of ophthalmology department.

References/further reading

Butler KH, et al. The red eye: A systematic approach to differential diagnosis and therapy. In *Emerg Med Reports*. March 7, 1994.

27 Seizure

Seet Chong Meng • Peter Manning

CAVEATS

- See Table 1 for common causes of seizures (or fits) in patients presenting to the ED.
- A history from a witness is vital to the diagnosis.
- Enquire about compliance to medication if a known epileptic develops a seizure.

> ☛ **Special Tips for GPs**
> - Always consider the possibility of meningitis if there is associated fever in a patient presenting with a seizure.
> - Refer all patients with seizures to the ED.
> - Do a bedside glucose level to exclude hypoglycaemia before referring the patient to the ED.

MANAGEMENT

Isolated seizure in an epileptic

- Take blood levels of anticonvulsants:
  1. If low, administer a double dose of medication.
  2. If the patient is non-compliant, strongly encourage compliance.
  3. If the patient is already compliant with medication, increase the dose if the maximum dose has not been reached.
  4. If the maximum dose has already been reached, consult neurologist for further anticonvulsants.

Table 1: Common causes of seizure

Idiopathic epilepsy
Scar epilepsy (secondary to previous stroke or head injury)
Meningitis or encephalitis
Brain tumour (primary or secondary)
Electrolyte imbalance such as hypoglycaemia, hypocalaemia, hypomagnesaemia
Drugs or alcohol
Convulsive syncope due to a cardiac dysrhythmia (ventricular fibrillation/tachycardia, torsades de pointes)
Febrile fits (in a child aged between 6 months and 5 years)

- **Disposition**: observe in ED for 2–3 hours; discharge if no further seizures. Refer to Neurology SOC.

First seizure in a patient not known to be an epileptic

Note: Seizure in the absence of a palpable major pulse should always be assumed to be due to ventricular fibrillation till proven otherwise.

- **With fever**
  1. Stat capillary blood sugar.
  2. Labs: FBC, urea/electrolytes/creatinine, ionized calcium, magnesium.
  3. **Disposition**: admit to exclude
     a. Meningitis
     b. Encephalitis
     c. Cerebral abscess
     d. Subarachnoid haemorrhage
- **Without fever**: exclude possible causes
  1. Stat capillary blood sugar.
  2. Labs: urea/electrolytes/creatinine, ionized calcium, magnesium.
  3. **ECG** in older patients to look for signs of ischaemia or dysrhythmias.
  4. Consider skull x-ray if history includes trauma.
  5. **Disposition**:
     a. Observe in ED for 2–3 hours. If the patient is well, and no abnormalities found in the lab investigations ordered above, patient can be discharged with referral to Neurology SOC.
     b. There is no need to commence antiepileptics.
     c. Warn the patient not to drive, ride a bicycle, drink alcohol, swim or climb heights.
     d. Admit if (1) a cause is found, eg positive risk factors for intracrannial abnormalities such as trauma, alcoholism, malignancy, shunts, HIV positive, old CVA; (2) abnormal neurological findings present; (3) patient is unreliable about follow-up; or (4) patient or patient's family insist on admission.

Status epilepticus

This is defined as ≥2 seizures without full recovery of consciousness between attacks or continuous seizure activity of ≥30 min.

- **Supportive measures**
  1. Airway measures: place patient in the recovery position.
  2. Open and maintain airway.
  3. Suction any vomitus with Yankauer catheter.

Note: If the patient is still convulsing, **do not** attempt to insert an oral airway, clear oral secretions or intubate the patient.

  4. Supplemental high-flow oxygen via reservoir mask.
  5. Prepare intubation equipment in case you are unable to maintain airway and adequate oxygenation.

6. Monitoring: vital signs, ECG, and pulse oximetry.
7. IV access.
8. Labs:
   a. **Stat capillary blood sugar**
   b. FBC, urea/electrolytes/creatinine, ionized calcium, magnesium, phosphate, arterial blood gas
   c. Consider liver function tests, individual anticonvulsants, serum toxicology screen including ethanol
   d. Chest x-ray and urinalysis to exclude causes
   e. Urinary catheter

- **Drug therapy**
  1. **Benzodiazepines**
     Dosage: for adults, IV Valium® 5 mg slow bolus at a rate not to exceed 2 mg/min; can be repeated at q 5 min (to a total of 20 mg)
     For infants and children, IV Valium® 0.02 mg/kg at a rate not to exceed 2 mg/min; can be repeated q 5 min (to a total of 10 mg), Rectal Valium® 5 mg suppository × 1 PR
  2. **Phenytoin**
     Dosage: IV phenytoin infusion at 18 mg/kg body weight at a rate not to exceed 50 mg/min. On the other hand, the infusion should not exceed 60 minutes since precipitation tends to occur after that. IV phenytoin is given neat without dilution (ECG and BP monitoring required)
  3. **Long-acting barbiturates: phenobarbitone**
     Dosage: IV phenobarbitone 10 mg/kg slow bolus at a rate of 100 mg/min, **followed by**, **if necessary**, IV phenobarbitone 10 mg/kg slow bolus at a rate of 50 mg/min
  4. **Consider rapid sequence intubation**: refer to *Airway Management/ Rapid Sequence Intubation*
- **Disposition**: admit to Neurology HD/MICU after appropriate consultation.

References/further reading

1. Bradford JC, Kyriakedes CG. Evaluation of the patient with seizures: An evidence based approach. *Emerg Med Clin North Am.* 1999;17(1):203–220.
2. Reuber M, Hattingh L, Goulding PJ. Epileptological emergencies in accident and emergency: A survey at St. James's University Hospital, Leeds. *Seizure*. 2000;9(9) 216–220.
3. Archibald-Taylor SK, Mills TJ. Seizures. In: Frank LR, Jobe KA, eds. *Admission and Discharge Decisions in Emergency Medicine*. Philadelphia: Hanley and Belfus 2002:165–170.

28 Shock/hypoperfusion states

Suresh Pillai • Shirley Ooi

Definition

- **Shock** is a pathophysiological condition with inadequate tissue and organ perfusion leading to a **hypoperfusion state** and eventual cellular hypoxia with all its attendant sequelae. The eventual outcome is common to all forms of shock (Table 1) irrespective of its cause.
- Generally, a systolic blood pressure less than normal for age with **classical signs of a hypoperfused** state like pallor, cool skin, tachycardia, diaphoresis or AMS constitutes shock. The only **exception** is **septic shock**, where in the early stages, there is hyperdynamic circulation with warm skin and bounding pulses. See Table 2 for how to recognize various types of shock.

CAVEATS

- **Hypovolaemic shock** is the **most common** type of **shock** encountered in the ED and all shock states should be treated as such initially until other aetiologies can be ruled out.
- Prompt recognition and initiation of treatment is paramount in trying to reduce mortality from shock. The evaluation of the cause of shock is done concurrently with the management.

Table 1: Types of shock

	Cause
Hypovolaemic	Haemorrhage secondary to multiple trauma Gastrointestinal haemorrhage Burns Ruptured aortic aneurysm Ruptured ectopic pregnancy Fluid loss from severe gastroenteritis or acute pancreatitis
Cardiogenic	Acute myocardial infarction Dysrhythmia
Obstructive	Tension pneumothorax Cardiac tamponade Pulmonary embolism
Septic	
Neurogenic	Spinal injury
Anaphylactic	

Table 2: How to recognize various types of shock

Diagnostic information	*Hypovolaemic*	*Cardiogenic*	*Neurogenic*	*Septic (Hyperdynamic state)*
Signs and symptoms	Pallor; skin clammy, cold; tachycardia; oliguria; hypotension; increased peripheral resistance	Skin clammy, cold; tachy- and brady-dysrhythmias; oliguria; hypotension; increased peripheral resistance	Skin warm, normal/low heart rate, normal/low urine output, hypotension, decreased peripheral resistance	Rigours, fever, skin warm, tachycardia, oliguria, hypotension, decreased peripheral resistance
Laboratory data	Low haematocrit (late)	Cardiac enzymes, ECG	Normal	Neutrophil count, Gram stain, cultures

- Shock is a clinical state. A patient with a normal blood pressure may still be in shock. This is especially so in patients with background hypertension. On the other hand, not all hypotensive patients are in shock. Nonetheless, they should be attended to immediately.
- Even if all the commonly-used clinical indicators of shock are normal, shock on a cellular, tissue or organ basis may still be present. There is a lot of literature discussing objective assessment of endpoints of shock resuscitation.

☛ **Special Tips for GPs**

- All patients in shock should be referred to hospital immediately for further evaluation.
- Beware of subtle signs in geriatric and paediatric patients who may present with subtle non-specific signs of septic shock. A high index of suspicion is needed.

MANAGEMENT

- All patients in shock should be managed in the critical care area.
- The patient should be put on continuous cardiac, BP, heart rate and pulse oximetry monitoring. Check for orthostatic hypotension if possible.
- The airway should be maintained and 100% oxygen by way of a non-rebreather mask should be administered. Consider intubation in any severely shocked patient with inadequate oxygenation and ventilation.
- Is there evidence of any blunt or penetrating injury to the chest to indicate the possibility of **tension pneumothorax** or **cardiac tamponade**?

1. Decompress a tension pneumothorax by inserting a 14G cannula over the 2nd intercostal space in the midclavicular line.
2. For suspected cardiac tamponade obtain an urgent cardiothoracic consult. Start IV fluid bolus with 500 ml normal saline and/or IV dopamine infusion at 5 μg/kg/min and prepare for pericardioentesis.

- For **hypovolaemic shock**:
  1. Set up two large bore (14G/16G) IV cannulae in both antecubital fossae
  2. Labs:
     a. FBC, urea/electrolytes/creatinine

Note: (1) Haematocrit (hct) is an extremely unreliable test. It may be normal during the early stages of acute blood loss. Alternatively, an elevated hct may be observed in trauma patients who are acute alcohol abusers because of the diuretic effect of alcohol. (2) Absolute neutrophil count is neither sensitive nor specific in septic shock as it may be elevated, normal or low.

     b. Troponin T and cardiac enzymes.
     c. Coagulation profile with a DIVC screen if necessary and GXM (6 units of whole blood in conditions with acute blood loss).
     d. Rapidly matched blood should be obtained from the Blood Bank if blood transfusion is urgent. An ABG should be obtained if necessary, especially in a severely shocked patient.

Note: Metabolic acidosis, elevated lactate and significant base deficit are markers of a poor prognosis. The ability to correct these abnormalities portends an improved outcome. However, sodium bicarbonate is not routinely used as it does little to positively affect morbidity and survival.

  3. At least 1 litre of crystalloid should be infused fast within one hour and the response assessed. Subsequently, colloids or whole blood (fully or rapidly matched depending on the urgency) can be infused as required. In paediatric patients fluid challenge with 20 ml/kg BW of Hartmann's solution.
  4. A central venous line is sometimes employed to guide continued fluid resuscitation.

- An ECG and chest x-ray should also be done. Is there chest pain and breathlessness suggestive of an acute **myocardial infarction** or **pulmonary embolism**? Refer to *Myocardial Infarction, Acute* and *Pulmonary Embolism*.

- Place an indwelling urinary catheter and do a urine dipstick looking for **urinary tract infection** or do a urine pregnancy test if an **ectopic pregnancy** is suspected. Is there abdominal pain in a female of reproductive age group who has missed her last menstrual period? (Document the last menstrual period.) Catheterize any female who is strongly suspected of having an ectopic pregnancy if she is unable to produce a urine specimen for pregnancy confirmation. Get an urgent Gynae consult for suspected ectopic pregnancies. Monitor urine output.

- In patients with a suspected **abdominal aortic aneurysm** look for a pulsatile abdominal mass. Get an urgent Cardiothoracic consult.
- Is there **fever** or any predisposition to sepsis due to the presence of an indwelling urinary catheter or an immunocompromised state in cancer patients undergoing chemotherapy? Refer to *Oncology Emergencies*.
  1. Intraabdominal sepsis due to gall bladder disease or peritonitis from a perforated appendix and pneumonia are not uncommon causes for septic shock. The elderly as well as the very young patient can present with non-specific signs and symptoms in septic shock.
  2. Blood (aerobic and anaerobic) and urine cultures should be obtained in patients with septic shock.
  3. Broad-spectrum antibiotics according to the possible source of infection should be commenced after appropriate cultures. Refer to *Sepsis/Septic Shock*.
- If **neurogenic shock** is suspected because of a possibility of spinal cord injury associated with vertebral fractures, get an urgent Orthopaedic consult. Refer to *Spinal Cord Injury*.
- Is there a history of bites or stings or exposure to potential allergens like drugs or food to indicate **anaphylactic shock**? Refer to *Allergic Reactions/ Anaphylaxis*.
- After appropriate evaluation and initial therapy, inotropic support may be instituted to maintain blood pressure as appropriate:
  1. IV dopamine 5–10 μg/kg/min
  2. IV dobutamine 5–10 μg/kg/min principally for cardiogenic shock
  3. IV norepinephrine 5-20 μg/min, titrated to effect

DISPOSITION

- All patients in shock should be admitted to the High Dependency Ward or to the ICU of the appropriate discipline after proper prior consultation.
- If there is associated multisystem trauma, the Trauma Team should be activated. Refer to *Trauma, Multiple*.

References/further reading

1. Monafo WW. Volume replacement in hemorrhagic shock and burns. *Adv Shock Res.* 1980;3:47.
2. Parrillo JE, et al. Septic shock in humans. *Ann Intern Med.* 1990;113:3.
3. Pennington DG. Emergency management of cardiogenic shock. *Circulation.* 1989; (suppl 1): 6.
4. Perkins RM, Levin DL. Shock in the paediatric patient. *J Paediatr.* 1982;101:163.
5. Lucke WC, Thomas H Jr. Anaphylaxis: Pathophysiology, clinical presentations and treatment. *J Emerg Med.* 1983;1(1):83–95.
6. Dabrowski GP, Steinberg SM, Ferrara JJ, Flint LM. A critical assessment of endpoints of shock resuscitation. *Surg Clin North Am.* 2000 Jun;80(3):825–844.
7. Rivers E, Nguyen B, Havstad S, et al. Early goal-directed therapy in the treatment of severe sepsis and septic shock. *N Engl J Med.* 2001 Nov 8;345(19):1368–1377.

29 Stridor

Peng Li Lee • Peter Manning

CAVEATS

- If the patient has an airway that is patent and maintained, **do not** disturb or manipulate the airway.
- Permit the patient to assume a position of comfort, eg a child will probably want to sit on mother's lap.
- **Do not** allow the patient to be unattended or to leave the department, eg to obtain x-rays.

> ☛ **Special Tips for GPs**
> - **Do not** stimulate the oropharynx in a futile attempt to make a definitive diagnosis.
> - Permit the patient to assume a position of comfort, eg a child will probably want to sit on mother's lap.
> - Organize transfer of patient to hospital by ambulance rather than private car.

MANAGEMENT

- Refer to Table 1 for features that differentiate croup/ALTB from epiglottitis.

Table 1: Differentiating croup/ALTB from epiglottitis in paediatrics

	Croup/ALTB	*Epiglottitis*
Age	3½–5 years	2–7 years
Organism	Usually viral: parainfluenza	Bacterial: *H. influenzae*
Onset	Days	Hours
Prodrome	Yes	Absent
Appearance	Non-toxic	Toxic
Fever	+/–	++
Cough	Barking	Nil
Voice	Hoarse	Muffled
Drooling	Nil	Yes
Severity	Variable	Usually severe
X-ray	Steeple sign	Thumb sign

Supportive care

- The moderate to severe cases should be managed in the critical care area. Only the milder cases of croup can stay in the intermediate acuity area (Table 2).
- See Table 3 for the do's and don'ts for child with stridor.
- Airway management equipment, including cricothyrotomy set, must be immediately available.
- Assemble immediately a team comprising registrars (or higher grade) in Anaesthesia and ENT surgery.
- Resuscitation drugs must be immediately available.
- Administer supplemental high-flow oxygen to maintain SpO_2 >95%.
- Monitoring: ECG, vital signs q 5–15 min, pulse oximetry.
- Establish peripheral IV line.
- **Labs**: optional
  1. FBC, urea/electrolytes/creatinine preoperative
  2. ABGs, COHb in smoke inhalation
  3. Blood cultures in suspected epiglottitis
- Lateral soft tissue x-ray of the neck and CXR if time and patient's condition permit.

Drug therapy

- **In angioedema**:
  1. **Adrenaline** 1:10,000 solution 5 μg/kg (0.05 ml/kg) IV or via ETT. To give the first half as a bolus and titrate the second half according to clinical response, or
  2. **Adrenaline** 1:1,000 solution 10 μg/kg (0.01 ml/kg) deep IM, to a maximum of 0.3 ml in children and 0.5 ml in adults.
  3. **Diphenhydramine** 2 mg/kg IV in infants/children and 12.5–25 mg IV in adults.
  4. IV **hydrocortisone** 5 mg/kg IV.
- **In suspected epiglottitis**: **ceftriaxone** (Rocephin®) 2 g IV for adults, **or** 100 mg/kg IV stat dose for children.
- **In croup** (mild/moderate): 5 ml of normal saline as cool mist nebulizer q 15 min.
- **In croup** (severe): **adrenaline** nebulized inhaled solution 5 ml of 1:1,000 solution in 2.5 ml of sterile water **once only**.
- **Disposition**: moderate to severe cases should be admitted to ICU or OT setting following consultation. Croup that clears with one saline neb can be discharged but follow up within 24 hours must be arranged.
- **Admission criteria for croup** include:
  1. A toxic appearance.
  2. Dehydration or inability to retain oral fluids.
  3. Worsening stridor or retractions at rest.

Table 2: Suggested management for croup based on clinical assessment of severity

Severity	*Clinical appearance*	*Treatment*
Mild	No retraction, normal LOC and colour	Treat with cool mist only; follow up as outpatient next day.
Mild to Moderate	Mild retractions, normal colour, restless if disturbed	Treat as outpatient only if patient improves after mist in ED, is older than 6 months and has a reliable family.
Moderate	Mild stridor at rest, cyanotic and lethargic	Admit and use adrenaline nebs
Severe	Cyanotic with severe retractions, severe stridor at rest	Treat with adrenaline nebs and admit to ICU

Table 3: Do's and don'ts for child with stridor

Do	*Don't*
Be gentle	Look into the throat
Allow child to assume most comfortable position	Force child to lie down
Give humidified oxygen	Perform venepuncture before airway assessment by anaesthetist
Assemble airway team: inform anaesthetist and ENT	Insist on lateral neck x-ray
Arrange for ICU bed if necessary	

4. Unreliable parents.
5. No improvement with adrenaline nebulization, or worsening at 2–3 hours following adrenaline administration.

SPECIFIC ENTITIES PRESENTING WITH STRIDOR

Epiglottitis

- Traditionally thought of as a childhood illness, but nowadays occurs more commonly in adults.
- Common causative organisms are *H. influenzae*, *S. pneumoniae*, and beta-haemolytic streptococcus.
- Clinical features
  1. Severe sore throat associated with odynophagia (painful swallowing)
  2. High fever
  3. Muffled voice
  4. Shortness of breath
  5. Stridor
  6. Tenderness on palpation of larynx
  7. Patient tends to sit erect and bends forward to reduce obstructive symptoms secondary to supra-glottic swelling
- If a film of neck lateral soft tissue is obtained, look for the following:
  1. An enlarged epiglottis: 'thumb sign'
  2. Enlarged aryepiglottic folds
  3. A ratio of epiglottic width/width of vertebral body of C3 of >0.5
  4. A ratio of aryepiglottic width/width of body of C3 of >0.35

Retropharyngeal abscess

- X-rays are optional and may waste valuable time. If a lateral soft tissue of neck film is obtained, look for the following:
  1. Soft tissue swelling anterior to vertebral bodies (**normal** is up to 1/3 width of vertebral body)
  2. Air-fluid levels in retropharyngeal space (uncommon)
- If immediate airway intervention is required, consider positioning the head in a downward and hyperextended position to avoid aspiration should the abscess rupture.
- Administer IV antibiotics effective against oral pathogens including anaerobes. Drug of choice is **penicillin** with **clindamycin** as an acceptable alternative.
- Specialist team should arrange immediate transfer to OT.

Tracheobronchial foreign body aspiration

- Tends to occur at the extremes of age with adults presenting more acutely with cardiopulmonary arrest; the FB is generally found during airway interventions.

- In children, pertinent facts are:
  1. 80% of cases occur in those under 3 years of age
  2. No more than 15% FBs lodge in or above the trachea
  3. Fewer than 10% of aspirated FBs are radiolucent
  4. 24% of children with aspirated FBs have previously been misdiagnosed as chest infections
  5. Oesophageal FBs can also cause airway compromise through tracheal compression
- Immediate treatment of patients with upper airway FB and respiratory failure consists of a series of 5 back blows and 5 chest thrusts in those under 1 year of age, and the Heimlich manoeuvre over 1 year, including adults. Directly inspect the oropharynx between thrusts and do not perform blind finger sweeps.
  1. If the above is unsuccessful, directly inspect the hypopharynx via laryngoscope. Remove the FB with Magill forceps if it is accessible.
  2. If the above is unsuccessful, consider endotracheal intubation or a surgical airway under controlled conditions.
  3. The specialist team should arrange for laryngoscopy or bronchoscopy.

Angioedema/anaphylaxis

- Airway patency and protection is the first priority in management.
- Administer supplemental oxygen taking care not to increase agitation and precipitate respiratory arrest.
- Establish peripheral IV access for fluid challenge with crystalloid solutions.
- **Drug therapy**: see main text on *Stridor.*

Smoke inhalation

- Injury is managed initially with cool mist oxygen therapy.
- An artificial airway may be needed as secretions may be copious.
- **Indications** for **endotracheal intubation**:
  1. Hypoxaemia unresponsive to supplemental oxygen
  2. Elevated PCO_2
  3. Worsening airway obstruction
- Draw arterial blood gas specimen (includes COHb). Refer to *Poisoning, Carbon Monoxide*.
- Perform ECG to exclude ischaemia.
- Perform chest x-ray to exclude barotraumas.

References/further reading

1. Gavalds M, Sadana A, Metcalf S. Guidelines for the management of anaphylaxis in the emergency department. *J Accid Emerg Med.* 1998;15(2):96–98.
2. Tausig LM, Castro O, Biandry PA, et al. Treatment of laryngotracheitis (croup): Use of intermittent positive pressure breathing and racemic epinephrine. *Am J Dis Child.* 1975;129:790–795.

30 Syncope

Francis Lee • Shirley Ooi

DEFINITION

Syncope is a sudden, **brief** loss of consciousness due to transient impairment of cerebral circulation from whatever the cause, usually occurring in the absence of organic or cerebrovascular disease.

CAVEATS

- There are many possible **causes** of syncope but the commonest, based on published evidence, are:
  1. Cardiac (4–25%)
  2. Vasodepressor vasovagal (8–37%)
  3. Orthostatic hypotension (4–10%)
  4. Micturition syncope (1–2%)
  5. Hypoglycaemia (2%)
  6. Unknown aetiology (13–41%)

  Refer to Figure 1 for the causes of syncope.
- Blood loss is a life-threatening cause of syncope. The possibility of GIT bleeding must be sought in all patients. For female patients who are pregnancy capable, ectopic pregnancy must be considered.
- The search for the cause of syncope should not necessarily end once postural hypotension is discovered.

> ☛ **Special Tips for GPs**
> - Although vasovagal mechanism is the most benign cause, it should be a diagnosis by exclusion. Consider other more serious causes first, such as cardiac, haemorrhage and ectopic pregnancy.

INITIAL MANAGEMENT OF PATIENTS WITH SYNCOPE

- In the hospital setting, such cases are usually brought to the attention of the triage nurse early. The patient should be transferred to the critical care area if his parameters are found to be unstable. Those who are stable should be rested in the intermediate care area.
- The patient should be placed on monitoring of pulse, blood pressure and cardiac rhythm.
- The patient's ABC is quickly assessed and low-flow oxygen via nasal prongs should be provided.

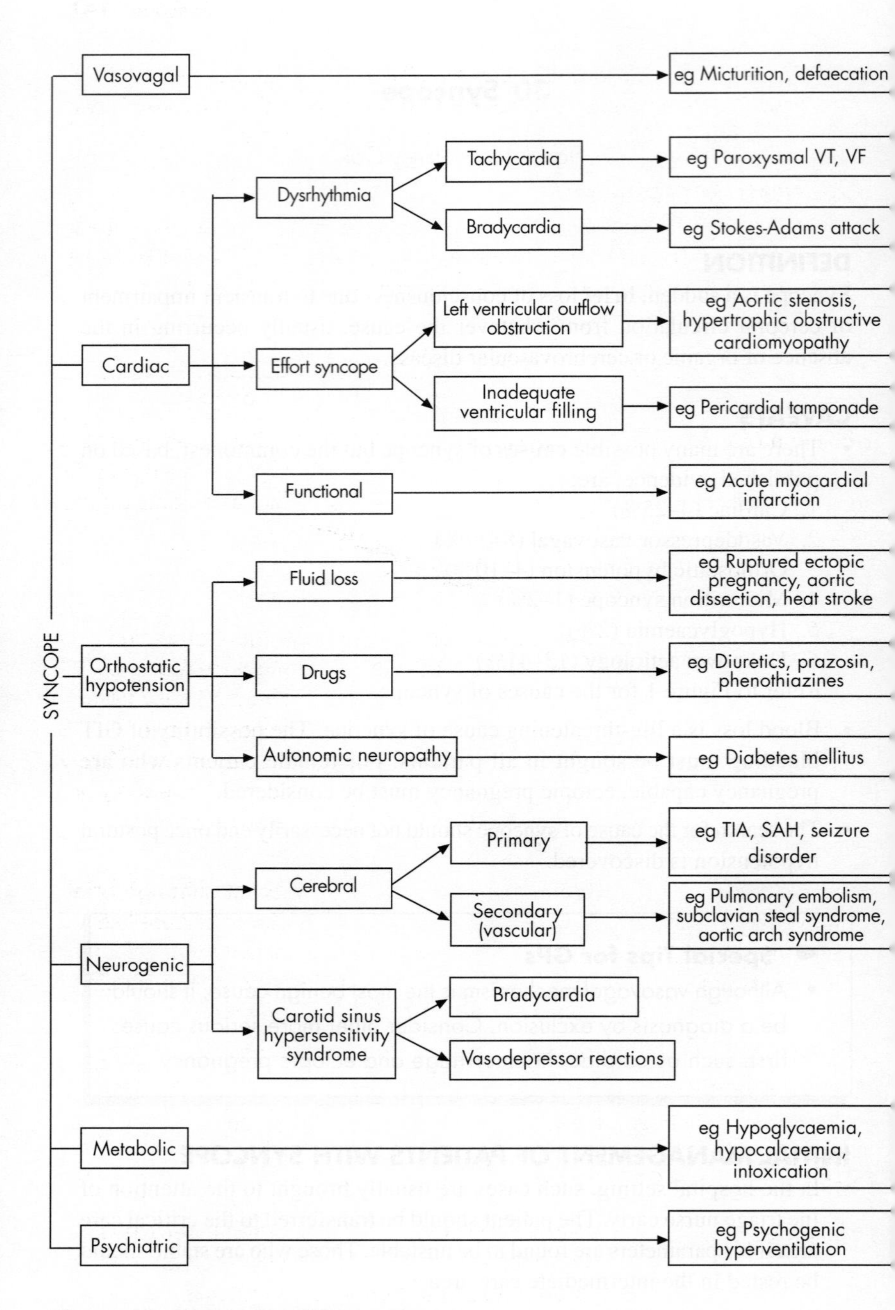

Figure 1: Causes of syncope

- IV line should be considered, especially if the initial parameters of the patient are not normal or if there is a high suspicion that the cause is due to a cardiac problem or volume loss (eg haemorrhage).

PATIENT ASSESSMENT

- A thorough history is difficult to obtain because very often, the patient cannot remember the details surrounding the event. It is also difficult at times to distinguish a syncopal event from a seizure (Table 1).

Table 1: Differential diagnosis of syncope

	Seizure	*Syncope*
Position of patient	Any position	Rarely in recumbent position except in Stokes-Adams attack.
Colour of patient	May not change, although there may be cyanosis.	Pallor
Onset	With aura. Injury from falling frequent.	Without aura and more deliberate. Hence, injury from falling is rare. However, more likely to have sweating or nausea prior to event.
Tonic-clonic movements with upturning eyes, tongue biting	Common	Absent although brief clonic seizure-like activity can accompany fainting episodes
Period of unconsciousness	Longer	Shorter
Urinary incontinence	Frequent	Seldom
Return of consciousness	Slow	Prompt
Sequelae	Mental confusion, headache, drowsiness, and aching muscles are common.	Physical weakness with a clear sensorium
Repeated spells of unconsciousness in a young person	May be present	Usually absent

- **Physical findings** important in the evaluation of syncope are:
  1. Signs of blood loss: pallor; tachycardia; erect and supine blood pressure
  2. Conscious state of patient: if drowsy, think of postictal state, subarachnoid haemorrhage or hypoglycaemia
  3. Cardiovascular examination for abnormal heart rhythm, murmurs and signs of heart failure
  4. Carotid bruit may suggest TIA as a cause
  5. Evidence of neurological deficit, indicating an ischaemic event
  6. Rectal examination for blood
- **Blood pressure** must be performed in all patients. It should be carried out in the following manner:
  1. 2 persons needed (to prevent patient from falling)
  2. Take supine BP and pulse after 10 minutes of supine positioning
  3. Stand patient up for 2 minutes
  4. Take standing BP and pulse
  5. If patient is not tolerant, take sitting parameters instead, with legs hanging down the side of trolley
  6. Definition of postural hypotension: decrease in SBP >20 mm Hg or increase in PR >20/min

INVESTIGATIONS

- **ECG** should be performed in all patients:
  1. Normal ECG makes cardiac ischaemia less likely as cause but does not exclude dysrhythmia.
  2. Abnormal ECG indicates the risk of association between the syncopal event and cardiovascular disease. Look for conditions which predispose to dysrhythmias, eg Wolff-Parkinson-White syndrome or prolonged QT syndrome.
- **Optional investigations** depending on index of suspicion include:
  1. Capillary blood sugar for hypoglycaemia
  2. Urine HCG for suspected ectopic pregnancy
  3. Head CT scan if a CNS pathology is suspected
  4. Electrolytes and FBC have low yield and should not be performed routinely

RISK STRATIFICATION

- Risk stratification allows a more objective approach towards the management and disposition of patients with syncope.

High risk category

- Acute myocardial infarction, myocarditis, dysrhythmias, 2nd and 3rd heart block, pacemaker dysfunction, ventricular tachycardia, prolonged QT syndrome, O&G problems, ectopic pregnancy, antepartum haemorrhage, severe GIT bleeding, pulmonary embolism, heat stroke, subarachnoid haemorrhage.

- Actions:
  1. Transfer to critical care area if not done so earlier
  2. Immediate resuscitation
  3. Consider admission to intensive care
  4. Contact relevant in-house discipline stat

Moderate risk category

- Clinical evidence of LV outflow obstruction, eg AS, suspected CVA or TIA, hypovolaemia, mild to moderately severe GIT bleeding, menorrhagia, severe GE, heat exhaustion, hypoglycaemia, patients with IHD, CCF or SVT and drug-induced syncope.
- Actions:
  1. Stabilize patient
  2. Consider admitting patient

Low risk category

- Vasovagal syncope, heat syncope, situation syncope (micturition syncope, postprandial, tussive), psychogenic syncope, anxiety and panic disorder, hyperventilation, supine hypotension of near term (after O&G review) and unexplained syncope (otherwise normal).
- Actions:
  1. Exclude all high and moderate risk conditions
  2. Observe for a period of at least 2 hours
  3. Discharge if patient is alert and attentive and parameters are stable
  4. For patients with recurrent vasovagal syncope, consider referral to Cardiology for tilt table test

References/further reading

1. Meyer M, Handler J. Evaluation of the patient with syncope: An evidence based approach. In: Masellis M, Gunn SWA, eds. *Emergency Clinics of North America.* Philadelphia: WB Saunders; 1999;17(1):189–201.

31 Trauma, multiple

Initial management

Shirley Ooi

INTRODUCTION

The treatment of the seriously injured patient requires rapid assessment of the injuries and initiation of life-preserving therapy. This is called **Initial Assessment** and includes:

- Preparation
- Triage
- Primary survey (ABCDE)
- Resuscitation of vital functions
- History of event
- Secondary survey (head-to-toe evaluation)
- Continued postresuscitation monitoring
- Reevaluation
- Definitive care

Note:

- Both primary and secondary surveys should be repeated frequently to ascertain any deterioration.
- This sequence is presented as a longitudinal sequence of events. In the actual clinical situation, many of these activities occur in parallel or simultaneously.
- Prehospital cardiac arrest is uniformly fatal if it persists for more than 5 minutes or is due to problems which cannot be rapidly corrected.

IN HOSPITAL PREPARATION

Advanced planning for the trauma patient's arrival is essential. Each hospital should have a Trauma Activation Protocol.

TRIAGE

Normally a prehospital phenomenon, but *could* be an ED factor occasionally:

- When facilities not over-extended: sickest seen first.
- When facilities are over-extended: most salvageable seen first.

PRIMARY SURVEY (ABCDE) and Resuscitation

During the **primary survey**, **life-threatening conditions** are identified and management is begun simultaneously. Remember that logical sequential

treatment priorities must be established based on overall patient assessment.
Note: Priorities for the care of paediatric patients are basically the same as for adults, although quantities of blood, fluids and medications may differ. Refer to *Trauma, Paediatric*.

Airway assessment with cervical spine control

- **Assessment**: **ascertain pathway and inspect for**:
  1. Foreign bodies
  2. Facial/mandibular fractures
  3. Laryngeal/tracheal fractures
- **Rapidly assess for airway obstruction**:
  1. Stridor
  2. Retractions
  3. Cyanosis
- **Management**: **establish a patent airway**
  1. Perform a chin lift or jaw thrust manoeuvre.
  2. Clear the airway of foreign bodies.
  3. Insert an oropharyngeal or nasopharyngeal airway.
  4. Establish a definitive airway.
     a. Orotracheal or nasotracheal intubation
     b. Needle cricothyrotomy with jet insufflation of the airway
     c. Surgical cricothyrotomy
- **Caveats**
  1. Assume a cervical spine injury in a multisystem trauma, especially with loss of consciousness or blunt injury above the clavide.
  2. The absence of neurologic deficit does not exclude injury to the cervical spine.
  3. Do not paralyse the patient immediately before assessing for the difficult airway. Refer to *Airway Management/Rapid Sequence Intubation*.
  4. Causes of **cardiac arrest** during or just after endotracheal intubation:
     a. Inadequate oxygenation of the patient before intubation
     b. Oesophageal intubation
     c. Mainstem bronchial intubation
     d. Excessive ventilatory pressures retarding venous return
     e. Excessive ventilatory pressures causing a tension pneumothorax
     f. Air embolism
     g. Vasovagal response
     h. Excessive respiratory alkalosis

Breathing (ventilation and oxygenation of airway pathway alone does not ensure adequate ventilation)

- **Assessment**
  1. Expose the neck and chest: ensure immobilization of the head and neck.
  2. Determine rate and depth of respiration.

3. Inspect and palpate the neck and chest for tracheal deviation, unilateral and bilateral chest movements, use of accessory muscles, and any signs of injury.
4. Auscultate the chest bilaterally: bases and apices.
5. If unequal breath sounds, percuss the chest for presence of dullness or hyperresonance to determine haemothorax or pneumothorax respectively:
   a. Tension Pneumothorax } may
   b. Flail chest with pulmonary contusion } acutely
   c. Open pneumothorax } impair
   d. Massive haemothorax } ventilation

- **Management**
  1. Attach the patient to a pulse oximeter.
  2. Administer high concentration of oxygen.

Note: FiO_2 >0.85 cannot be achieved with nasal prongs or a simple face mask. Non-rebreather mask with a reservoir is required to achieve FiO_2 100%.

  3. Ventilate with a bag-valve-mask.
  4. Alleviate **tension pneumothorax** by rapidly inserting a large bore needle into the second intercostal space in the midclavicular line of the affected hemithorax, followed by chest tube insertion into the fifth intercostal space, anterior to the midaxillary line.
  5. Seal **open pneumothorax** with sterile occlusive dressing, large enough to overlap the wound's edges, and taped securely on 3 sides to create a flutter-valve effect. Then insert a chest tube away from the wound site.
  6. Attach an end-tidal CO_2 monitoring device (if available) to the endotracheal tube.

- **Caveats**
  1. Differentiation of ventilation problems from airway compromise may be difficult, eg if a ventilation problem is produced by pneumothorax or tension pneumothorax but is mistaken for an airway problem and patient is intubated, patient could deteriorate further.
  2. Intubation and ventilation could produce a pneumothorax; hence chest x-rays should be performed as soon after intubation and ventilation as is practical.
  3. Do not force all trauma patients to lie flat on a trolley especially when they obviously breathe better sitting up.

Circulation with haemorrhage control

- Hypotension following injury must be considered to be hypovolaemic in origin until proven otherwise. Identify source of external, exsanguinating haemorrhage.
- Rapid and accurate assessment of the patient's haemodynamic status is essential. Three key elements of observation yield key information within seconds:

1. **Level of consciousness**: reduced cerebral perfusion pressure can result from hypovolaemia.
2. **Skin colour**: pinkness is helpful since it rarely goes with significant hypovolaemia. Ashen and grey skin of the face and white skin of the extremities are ominous signs of hypovolaemia; usually indicate a blood volume loss of at least 30%.
3. **Pulse**.
4. **BP if time permits at this stage**:
   a. If radial pulse present, blood pressure (BP) >80 mm Hg
   b. If only carotid present, BP >60 mm Hg
   c. Assess quality of pulse: full vs. thready and rapid
   d. Irregular pulse suggests possibility of cardiac impairment

- **Management**:
  1. Apply direct pressure to external bleeding site.
  2. Insert two large-calibre IV catheters, ie 14G or 16G.
  3. Bloods for GXM 4–6 units blood, FBC, urea/electrolytes/creatinine, coagulation profile and ABG if relevant.

Note: If no O negative blood is available, use type specific blood.

  4. Initiate vigorous IV fluid therapy with warmed crystalloids (normal saline or Hartmann's) and blood replacement.

Note: Do not resuscitate shock with glucose containing solutions as the fluids will leak into the extravascular space.

  5. Apply **ECG monitor**:
     a. Dysrhythmia: consider cardiac tamponade
     b. Pulseless electrical activity: consider cardiac tamponade, tension pneumothorax, profound hypovolaemia
     c. Bradycardia, aberrant conduction, ventricular ectopics: consider hypoxia, hypoperfusion
  6. Insert urinary and nasogastric catheters unless contraindicated.

Note: Urinary output is a sensitive indicator of the volume status of the patient. **Urinary catheterization** is **contraindicated** when urethral injury is suspected, ie if there is:

   a. blood at the urethral meatus
   b. scrotal haematoma
   c. prostate is high-riding or cannot be palpated

   A **gastric tube** is indicated to reduce stomach distention and decrease risk of aspiration. **Blood in the gastric aspirate** may represent:

   a. oropharyngeal (swallowed) blood
   b. traumatic insertion
   c. actual injury to the upper GI tract

   If there is epistaxis or cerebrospinal fluid rhinorrhoea suggestive of a cribriform plate fracture, insert gastric tube orally instead of nasally.

  7. Prevent hypothermia.

- **Caveats**:
  1. Persistent hypotension in trauma patients is usually due to hypovolaemia from continued bleeding.

2. The elderly, children, athletes and others with chronic medical conditions do not respond to volume loss in a similar manner. For example, elderly patients may not show a normal tachycardia response to blood loss, thus obscuring one of the earliest signs of volume depletion. This is worse if patient is on beta-blockers. Children have abundant physiologic reserve and often demonstrate few signs even of severe hypovolaemia.
3. Try not to insert an emergency subclavian line on the uninjured side of a patient with chest trauma. Femoral IV line can be used. If central lines are used for resuscitation they should be large bore in calibre (>8 Fr).

Disability (neurological evaluation)

Establishes the patient's level of consciousness, and pupillary size and reaction.

- **A simple mnemonic is the AVPUP method**
  A **A**lert
  V Responds to **V**ocal stimuli
  P Responds only to **P**ainful stimuli
  U **U**nresponsive
  P **P**upillary size and reaction

Note: Glasgow Coma Scale (GCS) is more detailed but comes as part of the secondary survey: unless rapid sequence intubation is planned whereupon assessment of GCS earlier is indicated.

1. Determine the level of consciousness using the AVPUP method.
2. Assess the pupils for size, equality and reaction.

- **Caveats**
  Do not assume that **altered mental state** in a trauma patient is due to head injury only. Consider the other causes such as:
  1. Hypoxia
  2. Shock
  3. Alcohol/drug intoxication
  4. Hypoglycaemia
  5. Conversely, do not assume that altered mental state is due to alcohol or drug intoxication. Brain injury needs to be excluded

Exposure/environmental control

Completely undress the patient by cutting off clothing, but prevent hypothermia by covering him/her with blankets and/or warmed IV fluids/ overhead lights.

- Continue **monitoring** the pulse rate, blood pressure, pulse oximetry, ECG and urinary output.
- Start taking **3 essential x-rays for all multiple trauma patients**:
  1. Lateral cervical spine
  2. Anteroposterior chest
  3. Anteroposterior pelvis

SECONDARY SURVEY

- This is a head-to-toe evaluation of the trauma patient, including vital signs assessment: BP, pulse, respiration and temperature.
- It does not begin until the primary survey is completed, resuscitation is initiated, and the patient's ABCs are reassessed.
- It may be summarized as '**tubes and fingers in every orifice**'.
- It starts with '**AMPLE history**':
  Allergies
  Medications currently taken
  Past illnesses
  Last meal
  Events/environment related to the injury

Head and face

- **Assessment**
  1. Inspect for lacerations, contusions and thermal injury
  2. Palpate for fractures
  3. Reevaluate pupils
  4. Cranial nerve function
  5. Eyes: haemorrhage, penetrating injury, visual acuity lens dislocation, contact lenses
  6. Inspect ears and nose for CSF leakage
  7. Inspect mouth for bleeding and CSF
- **Management**
  1. Maintain airway
  2. Haemorrhage control
  3. Prevent secondary brain injury. Refer to *Trauma, Head*
  4. Remove contact lenses

Neck

- **Assessment**
  1. Inspection: blunt and penetrating injury, tracheal deviation, use of accessory breathing muscles
  2. Palpation: tenderness, deformity, swelling, subcutaneous emphysema, tracheal deviation
  3. Auscultation: carotid arteries for bruits
  4. Lateral, cross-table cervical spine x-ray
- **Management**
  Maintain adequate in-line immobilization of the cervical spine.

Chest

- **Assessment**
  1. Inspection: blunt and penetrating injury, use of accessory breathing muscles, bilateral respiratory excursions

2. Auscultation: breath and heart sounds
3. Percussion: dull or resonant
4. Palpation: blunt and penetrating injury, subcutaneous emphysema, tenderness and crepitations

- **Management**
  1. Insertion of chest tube
  2. Needle decompression using 14G venula at the second intercostal space
  3. Correctly dress an open chest wound
  4. Perform chest x-ray

Note: Pericardiocentesis is not recommended these days. **Emergency room thoracotomy** is preferred in patients with evidence of cardiac tamponade. Salvage rates are low but best in patients with penetrating chest or abdominal wounds, and those who had witnessed recent cardiac arrest. Salvage rates are very low in patients who sustained blunt trauma. Therefore this procedure is generally not indicated in blunt trauma.

Abdomen

- **Assessment**
  1. Inspection: blunt and penetrating injury
  2. Auscultation: bowel sounds
  3. Percussion: rebound tenderness
  4. Palpation
  5. X-ray pelvis
- **Management**
  1. In a multiple-injured trauma patient, clinical exam is frequently not sufficient to rule out intraabdominal injury. Therefore further adjuncts such as Focused Assessment using Sonography in Trauma (FAST) exam, abdominal CT scan or peritoneal lavage are indicated: refer to *Trauma, Abdominal*.
  2. Transfer patient to operating room, if indicated.

Perineal and rectal exam

- **Evaluation**
  1. Anal sphincter tone
  2. Rectal blood
  3. Bowel wall integrity
  4. Prostate position
  5. Blood at the urinary meatus
  6. Scrotal haematoma
- **Perineal Assessment**
  1. Contusions, haematomas
  2. Lacerations

- **Vaginal Assessment**
  1. Presence of bleeding in vaginal vault
  2. Vaginal lacerations
- **Rectal Assessment**
  1. Rectal bleeding
  2. Anal sphincter tone
  3. Bowel wall integrity
  4. Bony fragments
  5. Prostate position

Back

- **Logroll patient to evaluate for**
  1. Bony deformity
  2. Evidence of penetrating or blunt trauma

Extremities

- **Assessment**
  1. Inspection: deformity, expanding haematoma
  2. Palpation: tenderness, crepitation, abnormal movement
- **Management**
  1. Appropriate splinting for fractures
  2. Relief of pain
  3. Tetanus immunization

Neurologic

- **Assessment**: **Reevaluate pupils and level of consciousness, GCS score**
  1. Sensorimotor evaluation
  2. Paralysis
  3. Paresis
- **Management**
  Adequate immobilization of entire patient.

DEFINITIVE CARE/TRANSFER

- If the patient's injuries exceed the institution's immediate treatment capabilities, the process of transferring the patient is initiated as soon as the need is identified.

References/further reading

1. American College of Surgeons Committee on Trauma. *Advanced Trauma Life Support for Doctors Manual*. 6th ed. Chicago: American College of Surgeons;1997.
2. Wilson RF, Walt AJ, eds. *Management of Trauma: Pitfalls and Practice*. Baltimore: Williams & Wilkins; 1996:10–11,24–27,46–47,346.

32 Urinary retention, acute

JP Travers • Peter Manning • Shirley Ooi

CAVEATS

- Some **common causes of urinary retention** in adult males include:
  1. Benign prostatic hypertrophy
  2. Constipation with impacted faeces
  3. Urethral stricture/bladder neck contracture
  4. Drugs: (a) antispasmodic agents; (b) tricyclic antidepressants; (c) antihistamines; (d) anticholinergic agents; (e) alpha-adrenergic stimulators, eg 'cold' tablets, ephedrine derivates
  5. Spinal cord problems
  6. Carcinoma of prostate
  7. Prostatitis

Note: In women, exclude pregnancy/pelvic mass as a cause of urinary retention!

- When catheterizing men who are likely to have **benign prostatic hypertrophy**, start with a size 14 Foley's catheter. If passage past the bladder neck cannot be achieved, repeat process with a size **larger**, not smaller, ie 16F. The additional rigidity often permits easy passage unlike the smaller sizes.
- Patients with **recurrent urethral strictures** should be approached with a small catheter.
- Patients with **prostatitis** (fever, chills, exquisitively tender prostate gland on digital rectal examination) are better served by a suprapubic catheter initially.
- Never force the passage of a urinary catheter. If unable to catheterize, seek help from a urology specialist or consider doing a suprapubic catheterization, only if experienced.
- **Urinary obstruction plus fever** is a **urological emergency** and mandates admission of patient. In this situation urinalysis may be unreliable and 'miss' pyuria.

☛ Special Tips for GPs

- A history of urinary obstruction and fever is a urological emergency and must be referred to the nearest hospital/ED immediately. Always assess the vital signs in such cases.
- In cases of chronic retention of urine (painless), do not place a urinary catheter without setting up an IV line first as the resulting diuresis may precipitate hypovolaemia and shock.

ACUTE OBSTRUCTION

- Assess vital signs: particularly important since **urologic obstruction plus fever is an emergency**.
- Labs: optional FBC, urea/electrolytes/creatinine, urinalysis looking for white blood cells and/or positive nitrites.
- Insert urinary catheter with sterile technique to relieve pain **after** allowing 5–10 minutes for the local anaesthetic gel to act and the patient to adapt/relax. Drain urine in 500–750 ml aliquots to reduce the possibility of severe bladder spasms, which can sometimes follow rapid decompression of the bladder. Allow 15–20 minute intervals between each aliquot. Pain will be reduced by the removal of the first aliquot.
- **Disposition**: can be discharged with indwelling cathether to early follow-up appointment in Urology Clinic if there is no haematuria, pyuria or fever while in the ED; otherwise admit to Urology.

Chronic obstruction with overflow

- Assess vital signs: look for fever.
- Place precautionary peripheral IV.
- Infuse crystalloid at maintenance rate.
- Labs: mandatory urea/electrolytes/creatinine, urinalysis.
- **Potential complications after release of obstruction**:
  1. Postobstruction diuresis: in chronic obstruction, there is the possibility of chronic backflow pressure on the renal tubule system due to hydronephrosis with subsequent chronic renal failure. Further, release of this pressure by urinary catheterization may result in a tremendous diuresis with subsequent dehydration and haemodynamic instability (the old postcatheterization shock).
  2. Hypotension secondary to vasovagal response or relief of pelvic venous congestion.
  3. Haemorrhage ex vacuo is uncommon; due to mucosal disruption post relief and usually resolves spontaneously.
- **Disposition**: observe in ED for 1–2 hours for diuresis. If diuresis does not ensue and there is no fever, haematuria or pyuria, patient can be discharged with indwelling cathether with urgent follow-up appointment in Urology Clinic.

References/further reading

1. Lawson DM. Urologic emergencies. *J Emerg Med Acute Pri Care*. 2001;5325(20):5991–6247.

33 Violent/suicidal patient

Peter Manning

Violent patients make their presence obvious, whereas suicide attempts may only be a suspected component of selected clinical presentations. Particularly important are cases such as single vehicle accidents, single driver accidents, accidental ingestions, risk-taking behaviour, and patients whose reasons for seeking care are unclear, eg vague somatic complaints such as persistent headache or chronic fatigue.

CAVEATS

- The principal role of the emergency physician is to delineate, if possible, organic from inorganic causes of psychosis.
- Never leave the patient alone: enlist the assistance of at least 5 uniformed security staff to stand in the background as a *show of force* if necessary. If the patient is female, at least one female staff member must be present at all times.
- Remember self-protection: the potential for a suicidal patient to be violent always exists.

> ☛ **Special Tips for GPs**
>
> - If you are evaluating such a patient in your office, do not allow yourself to become trapped by the patient being between you and the door.
> - Notify uniformed services according to local practice at the first hint of aggression; you may need their assistance sooner than you think.
> - Your patient may cooperate with **oral** doses of the drugs mentioned below should you have them available in your office. They can be given in larger doses than the parenteral route (eg 20 mg PO of either Valium® or Haldol®) and are less threatening to the patient than injections.

MANAGEMENT

- **Supportive care**
  1. Patient should be managed in either the intermediate or critical care area of the ED depending on the patient's general condition. Continual observation of the patient is maximized this way.

Table 1: Modified Sad Person's scale

	Factor	*Description*
S	Sex	Male
A	Age	<19 or >45
D	Depression or hopelessness	Admits to depression or decreased concentration, appetite, sleep, libido
P	Previous attempts or psychiatric care	Previous inpatient or outpatient psychiatric care
E	Excessive alcohol or drug use	Stigmata of chronic addiction or recent frequent use
R	Rational thinking loss	Organic brain syndrome or psychosis
S	Separated, divorced, or widowed	
O	Organized or serious attempt	Well thought-out plan or life-threatening presentation
N	No social support	No close family, friends, job or active religious affiliation
S	Stated future intent	Determined to repeat attempt or ambivalent

Note: Score as 1 point per positive description points.

Score of 9–10	=	High risk requiring emergency hospitalization. Notify Psychiatric staff.
Score of 6–8	=	Need for emergency psychiatric evaluation in ED.
Score of 5 or less	=	Possibility of home discharge in the care of competent individuals or family. Discuss the case with Psychiatric staff first.

2. Pay attention to the ABCs: hypoxaemia may be the cause of disruptive behaviour.
3. Take a full set of vital signs if patient permits: abnormalities may suggest an underlying organic, infectious or toxicological cause of the behaviour.
4. Monitoring: ECG, vital signs q 30–60 minutes, pulse oximetry, if patient permits.
5. Stat capillary blood sugar and serum electrolytes, if patient permits.
6. Urgent and standard approaches to ingestions or traumatic presentations must be undertaken.
7. Consider use of **restraints**: consideration of physical restraints to prevent self or other harm should be a recurrent thought process for the physician in charge.

8. Attempt to **build rapport** with the patient: patient privacy (the pulling of curtains partially around the cubicle), patient comfort, and an empathetic non-judgemental approach may elicit cooperation and enhance the ability of the team to gain accurate information, evaluate and effect appropriate interventions.
9. Evaluate **suicidal patient's risk assessment** utilizing the modified Sad Person's scale (Table 1).

- **Drug therapy**: if the patient is violent, consider the use of antipsychotic or tranquilizing agents, either singly, or better, in combination.
  Dosage: haloperidol (Haldol®) 5–10 mg IV; can be repeated 15 min later
  diazepam (Valium®) 5–10 mg IV; can be repeated 15 min later
- A useful alternative is oral administration since psychotic patients may be more aggressive when confronted with a needle.
  Dosage: haloperidol (Haldol®) 20 mg P.O. (concentrate form)
  diazepam (Valium®) 20 mg P.O.
- **Disposition**: make early Psychiatry consultation, preferably prior to sedation, though this may not always be possible due to the nature of the patient's presentation.

References/further reading

1. Hockberger RS, Rothstein RJ. Assessment of suicide potential by non-psychiatrists using Sad Person's Scale. *J Emerg Med.* 1988;6:100.

Specific conditions in adults

SECTION 2

34 Acid base emergencies

Benjamin Leong • Lee Kuan Wee

CAVEATS

- Symptoms and signs of acid base emergencies are often nebulous and wide ranging. Hence a high index of suspicion should be maintained.
- The role of the emergency physician in acid base emergencies is similar regardless whether it is acidosis, alkalosis, metabolic, or respiratory, ie to recognize that there is an acid base disorder, diagnose the cause where possible, and treat the patient in order to optimize resuscitation.
- Always consider acid base/electrolyte disorders in a patient with altered mental state.
- A PaO_2 level of 100 mm Hg in a patient on supplemental oxygen may not be normal. Always calculate the alveolar-arterial oxygen gradient (A-a gradient).

> **Special Tips for GPs**
> - Hyperventilation is a diagnosis of exclusion in tachypnoeic patients. Always exclude underlying metabolic acidosis with Kussmaul's breathing, pulmonary embolism and severe asthma. Refer to *Hyperventilation*.
> - Routine paper bag rebreathing for hyperventilation is potentially hazardous as it can cause significant hypoxia while raising PCO_2 only slightly.

DIAGNOSING ACID BASE DISORDERS

Important formulae

- The Henderson-Hasselbalch (H–H) Equation

$$pH = 6.1 + \log \frac{[HCO_3^-]\text{ (in mmol/L)}}{0.03 \times PaCO_2 \text{ (in mm Hg)}} \quad \text{(where } 6.1 = pK_A\text{)}$$

1. The **measured venous total CO_2** levels given in some electrolyte panels include $[HCO_3^-]$ and dissolved CO_2.

$$\begin{aligned}\text{Total } CO_2 &= [HCO_3^-] + \text{dissolved } CO_2 \\ &= [HCO_3^-] + 0.03 \times PaCO_2 \text{ (in mm Hg)} \\ &= [HCO_3^-] + 1.2 \text{ (if } PaCO_2 = 40 \text{ mm Hg)}\end{aligned}$$

2. Therefore the venous CO_2 may be used as an estimate of the serum bicarbonate level, bearing in mind that it is about 1 mm Hg higher than the actual bicarbonate level.

- **Anion gap (AG)**: $[Na^+] - [HCO_3^-] - [Cl^-]$
  1. **Normal = 3–11 mmol/L**. Recent changes in electrolyte measuring technique has resulted in a lowered normal range for the anion gap, and this has been validated in studies of normal healthy volunteers.
  2. An elevated AG suggests high anion gap metabolic acidosis (HAGMA).
  3. If the **AG** is **very low**, consider:
     a. Hypoalbuminaemia (the major unmeasured anion, most common cause of low anion gap)
     b. AG decreases by 2.5 mmol/L for every 1 g/dL decrease in albumin
     c. Paraproteinaemia
     d. Hyponatraemia
     e. Hypermagnesaemia
     f. Spurious hyperchloraemia
     g. Lab error (some authors quote this to be the commonest cause)

Steps in detecting an acid base disorder

- Look for abnormalities in **pH**, $[HCO_3^-]$, PCO_2, and **AG** corrected for albumin.
  1. Any abnormality in *any* of the 3 variables of the H-H equation (pH, $[HCO_3^-]$, PCO_2) is associated with an acid base disorder **without exception**.
  2. An elevated AG is a marker of high anion gap metabolic acidosis, **even in the presence of a normal pH or** $[HCO_3^-]$.
- **Check the internal consistency** of the results using the H-H equation if necessary.
- **Identify the primary abnormality** starting with the pH.
  1. pH < 7.35 and $[HCO_3^-] < 20$ mmol/L Acidosis, Metabolic
  2. pH < 7.35 and $PCO_2 > 45$ mm Hg Acidosis, Respiratory
  3. pH > 7.45 and $[HCO_3^-] > 24$ mmol/L Alkalosis, Metabolic
  4. pH > 7.45 and $PCO_2 < 35$ mm Hg Alkalosis, Respiratory
- **Identify any secondary abnormality** by checking adequacy of compensation.
  1. **Metabolic acidosis: expected $PCO_2 = (1.5 \times [HCO_3^-]) + 8$ mm Hg ($\pm$ 2)**
     a. If measured PCO_2 is lower than expected, concurrent respiratory alkalosis.
     b. If measured PCO_2 is higher than expected, concurrent respiratory acidosis.
     c. For HAGMA, account for excess or missing anions by calculating the **excess anion gap**

(1) Excess anion gap, $\Delta AG = AG - 11$
(2) Add ΔAG to measured $[HCO_3^-]$
(3) If total = normal $[HCO_3^-]$, simple HAGMA
(4) If total > normal $[HCO_3^-]$, there are too many HCO_3^- ions. Concurrent metabolic alkalosis
(5) If total < normal $[HCO_3^-]$, there are not enough HCO_3^- ions. Concurrent NAGMA

2. **Metabolic alkalosis: expected $PCO_2 = (0.6 \times [HCO_3^- - 24]) + 40$ mm Hg**
   a. If measured PCO_2 is lower than expected, consider concurrent respiratory alkalosis.
   b. If measured PCO_2 is higher than expected, consider concurrent respiratory acidosis.
3. **Respiratory acidosis or alkalosis**
   a. **Acute**
      (1) $[HCO_3^-]$ changes 1 to 2 mmol/L for every change in PCO_2 by 10 mm Hg
      (2) pH changes 0.08 for every change in PCO_2 by 10 mm Hg
   b. **Chronic**
      (1) $[HCO_3^-]$ changes 4 to 5 mmol/L for every change in PCO_2 by 10 mm Hg
      (2) pH changes 0.03 for every change in PCO_2 by 10 mm Hg
   c. If measured $[HCO_3^-]$ is lower than expected, consider concurrent metabolic acidosis
   d. If measured $[HCO_3^-]$ is higher than expected, consider concurrent metabolic alkalosis

- **If pH normal**, check for balanced acid base disorder.

1.	$[HCO_3^-] < 20$	$PCO_2 < 35$	metabolic acidosis + respiratory alkalosis
2.	$[HCO_3^-] > 24$	$PCO_2 > 45$	metabolic alkalosis + respiratory acidosis
3.	$[HCO_3^-]$, PCO_2 normal	$AG > 11$	HAGMA + metabolic alkalosis
4.	$[HCO_3^-]$, PCO_2 normal	AG normal	normal (unlikely NAGMA + metabolic alkalosis)

'Three Rules' at 3 am

- **Rule 1**: the direction of the pH change is the primary abnormality. Compensatory mechanisms do not 'overcompensate' nor even fully compensate to normal.
- **Rule 2**: the presence of a very high anion gap (>20) suggests a HAGMA even in the presence of a normal pH or $[HCO_3^-]$. The body does not generate an elevated anion gap just to compensate for alkalosis.

- **Rule 3**: the sum of the excess anion gap in HAGMA and the measured [HCO_3^-] should be equal to a normal [HCO_3^-]. If there is too much [HCO_3^-], then there is a concurrent metabolic alkalosis and if too little, there is a concurrent NAGMA.

INTERPRETING THE REST OF THE ARTERIAL BLOOD GAS RESULTS

- **Oxygen delivery and oxygenation**:
  1. It is important to document the amount of supplemental oxygen given to the patient in order to interpret the results properly.
  2. The FiO_2 delivered may be estimated by the following:
     a. Nasal prongs (2–4 L/min): 21% + 4% for every litre per minute
     b. Standard mask (6–8 L/min): FiO_2 50–60%
     c. Reservoir mask (Non-rebreather mask): 80–85%
  3. Oxygen delivered by low flow systems such as intra-nasal cannulae is significantly affected by entrainment of atmospheric air and hence FiO_2 delivered may be inconsistent and inaccurate.
  4. Ideally, supplemental oxygen should be delivered by a fixed system such as a Venturi mask, which allows accurate settings of FiO_2.
- The **Alveolar-arterial oxygen gradient (A-a gradient)** is a useful tool in evaluating how well a patient is oxygenating.
  1. $P(A\text{-}a)O_2 = PAO_2 - PaO_2$ (mm Hg)
     $= \mathbf{[(760 - 47) \times FiO_2 - PaCO_2/0.8] - PaO_2}$
     where FiO_2 is expressed as a decimal
  2. Normal = 10 to 20 mm Hg. Levels >50 mm Hg suggest severe pulmonary dysfunction.
  3. The A-a gradient is known to rise with a patient's age and the FiO_2.
     a. Add 3.5 mm Hg for every decade of life, or use the formula $\mathbf{[normal = \frac{Age}{4} + 4]}$.
     b. Add 5–7 mm Hg for every 0.1 increase in FiO_2.
     c. Note that there is **no** correction for smokers.
  4. Causes of an elevated A-a gradient include V/Q mismatch, right to left shunt, and diffusion abnormalities.
  5. However, the literature is unclear about interpretation of normal A-a gradient in a suspected PE patient.
  6. Another tool for quick estimation of oxygenation is the **PaO_2/FiO_2 ratio**.
     a. Normal = 500–600.
     b. Levels <300 suggest ARDS in patients with alveolar infiltrates in 3 of 4 pulmonary quadrants and normal pulmonary capillary wedge pressure.
- **Action for all acid base derangements**:
  1. Transfer patient to monitored area as necessary.
  2. Resuscitate as necessary.

3. Review patient for clinical effects and causes.
   a. History and physical examination.
   b. Review the ABG, electrolyte panels.

Metabolic acidosis

- **Definition**: pH <7.35 and $[HCO_3^-]$ <20 mmol/L
  1. **High Anion Gap Metabolic Acidosis (HAGMA)**: $[HCO_3^-]$ <20 mmol/L and Anion Gap >11 mmol/L
  2. **Normal Anion Gap Metabolic Acidosis or NAGMA (Hyperchloraemic metabolic acidosis)**: $[HCO_3^-]$ <20 mmol/L and Anion Gap <11 mmol/L
- **Causes**: the causes of HAGMA may be summarized by the mnemonics SULK (somewhat more reflective of pathogenic mechanisms) or CATMUDPILES, and the causes of NAGMA may be summarized by the mnemonic USEDCARP. See Table 1 for causes of HAGMA and Table 2 for causes of NAGMA.
- **Treatment of metabolic acidosis** is essentially targeted at the **underlying cause**, eg:
  1. DKA (hydration and insulin therapy)
  2. Shock (hydration, inotropes, treatment for sepsis)
  3. Renal failure (dialysis)
  4. Methanol/ethylene glycol ingestion (ethanol)
- **Bicarbonate therapy** is controversial.
  1. Potential adverse effects include electrolyte disturbances (eg hypokalaemia, hypocalcaemia), paradoxical intracerebral and intracellular acidosis, post treatment alkalosis, hypernatraemia/hyperosmolality and fluid overload. Furthermore, bicarbonate therapy has **not** been shown to improve survival.

Table 1: Causes of high anion gap metabolic acidosis

S	Salicylates, exogenous toxins (eg metformin, methanol, toluene, ethylene glycol, iron, paraldehyde)	**C**	Cyanide, Carbon monoxide
		A	Alcoholic ketoacidosis
		T	Toluene
		M	Methanol, methaemoglobin
U	Uraemia	**U**	Uraemia
L	Lactic acidosis (eg any cause of shock, hypoxia, metformin, phenformin, cyanide and CO poisoning, INH, iron)	**D**	Diabetic ketoacidosis
		P	Paraldehyde
		I	INH/Iron (via lactic acidosis)
		L	Lactic acidosis (eg any cause of shock, hypoxia, metformin, phenformin, cyanide poisoning)
K	Ketoacidosis (diabetic, alcoholic, starvation)	**E**	Ethylene glycol (**not** ethanol)
		S	Salicylates, solvent

Table 2: Causes of normal anion gap metabolic acidosis

Hyperkalaemic type	*Renal*	**U**	Ureterosigmoidostomy
	Renal tubular acidosis (type IV)	**S**	Small bowel fistula
	Potassium sparing diuretics	**E**	Extra chloride
	Hypoaldosteronism/Addison's disease	**D**	Diarrhoea
	Early obstructive uropathy	**C**	Carbonic anhydrase inhibitor
	Early uraemic acidosis	**A**	Adrenal insufficiency
	Resolving DKA	**R**	Renal tubular acidosis
	Exogenous Cl^- gain	**P**	Pancreatic fistula
	Hydrochloric acid (HCl)		
	Ammonium chloride (NH_4Cl)		
	Lysine-HCl, arginine-HCl		
Hypokalaemic type	*Gastrointestinal*		
	Diarrhoea (HCO_3^- loss > Cl^- loss)		
	Urinary to bowel diversion (eg ureterosigmoidostomy)		
	Surgical fistulae, drains		
	Renal		
	Renal tubular acidosis (types I, II)		
	Acetazolamide (functional RTA)		
Dilution acidosis	Excessive NaCl infusion dilutes plasma HCO_3^-		

2. Possible benefits are improved myocardial contractility, response to catecholamines and haemodynamic status.
3. Pathophysiologically, bicarbonate therapy is more likely to benefit a patient with NAGMA than one with HAGMA, because in NAGMA it takes days before renal recovery of bicarbonate ions can be significant, and in HAGMA, treatment of the underlying cause promotes conversion of the excess anions to bicarbonate.
4. A patient should be able to ventilate the increased CO_2 load before bicarbonate therapy is given.
5. Current recommendations do not advocate routine bicarbonate therapy unless pH <7.1 and patient is in haemodynamic compromise.
   a. Suggested targets include pH >7.1, $[HCO_3^-]$ >5 mmol/L
   b. Titrate in aliquots of 50 to 100 mls of 8.4% $NaHCO_3$ (by slow infusion diluted in D5%) and check 30 min after completion.

Note: There is no perfect formula to calculate the amount of bicarbonate needed to correct the pH as the acid base status is constantly changing with disease progression and therapy.

   c. A suggested rough rule of thumb is:

$$\mathbf{HCO_3^-\ (mmol)\ needed = 0.5 \times body\ wt\ (kg) \times [Target - measured\ HCO_3^-]\ (mmol)}$$

Respiratory acidosis

- **Definition**: pH <7.35 and PCO_2 >45 mm Hg.
- **Causes**: Respiratory acidosis arises when there is reduced exhalation of CO_2. See Table 3 for the causes.

Table 3: Causes of respiratory acidosis

Central causes of reduced respiratory drive	Drugs (eg sedatives, opiates) Head injury CNS lesions Metabolic alkalosis Loss of hypoxic drive in chronic type II respiratory failure treated with oxygen
Airway obstruction	Asthma COLD
Thoracic cage abnormalities	Kyphoscoliosis Morbid obesity Chest trauma
Neurological/neuromuscular abnormalities	Myasthenia gravis Guillain-Barré Syndrome Cervical/high thoracic spine injury

- **Treatment of respiratory acidosis** is targeted at the underlying cause:
  1. Ventilatory support may be necessary. Options include intubation or non-invasive positive pressure ventilation (NIPPV).
  2. Bicarbonate therapy is not usually required.
  3. Supplemental oxygen for patients with known Type II respiratory failure should be delivered by fixed systems to allow accurate titration and prevent suppression of hypoxic drive.

Metabolic alkalosis

- **Definition**: pH >7.45 and [HCO_3^-] >25 mmol/L
- **Causes**: the excess bicarbonate generated in metabolic alkalosis is usually rapidly removed by the kidneys. For metabolic alkalosis to persist, the acute cause must continue, or the renal compensatory mechanism must be impaired by a perpetuating mechanism (Table 4).

Table 4: Causes of metabolic alkalosis

Acute causes (initiating mechanisms of metabolic alkalosis)	
Increased HCO_3^- intake	• Antacid abuse • Excessive $NaHCO_3$ intake • Massive blood transfusion (due to breakdown of citrate)
Acid loss	• Upper gastrointestinal tract losses, such as severe vomiting (eg hyperemesis gravidarum, bulaemia), nasogastric suction, gastric outlet obstruction • Lower gastrointestinal tract losses, such as severe diarrhoea (eg gastroenteritis, laxative abuse) when HCO_3^- loss $<$ Cl^- loss, villous adenoma, rare causes such as chloride diarrhoea • Renal losses, such as loop and distal diuretics
Acid shifts	• Hypokalaemia
Perpetuating mechanisms of metabolic alkalosis	
Hypovolaemia	• Contraction alkalosis (due to reduced volume of distribution for bicarbonate and paradoxical renal H^+ loss)
Hypochloraemia (saline responsive)	• Causes of acute HCl losses (as above). • Rare causes of Cl^- depletion, such as achlorhydria and cystic fibrosis
Hypokalaemia (saline unresponsive)	• Increased mineralocorticoid activity, such as primary hyperaldosteronism, Cushing's disease, liquorice abuse, Liddle's syndrome • Renal potassium losses, such as diuretic use or abuse, rare congenital diseases (Bartter's and Gitelmann's syndromes)

- **Treatment of metabolic alkalosis:**
  1. Provide supplemental oxygen, a readily available resource in the ED.
  2. Treat acute causes
     a. Stop increased bicarbonate intake
     b. Reduce acid loss
        (1) Stop NG suction.
        (2) Give H2-blockers or proton pump inhibitors.
        (3) Stop loop or distal diuretics, change to potassium-sparing diuretics.
     c. Reduce acid shift by correcting hypokalaemia.
  3. Chloride sensitive type (saline responsive)
     a. Chloride replacement, usually with saline infusion:
        (1) Chloride deficit (mmol/L) = 0.3 × body wt (kg) × (100 − [Cl^-])
        (2) 1L of 0.9% NaCl contains 154 mmol of Na^+ and Cl^-.
        (3) Therefore amount required (L) = Cl^- deficit/154.
     b. Potassium replacement as necessary.
     c. Reduction of gastric acid loss with proton pump inhibitors or H2 antagonists.
  4. Chloride resistant type (saline unresponsive)
     a. Potassium replacement to limit renal preferential H^+ excretion.
     b. Mineralocorticoid antagonism with spironolactone or triamterene.
  5. Suggested targets of therapy include pH <7.55, HCO_3^- <40 mmol/L.

Respiratory alkalosis

- **Definition**: pH >7.45 and PCO_2 <35 mm Hg.
- Causes: see Table 5.

Table 5: Causes of respiratory alkalosis

Increased respiratory drive	Pain, anxiety (hyperventilation) Fever Primary CNS lesions (eg tumours, infection, CVA) Drugs (eg salicylates) Pregnancy
Hypoxia	Pulmonary embolism Pneumonia Pneumothorax Mild asthma Severe anaemia High altitude Carbon monoxide poisoning

- **Treatment of respiratory alkalosis** is targeted at the underlying cause, eg
  1. Oxygen for hypoxic conditions
  2. Analgesia for pain
  3. Antibiotics for pneumonia
  4. Chest tube for pneumothorax

  The respiratory alkalosis by itself does not usually require treatment, and should resolve with management of the underlying condition.
- **Clinical effects of acid base derangements**: the commonest encountered acid base derangement is metabolic acidosis. The clinical effects of acid base derangements are similar whether acidosis or alkalosis with only minor differences in their manifestations:
  1. **Altered mental states**
     a. Lethargy, drowsiness.
     b. Irritability, confusion.
     c. Obtundation, coma.
     d. In addition, alkaloses may result in giddiness and headache from cerebral vasoconstriction due to hypocarbia. Carpopedal spasm, tetany, peri-oral numbness and peripheral numbness, even seizures may result from the associated ionic hypocalcaemia.
  2. **Cardiovascular**
     a. Myocardial depression, hypotension
     b. Impaired response to catecholamines
     c. ECG changes and dysrhythmias due to electrolyte abnormalities
     d. Hypocalcaemia in alkaloses may have an additive cardiodepressive effect
     e. Cardiovascular collapse
  3. **Respiratory**
     a. Hyperventilation in metabolic acidosis and respiratory alkalosis.
     b. Hypoventilation in metabolic alkalosis.
     c. There may be tachypnoea and a sensation of shortness of breath associated with respiratory acidosis.
     d. There may be a fruity odour associated with the ketonaemia of DKA.
     e. Acidosis causes a right shift of the haemoglobin oxygen dissociation curve, resulting in poorer pulmonary uploading of oxygen to haemoglobin with downstream tissue hypoxaemia.
     f. Alkalosis causes a left shift of the haemoglobin oxygen dissociation curve, with decreased peripheral oxygen unloading and tissue hypoxaemia.
  4. **Electrolyte imbalances**
     a. Acidosis is associated with hyperkalaemia due to competitive preferential excretion of hydrogen ions.
     b. Alkalosis is associated with hypokalaemia due to preferential renal excretion of potassium ions. Further, alkalosis induces increased calcium binding to proteins, resulting in decreased fraction of free ionic calcium.

5. **Gastrointestinal**
   a. Nausea/vomiting
   b. Diarrhoea
   c. Abdominal pain in DKA

- **Disposition**: depending on the underlying cause, haemodynamic status and electrolyte abnormalities, patient should be admitted to the Medical ICU, High Dependency unit, or if clinically well and stable, to a general ward.

References/further reading

1. Nicolau DD, Kelen GD. Acid Base Disorders. In: Tintinalli JE, Kelen GD, Stapczynski JS, et al, eds. *Emergency Medicine: A Comprehensive Study Guide*. 5th ed. New York: McGraw-Hill; 2000:128–140.
2. Kwek TK. Acid Base Disorders. In: Tai D, Lew T, eds. *Bedside ICU Handbook*. Singapore: Tan Tock Seng Hospital; 2000:20–25.
3. Lolekha PH, Lolekha S, et al. Update on value of the anion gap in clinical diagnosis and laboratory evaluation. *Clin Chim Acta*. 2001:307(1–2):33–36.

35 Abdominal aortic aneurysm (AAA)

JP Travers • N Sanjay • Alex Chao

DEFINITION

A localized dilatation of an artery of greater than 50% of the normal diameter. A dilatation of less than 50% of the normal arterial diameter is termed *ectasia*.

CAVEATS

- Occurs in 5–7% people over 60 years old.
- In Singapore, the male:female ratio approximates 2:1, with an apparent lower incidence in Indians.
- May **present** as:
  1. Catastrophic intraperitoneal rupture causing collapse, shock and death. Most have a sentinel bleed into retroperitoneum, which then ruptures intraperitoneally.
  2. Abdominal, flank or back pain (sometimes mimicking ureteric colic).

Note: The back pain coud be either due to the expansion of the AAA with erosion of the spinal vertebrae or it could represent rupture of the aneurysm, which is a surgical emergency.

  3. Abdominal mass, often pulsatile, but occasionally not.
  4. Syncope with postural hypotension.
  5. Embolization causing acute ischaemic limb or mottling of the lower trunk and extremities. Peripheral embolization could cause **blue toe syndrome**.
  6. Aortoenteric fistula presenting as melaena.
  7. Compression of the bowel, stomach or oesophagus may lead to dysphagia, early satiety, nausea and/or vomiting.

Note: The majority (75%) are asymptomatic.

- Diffuse and non-specific nature of a symptomatic AAA may lead to errors in diagnosis. Any elderly patient presenting with hypotension, shock and back pain must have a ruptured AAA excluded. Most diagnostic **errors** are due to the **failure to palpate pulsatile mass**.
- Look for **expansile versus transmitted pulsation** by placing fingers alongside pulsation; deviation of the fingers laterally is due to aneurysm.
- All patients with a pulsatile mass >3 cm should have an ultrasound evaluation.
- Mortality rate from emergency surgery is 75–90%, whereas it is only 3–5% in an elective repair.

☛ Special Tips for GPs

- Aortic aneurysm may present as abdominal pain, back pain, colic or ischaemic leg pain.
- Diagnosis is often made by a physical examination of the abdomen.
- Diagnosis may be confirmed by B-Mode ultrasound.
- Elective surgical intervention is indicated for most patients with AAA >5 cm diameter to prevent rupture/death.
- Smaller aneurysms should be monitored by regular ultrasound measurements.

PATHOPHYSIOLOGY

- Most aortic aneurysms are associated with atherosclerosis, while other common aetiologies include cystic medial necrosis, Ehlers-Danlos syndrome, and dissection.
- Studies have shown decreased amounts of elastin and collagen in the walls of AAA.
- The immunologic component to atherosclerotic vascular disease has also been recognized, with infiltration of the aortic wall with macrophages and T&B lymphocytes: an important factor in the pathogenesis of AAA is an imbalance between aortic wall proteases and antiproteases.
- A genetic susceptibility exists with a 15–20% incidence of AAA among first-degree relatives.

RISK FACTORS

- Hypertension: seen in at least 40% of AAAs.
- Smoking: 8 times greater likelihood of having AAA compared with non-smokers.
- Hyperlipidaemia and hyperhomocysteinaemia.

RISK OF RUPTURE

- Aortic aneurysms have an exponential expansion rate and the risk of rupture is proportional to the diameter of the aneurysm:
  1. Aneurysms 4–5.5 cm diameter have 5% risk of rupture
  2. Aneurysms 6–7 cm have 33% risk of rupture
  3. Aneurysms >7 cm have 95% risk of rupture
- Some studies suggest hypertension and COLD are strong predictors of rupture in small aneurysms.

- Recent trials such as the UK Small Aneurysm trial and ADAM trial have shown no long-term survival benefit for surgery in aneurysms <4 cm diameter.

MANAGEMENT OF RUPTURED AORTIC ANEURYSM

General measures

- Manage patient in the critical care area.
- Intubation and resuscitation equipment must be immediately available.
- Inform appropriate surgical team stat according to local protocols.
- ABC primary survey, ensure patent airway and perform resuscitative measures as needed.
- Monitor ECG, vital signs, pulse oximetry.
- Establish at least 2 large-bore IV lines with normal saline as infusate but **do not** over-resuscitate patient. Permit hypotension of 90–100 mm Hg systolic.
- **Labs**: GXM 6 units whole blood, FBC, urea/electrolytes/creatinine, coagulation profile, ABG. Order group-specific blood as necessary if delay in full cross-match.
- Portable CXR (look for dissection/mediastinal widening).
- **Plain abdominal films** will show calcification in approximately 50% of cases, but needs to be seen in both lateral and AP films to diagnose an AAA. If the classical 'egg-shell' appearance is present, the degree of confidence in diagnosis is high. A negative plain x-ray does **not** exclude the diagnosis of AAA and limits the value of this study.
- Place urinary catheter.

Specific measures

- Do not allow repeated abdominal palpation once diagnosed.
- **Bedside ultrasound** is useful in the ED to diagnose the presence of an aneurysm but is operator-dependent. It may not detect a contained rupture.
- Ruptured AAA is a surgical emergency and the patient must be prepared for operation as soon as possible. There is no place for routine abdominal or CT films.
- However, if patient is **stable**, then **CT scan** has become the investigation of choice with regard to the diagnosis of AAA, but **must not delay definitive treatment** of a ruptured or leaking AAA.

Disposition

- Admit to Cardiothoracic Surgery or General Surgery according to local practice protocols.

References/further reading

1. Hals G. The clinical challenges of abdominal aortic aneurysm: Rapid, systematic detection and outcome-effective management. *Emerg Med Rep*. 2000;21(11):121–140.
2. UK small aneurysm trial. *Lancet*. 1998;352:1649–1655.
3. Noel AA, Cherry KJ. Ruptured abdominal aortic aneurysms. *J Vasc Surg*. 2001:34(1):41–46.
4. Powell JT, Brown LC. The natural history of abdominal aortic aneurysms and their risk of rupture. *Acta Chir Belg*. 2001;101(1):11–16.
5. Hsiang YN, Turnbull RG. Predicting death from ruptured abdominal aortic aneurysms. *Am Surg*. 2001;181(1):30–35.

36 Adrenal insufficiency, acute

Malcolm Mahadevan

CAVEATS

- Adrenal crisis may occur in the following situations:
  1. Following stress such as surgery or trauma in a patient with chronic adrenal insufficiency.
  2. Sudden withdrawal of steroids in a patient on long-term steroids.
  3. After bilateral adrenalectomy or damage to both adrenals after trauma, haemorrhage, etc.
- Clinical presentation is **subtle**:
  1. Non-specific weakness (99%), fatigue and weight loss are 3 cardinal features.
  2. GI upset: nausea and vomiting, abdominal pain (34%), diarrhoea (20%).
  3. Recent history of surgery or procedure, illness, injury, autoimmune disease, chronic steroid use or use of traditional Chinese medicine (TCM) for joint pains.
- **Physical examination** findings:
  1. Persistent hypotension and orthostatic hypotension.
  2. Dehydration: dry mucosae, reduced skin turgor.
  3. Hyperpigmentation in primary adrenocortical insufficiency: buccal mucosae, exposed areas or areas subject to friction.

> ☛ **Special Tips for GPs**
> - Methadone and ketoconazole may cause secondary adrenocortical insufficiency.
> - Initial diagnosis and treatment is presumptive; delays will result in poor clinical outcome.
> - Treat hypoglycaemia with dextrose and steroids concurrently.
> - Consider the diagnosis in patients who present with hypotension and increased pigmentation either in the buccal mucosa or over friction areas.

MANAGEMENT

Supportive measures

- Patient must be managed in the critical care area since this is a potentially life-threatening condition.

- Administer supplemental high-flow oxygen by non-rebreather reservoir mask.
- Monitor ECG, vital signs q 10–15 min, pulse oximetry.
- Establish 2 large-bore (14G/16G) peripheral IV lines.
- IV fluids: administer **IV 0.9% saline/D_5W** by rapid infusion till hypotension corrected (usual deficit approximates 2–3l).
- Investigations:
  1. Stat capillary blood sugar
  2. FBC
  3. Urea/electrolytes/creatinine **(mandatory)**, look for
     a. hyponatraemia
     b. hyperkalaemia
     c. metabolic acidosis
     d. elevated urea
     e. hypoglycaemia
  4. ABG
  5. Plasma cortisol (plain tube) and ACTH (EDTA tube on ice). **Send to lab as urgent**.
  6. ECG: may show low-voltage QRS tracing with non-specific ST–T wave changes and/or changes due to hyperkalaemia, reversible with glucocorticoid replacement.
  7. CXR may be normal, but often reveals a small heart. There may be stigmata of earlier infection or current evidence of TB or fungal infection, when this is the cause of Addison's disease.
  8. Urinalysis by urine stick reagent testing to exclude UTI.
- Correct precipitating factors, eg infection, AMI.

Drug therapy

- IV **D_{50}W** 40 ml to correct hypoglycaemia which may be refractory and require repeated boluses; feed with isocal if patient is alert.
- IV **hydrocortisone** 100 mg q 6 h: it is physiological, more rapidly acting than dexamethasone and has mineralocorticoid activity, especially in the case of suspected primary adrenocortical insufficiency. Draw blood for plasma cortisol and ACTH before treatment!
- IV **sodium bicarbonate** (if needed): 50 mmoles over 1–2 hours; monitor acid base status with serial ABGs.

Disposition

- Consult Endocrine/General Medicine regarding anticipated admission to MICU for close monitoring of vital signs.

References/further reading

1. Werbel SS, Ober KP. Acute adrenal insufficiency. *Endocrinol Metab Clin North Am.* 1993;22:303.

37 Alcohol intoxication

Peter Manning

CAVEATS

- Ethanol use is associated with a significantly increased risk of serious injury due to impaired motor control and judgement.
- Depression of the level of consciousness masks many of the usual responses to pain and underlying diseases.
- Ethanol consumption is often associated with respiratory depression and a depressed gag reflex.
- There is a significant **differential diagnosis** for the alcohol intoxicated patient (Table 1).
- Blood ethanol level falls at a rate of **20–30 mg % per hour**.
- **Glasgow Coma Scale (GCS)** is not statistically affected by alcohol until a blood alcohol level of >200 mg % is reached. Hence, do not attribute alterations in the conscious state to alcohol unless the patient has a minimal blood alcohol level of 200 mg %.[2,3]

Table 1: Differential diagnosis of altered mental state in the alcohol-intoxicated patient

CNS disorders	Convulsions or postictal state, strokes, subdural haematoma, tumours
Environmental disorders	Hypothermia
Infectious disorders	Meningitis/encephalitis, pneumonia, sepsis
Metabolic disorders	Diabetic ketoacidosis, hepatic encephalopathy, hypercalcaemia, hypoglycaemia, hyponatraemia, uraemia
Respiratory disorders	Hypoxaemia
Toxicological disorders	Benzodiazepines, carbon monoxide, ethanol, ethylene glycol, isopropyl alcohol, methanol, narcotics, sedative hypnotics
Traumatic disorders	Cerebral concussion, cerebral contusion, epidural haematoma, hypotension, subarachnoid haemorrhage

MANAGEMENT

Philosophies of Management

Goals are

- To protect the patient from hurting him/herself and others.
- To treat potentially **life-threatening conditions** without delay, ie reversible conditions such as hypoxaemia, dehydration, hypoglycaemia, and hypothermia.
- To ensure appropriate disposition and follow up.
- To examine for **injuries** which might otherwise be ignored.
- Search actively for the existence of **Wernicke's encephalopathy**: classic triad that presents in only 10% cases. Look for mental changes of depression, apathy, confusion (80% of cases), ocular changes of horizontal nystagmus or lateral rectus palsy (30% of cases), and ataxia (20% of cases).

Goals achieved through several management principles

- Observation with frequent measurements of vital signs and neurological assessment.
- Aggressive evaluation of non-improving or deteriorating mental status.
- Continued observation until the patient is able to function independently and care for himself.
- Intravenous hydration and nutrition.
- Restraints by chemical or physical means when needed (to protect the patient and others).

Supportive care

- Unless the patient is alert and conversant, drunken patients must be evaluated in a **monitored location.**
- Maintain airway and C-spine evaluation.
- Oral/nasopharyngeal airway depending on the presence of a gag reflex.
- Suctioning equipment must always be immediately available.
- If a history of **trauma** is suspected, apply a **stiff collar with or without manual immobilization**.
- Establish peripheral intravenous access.
- IV crystalloids to be run at a rate appropriate for volume replacement. IV D_5W 500 ml over 3–4 hours is suitable for the normovolaemic patient.
- Use of **physical restraints**: in this way the patient can be controlled without adding medications which would complicate the assessment of a patient whose level of consciousness is already depressed.
- Undress patient.

- Measure accurate body temperature.
- **Labs**: the minimum, for a mildly obtunded or confused patient, is a **stat capillary blood sugar.** Since the history and physical findings are often limited, the intoxicated patient with **altered mental state** often requires laboratory and radiological evaluation:
  1. **Essential labs**
     a. FBC
     b. Urea/electrolytes/creatinine: calculate anion gap $[Na^+] - [HCO_3^-] - [Cl^-]$. Refer to *Useful Formulae*.
  2. **Optional labs**
     a. **Blood ethanol level**: the importance of this test lies in the situation where the level does not correlate as expected (eg where it is low or even zero) then an intensive search to explain the altered mental state is essential.

Note: (1) If you draw such a specimen do so using **non-alcohol skin preparations**, and (2) in drunk driving cases written, signed consent of the patient to take blood is **essential**.

  b. **Urinalysis**: for blood, sugar or ketones.
  c. **Serum amylase**.
  d. **Liver function tests (including PT & PTT)**.
  e. **Toxicology studies**: general screening tests are of limited value but should be ordered as directed by history and examination dictate.
  f. **Serum osmolality**: useful in suggesting the presence of other alcohols, eg methanol and ethylene glycol. Normal range is 286 ± 4 mOsm/kg H_2O. Calculate the osmolal gap (should not exceed 10 mOsm/kg).
  g. **Osmolal gap** = measured osmolality − calculated osmolality. Refer to *Useful Formulae*.
  h. **Arterial blood gas**: not necessary if SpO_2 is normal.

- **X-rays**:
  1. **CXR**: useful if history is one of chest trauma, or there is fever, or abnormal auscultatory finding.
  2. **Lateral C-spine, AP pelvis and extremities**: need is based on history and physical examination.
  3. **Head CT scan**: indicated in cases where:
     a. There is evidence of head trauma with persistent LOC or focal neurological findings.
     b. Patient's mental state is inconsistent with the blood ethanol level (see Caveats).
     c. There is no improvement in, or a worsening of, neurological status with time.
- **ECG**: useful in detection of concomitant cardiac disease, eg IHD or alcoholic cardiomyopathy.

Drug therapy

- **Thiamine** 100 mg IV: thiamine stores are often diminished in alcoholic patients.
- **D_{50}W** 40 ml IV bolus for documented hypoglycaemia.

Note: Theoretically, it is important to precede the dextrose with thiamine in a malnourished patient since giving dextrose first may precipitate a Wernicke's encephalopathy (triad of ataxia, global confusion and ocular abnormalities, primarily horizontal nystagmus or a bilateral sixth nerve palsy). This consideration is not supported by evidence. It is argued that it takes hours, if not days, for Wernicke's encephalopathy to develop clinically; also, thiamine can be administered immediately after the dextrose.

- **Haloperidol** 5 mg IV: can be repeated in 5–10 minutes. This drug is used in the severely agitated intoxicated patient in conjunction with physical restraints. Haloperidol produces minimal sedation with excellent behavioural control.
- If the history and physical examination suggest concomitant narcotic use, **naloxone** 2 mg IV will help to identify and reverse the CNS and respiratory depression.

Disposition

- **Admit to HD/ICU setting**, after appropriate consultation, for the following:
  1. Multiple trauma
  2. Ingestions of methanol and ethylene glycol
  3. Sepsis
  4. Gastrointestinal haemorrhage
  5. Acute myocardial infarction
  6. Major withdrawal syndromes
- Admit to **General Medicine** for concurrent pneumonia, hepatitis or pancreatitis. Admit to **General Surgery** or **Neurosurgery** for concurrent stable head injury depending on institutional practice.

Discharge criteria

- Capable of eating/drinking.
- Walking with a steady gait.
- Orientated to surroundings.
- Availability of friends or family to accompany the patient.

SPECIAL SITUATIONS

Children

- Children exposed to ethanol either by drinking alcoholic beverages or mouthwash. Respiratory depression is common even after small doses of ethanol.

- **Hypoglycaemia is common**: treat with 2–4 ml/kg of solution of $D_{25}W$ IV (dilute $D_{50}W$ 1:1 with sterile water since $D_{50}W$ is very hyperosmolar).

Note: Repeated administration is usually not required and may result in a hyperosmolar state.

Methanol and ethylene glycol

- Should be suspected in drunk patients who complain of abdominal pain or visual impairment, **or**, in whom there is a high osmolal gap.
- Differ in toxicity but treatment for either is essentially the same.
- Neither agent is itself dangerous producing only ethanol-like intoxication; it is the metabolites formed after metabolism with alcohol dehydrogenase that produce the toxicity some 6–12 hours after ingestion. This delay in onset of symptoms can be even greater with concurrent ethanol intoxication.
- Serum levels of either alcohol are not readily available so indirect measures such as anion and osmolal gaps are useful.

Note: Osmolal gap increases first before metabolism, only for the anion gap to increase later.

- **Methanol metabolites cause**:
  1. GI tract irritation: nausea, vomiting and abdominal pain.
  2. CNS intoxication: headache, confusion and decreased level of consciousness.
  3. Ocular toxicity: look for retinal oedema and hyperaemia of the disc, and document visual acuity.
  4. Metabolic acidosis.
- **Ethylene glycol metabolites cause**:
  1. Same as for methanol with the addition of renal failure.
- **Management**:
  1. **Supportive care** as for ethanol poisoning.
  2. **Drug therapy**.
     a. Aggressive treatment of metabolic acidosis with sodium bicarbonate.
     b. Block metabolism of parent compounds to their toxic by-products by the administration of ethanol since alcohol dehydrogenase has a greater affinity for ethanol than methanol or ethylene glycol.
     c. **Ethanol therapy**:
     To **maintain** an ethanol level of 100–120 mg/dl
     Load 0.6–0.8 g/kg
     Maintain 0.11 g/kg/h
     Dialysis 0.24 g/kg/h
     Oral methods: not to be used if patient is obtunded and has no gag reflex
     Load use 50% solutions for load by Ryle's tube: 2 ml/kg of 50% gives 0.8 g/kg
     Maintain 0.11–0.13 g/kg/h

Use 0.16 ml/kg/h of 95% solution but dilute with water 1:1 to avoid gastritis and give 0.33 ml/kg/h

Increase proportionately with dialysis.

IV methods

Load use 10% concentration in D_5W through a central line at 10 ml/kg

Maintain use 1.6 ml/kg/h of 10% solution

Increase proportionately with dialysis

d. **Fomeprizole** (a synthetic alcohol dehydrogenase inhibitor) **therapy**: for suspected or confirmed ingestion and intoxication with ethylene glycol or methanol.

Without haemodialysis

Load IV fomeprizole 15 mg/kg, followed by doses of 10 mg/kg q 12 h × 4 doses, then 15 mg/kg q 12 h thereafter

Note: All doses to be administered as a slow intravenous infusion with **normal saline as diluent** over 30 minutes. Do not administer undiluted or by bolus injection.

During haemodialysis: The frequency of dosage should be increased to every 4 hours with the same rate constraints as mentioned above. Therapy should be continued until ethylene glycol or methanol concentrations are less than 20 mg/dl and the patient is asymptomatic.

Oral use of fomeprizole: suitable for cases in which the ingestion was very recent and there is no vomiting.

Dosage: 15 mg/kg initially, followed by 5 mg/kg 12 h later; then 10 mg/kg q 12 h until ethylene glycol plasma levels are undetectable.

3. **Haemodialysis to remove both parent compounds and their toxic by-products**. **Indications** as follows:
   a. When blood levels exceed 25 mg/dl.
   b. When metabolic acidosis is not correctable.
   c. With impending renal failure.
   d. With visual symptoms in methanol poisoning.

Isopropanol

- Metabolized to acetone but there is little or no acidosis.
- Crosses blood-brain barrier much faster and is about twice as intoxicating as ethanol.
- **Toxic effects**:
  1. CNS depression
  2. GI tract irritation with gastritis, vomiting, and haemetemesis

  Treatment: A serum isopropyl alcohol level adds little to management. Treat as for ethanol toxicity.

Alcoholic ketoacidosis

- Seen classically in the chronic alcoholic who binges and then presents with nausea, vomiting, abdominal pain, and starvation with poor caloric intake.
- Ketoacidosis results from the accumulation of acetoacetate and beta-hydroxybutyrate.
- Labs reveal serum pH of about 7.1, serum bicarbonate of 10, low serum potassium and phosphate, and a normal or low serum glucose level.
- **Treatment**: rehydration with 5% dextrose saline solution, antiemetics if needed, benzodiazepines as needed for withdrawal symptoms (Table 2), potassium and phosphate replacement.

Note: Insulin therapy is contraindicated and bicarbonate is rarely required.

- The likelihood of developing severe withdrawal symptoms increases with concomitant infections or medical problems, a prior history of withdrawal seizures or delirium tremens, and a higher intake of alcohol.
- **Withdrawal seizures** (rum fits):
  1. Usually generalized seizures and self-limited.
  2. Onset: usually within 48 hours of last alcohol intake.
  3. It is usually not possible to differentiate withdrawal seizures from other aetiology from history and physical examination.
  4. Suggest:
     a. Focal seizure: head CT scan
     b. Febrile seizure: LP after head CT scan. Start antibiotics stat
     c. Status seizure: head CT scan and metabolic screen
- **Management**:
  1. Provide relief from anxiety and hallucinations.
  2. Halt progression of AWS.
  3. Supportive therapy:
     a. Secure ABCs.
     b. Volume replacement: IV dextrose 5%/saline alternating with dextrose 5%.
     c. Correct electrolyte and metabolic disorders: glucose, thiamine, potassium, magnesium.
     d. IV thiamine 100 mg and IV magnesium sulphate 1–2 g may be started empirically.
  4. Drug therapy:
     a. **Benzodiazepine**: (1) IV diazepam 5–10 mg slow bolus every 5–10 min titrated clinically (max. 20 mg), or (2) PO diazepam 10–20 mg for mild cases (may be repeated after 60 min).
     b. **Haloperiodol**: IM haloperiodol 5–10 mg for agitated patients.
     c. **Beta-blockers**: (1) Indicated if multiple doses of diazepam have been used and/or significant tachyarrhythmias, (2) IV propanolol 0.5 mg every 5–10 min.

Table 2: Alcohol withdrawal syndrome (AWS)

Stage	Onset	Duration	Symptoms	Signs
I *The shakes*	6–8 h	2–3 days	• Anxiety • Agitation • Fear • Loss of appetite • Loss of sleep • Tremor	• Tachycardia • Hypertension • Hyperreflexia
II *The horrors*	0–24 h	2–3 days	The above plus • Hallucinations	The above plus • Fever • Sweating
III *Withdrawal seizures*	7–48 h	6–12 h		The above plus • Grand mal seizures
IV *Delirium tremens*	3–5 days	2–5 days	The above plus • Confusion • Nightmares	The above plus • Fever • Mydriasis

d. **IV phenytoin has no/little role in AWS**.

5. **Disposition**:
   a. All cases should be admitted to GM except for the mild cases that may be discharged with oral benzodiazepine and Psychiatry to follow up.
   b. Delirium tremens should be admitted to ICU for close monitoring.

References/further reading

1. Lindblad R, Galesh G. Alcohol intoxication. In: Hamilton GC, Sanders AB, Strange GR, Trott AT, eds. *Emergency Medicine: An Approach to Clinical Problem Solving*. Philadelphia:WB Saunders; 1991;20:378–393.
2. Galbraith S, Murray WR, Patel AR, et al. The relationship between alcohol and head injury and its effect on the conscious level. *Br J Surg*. 1976;63:128–130.
3. Jagger J, Fife D, Vernberg K, et al. Effect of alcohol intoxication on the diagnosis and apparent severity of brain injury. *Neurosurgery*. 1984;15:303–306.

38 Allergic reactions/anaphylaxis

Peter Manning • Peng Li Lee

DEFINITIONS

- **Urticaria**: oedematous and pruritic plaques with a pale centre and raised borders.
- **Angioedema**: oedema of the deeper layers of the skin that is non-pruritic but may cause burning, numbness or pain.
- **Anaphylaxis**: a severe systemic allergic reaction to an antigen that is precipitated by the abrupt release of chemical mediators in a previously sensitized patient. Prior exposure to the antigen is necessary for anaphylactic shock to occur.
- **Anaphylactoid reactions** resemble anaphylactic reactions but do not require prior exposure because they are not immunologically mediated. Rather, they are due to direct histamine release from mast cells and macrophages.

CAVEATS

- These states represent a spectrum of hypersensitivity reactions ranging from mild urticaria to the life-threatening anaphylaxis; progression from a milder form to full-blown anaphylaxis may occur.
- **Frequency**

Urticaria	*Angioedema*	*Anaphylaxis*
200 cases	20 cases	1 case

- These reactions are IgE or IgG_4-mediated and are responsible for the majority of anaphylactic reactions that occur, eg drug-induced reactions (penicillin and NSAIDs are the most common) and the following:
  1. Foods (shellfish, egg white, peanuts)
  2. Hymenoptera venoms (bees, wasps and hornets)
  3. Environmental reactions (dust, pollen, etc).

ANAPHYLAXIS

Shock/stridor/bronchospasm: a deadly but often preventable emergency.

Clinical evolution of symptoms

- **Early signs of impending anaphylaxis**
  1. Nasal itching or stuffiness.
  2. A lump in the throat (laryngeal or uvular oedema) or hoarseness.
  3. Lightheadedness and syncope.
  4. Chest pain, shortness of breath and tachypnoea.
  5. Skin complaints: warmth and tingling of the face (especially the mouth),

☛ **Special Tips for GPs**

- It is safer to refer all patients with various presentations of allergic reactions to the ED, except for those with a mild and isolated urticarial rash.
- Always ask the patient regarding '**a lump in the throat**' and treat with **SQ adrenaline** (assuming there are no contraindications such as IHD), **before** sending the patient to the ED by ambulance, as this is an early sign of laryngeal or uvular oedema.
- Adrenaline is the mainstay of treatment in anaphylaxis. In normotensive patients, administer SQ or IM adrenaline 1:1,000 0.01 ml/kg (up to 0.3 ml). In hypotensive patients, administer 0.1 ml/kg (up to 0.5 ml) of a 1:10,000 solution IV over 5 minutes, or by deep IM injection if IV access unavailable.
- Set up a peripheral IV line and give crystalloid infusions and antihistamines before sending an anaphylactic patient to the ED by ambulance.

upper chest, palms or soles are usually the first clinical manifestations of anaphylaxis.

6. GI complaints: nausea, vomiting, diarrhoea with tenesmus or crampy abdominal pain.

- **Full-blown anaphylaxis**
  1. Angioedema of the tongue, soft palate and larynx that can lead quickly to acute upper airway obstruction with stridor.
  2. Hypotension, tachycardia (or other dysrhythmias), AMS, dizziness, wheezing and cyanosis that can lead quickly to cardiopulmonary arrest.

Note: Coughing is an ominous sign that often portends the onset of pulmonary oedema.

3. The skin may or may not show the classic wheal-and-flare reaction. If the patient has poor skin perfusion or is dark-skinned, a skin reaction may be difficult to see.

Management

- **Supportive measures**
  1. If relevant, stop administration of suspected agent such as blood transfusion.
  2. If relevant, flick out insect stinger with a tongue blade. **Do not squeeze**, as this may result in further envenomation by the originally partially discharged sac.

3. If allergen was ingested, consider gastric lavage and activated charcoal.
4. If no pulse present, commence external cardiac massage.
5. Patient must be managed in a resuscitation area.
6. Provide supplemental high-flow oxygen.
7. Monitoring: ECG, pulse oximetry, vital signs q 5 min.
8. Establish large-bore IV × 1 (14/16G).
9. Circulatory support: 2l Hartman's or NS as bolus.
10. Be prepared for intubation or cricothyroidotomy.

Note: Extreme caution is indicated in the consideration of sedation and paralysis prior to intubation. Consider using 'Awake Oral Intubation'; refer to *Airway Management/Rapid Sequence Intubation* for details. Rosen states in his text that 'Sedation and paralysis are contraindicated because a distorted airway may preclude intubation after paralysis.'

11. Obtain immediate Anaesthesia/ENT consultations for assistance in airway management.
12. Labs: none immediately necessary.

- **Drug therapy**
  1. **Adrenaline**: the drug of choice:
     a. Normotensive patient: 0.01 ml/kg (up to 0.5 ml) of a **1:1,000 solution SC/deep IM**
     b. Hypotensive patient: 0.1 ml/kg (up to 5 ml) of a **1:10,000** solution given slowly **IV** over 5 minutes (or by deep IM injection if IV access unavailable)
     c. In either case half the calculated dose may be infiltrated around a causative sting
  2. **Glucagon**: consider use when adrenaline is relatively contraindicated, eg IHD, severe hypertension, pregnancy, patients on beta-blockers, or if there is no response to adrenaline. Dosage: 0.5–1.0 mg IV/IM: can be repeated once after 30 minutes.
  3. Choose one of the **antihistamines** in Table 1.

Tip: Dilute each ml of 25 mg of promethazine (Phenergan®) to 10 ml with normal saline and give IV at a rate not more than 2.5 mg/min to avoid the side effect of transient hypotension.

Table 1: Types of antihistamines and dosage

Types of antihistamines	*Dosage*
Diphenhydramine	Adult: 25 mg IM/IV Paediatrics 1mg/kg IM/IV
Chlorpheniramine (Piriton®: a H_1-blocker)	10 mg IM/IV
Promethazine (Phenergan®)	Adult: 25 mg IM/IV Child >6 yrs: 12.5 mg IM/IV Child <6 yrs: 6.25–12.5 mg IM/IV

4. **Cimetidine** (Tagamet®: a H_2-blocker) for persistent symptoms unresponsive to above treatment. Dosage: 200–400 mg IV bolus.
5. **Nebulized bronchodilators** for persistent bronchospasm. Administer salbutamol (Ventolin®) 2:2 via nebulizer q 20–30 minutes.
6. **Corticosteroids** to potentiate the effects of adrenaline and decrease capillary permeability: effects are not immediate. Dosage: hydrocortisone 200–300 mg IV bolus; can be repeated q 6 h.

- **Disposition**:
  Patients should be admitted to ICU/HD following appropriate consultation, for observation and repeated doses of antihistamines and steroids.

ANGIOEDEMA

Drug-induced angioedema

ACE-inhibitors are a common cause; other causes are those of urticaria (see below).

- **Clinical presentation**: body areas that are typically affected include
  1. face and neck (with a predilection for the lips, soft palate and laryngeal structures)
  2. foreskin and scrotum
  3. hands and feet
- **Management** is symptomatic but one must be ready to establish a definitive airway since deterioration to anaphylaxis can occur at any time.
- **Supportive measures**
  1. Patient should be managed in at least the intermediate care area.
  2. Monitoring: vital signs q 15 min, pulse oximetry, ECG.
  3. Establish peripheral IV plug as a precaution.
  4. Supplemental oxygen to maintain SpO_2 >94%.
  5. Be prepared for intubation or cricothyroidotomy: see cautionary note above regarding sedation and paralysis. Consider using 'Awake Oral Intubation'; refer to *Airway Management/Rapid Sequence Intubation* for details.
- **Drug therapy**
  1. **Adrenaline**
     a. IM 0.3–0.5 ml 1:1,000 solution SQ q 20 min in adults >45 kg body weight
     b. IM 0.01 ml/kg (up to 0.3 ml) 1:1,000 solution SQ q 20 min in children and adults <45 kg
  2. **Antihistamine**: refer to the dosage in Table 1.
     a. Diphenhydramine
     b. Chlorpheniramine
     c. Promethazine

3. **Prednisolone**
   a. Dosage: 40–60 mg PO in adults
   b. 2 mg/kg body weight PO in children

- **Disposition**: admit for 12–24 hours observation since a rebound may occur 6–12 hours after the initial onset and apparently successful treatment. If eyelid swelling is the sole symptom/sign, then patient may be discharged following resolution.

Hereditary angioedema (HAE)

Caused by a deficiency of C_1-esterase inhibitor and is precipitated in most cases by trauma or stress.

- **Clinical presentation**
  - Marked facial oedema, swelling of lips and tongue, soft palate and laryngeal structures
  - Abdominal pain with nausea, vomiting and diarrhoea are common
- **Management**
  1. Treat with fresh frozen plasma (contains C_1 inhibitor)
  2. Adrenaline as above may also be effective

Note: Cases of HAE often do not respond to corticosteroids, antihistamines or standard doses of adrenaline, and a definitive airway may be needed.

- **Disposition**: admit all such cases to a high dependency unit for 12–24 hours given the tendency for resistance to treatment.

URTICARIA

Refer to Table 2 for common causes of urticaria.

Table 2: Common causes of urticaria

Drug reaction	Penicillin Aspirin Sulpha drugs NSAIDs TCMs
Infection	Infectious mononucleosis Hepatitis B Coxsackie virus Parasitic infestations
Others	Food: peanuts, food dyes and flavourings Exposure to sun, heat and cold Malignancies Pregnancy

- **Management**: this is symptomatic in most cases but be aware that progression to anaphylaxis has been known.
- **Supportive measures**: the patient should preferably be managed in the intermediate care area of the ED; management in the low acuity area is feasible but frequent reevaluations are necessary to detect deterioration early.
- **Drug therapy**
  1. **Antihistamines**: refer to the dosage in Table 1.
     a. Diphenhydramine
     b. Chlorpheniramine
     c. Promethazine
  2. **Prednisolone**: dosage: 40–60 mg PO in adults if lesions are extensive, or this is a recurrent episode, or patient has had angioedema before. Prescribe a 5-day home course and no tapering of dose required.
- **Disposition**
  1. Patient can be discharged if the response to treatment is prompt and there is no angioedema.
  2. Discharge with a course of antihistamines for at least 3 days.
  3. Consider admission if patient has a past history of admission for urticaria.

ANAPHYLACTOID REACTIONS

Anaphylactoid reactions resemble anaphylactic reactions but do not require prior exposure because they are not immunologically mediated. They are due to direct histamine release from mast cells and macrophages.

Management

- **Commonly implicated agents include**: radiographic contrast media, aspirin, NSAIDs, opiates.
- **Treatment**: the same as that for anaphylaxis.

References/further reading

1. Gavalas M, Sadana A, Metcalf S. Guidelines for the management of anaphylaxis in the emergency department. *J Acc Emerg Med*. 1998;15:96–98.
2. Rosen P, Barkin R, Danzyl DF, et al. *Emergency Medicine: Concepts and Clinical Practice*. 4th ed. St. Louis, MO: Mosby; 1998.
3. Hamilton G. *Presenting Signs and Symptoms in the Emergency Department: Evaluation and Treatment*. Baltimore: Williams & Wilkins; 1993:194–201.

39 Aortic dissection

Shirley Ooi

DEFINITIONS

- Aortic dissection is intimal tear, intramural haematoma or separation of the tunica media that occurs usually in patients with risk factors such as Marfan's syndrome, hypertension, smoking, atherosclerotic aorta or pregnant patients.
- Two primary types of classifications have been in use: the DeBakey and Stanford classifications.
- The **DeBakey system** is divided into:
  1. Type I involving the ascending aorta, aortic arch and the descending aorta.
  2. Type II involving the ascending aorta, but does not extend beyond the left subclavian artery.
  3. Type III involving only the descending aorta, starting at, or distal to, the left subclavian artery.
- The **Stanford system** is divided into:
  1. Type A involving the ascending aorta (with or without descending aorta involvement).
  2. Type B involving only the descending aorta.

  The Stanford classification is simpler and is related to treatment. See p. 93 for details.

CAVEATS

- Consider the **diagnosis of aortic dissection** in any patient with:
  1. Sudden, severe, tearing chest pain/upper abdominal pain radiating to the back, maximal at the outset and migrating over time. As a rule, the pain of acute MI is *not* migratory, and when the two occur together, the dissection typically begins first and leads to the MI.
  2. Chest pain with associated neurological symptoms, syncope, TIA, stroke or paraplegia.
  3. Chest pain with increased risk of aortic dissection, eg hypertension, Marfan's syndrome.
  4. Pulse deficits or difference in systolic blood pressure in both arms >20 mm Hg or BP in lower limbs is lower than in upper limbs.
  5. Chest pain with new onset aortic regurgitation murmur.
  6. Chest pain with widened mediastinum of >8 cm on PA CXR.
- **Diagnoses** that may be **confused** with **thoracic aortic dissection** include:
  1. Myocardial infarction or unstable angina
  2. Abdominal disease

3. Stroke
4. Lower extremity ischaemic thrombosis
5. Pneumonia
6. Pericardial disease

Note: Aortic dissection can occur together with any of the above diagnoses.

- When a patient is **initially evaluated for aortic dissection** and the entity is not found, **remember** the following points:
  1. In some cases, multiple tests (ie transoesophageal echocardiography [TEE] followed by CT scan, etc.) are needed to detect the disease.
  2. The next most likely cause of the patient's complaints may be another type of serious cardiac disease.
  3. If a patient needs to be evaluated for aortic dissection, it is usually done with admission as the ultimate disposition, regardless of the diagnostic test results.
  4. Patients with a negative evaluation for aortic dissection have a high rate (23%) of acute MI or unstable angina, both of which should not be overlooked even if dissection is excluded.
- Remember that acute aortic dissection is 2–3 times more common than ruptured abdominal aneurysm, and the misdiagnosis rate is as high as 90%. Furthermore, the mortality of untreated type A dissection is 1% per hour in the first 48 hours.

☛ Special Tips for GPs

- Aortic dissection is a serious condition that is very easily missed unless one specially looks for it. It should be considered very seriously if the ECG done for a suspected acute MI is normal or in chest pain patients with concomitant neurological deficits. Remember that it is one of the 6 life-threatening causes of chest pain!
- Once the diagnosis is suspected, do not send the patient to the ED in his own transport. Call the ambulance. Meanwhile, if possible, set up 1–2 IV lines, control patient's BP and alleviate pain.
- If aortic dissection is suspected, remember that antiplatelet agents and thrombolytic therapy are contraindicated.

MANAGEMENT

Note: The **goal of treatment** is to prevent death and irreversible end-organ damage. The **aim of medical therapy** is to lower the rate of rise of blood pressure (dP/dT) and to lower the mean BP and heart rate.

- Monitor vital signs (including cardiac monitoring) in the critical care area.
- Give high-flow supplemental oxygen.
- Set up 2 large bore IV lines. Send **blood** for:
  1. FBC
  2. Urea/electrolytes/creatinine
  3. Coagulation profile
  4. GXM 4–6 units packed cells; if hypotensive, 2 units rapid match blood as well.
  5. Cardiac enzymes
- Do 12-lead **ECG** to exclude concomitant acute MI.
- Order **chest x-ray**. See Table 1 for features suggestive of aortic dissection.

Note: The screening upright CXR will be abnormal in 80–90% of cases of aortic dissection. However, a normal CXR does *not* exclude the diagnosis.

- Give **pain relief** with IV morphine 2.5–5.0 mg titrated to clinical need.
- Insert **urinary catheter** to monitor urine output and to exclude anuria/oliguria suggesting possible involvement of both renal arteries.

Note: Most patients with acute aortic dissection present with significant hypertension. A small percentage will present with hypotension from aortic rupture into the pleural space or into the pericardium with subsequent tamponade.

Table 1: Chest x-ray findings in aortic dissection

1. Widened superior mediastinum (>8 cm on PA film; most common, ie 75% of CXRs).
2. Extension of aortic shadow >5 mm beyond its calcified wall ('eggshell' or 'calcium' sign; this is due to the acute dissection separating the adventitia and the calcified intima; most specific although not common).
3. Obliteration of aortic knob or localized bulge.
4. Aortic enlargement.
5. Double density of the aorta (false lumen less radio opaque).
6. Loss of space between aorta and pulmonary artery.
7. Widening of the paravertebral stripe.
8. New pleural effusion (free haemothorax).
9. Apical pleural cap (localized apical haemothorax).
10. Depression of left mainstem bronchus to >140°.
11. Shift and elevation of right mainstem bronchus.
12. Deviation of trachea/endotracheal tube/NG tube to the right (away from developing haematoma).

- Put the patient on circulation and neurological observation chart.
- Start **hypotensive therapy** if patient is hypertensive. Aim to **reduce systolic BP to 100–120 mm Hg**, providing the urine output remains >30 ml/h. Give:
  1. IV **nitroprusside infusion plus IV propranolol**
     Make a solution of 100 μg/ml nitroprusside by adding 50 mg to 500 ml 5% dextrose. Start infusion at 6 ml/h (10 μg/min) and increase it by steps of 10 μg/min every 5 minutes as necessary, and give IV propranolol 1 mg every 5 minutes until a **target heart rate of 60–80 beat/minute** is achieved (give **before** or **simultaneously** with nitroprusside as nitroprusside may produce reflex tachycardia).

  or

  2. IV **labetalol infusion**: IV labetalol may be more readily accessible and is a good alternative as it produces both alpha- and beta-adrenergic block. Make up a solution of 1mg/ml by diluting 200 mg to 200 ml N/S or 5% dextrose solution. Start infusion at 15 ml/h and increase it every 15 minutes as necessary. Alternatively, give IV labetalol 20 mg bolus initially followed by 20–80 mg every 5–10 minutes until target heart rate is reached, then start continuous infusion at 1–2 mg/h.
     Contraindications for beta-blocker use include patients with history of congestive heart failure, heart block, asthma, or chronic obstructive lung disease. IV diltiazem can be given in such cases in place of beta-blockers. Mix 125 mg in 100 ml 5% dextrose (1 mg/1ml) and give as 20 mg bolus followed by rebolus in 15 minutes or start infusion at 5–15 mg/h.
- If hypotensive, start IV fluid resuscitation. Treatment for cardiac tamponade not responding to fluid resuscitation is immediate pericardiocentesis.

Note: All patients receive medical therapy initially, regardless of dissection type.

- Patients with documented aortic dissection who are **normotensive** or have no pain should still be treated with a medical regimen. Further decreases of their blood pressure and heart rate to the aforementioned ranges are unlikely to cause harm and will help stop progression of the dissection in the same manner as in hypertensive patients.
- The **indications for surgical repair** of aortic dissection include:
  1. All Stanford type A dissections.
  2. Type B dissections with complications (rupture, severe distal ischaemia, intractable pain, progression, uncontrolled hypertension). Otherwise Type B dissections can be managed medically.
  3. Uncontrolled hypertension.
  4. Progression of dissection.
- Contact cardiologist-on-call for TEE or arrange for thorax CT if diagnosis is suspected but not very clear on pure clinical grounds.

Note: TEE is the definitive diagnostic study of choice in aortic dissection in an unstable patient.

- Contact cardiothoracic surgeon as soon as diagnosis is suspected and while medical therapy is being instituted.

References/further reading

1. Hals G. Acute thoracic aortic dissection: Current evaluation and management. Part I: Pathophysiology, risk factors, and clinical presentation. *Emerg Med Rep*. 2000;21(1):1–10.
2. Hals G. Acute thoracic aortic dissection: Current evaluation and management. Part II: Definitive diagnosis, patient evaluation, and outcome optimizing management in the emergency department. *Emerg Med Rep*. 2000;21(2):11–22.

40 Appendicitis, acute

Malcolm Mahadevan

CAVEATS

- The **classical presentation** of pain beginning periumbilically and moving to the right lower quadrant (RLQ) associated with vomiting, anorexia, rebound and fever are reported in only 50–60% of patients.
- Vomiting following the onset of abdominal pain is more consistent with appendicitis than other diagnosis. See Table 1 for differential diagnosis of appendicitis.
- All patients with RLQ tenderness should be diagnosed as having appendicitis until proven otherwise. Special groups of patients to be particularly vigilant include children, the elderly, women, pregnant women and the immunocompromised.
- **Atypical presentations** are actually more common. Healthy adult males are the only group of patients considered to be at low risk for misdiagnosis, and the only patient who is safe from appendicitis is the patient who has already had his or her appendix removed!
- **Right lower quadrant pain** (80%) and **pain before vomiting** (100%) are more consistent for appendicitis compared with fever (67%) and nausea (58%).
- Rectal tenderness on rectal examination has only a sensitivity of 41% and a specificity of 77%. Although it used to be taught that appendicitis is very unlikely in the absence of **anorexia,** anorexia is present only in 68% of patients with appendicitis.

Table 1: Differential diagnosis of appendicitis

GE	Pancreatitis
Non-specific abdominal pain	Biliary tract disease
Intestinal obstruction	Endometriosis
Inflammatory bowel disease	Ovarian cyst
Diverticulitis	PID
	Mid cycle
Adenitis	
Henoch Schönlein purpura	Renal colic
	UTI
	Torsion testis

- Temperatures >39°C are uncommon in the first 24 hours of illness but not uncommon after the rupture of appendix. Think of other diagnosis (eg acute pyelonephritis, PID) in a patient with a high fever (>39°C) early in the onset of abdominal pain.
- **No** laboratory test can establish the diagnosis of acute appendicitis with 100% accuracy. Serial clinical examination is the key to diagnosis.
- Leukocytosis with 'left shift' is seen in 75–80% of patients with acute appendicitis. Both of these values alone have been shown not to be useful in ruling out appendicitis as they are too non-specific; they can be seen in many of the diseases that are confused with appendicitis as well.
- The only finding specific for appendicitis on abdominal x-ray is the faecolith but this is rarely seen on plain films (2% incidence) and does not justify the cost of obtaining the study.

☛ Special Tips for GPs

- Appendicitis is most commonly seen in 10–30 year olds, although it can also be seen in patients of any age. Although rare in infants, it has been reported.
- Recurrent and chronic appendicitis are recognized clinical entities and do occur, albeit not frequently.
- It should be included in the differential of *any* patient seen with abdominal pain. See Table 1 for a differential diagnosis of appendicitis.

MANAGEMENT

High clinical probability of acute appendicitis

- History and physical examination (including pelvic and rectal).
- Nil by mouth.
- Set up IV lines and send blood for FBC, urea/electrolytes/creatinine.
- Urinalysis.
- Urine pregnancy test, if applicable.
- Analgesia: titrated IV analgesia, eg opiates together with an antiemetic, can be safely administered as it improves symptoms but does not mask the signs of peritonism.[7,8,9,10,11]
- Surgical consultation.
- Give IV ceftriaxone 1g and IV Flagyl® 500 mg if there are signs of appendiceal perforation.
- Admit to General Surgery for appendectomy.

Borderline cases of appendicitis

- History and physical exam (including pelvic and rectal).
- FBC.
- Urinalysis.
- Urine pregnancy test, if applicable.
- Surgical consultation for follow-up, if follow-up in ED, see in 12–24 hours for repeat examination, with earlier return for increased symptoms.

References/further reading

1. Hals G. Acute appendicitis: Meeting the challenge of diagnosis in the ED. *Emerg Med Rep.* 1999;20(8):71–86.
2. Coleman C, Thompson JE, Bennion RS, et al. WBC count is a poor predictor of severity of disease in the diagnosis of appendicitis. *Am Surg.* 1998;64:983–985.
3. Dueholm S, Bagi P, Bud M. Laboratory aid in the diagnosis of acute appendicitis: A blinded, prospective trial concerning the diagnostic value of leukocyte count, neutrophil differential count, and C-reactive protein. *Dis Colon Rectum.* 1989;32:855–859.
4. Malone AJ, Shetty MR. Diagnosis of appendicitis. *Lancet.* 1997;14:349.
5. Hoffman J, Rasmussen AB. Aids in the diagnosis of acute appendicitis. *Br J Surg.* 1989;76:774–779.
6. Does this patient have appendicitis? *JAMA.* 1996;276:1589.
7. Zollie N, Cust MP. Analgesia in the acute abdomen. *Ann Royal Coll Surg Edin.* 1986;68:209–210.
8. Attard AR, Corlett MJ. Safety of early pain relief for acute abdominal pain. *BMJ.* 1992;305:554–556.
9. LoVecchio F, Oster N. The use of analgesics in patients with acute abdominal pain. *J Emerg Med.* 1997;15;6:775–779.
10. Pace S, Burke TF. Intravenous morphine for early pain relief in patients with acute abdominal pain. *Acad Emerg Med.* 1996;3:1086–1092.
11. Mahadevan M, Graff L. Prospective randomized study of analgesic use for ED patients with right lower quadrant abdominal pain. *Am J Emerg Med.* 2000;18:753–756.
12. Fitzgerald DJ, Pancioli AM. Appendicitis. In: Tintinalli JE, Kelen GD, Stapczynski JS, et al, eds. *Emergency Medicine: A Comprehensive Study Guide.* 5th ed. New York: McGraw-Hill; 2000;535–539.

41 Assault (non-sexual)

JP Travers • Peter Manning

DEFINITIONS

- **Abrasion**
  1. The most superficial type of injury, ie scratch or graze.
  2. Confined to the epidermis or most superficial of dermis.
- **Contusion, ie bruise**
  1. Blunt injury to the tissues damages blood vessels beneath the surface, allowing blood to extravasate (leak) into the surrounding tissues.
  2. May be associated with overlying lacerations or abrasions.
  3. May be flat or elevated.
- **Laceration, ie cut, gash or tear**
  1. A splitting or tearing wound caused by blunt injury that passes through the full thickness of the skin and thus bleeds profusely.
  2. Should not be confused with an incised wound.
- **Incised wounds**, ie 2 types of sharply-cut wounds, caused by object with a cutting edge
  1. Slash wound in which length > depth.
  2. Stab wound in which depth > length.

CAVEATS

- Assume that all assault cases will come to court and that you may be called upon to give evidence, whereupon your opinion becomes public knowledge. The case may come to court several years after the attack. You will have to rely on your written notes taken at the time of the examination in addition to any diagrammatic or photographic evidence that you obtained.
- Therefore, your medical records should be thorough and accurate.
- There is no such thing as a 'medicolegal' x-ray. X-rays should be ordered, or not ordered, based on clinical grounds only. It is the documentation that is critical medicolegally.

HISTORY

- Record accurately with, wherever possible, the patient's own words, including:
  1. **Time** of the assault.
  2. **Method** of the assault, ie kicking, punching, beating with weapon, etc.
  3. **Weapon(s)** used, eg knife, *parang*, gun.

EXAMINATION

- Record all major and minor injuries.
- Include shape, size, depth, colour, diameter (see comments below on use of cameras).
- Photograph all lesions (a Polaroid camera is useful, though better images are now available via digital cameras with attached printers):
    1. Use the photos as an *aide-mémoire* so that you can accurately record all injuries without wasting your time making multiple trips to the patient.
    2. Label and date all photos with the initials of the person who took them using an addressograph label.
    3. File the photos with the ED record.

POST-EXAMINATION

- Fill in all details required in any requested **Police Report**, including whether or not the lesion(s) is/are consistent with the mode and time of injury. If requested to give an opinion on 'Fitness for detention', state 'Don't know'.
- If your department's work flow permits, recall the patient for **review in approximately 24–48 hours** (your next shift would be ideal). This serves for reevaluation and photography of previously injured areas which might have changed in appearance **and** for evaluation of areas which only at the time of the review are showing signs of injury.

References/further reading

1. Knight B. *Simpson's Forensic Medicine*. 11th ed. London: Arnold; 1997:44–45.

42 Asthma

Malcolm Mahadevan

CAVEATS

- **'All that wheezes is not asthma': differentials** to consider include congestive cardiac failure, upper airway obstruction, bronchogenic carcinoma with obstruction or metastatic carcinoma with lymphangitic metastasis.
- Asthma is a chronic inflammatory disorder characterized by increased responsiveness of the airway to multiple insults and hence the cornerstone of therapy is steroids.
- The **triad of asthma symptoms** are dyspnoea, wheezing and cough.
- The **aims of ED therapy** for asthma is to reverse airflow obstruction, ensure adequate oxygenation and relieve inflammation.

> ☛ **Special Tips for GPs**
>
> - During an acute asthma attack, the early use of an **oral corticosteroid** will reduce the risk of asthma death. Thus, nearly all patients who need nebulized treatment for acute severe asthma in the clinic need a course of oral prednisolone approximately 0.5 mg/kg/day for 7–10 days without the need to tail down.
> - Patients who need frequent (more than once in 6–12 months) nebulizations for acute asthma are at high risk of dying from it.
> - Daily use of a **low dose inhaled corticosteroid** will reduce the risk of severe exacerbations and thus reduce asthma deaths in high-risk patients very cost effectively.

MANAGEMENT

- In the ED, signs and symptoms of a severe asthmatic attack are first sought for. If any of these are present, manage the patient in the critical care area.
- Severity of exacerbation is summarized in Table 1.
- Table 2 shows risk factors of dying from asthma.
- **Management** consists of two arms: supportive and therapeutic. **Initial therapy** for non-life-threatening asthmatics with mild to moderate exacerbation includes inhaled beta agonist/anticholinergic combination and oral steroids. See flow chart in Figure 1 and p. 602 for PEFR nomogram.

Table 1: Classifying severity of asthma exacerbations

	Mild	*Moderate*	*Severe*	*Respiratory arrest imminent*
Symptoms				
Breathlessness	While walking Can lie down	While talking Prefers sitting	While at rest Sits upright	Exhausted Feeble respiratory effort
Speech	Sentences	Phrases	Words	Hardly able to talk
Mental state	May be agitated	Usually agitated	Usually agitated	Drowsy or confused
Signs				
Respiratory rate	Increased	Increased	Often >30/min	Decreased
Use of accessory respiratory muscles	Usually not	Commonly	Usually	Paradoxical thoracoabdominal movement
Wheeze	Moderate, often only end expiratory	Loud; throughout exhalation	Usually loud; throughout inhalation and exhalation	No wheeze ('silent chest')
Pulse/minute	<100	100–120	>120	Bradycardia
SaO_2% (room air)	>95%	91–95%	<91%	Clinically cyanosed

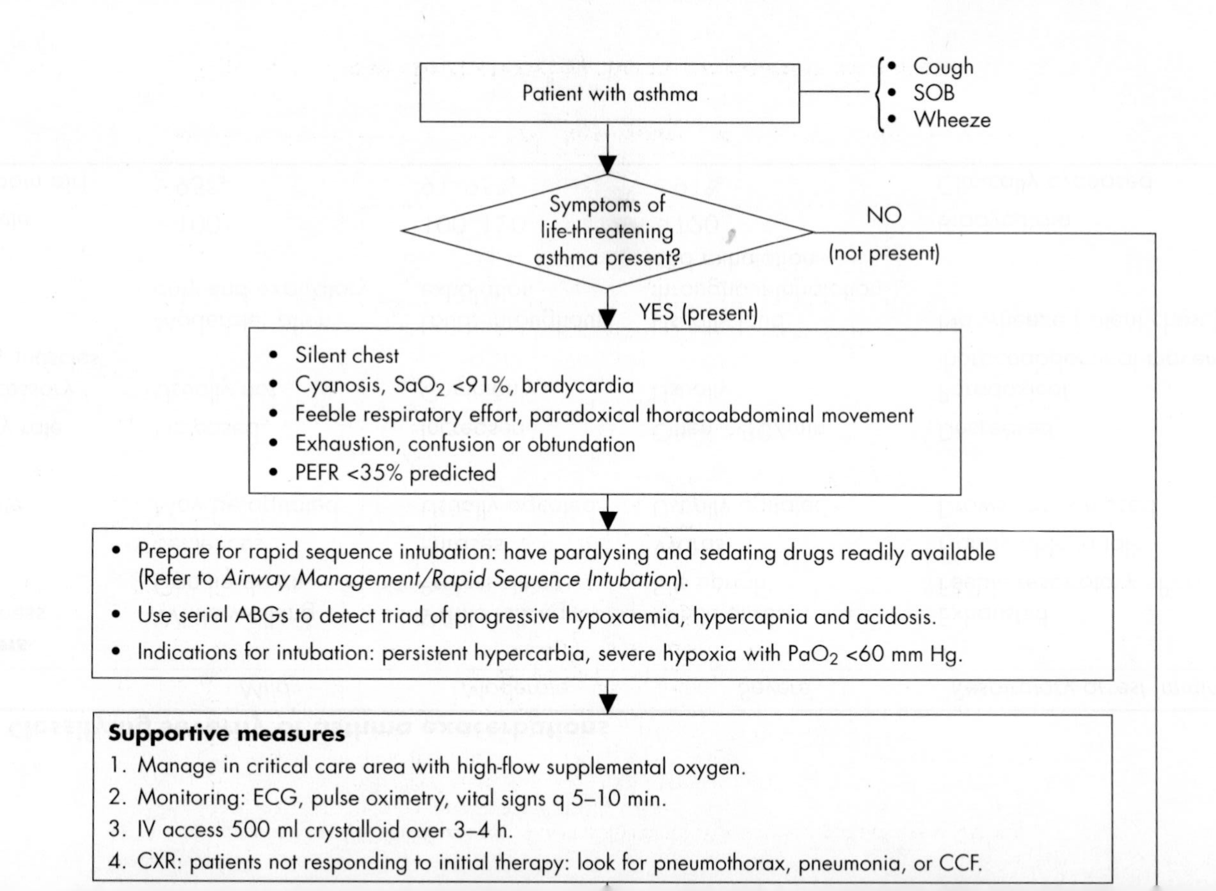

Patient with asthma
Cough
SOB
Wheeze
Symptoms of life-threatening asthma present?
NO (not present)
YES (present)
Silent chest
Cyanosis, SaO_2 <91%, bradycardia
Feeble respiratory effort, paradoxical thoracoabdominal movement
Exhaustion, confusion or obtundation
PEFR <35% predicted
Prepare for rapid sequence intubation: have paralysing and sedating drugs readily available (Refer to *Airway Management/Rapid Sequence Intubation*).
Use serial ABGs to detect triad of progressive hypoxaemia, hypercapnia and acidosis.
Indications for intubation: persistent hypercarbia, severe hypoxia with PaO_2 <60 mm Hg.
Supportive measures
1. Manage in critical care area with high-flow supplemental oxygen.
2. Monitoring: ECG, pulse oximetry, vital signs q 5–10 min.
3. IV access 500 ml crystalloid over 3–4 h.
4. CXR: patients not responding to initial therapy: look for pneumothorax, pneumonia, or CCF.

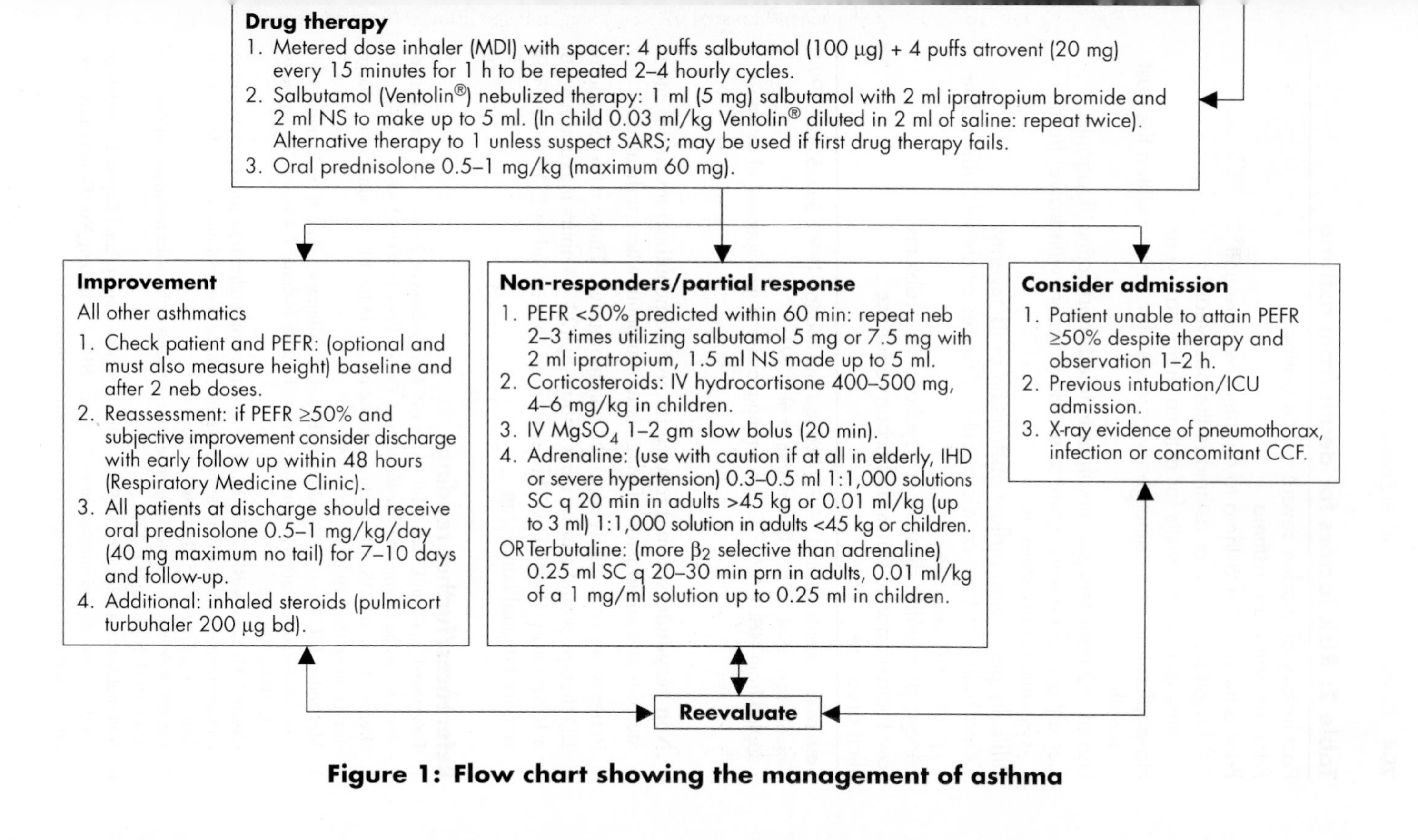

Figure 1: Flow chart showing the management of asthma

Table 2: Risk factors for death from asthma

Past history of sudden severe exacerbations
Prior intubation for asthma
Prior admission for asthma to an intensive care unit
≥2 hospitalizations for asthma in the past year
≥3 emergency care visits for asthma in the past year
Hospitalization or an emergency care visit for asthma within the past month
Use of >2 canisters per month of inhaled short-acting β_2-agonist
Current use of systemic corticosteroids or recent withdrawal from systemic corticosteroids
Difficulty perceiving airflow obstruction or its severity
Comorbidity, as from cardiovascular diseases or chronic obstructive pulmonary disease
Serious psychiatric disease or psychosocial problems
Low socioeconomic status and urban residence
Illicit drug use

Sources: Kallenbach et al. 1993; Rodrigo and Rodrigo 1993; Suissa et al. 1994; Greenberger et al. 1993; O'Hollaren et al. 1991.
Adapted from NHLBI MAEP Guide for diagnosis and management of asthma.

- **Non-responders** would require intensified nebulizations, intravenous steroids and an infusion of magnesium sulphate where indicated.
- Patients are continually assessed and monitored. Those who respond to ED therapy would require early follow-up (24–48 hours maximum) with a Respiratory Physician. Those who fail to respond to ED therapy will require hospital admission.

References/further reading

1. Emerman CL, Cydulka RK, McFadden ER. Comparison of 2.5 mg vs 7.5 mg inhaled albuterol in the treatment of acute asthma. *Chest.* 1999;115(1):92–96.
2. Brenner B, Kohn MS. The acute asthmatic patient in the ED: to admit or discharge. *Am J Emerg Med.* 1998;16(1):69–75.
3. McFadden ER, Casale TB, Edwards TB, et al. Administration of budesonide once daily by means of turbuhaler to subjects with stable asthma. *J Allergy Clin Immunol.* 1999;104(1):46–52.
4. Quadrel M, Lavery RF, Jaker M, et al. Prospective randomized trial of epinephrine, metaproterenol and both in the prehospital treatment of asthma in the adult patient. *Ann Emerg Med.* 1995;26(4):469–473.
5. Lin RY, Rehman A. Clinical characteristics of adult asthmatics requiring intubation. *J Med.* 1995;26(5–6):261–277.
6. National Asthma Education and Prevention Program Expert Panel Report 2. Guidelines for the diagnosis and management of asthma. NIH. Publication No. 97-4051 July 1997 http://www.nhlbi.nih.gov/guidelines/asthma/asthgdln.pdf

43 Bites, mammalian and human

Shirley Ooi

CAVEATS

- Human bites have a higher risk of infection compared to dog or cat bites.
- Think of **punch bite cellulitis**/clenched fist injury in puncture wounds or infections at the 4th or 5th metacarpophalengeal joints.
- Puncture wounds may look innocuous but there is a higher risk of wound infection compared to larger wounds.
- Dogs have larger teeth and hence cause tearing of tissues. In contrast, cats have fine, sharp teeth and weaker biting forces causing puncture wounds. Hence the infection rate for cat bite wounds is higher at 50% compared to 2–5% for dog bite wounds (Table 1).
- Wound infections due to ***P. multocida*** are characterized by a rapidly developing (**within a few hours** after animal bite) inflammatory reaction. In contrast, dog and cat bite wound infections occurring **after 24 hours** are more likely to contain ***Staphylococcus*** or ***Streptococcus* sp**. from the patients' own flora.

Table 1: Some common microorganisms in dog and cat bite wounds

	Dog bite (%)	*Cat bite (%)*
Aerobic		
Pasteurella sp. (especially *P. multocida*)	50	75
Streptococcus sp.	46	46
Staphylococcus	46	35
Neisseria	16	19
Corynebacterium	12	28
Moraxella	10	35
Enterococcus	10	12
Bacillus	8	11
Anaerobes		
Fusobacterium sp.	32	33
Bacteroides sp.	30	28
Porphyromonas	28	30
Prevotella	28	19
Propionibacterium	20	18
Peptostreptococcus sp.	16	5

Source: Adapted from Talan et al.[4]

- ***Capnocytophoga canimorsus***, formerly known as 'dysgonic fermenter – 2' (DF-2), is a fastidious and thin gram-negative bacillus associated with a severe infection, ie sepsis with DIVC, acute renal failure, endocarditis, peripheral gangrene and cardiopulmonary failure. The clinical picture may be more severe in immunocompromised patients, with 25% fatality. **Penicillin** is the drug of choice and should be used prophylactically in high-risk patients. Alternatives are cephalosporins, tetracyclines, erythromycin and clindamycin.

> ☛ **Special Tips for GPs**
> - Human bites are often unreported. Therefore, when treating cuts, scratches and lacerations of scalp, dorsum of hand or genitalia, consider the possibility of a human bite.
> - Local dogs and cats in Singapore are free of rabies.
> - In Singapore, if bitten by a 'foreign dog', refer to the Communicable Disease Centre for antirabies prophylaxis.

DOG AND CAT BITE

Management

- Life-threatening injuries must be excluded first when there is severe animal attack. However, most bite wounds are minor.

Principles of wound care

Thorough evaluation of injury

- Wounds
  1. Location
  2. Number
  3. Type
  4. Depth
  5. Overt signs of infection

Note: As bite wounds are frequently punctures, they may be more extensive than they appear.

- Injuries of deeper structures
  1. Tendons
  2. Joint spaces
  3. Blood vessels
  4. Nerves
  5. Bones

Note: Use local or regional anaesthesia and a proximal tourniquet to facilitate wound exploration.

Do x-rays if

- Considerable oedema and tenderness about wound
- Bony penetration (suspected)
- Foreign bodies (suspected)
- Note the following on x-rays:
  1. Fracture
  2. Foreign body
  3. Tooth
  4. Subcutaneous emphysema (necrotizing infections or air introduced during wound manipulation)

Meticulous wound care with

- Thorough cleansing.
- Debridement of devitalized tissues.
- Copious high-pressure irrigation with normal saline solution. This markedly decreases the concentration of bacteria in contaminated wounds. To irrigate puncture wounds, use an 18-gauge needle or plastic catheter tip with a 20 ml syringe inserted into the wound in the direction of the puncture. Care should be taken not to inflict additional trauma or to inject fluid into the tissues. If an eschar is present, it should be removed so that any abscess or exudate that has developed beneath it can be detected and treated.

Note: Cultures from bite wounds obtained at the time of injury are of little value because they cannot be used to predict whether infection will develop, or, if it does, the causative pathogens. Hence, aerobic and anaerobic bacterial culture should only be obtained from an infected bite wound.

Controversy: Primary closure or not

- Historically, such wounds were not closed primarily (except for face and scalp). However, more recent literature supports primary closure after adequate wound preparation except for:
  1. Puncture wounds (because they cannot be cleaned adequately)
  2. Bite wounds with extensive crush injury
  3. Wounds requiring considerable amount of debridement
  4. Hand wounds (because of concerns about serious complications)
  5. Bites to the arms and legs occurring more than 6 to 12 hours earlier
  6. Bites to the face occurring 12 to 24 hours earlier

Note: Delayed primary suture should be done for the latter 3 situations. Subcutaneous sutures should be used sparingly because any foreign material in a contaminated wound increases the risk of infection.

Bite wounds of hands

- Treatment
  1. Thorough cleansing and irrigation

2. Debridement
3. Splinting with a bulky immobilization dressing
4. Elevation for several days until oedema has mostly resolved: this must be emphasized to the patient
5. Prophylactic antibiotics
6. Tetanus prophylaxis

Drug therapy

- Whether antibiotics prevent infection in bite wounds remains controversial.
- Currently, antibiotics are not given routinely. Instead give prophylactic antibiotics only in cases where the probability of infection is >5–10%, i.e:
  1. Dog or cat bites with full-thickness puncture
  2. Hand wounds
  3. Lower extremity wounds
  4. Wounds requiring surgical debridement
  5. Wounds involving joints, tendons, ligaments or fractures
  6. Wounds in high-risk hosts
  7. Wounds with an adjacent prosthetic joint

  Give prophylactic antibiotics for 3–5 days. Refer to Table 2 for factors affecting the risk of infection in dog and cat bite wounds.
- **Choice of antibiotics**
  1. **Augmentin** has been shown in randomized controlled trials to be superior to placebo in 'uninfected wound'. It is also cheap and easily tolerated.
  2. Give **augmentin** alone either PO or IV, depending on the severity of the bite. For penicillin allergic patients, give **clindamycin** or **ciprofloxacin**.
- **Disposition**
  1. Outpatient treatment for local cellulitis only and no deep structure involvement.

Table 2: Factors affecting the risk of infection in dog and cat bite wounds

Increased risk	*Decreased risk*
1. Age <2 years; >50 years	1. Face and scalp wounds
2. Diabetes mellitus	
3. Chronic alcoholism	
4. Immunosuppression	
5. Extremities	
6. Exposure >24 hours	
7. Puncture wounds (40% of all infections)	

2. Admit for IV therapy and surgical consultation:
   a. severe cellulitis
   b. systemic signs, eg fever or chills
   c. has advanced past a joint
   d. has spread rapidly
   e. has not responded to oral or outpatient therapy
   f. when wounds or infections are thought or known to involve a bone, joint, tendon or nerve
   g. unreliable or incompetent patients

- **Tetanus immunoprophylaxis**: dog and cat bites are tetanus-prone wounds
- **Rabies immunoprophylaxis**
  1. Local dogs and cats in Singapore (rabies free)
  2. In Singapore, if bitten by 'foreign' dogs, refer to local health authority for rabies prophylaxis

HUMAN BITES

Management

- As in animal bites.
- **Bacteriology**: infections of human bites are associated with α-haemolytic *streptococci*, *S. aureus*, *Eikenella corrodens*, *Haemophilus* sp. and in >50% of cases anaerobic bacteria.

Note: Most human bite wounds are usually not closed primarily except for cosmetic purposes, eg face and neck in females.

- If wound appears minor, antibiotics can be withheld.
- For more extensive wounds, give penicillinase-resistant penicillin or broad spectrum second generation cephalosporins:
  1. Prophylaxis in uninfected bites: oral augmentin 375 mg 8 h × 2–3 days
  2. Superficial infections: oral augmentin 375 mg 8 h × 5–7 days
  3. Deeper infections: admit for IV antibiotics
- Remember that human bites can transmit organisms such as the human immunodeficiency virus, hepatitis B virus and even syphilis (refer to *Needlestick/Body Fluid Exposure* for further details on prophylaxis).
- **Disposition**:
  1. Discharge patients with wounds seen within 24 hours that show superficial infection. These may be treated as outpatients with follow-up within 24–48 hours.
  2. Admit if:
     a. Any degree of infection occurs beyond limited local wound cellulitis
     b. Wound seen >24 hours after bite
     c. Immunocompromised patient
     d. Human bites of hands and genitalia

References/further reading

1. Ooi BSS. Dogs, cat and human bites. *Singapore Family Physicians*. 1999;25(4):9–14.
2. Dire DJ. Emergency management of dog and cat bite wounds. *Emerg Med Clin North Am*. 1992;10(4):719–736.
3. Eckerline CA, Blake J, Koury RF. Puncture wounds and bites. In: Tintinalli JE, Kelen GD, Stapczynski JS, et al, eds. *Emergency Medicine: A Comprehensive Study Guide*. 5th ed. New York: McGraw-Hill; 2000;333–335.
4. Talan DA, Citron DM, Abrahamian FM, et al. Bacteriologic analysis of infected dog and cat bite wounds. *N Eng J Med*. 1999;340(2):85–92.
5. Fleisher GR. The management of bite wounds (editorial). *N Eng J Med*. 1999:340(2);138–140.
6. Goldstein EJ. Bite wounds and infection. *Clin Infect Dis*. 1992;14(3):633–638.

44 Bites, snake

Shirley Ooi • Peter Manning • Suresh Pillai

CAVEATS

- One of the most important issues in snake bites is to try to ascertain if the snake is venomous as it is usually quite difficult for the victim or bystander to be able to identify the snake.
- The best clues to a **venomous bite** are:
  1. The presence of intense local pain.
  2. Oedema surrounding a puncture wound and gradually spreading proximally.
  3. The presence of petechiae, ecchymoses, and serous or haemorrhagic bullae.
  4. The presence of systemic effects like nausea, vomiting, diarrhoea, severe abdominal pain, restlessness, hypotension, haemorrhagic manifestations (epistaxis, gum bleeding, GI bleeding), neurological symptoms (paralysis, ptosis, impairment of eye movements, speech and swallowing difficulty, unsteady gait, seizures), respiratory paralysis and dark coloured urine (from myoglobinuria).
- If the snake is available for inspection, contact the local zoo or herpetologic society, according to local practice, whose members can be asked to assist in the identification of the snake. See Figure 1 for identification of snake bites.
- Be careful **not to handle a 'dead' snake** as reflex envenomation by a decapitated head of a snake can still occur several hours after its death.
- Only a small minority of land snakes are venomous.
- **All sea snakes** are **venomous**. Suspect if there is a history of **painless bite** occurring while swimming in the sea or during sorting of the fishing net. Generalized muscle aches and pains, and stiffness when attempting to move, usually occur within half to one hour after the bite.
- **Snake venom** may be broadly **classified** into:
  1. Haematotoxins or cardiovascular toxins (as in Crotalidae)
  2. Neurotoxins (as in Elapidae and Hydropiidae)
  3. Myotoxins (as in Hydropiidae)
- See Table 1 for grades of envenomation.
- Antivenin should only be administered in hospital if there is moderate to severe envenomation.

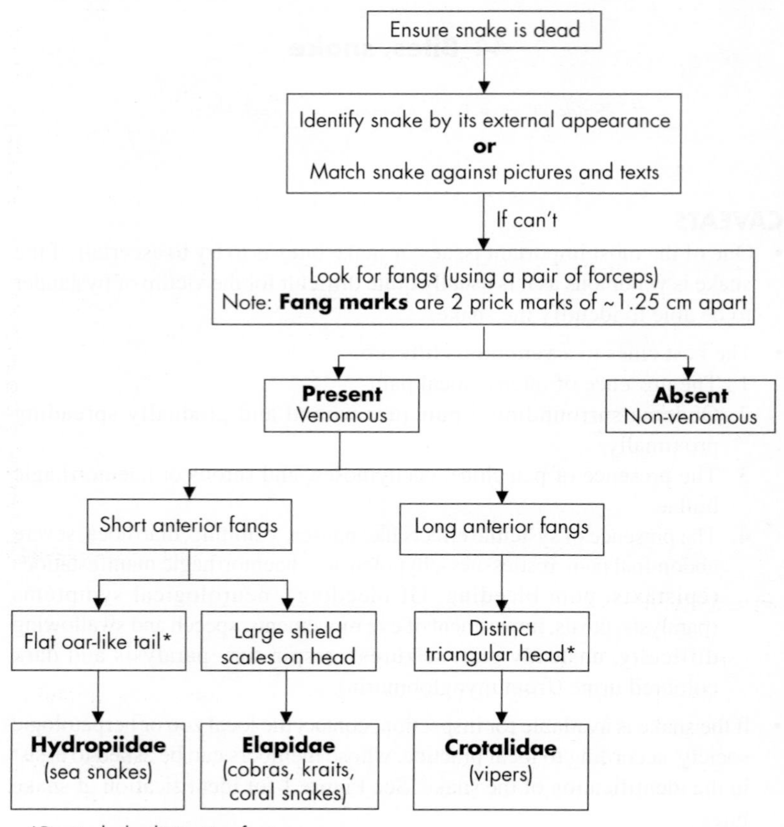

Figure 1: Identification of snake bites

Table 1: Grades of envenomation

Minimal	No pain to moderate pain, erythema, oedema 2.5–15 cm, no systemic symptoms
Moderate	Severe pain, tenderness, oedema 25–40 cm, erythema, petechiae, vomiting, fever and weakness
Severe	Widespread pain, oedema 40–50 cm, ecchymosis, systemic signs
Very severe	Rapid swelling, ecchymosis, CNS symptoms, visual disturbance, shock, convulsions

> ☛ **Special Tips for GPs**
> - Try to get the snake identified or bring it along to the hospital, taking special precautions when handling a 'dead' snake.
> - Immobilize the bitten extremity to decrease metabolism, absorption and spread of venom.
> - Never use tourniquets; squeeze or apply suction to wound. Apply a constricting band proximal to the wound. It should be loose enough to admit a finger between the band and the area of the wound. It is useful if applied within 30 minutes of the bite.
> - Look for signs of envenomation.
> - Antivenin should be administered only in an area with full resuscitation facilities like the ED or ICU.

MANAGEMENT

Supportive measures

- Manage patient in resuscitation area. Place patient supine and immobilize bitten extremity in a dependent position.
- Maintain clear airway. If danger of bulbar or respiratory paralysis exists, intubate or ventilate via surgical airway if intubation is not possible for any reason.
- Give supplemental high-flow oxygen.
- Do complete set of vital signs.
- Monitoring: ECG, vital signs q 5–10 min, pulse oximetry.
- **Labs**: mandatory FBC, coagulation profile, urinalysis, urea/electrolytes/creatinine, ECG. Severe cases: urine myoglobin, DIC screen, creatinine phosphokinase. Shock or respiratory depression: ABG.
- If patient arrives with **tourniquet in place**, ensure the following before you release it, anticipating sudden envenomation from the snake bite:
  1. Peripheral IV line in place with normal saline
  2. Resuscitation equipment immediately available
  3. Full monitoring in place
- Urinary catheter to monitor urine output (if patient unstable).
- Keep patient nil by mouth: nausea and vomiting occur following haematotoxic venomous bites.

Table 2: Guidelines for dosage of antivenin

Grade of envenomation	*Dosage*
Minimal envenomation	Antivenin **not** indicated
Moderate envenomation	20–40 ml (2–4 vials)*
Severe	50–90 ml (5–9 vials)
Very severe	100–150 ml (10–15 vials)

* Controversial

- Irrigate eyes in cases of snake bite ophthalmia (eg some cobras will spit in the eyes of a victim).
- **Do not** apply a tourniquet to the affected extremity.
- **Do not** apply ice packs to the wound since, upon removal, reflex vasodilatation may result in rapid absorption of venom.
- **Do not** incise or suck the wound.

Specific measures

- **Use of antivenin to neutralize the snake venom**: polyvalent antivenin should be kept in the critical care area and stored in the refrigerator at 2–6°C. When used, the antivenin must be constituted quickly since it deteriorates and loses its effectiveness at room temperature.
- **Indications for use should be according to the grades of envenomation** (Table 2).
- **Prevention of serum reaction**: before injecting the antivenin,
  1. Enquire whether patient has been given serum injections before (eg the old ATS, but not ATT).
  2. Patient has personal or family history of allergy:
     a. Test sensitivity of patient to serum by intradermal injection of 0.1 ml of serum diluted 1:10. Observe for 30 minutes for local and general reactions. If these occur, consider giving IV diphenhydramine, IV corticosteroids and/or IM adrenaline 1:1,000 or IV adrenaline 1:10,000.
     b. Inject antivenin in allergic or sensitive patients under cover of antihistamines and hydrocortisone given 15–30 minutes before administration of the antivenin.
- **Anticholinesterases**: For patients with severe neurotoxic symptoms, administer test dose of IV edrophonium chloride (Tensilon) 10 mg with IV atropine 0.6 mg. If response is convincing, administer IV neostigmine.
- **Analgesia/sedation**: Pain and agitation may be severe. Administer morphine or diazepam, or both, in small doses IV titrating to effect. Be prepared to intubate since some degree of respiratory depression may already exist due to muscular weakness resulting from toxicity from the snake venom.

Disposition

- Admit all snake bites for observation. If severe, seek ICU medical team consultation.

References/further reading

1. Gopalakrishnakone P, Chou LM, Aye MM, et al. *Snake Bites and their Treatment.* Singapore: Singapore University Press; 1990.
2. Gopalakrishnakone P, How J. A field guide to dangerous snakes. Headquarters Medical Services.
3. Gopalakrishnakone P, Chou LM. *Snakes of Medical Importance (Asia-Pacific Region).* Venom and Toxin Research Group National University of Singapore and International Society on Toxinology (Asia-Pacific Section). Singapore: Singapore University Press; 1990.
4. Podgorny G. Reptile bites and scorpion stings. In: Tintinalli JE, Ruiz E, Krome RL, eds. *Emergency Medicine: A Comprehensive Study Guide*. 3rd ed. New York: McGraw-Hill; 1992:660–665.
5. Kunkel DB. Bites of venomous reptiles. *Emerg Med Clin North America.* 1984;2:563.
6. Nelson BK. Snake venomation, incidence, clinical presentation and management. *Med Toxicol*. 1989;4:17.
7. Podgorny G. Treatment of snake bite. In: Hadad LM, Winchester JF, eds. *Clinical Management of Poisoning and Drug Overdose.* Philadelphia: Saunders; 1983.
8. Wythe ET. Snakebite. In: Olson KR, ed. *Poisoning and Drug Overdose*. 2nd ed. Connecticut: Prentice-Hall; 1994:285–288,312–313.
9. Kearney TE. Antivenin, Crotalidae (rattlesnake). In: Olson KR, ed. *Poisoning and Drug Overdose.* 2nd ed. Connecticut: Prentice-Hall; 1994:312–313.
10. Hurlbut KM, Dart RC, Spaite D. Reliability of clinical presentation for predicting significant pit viper envenomation. *Ann Emerg Med.* 1988;12:438.
11. White RR, Weber RA. Poisonous snakebite in central Texas: Possible indications for antivenin treatment. *Ann Surg.* 1991;213:466–471.
12. Otten EJ. Venomous animal injuries. In: Rosen R, Barkin RM, Braen CR, et al, eds. *Emergency Medicine: Concepts and Clinical Practice*. 3rd ed. St. Loius: Mosby Year Book; 1992.
13. Dart RC, Sullivan Jr. JB. Elapid snake envenomations. In: *The Clinical Practice of Emergency Medicine*. 2nd ed. Philadelphia: Lippincott-Raven; 1996.

45 Burns, major

Francis Lee • Shirley Ooi

CAVEATS

- **Definition of major burns** requiring admission to a **burns centre**:
  1. Partial thickness and full thickness of burns >10% body surface area (BSA) in children <10 years or adults >50 years.
  2. Partial thickness and full thickness of burns >20% BSA of adults in the other age groups.
  3. Partial thickness and full thickness of burns involving special areas: face, eyes, ears, head, neck, perineum, genitalia, hands, feet or those that involve skin overlying major joints.
  4. Full thickness burns >5% BSA in any age group.
  5. Significant electrical burns including lightning injury.
  6. Significant chemical burns.
  7. Suspected inhalation injury.
  8. Circumferential burns.
  9. Burn injury in patients with preexisting illness that could complicate management, prolong recovery or affect mortality.
- Assessment of a patient with major burns follows Advance Trauma Life Support (ATLS) principles. The primary survey stage screens for life-threatening injuries, such as airway problems and respiratory difficulties. The secondary survey involves a thorough examination of the patient. It is at this juncture that the extent of burns is assessed and fluid regime calculated.

INITIAL MANAGEMENT

- The burns patient should be assessed in the critical care or resuscitation area.
- After primary ABC assessment, an airway risk assessment is carried out and a decision could be made for prophylactic intubation. The **risk factors** arranged in increasing probability of **upper airway obstruction** are:
  1. Burns and scalds around the nose or mouth
  2. Soot in the nostrils or singed nasal hairs
  3. Burns of the tongue
  4. Swelling of the intraoral tissues
  5. Voice becoming hoarse
  6. Laryngeal oedema visible on laryngoscopy
  7. Inspiratory stridor

- Consider **intubation** if airway is at risk. Refer to *Airway Management/ Rapid Sequence Intubation*:
    1. As it is a potentially difficult airway, 'awake intubation technique' may be used first before RSI.
    2. Get cricothyroidotomy set to be on standby just in case intubation fails.
    3. All monitoring devices must be in place before RSI is commenced.
    4. Intubation should be carried out in the presence of a senior emergency physician or anaesthetist.
    5. Suxamethonium is **not** contraindicated in acute burns.
- 100% oxygen is given to those patients who do not require intubation.
- Establish IV access. Start a crystalloid infusion.
- **Investigations** are ordered:
    1. Mandatory blood investigations: FBC, urea/electrolytes/creatinine, liver function test, coagulation studies, capillary blood glucose
    2. Optional blood investigations: carboxyhaemoglobin level, ABG
    3. ECG and CXR should be performed
- Patient should be catheterized to assess urine output.
- Care should be taken to prevent hypothermia.

BURNS ASSESSMENT AND FLUID REGIME

- The severity of burns should be assessed. The depth of burn is documented as partial or full thickness. The extent of burns is assessed using the **Wallace Rule of 9** in adults (see Figure 1). For children, the differences in body proportion according to age mandates assessment with a **Lund-Browder chart** (see Figure 2).
- Remember the palm (excluding the fingers) of the patient's hand represents approximately 1% of the patient's BSA.
- Based on the size of burns wound assessed, the fluid regime is calculated. Any patient with burns >20% BSA needs circulatory volume support. Establish large bore (at least 16G) IV catheter in a peripheral vein. If the extent of burn precludes catheter placement through unburned skin, overlying burned skin should not deter catheter placement in an accessible vein. The upper extremities are preferable to lower extremities for venous access because of the high incidence of phlebitis and septic phlebitis in the saphenous veins. Many formulae have been developed using various combinations of crystalloids and colloids. The Parkland's formula in Table 1 is an example.

PAIN RELIEF

- Adequate pain relief should be given:
    1. IV Pethidine® 1 mg/kg or

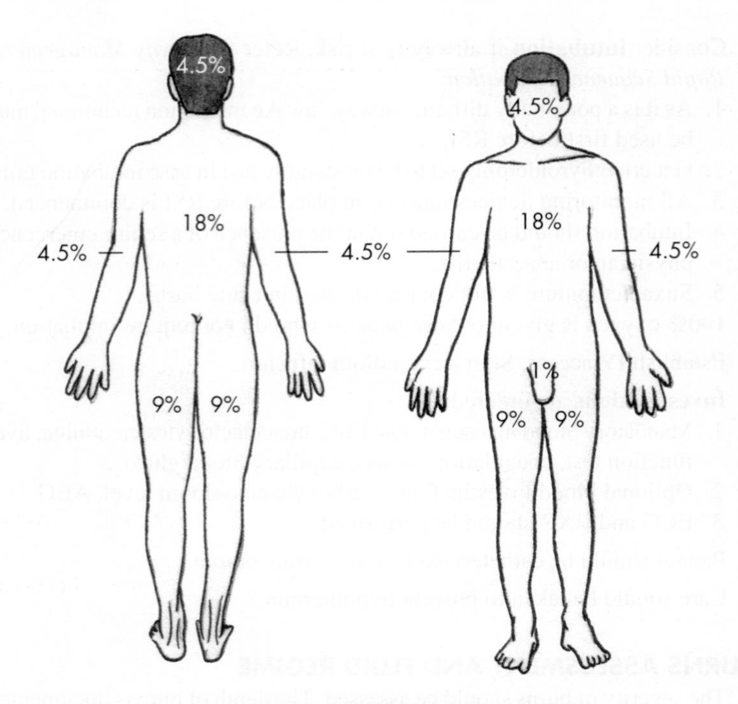

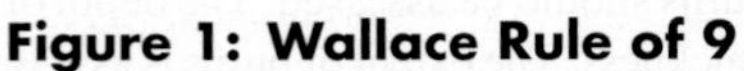
Figure 1: Wallace Rule of 9

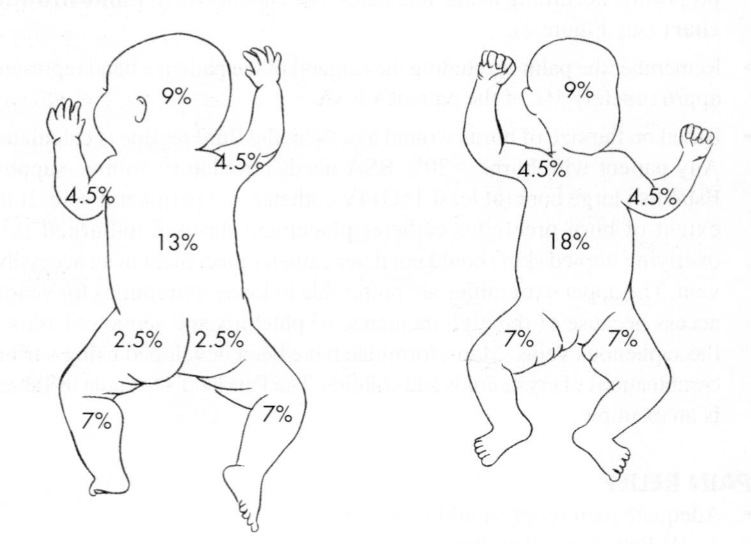

Figure 2: Lund-Browder chart

Table 1: The Parkland's formula

Total fluid requirements in the first 24 h = 2–4 ml/kg/% total BSA • Divide total volume into 2 halves • Infuse the first half in the first 8 h • Infuse the rest in the next 16 h **Start time = Time of burn injury** Fluid of choice = Hartmann's solution

2. IV morphine 2 mg every 30 min till pain relief achieved (maximum of 10 mg) or
3. IV tramadol 50 mg followed by an infusion
4. Entonox inhalation may be used during dressing

BURN WOUND MANAGEMENT

- The burns should be cooled, clean and covered with a dressing. Refer to *Burns, Minor*.
- **Escharotomy** should be performed for full thickness, circumferential burns of the trunk and limb:
  1. Escharotomy could be carried out without analgesia.
  2. A sterile knife is used.
  3. Incision should be carried out along anatomical lines, starting with a few lines and increasing when necessary. The incision must extend across the entire length of the eschar in the lateral and/or medial line of the limb including the joints. For circumferential burns of the thorax, bilateral escharotomy incisions in the anterior axillary lines should be considered if respiratory excursions are limited.
  4. The end point is that the depth of incision should reach the fat layer. Cutting till bleeding is seen is not recommended.

References/further reading

1. Settle J, ed. *Principles and Practise of Burns Management.* New York: Churchill Livingston; 1996.
2. Masellis M, Gunn SWA, eds. *The Management of Burns and Fire Disasters: Perspectives 2000.* Dordrecht: Kluwer Academic Publishers; 1995.
3. Herndon DN. *Total Burns Care.* Philadelphia: W.B. Saunders; 1996.
4. Committee on Trauma of the American College of Surgeons. *Advanced Trauma Life Support for Doctors Manual.* 6th ed. Chicago, American College of Surgeons: 1997:273–83.

46 Burns, minor

Francis Lee • Peter Manning

DEFINITIONS

- **First-degree burns** (eg sunburn) are characterized by erythema, pain, and the absence of blisters. They are not life-threatening, and generally do not require intravenous fluid replacement.
- **Second-degree burns or partial-thickness burns** are characterized by a red or mottled appearance with associated swelling and blister formation. The surface may have a weeping, wet appearance and is painfully hypersensitive, even to air currents.
- **Full-degree or third-degree burns** usually appear dark and leathery. The skin also may appear translucent, mottled or waxy white. The surface may be red and does not blanch with pressure. The surface is painless and generally dry.

CAVEATS

- Burn wounds can be managed on an outpatient basis provided they do not fall into the following categories:
  1. Burns >15% body surface area (BSA) in adults, >10% in children
  2. Burns involving special areas: eyes, ears, face, hands, buttocks and perineum
  3. Suspected inhalation injury
  4. Circumferential burns
  5. Poor home support and poor patient compliance
  6. Electrical injury
  7. Full thickness burns
- **Cooling** is an important facet in the management of burn wounds that is seldom remembered. This action limits the damage produced by heat that is retained in the skin tissues, reduces swelling and relieves pain.
- **Alkali burns** are generally of greater significance than acid burns due to the former's tendency to penetrate into deeper tissues by liquefactive necrosis.

INITIAL MANAGEMENT OF MINOR BURNS

- Ensure that ABC is secure and vital signs are stable.
- Remove all burning objects from the wound.
- Remove all potentially constricting objects from the affected body region, eg bangles, rings.

☛ **Special Tips for GPs**

- Very often burn injuries warrant a referral to the ED. The quick management steps include:
  1. Quick assessment of patient's conscious state, airway, breathing and circulation to determine whether ambulance transport is needed.
  2. Quick cooling of burn wounds, as described below.
  3. If dressing cannot be performed, the burn area can be protected with a clean dry sheet of cloth or plastic wrap (clingfilm is a possible improvisation) and bandaged.
- **Hydrofluoric acid (HF) burns** are highly significant, regardless of size and must be referred to the ED.

- Cooling burns. This can be achieved using a '10–15' rule:
  1. Cooling of burns within 10–15 min of incident
  2. Using cold water (approximately 10–15°C)
  3. For 10–15 min
  4. From a distance of 10–15 cm
- The burn wound is then cleansed gently with a mild chlorhexidine solution or normal saline.
- The wound size should be documented for the purpose of follow-up (refer to *Burns, Major*).
- A dressing is then applied to the skin. There are various commercial preparations but a good burns dressing should consist of 3 layers:
  1. An inner non-adherent layer (eg gauze, Tulle-gras, Opsite)
  2. Middle absorbent layer (eg cotton wool, Gamgee)
  3. Outer protective layer (eg plastic wrap, bandage)
- Oral pain relief should be given.
- **Blisters** should be left alone unless they are large and tense. These should be aspirated using a clean needle. Blisters should not be deroofed as the skin layer acts as a good protective cover and natural dressing.
- **Minor facial burns** can be managed without the need for a dressing. The good circulation of the face contributes to good healing and low risk of infection:
  1. Cold saline is applied to the burn areas for 1–2 hours.
  2. Wounds are washed with mild antiseptic solution and then left to air.
  3. The patient is advised to wash his/her face twice daily with soap and water.

4. Avoidance of sun exposure for 15 days is necessary to prevent hyperpigmentation.
5. Patient should also be warned of possible swelling occurring in the first 3 days.

- **Antibiotic cream** is helpful but oral prophylaxis is unnecessary. A commonly used topical preparation is 1% silver sulphadiazine that can be applied onto the wound before dressing. Avoid the use of silver sulphadiazine in the following situations:
  1. Known allergy to sulpha drugs
  2. G6PD deficiency
  3. Late pregnancy
  4. Children <2 years old
  5. Sun-exposed areas, eg face and neck (silver tarnishes and leaves a black stain)

Note: It is unnecessary to use 1% silver sulphadiazine in superficial partial thickness burns.

- **Tetanus immunization** status should be checked and tetanus toxoid administered.

Follow-up care of patients

- All patients treated as outpatients should be seen again in 24 hours. At this point, the wound is checked for extension of burns injury and presence of exudate strikethrough. If exudate is present, the following could be done:
  1. If excessive oozing occurs, another layer of dressing could be applied onto the existing one.
  2. If Opsite is the primary dressing, any exudate could be aspirated with a clean needle. An additional layer of Opsite is then applied onto the existing one.
  3. The attempt to remove dressing for the purpose of changing may affect wound healing as the peeling action disrupts newly formed epithelium and granulation tissues.
- A review in 72 hours is necessary for the purpose of detecting early signs of infection. Signs of infection include:
  1. Serosanguinous, pus-like or foul-smelling discharge
  2. Inflamed wound margins
  3. Wound tenderness
  4. Fever and chills
- If wound healing is uncomplicated, the patient could be referred to an appropriate physician (GP, outpatient service, etc) for follow-up in 5 days. During the follow-up, a change of the outer layer and middle absorbent layer of dressing may be necessary. A partial thickness burn wound generally heals in 10–15 days and the inner layer separates from the wound when new epithelium is formed.

SPECIAL BURNS

Tar or asphalt burns

- Superficial black tar can be removed 30–45 minutes after applying a layer of white paraffin or Neosporin ointment.
- Embedded tar should be left alone as attempts at removal often cause more damage.
- The embedded tar will separate when new epithelium is formed.

Acid/alkali burns

- Burn wounds by chemicals should be thoroughly irrigated with water.
- Adequacy of decontamination could be assessed with litmus paper.
- No attempt should be made to neutralize the opposite chemicals. The exothermic reaction produced by neutralization causes thermal injury to the wound.

Hydrofluoric acid burns

- Hydrogen fluoride (HF) is primarily an industrial raw material. It is used in separating uranium isotopes, as a cracking catalyst in oil refineries, and for etching glass and enamel, removing rust, and cleaning brass and crystal. It is also used in manufacturing silicon semiconductor chips. Some consumer products that may contain HF include automotive cleaning products, rust inhibitors, rust removers and water-spot removers.
- HF acts like alkalis and will cause progressive tissue loss including bony destruction.
- HF is one of the strongest inorganic acids, causing tissue damage by two mechanisms: a corrosive burn from the free hydrogen ions, and a chemical burn from tissue penetration of the fluoride ions. Fluoride ions penetrate and form insoluble salts with calcium and magnesium, and poison cellular enzymatic reactions. Soluble salts are also formed with other cations but dissociate rapidly, releasing the fluoride ions, and causing further tissue destruction.
- Absorption of fluoride ions can result in hypocalcaemia, hypomagnesaemia, hyperkalaemia and cardiac arrest.
- Dysrhythmias are a primary cause of death.
- Hypocalcaemia should be considered in all instances of inhalation and ingestion exposure and whenever skin burns exceed 60 cm^2.
- Patients exposed to solution of 7% or less may take 12–24 hours before onset of symptoms.
- The adverse action of fluoride ions may progress for several days.

- **Potential sequelae**:
  1. Fingertip injuries cause persistent pain, bone loss and nail bed injury.
  2. Skin burns heal slowly with extensive scarring.
  3. Eye exposure can lead to prolonged or permanent visual defects, blindness or total eye destruction.
  4. Ingestion exposure may lead to oesophageal strictures.
- **Exposure to skin**:
  1. HF burns are a unique clinical entity; burns to the fingers and nail beds may leave the overlying nails intact.
  2. Contact with <7% concentration produces no immediate pain on contact. Delayed serious injury may occur up to 24 hours later.
  3. Contact with 12% concentration causes a throbbing pain and swelling, often delayed up to 8 hours.
  4. Contact with >14% causes immediate severe throbbing pain and a whitish skin discolouration and blisters.
- **Exposure to eyes**: range from eye irritation to death of superficial cells leading to permanent clouding.

Management of HF burns

- Consists of supportive care and the use of specific antidotes in the form of calcium-containing medications. **Calcium gluconate** is given to bind the enzyme-poisoning fluoride ion and curtail its toxic effects. It can be given topically, subcutaneously, intradermally, by intraarterial infusion or by intravenous regional perfusion technique based on Bier's method.

Note: A hydrogen fluoride antidote should be kept in the ED pharmacy. Liberal consultations with multiple specialties are encouraged.

- Decon: rapid skin decontamination is critical.
- ABCs:
  1. Evaluate and support airway.
  2. Intubate orotracheally if ventilation/oxygenation is compromised.
  3. Get cricothyroidotomy set to be on standby in case intubation is not achieved.
  4. Administer 100% supplemental oxygen in patients with respiratory symptoms.
  5. Monitoring: ECG, vital signs q 5–15 min, pulse oximetry.

Note: Hypocalcaemia may cause a prolonged Q-T interval and dysrhythmias.

- Inhalation exposure: administer calcium gluconate nebulizer therapies (25 ml of calcium gluconate diluted to 100 ml of water) for patients with severe respiratory distress.
- **Blisters**:
  1. Open and drain, and debride necrotic tissue before treatment.
  2. Then, continuously massage the burned area with calcium gluconate gel until the pain is relieved.

Note: The main limitation of topical therapy is the impermeability of the skin to calcium.

3. The gel is available in the hydrogen fluoride antidote kit or can be constituted by dissolving 10% calcium gluconate solution in 3 times the volume of water-soluble lubricant, eg KY gel.
4. Ensure that staff wears rubber gloves during this procedure.
5. If some pain relief is not obtained within 30 to 60 minutes, consider calcium gluconate injections.

- **Large burns or deeply penetrating burns**:
  1. Inject sterile aqueous calcium gluconate into and around the burned area.
  2. Technique: inject 5% calcium gluconate using a small gauge needle (#27–30G). Do not inject more than 0.5 ml per cm^2.
  3. **Do not inject calcium chloride** to treat skin burns. It will cause extreme pain and cause further tissue injury.
- **Hand exposure**:
  1. Subungual burns often do not respond to immersion treatment.
  2. Consider nail avulsion to expose the area in contact with the acid.

Note: Digital block may be necessary but be aware that it may interfere with determining the adequacy of therapy.

3. Calcium gluconate may be injected in very small amounts into the involved digit using a very small gauge needle (#27–30G). Care must be taken since multiple injections into the fingers can lead to tissue ischaemia.
4. An alternative to digital block is IV regional calcium gluconate. Technique: using a Bier's ischaemic arm block technique, infuse an IV solution of 10–15 ml of 10% calcium gluconate plus 5,000 units of heparin diluted up to 40 ml in 5% dextrose saline. Endpoint is:
   a. Pain relief in the digit(s).
   b. The cuff is more painful than the burn.
   c. 20 minutes of ischaemic time has elapsed.
5. Consult Hand Surgery for all cases except those where pain disappears completely with treatment.

- **Eye exposure**
  1. **Do not use oils, salves or ointments** for injured eyes.
  2. Continuous irrigation with sterile water or saline for 15 minutes.
  3. If pain persists, irrigate with 1% solution of calcium gluconate (50 ml of 10% solution in 450 ml of sterile saline).

Note: Do **not use** the **10% solution for eye irrigation**.

4. Test visual acuity:
   a. Instil fluorescein stain and perform slit lamp examination.
   b. Obtain opthalmoscopy consultation if corneal defects are noted.

- **Disposition**: admit all cases of HF acid burns.

References/further reading

1. Richter F, Fuilla C, et al. The early cooling of burns. In: Masellis M, Gunn SWA, eds. *The Management of Mass Burn Casualties and Fire Disasters.* London: Kluwer Academic Publishers; 1992:273.
2. Jeffcott M. The nursing of the burned patient. In: *Burncare*. Hull: Smith & Nephew Limited & British Burn Association; 1986:87.
3. Wilson G, French G. Plasticised polyvinyl chloride as a temporary dressing for burns. *British Medical Journal.* 1987;294:556–567.
4. U.S. Department of Health and Human Services. Public Health Service Agency for Toxic Substances and Disease Registry. Hydrogen fluoride. In: *Medical Management Guidelines for Acute Chemical Exposure*. Volume III. California: 1994:11–15.

47 Chronic obstructive lung disease

Quek Lit Sin • Malcolm Mahadevan

DEFINITION

- Chronic obstructive lung disease (COLD), or chronic obstructive pulmonary disease (COPD) is characterized by partially reversible airflow limitation which is progressive and associated with an abnormal inflammatory response of the lungs to noxious particles or gases.

CAVEATS

- **Characteristic symptoms** include cough, chronic sputum production and exercise-induced dyspnoea with a majority of patients having been exposed to tobacco.
- About 10% of COLD patients have no smoking history.
- 10% of COLD patients have clinical features of asthma and should be treated as asthma.

> **☛ Special Tips for GPs**
>
> - Advise all patients with COLD to quit smoking as this is the most important intervention.
> - Flu vaccination should also be considered as it has been shown to reduce exacerbations.

DIFFERENTIAL DIAGNOSIS

- Congestive heart failure (CHF): beta natriuretic peptide may be one of the best ways to distinguish COLD from CHF
- Acute coronary syndrome
- Pulmonary embolism (PE)
- Pneumothorax/lung collapse
- Pneumonia

MANAGEMENT

- **Supplemental low-flow controlled O_2** for all patients with respiratory distress or SpO_2 <90% aiming for a saturation of 90–95%. Oxygen delivery may be by nasal prongs or venturi mask (venti mask).
- **Indications for RSI and ventilation**:
  1. Imminent respiratory arrest.
  2. Severe or profound dyspnoea.

Table 1: Classification of COLD by severity according to global initiative for chronic obstructive lung disease (GOLD)

0: At risk	Normal spirometry Chronic symptoms (cough, sputum production)
I: Mild	FEV_1/FVC <70% FEV_1 ≥80% predicted With or without chronic symptoms (cough, sputum production)
II: Moderate	FEV_1/FVC <70% 30% ≤ FEV_1 <80% predicted
III: Severe	FEV_1/FVC <70% FEV_1 <30% predicted or FEV_1 <50% predicted plus respiratory failure* or clinical signs of right heart failure

* Respiratory failure = arterial partial pressure of oxygen (PaO_2) <8.0 kPA (60 mm Hg) with or without arterial partial pressure of CO_2 ($PaCO_2$) >6.7 kPa (50 mm Hg)

3. Severe acidosis or hypercapnia.
4. Altered mental state.
5. Shock.

Note: Ventilatory settings should be low rates, low tidal volumes and prolonged expiratory phase.

- **Medications** include:
  1. β_2- agonists: salbutamol 5 mg (1 ml) nebulized. The efficacy of this depends on the reversibility of the patient's COLD.
  2. Anticholinergics: ipratropium bromide 2 ml (0.5 mg). Combining 1 and 2 has no additional side effects and provides superior bronchodilation compared with using either alone.
  3. Corticosteroids: 0.5–1.5 mg/kg of oral prednisolone for 10 days to 2 weeks.
  4. Methylxanthines (aminophylline) have NOT been shown to improve FEV_1 or affect hospital admission.
  5. Antibiotics: indications include increased SOB, increased sputum levels and increased sputum purulence. Common colonizers of respiratory tract include *Strep pneumoniae, Haemophilus influenzae, Moraxella catarrhalis, Klebsiella, Mycoplasma, Pseudomonas* and *Streptococcus*. Useful antibiotics include the advanced generation macrolides and quinolones.

Note: Magnesium sulphate has not been found to be useful for COLD.

- **Non-invasive ventilation (NIV)**, the new standard in care, will reduce mortality, the need for intubation, complications and length of stay when compared with the usual medical treatment. The **indications for NIV** are:
  1. Moderate respiratory acidosis (**pH 7.26–7.32**).
  2. Persistent respiratory distress (RR >22/min) following the initial treatment of acute exacerbation of COPD.

- Patients **not suitable for NIV** are those with:
  1. Respiratory arrest.
  2. Cardiovascular instability (hypotension, arrhythmias, myocardial infarction).
  3. Impaired mental state and increasing drowsiness.
  4. High aspiration risk.
  5. Recent facial or gastroesophageal surgery.
  6. Craniofacial trauma and fixed nasopharyngeal abnormalities.
  7. Extreme obesity.
- **Discharge criteria** include:
  1. Inhaled β_2-agonist therapy required no more frequently than every 4 hours.
  2. The patient who is previously ambulant is able to walk comfortably.
  3. The patient has been clinically stable for 12–24 hours.
  4. ABGs have been stable for 12–24 hours.
  5. The patient or caregiver fully understands the correct use of medications.
  6. Follow-up and home care arrangements have been completed.
  7. The patient, his/her family and the physician are confident that the patient can manage successfully.

References/further reading

1. Barnes PJ. New therapies for COPD. *Thorax*. 1998;53(2):137–147.
2. Barnes PJ. Mechanism in COPD: Differences from asthma. *Chest*. 2000;117(2 suppl):10s–14s.
3. Pauwels RA, Buist AS, Calverley PM, et al. Global strategy for the diagnosis, management, and prevention of chronic obstructive pulmonary disease. NHLBI/WHO Global Initiative for Chronic Obstructive Lung Disease (GOLD) Workshop summary. *Am J Respir Crit Care Med*. 2001;163(5):1256–1276. Review.
4. Dao Q, Krishnasuramy P, Kazanegra R, et al. Utility of β-type natriuretic peptide in the diagnosis of CHF in an urgent care setting. *J Am Coll Cardiol*. 2001;37(2):379–385.
5. Friedman M. Combined bronchodilator therapy in the management of chronic obstructive pulmonary disease. *Respirology*. 1997;2 Suppl 1:S19–S23. Review.
6. Campbell S. For COPD a combination of ipratropium bromide and albuterol sulfate is more effective than albuterol base. *Arch Intern Med*. 1999;159(2):156–160.
7. Gross N, Tashkin D, Miller R, et al. Inhalation by nebulization of albuterol-ipratropium combination (Dey combination) is superior to either agent alone in the treatment of chronic obstructive pulmonary disease. Dey Combination Solution Study Group. *Respiration*. 1998;65(5):354–362.
8. Routine nebulized ipratropium and albuterol together are better than either alone in COPD. The COMBIVENT Inhalation Solution Study Group. *Chest*. 1997;112(6):1514–1521.
9. Wood-Baker R, Walters EH, Gibson P. Oral corticosteroids for acute exacerbations of chronic obstructive pulmonary disease. *Cochrane Database Syst Rev*. 2001;(2);CD001288.
10. Barr RG, Rowe BH, Camargo CA Jr. Methylxanthines for exacerbations of chronic obstructive pulmonary disease. *Cochrane Database Syst Rev*. 2001;(1):CD002168.

11. Kramer N, Meyer TJ, Meharg J, et al. Randomized, prospective trial of non-invasive positive pressure ventilation in acute respiratory failure. *Am J Respir Crit Care Med.* 1995;151(6):1799–1806.
12. Bott J, Carroll MP, Conway JH, et al. Randomized controlled atrial of nasal ventilation in acute ventilatory failure due to chronic obstructive airway disease. *Lancet.* 1993;341(8860):1555–1557.
13. Mehta S, Hill NS. Noninvasive ventilation. *Am J Respir Crit Care Med.* 2001;163(2):540–577.

48 Coronary syndromes, acute

Shirley Ooi

DEFINTION

Acute coronary syndromes (ACS) include conditions that share the same pathophysiology of coronary occlusion, ie unstable angina, non-ST elevation MI (NSTEMI) and ST-segment elevation MI (STEMI). However, as the management of **unstable angina** and **NSTEMI** are basically somewhat similar, the management will be covered in this chapter. The management of STEMI is covered in *Myocardial Infarction, Acute*.

CAVEATS

- **Patients usually present** with one of the following patterns of symptoms:
  1. New onset (<2 months) of severe angina.
  2. Abrupt worsening of previous angina, with symptoms becoming more frequent, more severe, or more prolonged and less responsive to glyceryl trinitrate (GTN).
  3. Prolonged (>15 minutes) angina occurring at rest.

Note: Non-STEMI should be diagnosed in any patient whose cardiac enzymes are raised without evidence of acute Q-wave MI. A NSTEMI does not need to have ECG changes present.

- **The ECG** may show:
  1. ST segment depression.
  2. Transient ST segment elevation that resolves spontaneously or after GTN.
  3. T wave inversion.
  4. Evidence of previous myocardial infarction.
  5. Left bundle branch block.
  6. Minor non-specific changes.
  7. Or it can be normal.

  The ECG should **not** show persistent acute ST segment elevation.
- Conventional **cardiac enzymes** (CK, CK-MB, AST, LDH) may be normal or elevated. Elevated **troponin T** or **I** concentrations are highly specific for myocardial damage and identify patients at high risk for complications. Troponin T >0.1 μg/l, positive qualitative troponin T test and troponin I >0.4 μg/l are independent markers associated with an increased risk of early death in patients with an ACS without ECG ST segment elevation. The higher the troponin concentration the greater the risk of death within 30–42 days of presentation. Normal or undetectable troponin concentrations >12 hours after the onset of symptoms identify patients with a low risk of early complication.

- Studies of troponin T compared with troponin I indicate that the two markers are equally sensitive and specific, have similar prognostic significance, and support their role in risk stratification.
- For those with ACS, **the risk of an early adverse outcome is increased** in the following circumstances:
  1. Age >65 years old.
  2. Comorbidity, especially DM.
  3. Prolonged (>15 minutes) cardiac pain at rest.
  4. Ischaemic ECG ST segment depression on admission or during symptoms.
  5. ECG showing T wave inversion (associated with a risk intermediate between that associated with ST segment depression and a normal ECG).
  6. Evidence of impairment of left ventricular function (either preexisting or during myocardial ischaemia).
  7. Positive cardiac troponin release.
  8. Elevated C-reactive protein (determined by specific high sensitivity assay).
- **Low risk categories**: a normal cardiac troponin at 12 hours after the onset of symptoms can identify a group of people at low risk of immediate cardiac events; furthermore these patients who also have a normal ECG and normal cardiac enzymes (CK-MB) do not need admission to CCU or high dependency unit.
- **Treatment** aims consist of control of symptoms and prevention of MI and death. This can be achieved by instituting **antiischaemic** and **antithrombotic therapy** in the first instance, and if this is not successful, follow up with mechanical revascularization.
- It is important to manage **hypertension and heart failure** in the acute phase of ACS, as treatment can diminish wall stress and myocardial ischaemia, and can help to stabilize the patient.
- **Thrombolytic treatment** has **not** been shown to be of benefit in patients with ACS without ECG ST segment elevation (except for those with suspected acute MI and left bundle branch block).

> ☛ **Special Tips for GPs**
> - Refer all cases of ACS to the emergency department.
> - Give aspirin 300 mg stat before sending the patient to hospital.

MANAGEMENT

Continuing ischaemic chest pain/ECG changes suggestive of unstable angina or NSTEMI

- Monitor vital signs in the critical care area.

- Give oxygen via mask.
- Oral **aspirin** 300 mg.

Note: This is the mainstay of ACS therapy. It achieves platelet inhibition within 1 hour. Avoid enteric-coated aspirin because its onset of action is delayed 3–4 hours. Aspirin reduces the risk of cardiac death and non-fatal myocardial infarction by about 50% at 3 months.

- **IV plug** and **blood tests,** ie FBC, urea/electrolytes/creatinine, cardiac enzymes, cardiac troponin T or I, coagulation profile, GXM 2 units packed cells.
- Give **IV GTN** 20–200 μg/min to relieve pain or ischaemia. Increase in increments of 5–10 μg/min at 5–10 min intervals until chest pain resolves or mean arterial pressure decreases by 10%. Discontinue if hypotensive.

Note: IV GTN is especially useful in patients with ACS and hypertension/heart failure. There is no evidence that administration by IV infusion is more efficacious than equipotent doses of long-acting nitrates given by other routes, but titration of dose may be quicker and easier to manage with IV administration. GTN is contraindicated in right ventricular infarction.

- Give **IV morphine** in titratable doses for pain relief if chest pain persists despite IV GTN.
- Give **beta-blockers** to reduce risk of infarction if no contraindications, eg heart failure, respiratory failure, more than or equal to 2nd degree heart block, systolic blood pressure <90 mm Hg.
  Eg: Oral atenolol/metoprolol 50–100 mg/day.
- Give **calcium channel blockers** in conjunction with beta-blockers or in patients with contraindications to beta-blockers but with no heart failure or left ventricular dysfunction. Titrate to HR ~ 60/min.
  Eg: IV diltiazem 5 mg over 2–5 min, repeated every 5–10 min up to total dose of 50 mg. Follow by infusion of 5 mg/min up to 15 mg/min.
- **Heparin**, when used IV, reduces the incidence of recurrent ischaemia and progression to Q-wave MI.
  Use of IV heparin requires careful monitoring of the level of anticoagulation and is relatively labour-intensive. Monitoring is not necessary in low molecular weight heparins and their action is more predictable because of their almost complete bioavailability. They must be given twice daily by subcutaneous injection for at least 3 days and they appear to have similar efficacy to IV heparin.

Note: The following have been shown to reduce the risk of complications in patients with unstable angina and non-STEMI:

1. Unfractionated heparin without aspirin is more effective than placebo.
2. Unfractionated heparin combined with aspirin may be more effective than aspirin alone.
3. Low molecular weight heparin combined with aspirin is more effective than aspirin alone.

- High risk cases should be treated with an **intravenous small molecule platelet glycoprotein IIb/IIIa inhibitor** for up to 96 hours. It should also be given to those with elevated troponin T who are scheduled to undergo percutaneous coronary intervention using unfractionated heparin. This should commence before intervention. The three currently available agents are abciximab, tirofiban and eptifibatide.
- **Detection and correction of an obvious precipitating factor**, eg anaemia, fever, thyrotoxicosis, hypoxia, tachydysrhythmias, aortic stenosis or sympathomimetic drugs.
- Do chest x-ray.
- Admit to CCU.

Diagnosis of unstable angina made on clinical grounds without ECG changes/non-specific ECG changes present and patient already free of chest pain

- Monitor in the intermediate area.
- Give oral **aspirin** 300 mg.
- Set up **IV plug and take blood for tests**, ie FBC, urea/electrolytes/creatinine, cardiac enzymes, cardiac troponin T or I, coagulation profile, group and cross match 2 units packed cells.
- Apply **nitroderm patch** 5–10 mg depending on BP.
- Do chest x-ray.
- Admit to **Cardiology general ward**.

References/further reading

1. Guidelines for the management of patients with acute coronary syndromes without persistent ECG ST segment elevation by the British Cardiac Society Guidelines and Medical Practice Committee, and Royal College of Physicians Clinical Effectiveness and Evaluation Unit. *Heart* 2001;85:133–142.
2. Acute myocardial infarction and unstable angina: Acute coronary syndromes. In: McConachie I, Roberts DH, eds. *Handbook of Cardiac Emergencies*. London: Greenwich Medical Media Ltd; 2000:168–173.
3. Kleinschmidt K. Acute coronary syndromes (ACS): Pharmacotherapeutic interventions – Treatment guidelines for patients with and without procedural coronary intervention (PCI). Part I: Clinical pathophysiology and antiplatelet agents. Part II: Evidence-based analysis of antithrombin therapy – Standard heparin vs low molecular weight heparins. Part III: Fibrinolytic therapy, procedural coronary. *Emerg Med Rep.* Nov 6, Nov 20, Dec 4, 2000.

49 Crush syndrome

Irwani Ibrahim

CAVEATS

- Failure to recognize this condition results in full-blown crush syndrome, which has high mortality.
- Toxic metabolites released from the crushed muscle result in:
  1. Blocked renal tubules leading to renal failure.
  2. Electrolyte and acid base imbalance causing dysrhythmias followed by DIVC.
- **Causes**:
  1. Burns.
  2. Prolonged entrapment >60 minutes involving large muscle mass, eg in crush injuries, alcoholics or drug abusers who have lain on a limb during a period of prolonged unconsciousness.
  3. Non-traumatic neuroleptic malignant syndrome.
  4. Exertional prolonged grand mal fits.
- **Problems of crush syndrome**: hypovolaemia, hyperkalaemia, hypocalcaemia, myoglobinuria, renal failure, ARDS, DIVC.

> ☛ **Special Tips for GPs**
> - Vigorous fluid resuscitation as early as possible preferably at the scene is beneficial.

MANAGEMENT

- ABC as in major trauma protocol.
- Establish 2 large bore intravenous lines and **vigorous** fluid resuscitation **immediately** at least 1.5l/h preferably at the scene.
- Labs: FBC, urea/electrolytes/creatinine, serum calcium, coagulation profile.
- Do urinalysis for myoglobin.
- ECG to detect arrhythmia as a result of hypocalcaemia and hyperkalaemia.
- Monitor urine output closely: consider inserting urinary catheter. If urine output is poor, consider forced mannitol-alkaline diuresis till urine reaches pH >6.5.
- Consider antitetanus prophylaxis if there are open wounds.
- Inform Orthopaedic Registrar who may arrange for immediate fasciotomy.

References/further reading

1. Greaves I, Porter K, Burke D. *Key Topics in Trauma.* Oxford: Bios Scientific Publishers; 1997:74–75.
2. Michaelson M. Crush injury and crush syndrome. *World J of Surgery*. 1992;16(5): 899–903.

50 Dengue fever

Quek Lit Sin

DEFINITION

Dengue fever is an acute febrile infectious disease, caused by a virus from the genus Flavivirus, vector: *Aedes aegypti*. The pathophysiology of the disease is the result of an abrupt increase in capillary permeability, with diffuse capillary leakage of plasma, haemoconcentration and, in some cases, non-haemorrhagic hypovolaemic shock. Incubation period: 3–6 days; some cases may reach 15 days.

CLINICAL MANIFESTATIONS

Dengue fever (DF)

- The clinical symptoms of dengue fever in its early stages are similar to those of a patient with a viral infection.
- It is characterized by fever and thrombocytopaenia.

Dengue haemorrhagic fever (DHF)

- The early phase of illness is indistinguishable from dengue fever.
- After 2–5 days, a few cases in the first infection, or more commonly after reinfection by another serotype, patient may present with **thrombocytopaenia (<100,000/mm^3)** and **haemoconcentration** (haematocrit elevated by >20% or haematocrit >45%).
- Haemorrhagic manifestations may or may not occur; the spleen is not palpable, but hepatic enlargement and tenderness are signs of bad prognosis.
- Other manifestations include: **pleural effusion, hypoalbuminaemia, and encephalopathy with normal cerebrospinal fluid**.
- **Acute liver failure** with unusual change in consciousness or abnormal neurological signs (hyperreflexia) may occur. Such patients succumb quickly from severe haemorrhage, renal failure, brain oedema, pulmonary oedema and superimposed infection. Early intervention is necessary. Diffuse capillary leakage of plasma is responsible for the haemoconcentration.
- **Dengue haemorrhagic fever** is classified according to the following by the **World Health Organization classification**:

  Grade I Fever, constitutional symptoms and a positive tourniquet test
  Grade II Grade I and presence of spontaneous bleeding
  Grade III Grade II and haemodynamic instability with mental confusion
  Grade IV Grade III with profound shock

  Cases are accompanied by thrombocytopaenia and haemoconcentration. Grades III and IV denote **dengue shock syndrome (DSS)**.

CAVEATS

- The diagnosis of dengue fever at the ED is clinical and often the first diagnosis that crosses the emergency physician's mind when the fever persists >3 days and is recalcitrant to treatment.
- Abdominal symptoms like nausea, vomiting, epigastric pain and diarrhoea often mislead us into making a diagnosis of gastroenteritis or viral gastritis. This is especially true in children.
- It is often the persistent high and prolonged fever that is resistant to treatment that leads us to investigate further. This is particularly true for patients living or working in dengue prone areas.
- Some patients may also present with severe backaches.
- Patients who have family members with suspected dengue infection run a higher risk of having the same infection. With this history in a symptomatic patient, it is necessary to monitor platelet counts.

> ☛ **Special Tips for GPs**
>
> - Skin rash of *generalized erythema with pockets of sparing over the lower limbs* is not consistent. However, patients with dengue often appear to be flushed over the face. Occasionally, patients may come with a history of bleeding from the gums.
> - Refer all cases of suspected or confirmed DHF or DSS immediately to the hospital for inpatient management.

MANAGEMENT

- No specific treatment of dengue is available. Early institution of supportive treatment (fluids replacement and correction of electrolyte imbalances) is the key to managing patients with dengue in all its forms.
  1. Monitor platelet counts daily till they show an upward trend.
  2. Monitor coagulation profile closely; repeat test if necessary.
- Ill patients must be managed in the critical care area where they can be monitored.
- **A FBC is essential for any patient who presents with persistently high fever with no definite focus of infection. Important lab findings in a patient who has dengue** are:
  1. Leukopaenia: the presence of leukocytosis and neutrophilia excludes the possibility of dengue, and bacterial infections must be considered.
  2. Thrombocytopaenia (<100,000/mm^3): leptospirosis, measles, rubella, meningococcaemia, septicaemia, malaria and Severe Acute Respiratory Syndrome (SARS) may also cause thrombocytopaenia but rash is unusual in uncomplicated malaria.

3. Haematocrit showing haemoconcentration.
4. Urea and electrolytes: may show hyponatremia.
5. Liver function test: abnormal liver enzymes.

- Intensive monitoring of vital signs and markers of haemoconcentration, replacement of intravascular volume with lactated Ringer solution or isotonic saline, correction of metabolic acidosis, and oxygen therapy are life saving in patients with DSS. Once the patient is stabilized, capillary leakage stops and resorption of extravasated fluid begins, care must be taken not to induce pulmonary oedema with continued intravenous fluid administration.
- Salicylates should be avoided for symptom relief because of the potential bleeding diathesis and because dengue has been associated with Reye's syndrome in a few cases. Hepatotoxic drugs and long-acting sedatives should be avoided.
- **Disposition**: hospitalization for intravenous fluid therapy is necessary in cases where there are:
  1. Significant dehydration (>10% of normal body weight) has occurred and rapid volume expansion is needed or when there is spontaneous bleeding. This would mean that only patients in Grade I who are responding to oral fluid rehydration and who have no associated complications can be sent home.
  2. Clinical bleeding tendency.
  3. Severe thrombocytopaenia (ie platelets <100,000).
  4. A platelet count of <20,000 will necessitate bed rest for fear of spontaneous bleeding and accidental trauma.
  5. Patients who are elderly, very young and those with concomitant illness (ie allergies, diabetes mellitus, ischaemic heart disease).

Note: Those with a platelet count between 100,000–140,000 can be discharged but to return for serial FBC checks until platelet counts normalize.

References/further reading

1. World Health Organization (WHO). *Dengue Haemorrhagic Fever: Diagnosis, Treatment, Prevention and Control*. 2nd ed. Geneva: WHO; 1997.
2. Singapore Ministry of Health Clinical Guidelines on Dengue Fever/Dengue Haemorrhagic Fever. 2002.

51 Dermatology in emergency care

Peng Li Lee • Shirley Ooi

CAVEATS

- In a febrile patient with purpuric rash, consider **meningococcaemia**.
- In an ill patient with petechial rash, think of the possibility of DIVC from sepsis.
- In a hypotensive patient with joint pain and 'bruising', consider the possibility of **necrotizing soft tissue infections** which can be very deceptive in their initial presentation.
- It is still possible for a vaccinated person to have chicken pox although it is often very mild and may be mistaken for a 'viral fever'.
- Think of **varicella pneumonitis** if a patient has tachypnoea, cough and high fever 3–5 days into the course of illness.

> ☛ **Special Tips for GPs**
> - Quick reference for **meningococcaemia prophylaxis**: Single dose of ciprofloxacin 500 mg.

VARICELLA (CHICKEN POX)

Agent: varicella zoster virus (VZV).

Clinical features

- **Incubation period**: 10–21 days but is usually between 14 and 17 days.
- Usually preceded by prodrome: low-grade fever, malaise, myalgia (can be absent in young children).
- Early lesions may be macular or papular before the vesicles appear, followed by crusting.
- Generalized distribution including scalp, genital areas, oral mucosa and conjunctiva but predominantly in the trunk.
- Lesions appear in crops with differing stages of vesicles and crusting.
- Patients are **infectious** approximately 48 hours prior to onset of vesicular rash, during period of vesicle formation, generally 4–5 days, and until all vesicles are crusted.

Management

- Consider **acyclovir** if patient is seen within the first 24–72 h of onset of rash.
  Dosage: 800 mg (adults) or 20 mg/kg (paediatrics) 5× per day × 5 days.
- Antihistamine for control of itch may be considered, eg chlorpheniramine 4 mg tds.
- **Do not give aspirin** as an antipyretic as it may cause Reye's syndrome.
- Consider oral antibiotics if there are signs of bacterial infection, eg penicillin V (Group A *streptococcus* is a common causative organism)/cephalexin/ doxycycline (if penicillin/cephalexin allergic) or cloxacillin if *staphylococcus aureus* suspected.
- Immunocompromised patients should be admitted.

Complications

- Occur more commonly in adults and immunocompromised patients: aseptic meningitis, encephalitis, pneumonia, pneumonitis, transverse myelitis and Reye's syndrome.
- **Foetal varicella syndrome** is associated with phocomelia; **neonatal varicella** can be fatal and can be transmitted intrapartum.
- Immunity can be rapidly determined by IgG.

Isolation

- Advise isolation until no new vesicles erupt and all lesions are crusted.
- Pregnant women who are not immune should consider VZIg.

HERPES ZOSTER ('SHINGLES')

Represents reactivation of latent varicella zoster virus.

Clinical features

- Painful vesicles in unilateral dermatomic distribution.
- Common **sites** are torso, scalp and face.
- The **onset** of herpes zoster is heralded by pain within dermatome that may precede lesions by 48–72 hours, followed by an erythematons maculopapular rash which evolves rapidly to vesicular lesions.
- The total **duration** of disease is generally between 7 and 10 days; however it may take as long as 2–4 weeks before skin returns to normal.
- **Atypical presentations**:
  1. Pain unaccompanied by typical lesions.
  2. It may disseminate in immunocompromised patients.

- **Trigeminal herpes zoster** with involvement of the opthalmic nerve (**zoster ophthalmicus**) may result in corneal ulcers and loss of vision. Always do a fluorescein staining to exclude corneal ulcers when vesicles are seen on the bridge of the nose and around the eye and forehead.
- The most debilitating **complication** of herpes zoster is **pain** associated with acute neuritis and postherpetic neuralgia.

Management

- **Pain control** with analgesia in acute phase. Tricyclic antidepressants, eg amitriptyline 10 mg ON, may be considered for patients with persistent pain despite apparent healing of the lesions (**postherpetic neuralgia**); other agents include gabapentin and narcotics (used in severe cases).
- **Antiviral agent**, eg Acyclovir:
  1. Shown to shorten course of herpes zoster if given within first 48–72 h of rash onset.
  2. Dosage: Tab 800 mg 5 times a day for 7–10 days.
  3. Admit for intravenous acyclovir for immunocompromised patients who are ill or with extensive disease.
- **Steroids** may prevent postherpetic neuralgia.[5]
- Refer to Opthalmologist if there is corneal involvement.

PEMPHIGOID AND PEMPHIGUS

- Both are bullous diseases due to an autoimmune process.
- The mainstay of treatment for both bullous diseases is antiinflammatory.
- Skin biopsy is often indicated to confirm diagnosis.
- The differentiating clinical features are shown in Table 1.

Table 1: Differentiating features between pemphigoid and pemphigus

Features	*Pemphigoid*	*Pemphigus*
Age	Elderly	Young/middle-aged
Lesions	Tense blisters	Flaccid blisters that break easily to leave erosions
	Itchy	Painful
	Mucous membrane often spared	Mucous membrane commonly involved; often the presenting feature
Prognosis	More benign	Potentially lethal

Management

- Generally both **require inpatient management** for:
  1. Systemic steriods ± immunosuppressives
  2. Local wound care
  3. Treatment of infection
  4. Correction of fluid and electrolyte loss from large denuded skin

NECROTIZING SOFT TISSUES INFECTIONS

- A group of rapidly life-threatening bacterial infections of soft tissues characterized by tissue necrosis.
- Specific terms used depend on the tissues involved and causative organisms:
  1. Necrotizing fasciitis
  2. Necrotizing myositis
  3. Fournier's gangrene (genitalia)
- **Organisms**:
  1. Group *A Streptococci*
  2. Polymicrobial
  3. *Staphylococcus aureus*

Clinical features

- Toxic, febrile and often hypotensive ± confusion and delirium.
- The skin findings may be deceptively minor compared to the systemic toxicity of the patient.
- There is oedema and erythema initially, progressing to pallor and greyish discolouration with haemorrhagic bullae (due to ischaemia when blood vessels are destroyed) or gangrene.
- Abdominal pain is a common presenting complaint.

Differential diagnosis

- Cellulitis and other non-necrotizing soft tissue infections.
- *Erysipelas* has clearly demarcated margins and streaking in lymphangitis is prominent; vesicles and bullae may develop in severe infection (common organism: Group A beta-haemolytic *Streptococci*).

Management

- Patient should be managed in the critical care area with close monitoring.
- Fluid resuscitation and inotropic support if neccesary.
- Consider x-ray of the soft tissue area involved to look for free air in the subcutaneous tissue.

Note: Absence of it does not rule out the diagnosis.

- Do blood culture.

- Start broad spectrum antibiotics, eg IV **crystalline penicillin + clindamycin (for Group A *Streptococci* + Anaerobes with some *Staphalococcus* coverage) + ceftazidime (for gram-negative rods and meliodosis)**.
- Refer to Orthopaedic/General Surgeon (depending on the site involved) for immediate surgical exploration and debridement of necrotic tissue.
- **Disposition**: HD or ICU depending on the stability of the patient.

MENINGOCOCCAEMIA

Causative organism: *N. meningitidis* (gram-negative diplococci on initial CSF gram stain result).

Clinical features

- Abrupt onset of fever, malaise, myalgia, arthralgia, headache, nausea and vomiting.
- Generally toxic with rapid progression to obtundation and signs of meningitis.
- Associated cutaneous findings: scattered pink or purpuric papules (palpable lesions <1.5 cm) that may become vesicular or pustular.
- May progress to **purpura fulminans**: irregular but well-demarcated plaques of purple purpura with central grey, dusky, deep purple or black necrosis.

Management

- Patient should be managed in the critical care area with close monitoring.
- Fluid resuscitation and inotropic support if necessary.
- Do blood culture.
- Antibiotic may be started before lumbar puncture.
- Antibiotic of choice: IV **penicillin G 4 million units** 4 hourly (consider chloramphenicol if allergic to penicillin) or ceftriaxone 2 g bd.
- **Disposition**: HD or ICU (request for isolation).

Prophylaxis

- **Indications**:
  1. Close contacts for at least 4 hours during the week before illness onset, eg housemates, day care contacts, cellmates.
  2. Exposure to patient's nasopharyngeal secretions, eg via kissing, mouth-to-mouth resuscitation, intubation, nasotracheal suctioning.
- **Regime**:
  1. Ciprofloxacin 500 mg po single dose or rifampicin 600 mg po bd × 4 doses (adults).
  2. Rifampicin 10 mg/kg po bd × 4 doses (paediatrics).

ACUTE URTICARIA

A fairly common condition seen at ED due to the intense itch and sudden generalized rash that patients experience.

Clinical features

- Pink, non-scaling, flat-topped weals that are migratory.
- Lesions are pruritic.

Common causes

- Viral: suggested by recent history of fever, myalgia and URTI symptoms.
- Drugs: penicillin, sulfa, NSAIDs.
- Food allergies.
- Environmental factors: eg cold, sunlight, pressure.
- Unknown: there is often no obvious cause.

Management

- Identify and eliminate causative factors if possible.
- Symptomatic treatment.
- **Antihistamine**
  1. Parenteral route choices:
     - Promethazine: IM 25 mg (adults) or 0.5 mg/kg (paediatrics)
     - Diphenhydramine: IM 25 mg (adults) or 1 mg/kg (paediatrics)
  2. Oral route choices:
     - Chlorpheniramine (Piriton®): Tab 4 mg tds
     - Hydroxyzine (Atarax®): Tab 25 mg tds
     - Newer less sedative options: cetirizine (Zyrtec®), loratadine (Clarityne®)
- **Steroids**:
  1. To be considered if lesions are extensive and recurrent, or associated with angioedema.
  2. Prednisolone tab 1 mg/kg OM for 5 days
- **Disposition:** Can be discharged if the response to treatment is prompt and there is no associated angioedema.

ERYTHEMA MULTIFORME

A hypersensitivity reaction, classified as:

- EM minor: milder and more common form.
- EM major/bullous EM/Stevens–Johnson syndrome: significant blistering and erosions of mucous membranes.

Clinical features

- Red, flat-topped papule 1–3 cm.
- Non-pruritic and non-scaling.
- Bull's eye or target lesions: dusky, violaceous or brown centre.
- Fixed lesions.
- Usually starts in the hands and feet, including the palms and soles, before becoming generalized.
- Blistering can occur within the target lesions.
- Erosion of mucous membranes may be present.

Causes

- Infection: HSV, EBV, *Streptococcus*, *Mycoplasma* are common causes.
- Drugs: sulfa drugs, penicillin, tetracycline, anticonvulsants, (eg phenytoin, carbamazepine, barbiturates), NSAIDs, allopurinol, hydrochlorothiazide, procainamide,
- Other: autoimmune causes.

Management

- Determine **cause** and eliminate allergens if possible:
  1. Medication review
  2. Symptomatology review for common infectious diseases
  3. Food allergies
  4. Insect bites/stings
  5. Autoimmune diseases
- **EM minor**
  1. Provide reassurance if cause is proven and no evidence of progression.
  2. Medications generally are not required as the rash is generally not pruritic or painful.
  3. Follow-up in Dermatology/General Medicine clinic.
- **EM major**
  1. Admit for inpatient care.
  2. Provide general supportive care of fluid and electrolytes maintenance.
  3. Provide wound care.
  4. Control infection.
  5. Note that systemic steroids are controversial.
  6. Admit to Burn Unit or HD if significant skin loss or toxic epidermal necrolysis occurs.

ERYTHEMA NODOSUM

A hypersensitivity reaction.

Clinical features

- Acute onset of red tender nodules.
- Distributed mainly on the lower leg, especially the shins.

Causes

- Infections: *Streptococcus*, tuberculosis, infectious mononucleosis, *chlamydia*, *yersinia*.
- Associated with sarcoidosis, Hodgkin's disease, ulcerative disease.
- Drugs: oral contraceptives, sulphonamides, penicillin, tetracyclines.

Management

- Conduct systemic review for possible infections.
- Eliminate any precipitating cause.
- Symptomatic treatment, eg NSAIDs for pain relief.
- Refer to Dermatology for follow-up.

References/further reading

1. Edward L. *Dermatology in Emergency Care*. New York: Churchill Livingston; 1977.
2. Buton PK, et al. *ABC of Dermatology*. London: BMJ; 1998.
3. Gilbert DN, Moellering RC, Sande MA. *The Sanford Guide to Antimicrobial Therapy*. 30th ed. USA: Jeb C. Sanford; 2000.
4. Keczkes K, Basheer AM. Do corticosteroids prevent post-herpetic neuralgia? *Br J Dermatol.* 1980 May;102(5):551–555.

52 Diabetic ketoacidosis (DKA)

Peter Manning • Chong Chew Lan • Sim Tiong Beng

CAVEATS

- DKA is caused by an absolute or relative decrease in insulin levels in the presence of excessive glucagons. **Diagnostic criteria** are:
  1. Hyperglycaemia with blood glucose ≥14 mmol/l
  2. Acidaemia with arterial pH <7.3, bicarbonate <15 mmol/l
  3. Ketonaemia or ketonuria
- High plasma glucose level leads to osmotic diuresis with sodium and water loss, hypotension, hypoperfusion and shock. Patients present with significant polyuria, polydipsia, weight loss, dehydration, weakness and clouding of sensorium.
- Younger undiagnosed diabetics frequently present with DKA developing over 1–3 days. Plasma glucose level may not be grossly raised.
- GI complaints are common presenting symptoms, especially in the young. There may be nausea, vomiting and abdominal pain. This can be severe and misdiagnosed as 'acute surgical abdomen'. Serum amylase level is often elevated in the absence of pancreatitis.
- Hyperventilation with deep rapid breathing ('air hunger') and the smell of acetone on the breath is characteristic of DKA.
- **Causes**:
  1. Infection: common foci are UTI, respiratory tract, skin
  2. Infarction: myocardial, CVA, GIT, peripheral vasculature
  3. Insufficient insulin
  4. Intercurrent illness
- Signs of infection are often masked or deceptive. Temperature is rarely raised and increased total white count may only reflect ketonaemia; however, any fever, even low grade, indicates sepsis. If in doubt, it is probably safest to treat with a broad spectrum antibiotic.
- Over-rapid fluid replacement can cause cardiac failure, cerebral oedema, and ARDS, especially in patients with underlying cardiac disease or the elderly. CVP monitoring may be needed.

MANAGEMENT

Supportive measures

- Patient must be managed in a monitored area.
- Supplemental high-flow oxygen.

☛ **Special Tips for GPs**

- Have a high index of suspicion when seeing patients with complaints of nausea and vomiting, with or without abdominal pain. The 'viral gastritis' may turn out to be DKA.
- Check bedside blood sugar level for all toxic-looking febrile patients.
- Check bedside blood sugar level and urine dipstick for ketones if the diagnosis is suspected.
- Put up a normal saline infusion and give IV/IM insulin stat before sending to hospital by ambulance.

- Monitoring: ECG, pulse oximetry, vital signs q 15–30 min, blood levels of glucose, ketones, potassium and acid base balance q 1–2 hours.
- Labs: FBC, urea/electrolytes/creatinine/calcium/magnesium/phosphate (to include venous glucose), cardiac enzymes, DIC screen (if septic), urinalysis (for ketones and leucocytes), serum ketones (beta-hydroxybutyrate) and arterial blood gas.
- Consider blood culture (**at least** 7.5 ml blood per bottle).
- 12-lead ECG, CXR, urine dipstick: look for a cause of the DKA.
- Circulatory support: IV normal saline as the basic resuscitation fluid, switching to 0.45% NS as perfusion improves and BP normalizes, then D_5W/0.45% NS as serum glucose level drops. Total fluid loss in DKA averages 4–6 litres.
- Urinary catheter to monitor urine output.

Specific measures

- **IV volume replacement**: administer normal saline at 15–20 ml/kg/h in the first hour, with recourse to colloids if patient is still hypotensive. Then, if patient is **not** hypotensive or hyponatraemic, administer 0.45% normal saline at 10–20 ml/kg/h over the next 2–4 hours with careful monitoring of the serum glucose level. Switch to D_5W/0.45% NS when serum glucose level falls below 14 mmol/l. Normal or half strength NS may be continued in conjunction with IV dextrose 5% to correct fluid/electrolyte derangements. Monitor urine output hourly, and check electrolytes and creatinine every 2–4 hours till stable.

Note: Fluid replacement should correct estimated deficits (4–6 litres) within the first 24 hours, but serum osmolality should not decrease by more than 3 mOsm/kg/h to avoid cerebral oedema.

- **Restoration of electrolyte balance**: early potassium replacement is now standard. If oliguria is present, renal function studies may be elevated. If abnormal, potassium replacement must be decreased. Establish that there is urine output first, then replace as follows:
  1. Serum K^+ <3.3 mmol/l, give 20–40 mEq KCl per hour.

Note: A concurrent low-dose insulin infusion will not reduce the serum potassium appreciably.

  2. Serum K^+ 3.3–4.9 mmol/l, give 10–20 mEq K^+ per hour (can be given as 2/3 KCL and 1/3 $KHPO_4$; phosphate replacement is indicated when serum phosphate <0.3 mmol/l) or if patient is anaemic or in cardiorespiratory distress.
  3. Serum K^+ >5.0 mmol/l, withhold potassium but check serum potassium every 2 hours.

- **Restoration of acid base balance**: sodium bicarbonate is to be given only if severe hyperkalaemia or if the arterial pH is <7.0, since IV volume replacement and, later, insulin will improve the metabolic acidosis. If pH is 6.9–7.0, give IV 8.4% $NaHCO_3$ 50 ml dilute in 200 ml NS and run over 1 h. If pH is <6.9, give 100 ml 8.4% $NaHCO_3$ dilute in 400 ml NS and run over 2 h.

Note: No beneficial but deleterious effects can occur when given at higher pH. Repeat the ABG after 1 hour of hydration and bicarbonate therapy; if pH still <7.0, administer 8.4% $NaHCO_3$ 50 ml in 200 ml NS over 1–2 hours as an infusion.

- **Insulin administration**: large doses are not needed to reverse DKA. In addition, hypoglycaemia and hypokalaemia are more likely to occur with large-dose insulin therapy.
  1. Administer a bolus dose of 0.15 units/kg body weight of IV SI in adults, followed by a low-dose continuous infusion of 0.1 units/kg body weight/hour in both adults and children. Adjust the infusion rate to obtain a drop serum glucose level by approx. 3–4 mmol/l per hour. Monitor blood glucose hourly.
  2. When blood glucose level falls below 14 mmol/l, **halve** the IV SI infusion rate to 0.05–0.1 units/kg/h and add dextrose in the IV fluids to aim for blood glucose level of 8–12 mmol/l. Maintain the SI infusion until acidosis clears (pH >7.3 and HCO_3 >15). SC SI q 4 h can then be instituted within an overlap period of 1–2 hours. Do **not** stop IV SI simply because blood glucose has normalized.
- **Treat precipitating factor**, eg sepsis, AMI.

Disposition

- Admit all cases of DKA.
- Patients with hypotension or oliguria refractory to initial rehydration, or who have mental obtundation/coma, with total serum osmolality >340 mOsm/kg, should be considered for HD or MICU.

- More mild cases can be admitted to a general ward or managed in the ED with input from the General Medicine registrar.

References/further reading

1. Wyatt JP, Illingworth RN, Clancy MJ, et al, eds. *Oxford Handbook of Accident and Emergency Medicine*. Oxford: Oxford University Press; 1999:152–153.
2. Singapore Ministry of Health Clinical Guidelines on Diabetes Mellitus 1999.
3. American Diabetes Association Position Statement. Hyperglycemic crises in patients with diabetes mellitus. *Diabetes Care*. 2003:26:S109–117.
4. Kitabchi AE, Umpierrez GE, Murphy MB, et al. Management of hyperglycemic crises in patients with diabetes (technical review). *Diabetes Care*. 2001;24(1):131–153.

53 Diving emergencies

Francis Lee

CAVEATS

- Two major diving emergencies may be seen in the ED:
  1. Decompression Illness (DCI)
  2. Cerebral arterial gas embolism (CAGE)
- **Diagnosis** requires a high index of suspicion:
  1. Recent (<24 h) participation in compressed air diving (using scuba or other types of breathing apparatus).
     plus
  2. Onset of new symptoms (a combination of any of these):
     General: malaise, unusual fatigue, amnesia, sense of ill-being
     Musculoskeletal: joint pains, myalgia, back pain
     Neurological: patchy numbness, weakness, gait, visual problems
     Chest: chest pain, dyspnoea, persistent coughing
     Skin: pruritic rash
- Table 1 shows the distribution of symptoms in 1,249 cases of decompression illness in recreational divers reported to the Divers Alert Network (DAN).

Table 1: Symptoms of decompression illness

Initial symptoms	*%*
Pain	40.7
Altered skin sensation	19.2
Dizziness	7.8
Extreme fatigue	5.7
Headache	5.7
Weakness	4.8
Nausea	2.9
Difficulty in breathing	2.5
Altered level of consciousness	2.1
Itching	1.6
Visual disturbance	1.5
Rash	1.1
Paralysis	1.0

> ☛ **Special Tips for GPs**
> - Think of diving emergencies in patients presenting with new vague symptoms but with a history of recent (<24 h) participation in compressed air diving.

MANAGEMENT

- Immediate: if patient is **stable** (most common presentation),
  1. Place patient at the intermediate area.
  2. Nurse in a head-down position.
  3. Give 100% oxygen.
  4. Set up IV drip.
  5. Run IV NS 500 ml over 1h followed by 500 ml over 4 h.
  6. If patient is unstable, management should be carried out in the critical care area. Patient's ABC should be assessed and monitoring is required. In very severe cases with cardiopulmonary complications or arrest, manage according to standard ACLS regime.
  7. Patient should also be checked for any physical trauma sustained concomitant to diving complications.
- **Investigations**
  1. CXR to look for pneumothorax or pneumomediastinum.
  2. ECG to exclude cardiac cause of chest pain if this is a primary symptom.
  3. ABG if patient is breathless or has low oxygen saturation.
- **Definitive**: the definitive treatment for diving emergencies is **immediate** recompression therapy.
  1. If you suspect that a patient has DCI or CAGE, you should seek advice from a diving medicine specialist, after initial stabilization of the patient.
  2. **If the diagnosis of a diving injury is certain, do not admit such patients to neurology or medical units 'for investigation' because**
     a. these departments have no recompression facility
     b. delay in treatment of DCI and CAGE increases morbidity or even mortality

COMPARISONS BETWEEN DCI AND CAGE

- Generally, the characteristics of **CAGE** can simply be described as **'fast, short and shallow'** and that of **DCI** as **'slow, long and deep'** (Table 2).

Table 2: Characteristics of CAGE and DCI

Factors	*CAGE*	*DCI*
Precipitating factors	Panic underwater, resulting in rapid uncontrolled ascent	Poor dive profile. Diving longer and deeper than recommended safety limits
Diving depth	Generally shallow. Can occur with depth as shallow as 3 metres	Usually deep, beyond limits
Time course/onset of symptoms	A rapid event, seconds to minutes Tends to be immediate, after surfacing	A slow event, few minutes to hours Delayed
Loss of consciousness	Frequent	Infrequent
Non-specific symptoms	Infrequent	Frequent
Joint pains	Uncommon	Very common
Neurological symptoms	Tends to be unilateral like a CVA	Tends to be bilateral and patchy
Sensory loss	Unilateral, focal	Common, patchy

References/further reading

1. Bennett P, Elliot D. *The Physiology and Medicine of Diving*. 4th ed. London: WB Saunders; 1993.
2. Edmonds C, Lowry C, Pennefather J. *Diving and Subaquatic Medicine*. 3rd ed. Boston: Butterworth-Heinemann; 1992.
3. Kindwall E, Whelan T. *Hyperbaric Medicine Practice*. 2nd ed. Flagstaff, AZ: Best Pub Co.; 1999.
4. Schilling CW, Carlston CB, Mathias RA. *The Physician's Guide to Diving Medicine*. New York: Plenum Press; 1984.

54 Eclampsia

Peter Manning

DEFINITIONS

- **Preeclampsia**: elevation of the systolic or diastolic BP that occurs after the 20th to 24th week of pregnancy in a previously normotensive or hypertensive woman.
- **Eclampsia**: preeclampsia and grand mal seizures (fits) or coma.

CAVEATS

- The aim of management is, first of all, to stabilize the mother and then deliver the baby:
  1. Maternal airway management.
  2. Prevention and control of convulsions with magnesium sulphate therapy.
  3. Restoration of intravascular volume.
  4. Control of BP.
- Delivery of baby: how and when the baby is delivered is a decision to be made by an O&G specialist.
- Immediate O&G consultation to be made when diagnosis is evident.
- **HELLP** syndrome is a very severe form of preeclampsia characterized by:
  1. **H**aemolysis
  2. **EL**evated liver enzymes and
  3. **L**ow **P**latelets (<100,000/mm^3).

  Symptoms: RHC pain with nausea and vomiting are the most common. Signs commonly include generalized oedema, RHC tenderness, jaundice, GIT bleeding and haematuria.

> ☛ **Special Tips for GPs**
> - 60% of cases occur during the first pregnancy.
> - Primagravidas at the extremes of age (<17 or >35 years old) are at increased risk.
> - Patients with a history of chronic hypertension are more prone to preeclampsia and eclampsia.

MANAGEMENT

Supportive measures

- Patient must be managed in the critical care area.

- Airway management equipment must be immediately available.

Note: The patient who does not require intubation should be nursed in the left lateral position.

- Resuscitation drugs must be immediately available.
- Calcium chloride (antidote for magnesium toxicity) must be immediately available.
- Administer supplemental high-flow oxygen via reservoir mask.
- Monitoring: ECG, vital signs q 5 min, pulse oximetry.
- Establish peripheral IV line and commence Hartmann's solution: give bolus of 250 ml stat followed by infusion at 100 ml/h.
- Labs: FBC, urea/electrolytes/creatinine, liver function tests, and GXM, PT/PTT.
- ECG (optional).
- Place urinary catheter: measure hourly urine output.

Drug therapy for convulsions

- **Magnesium sulphate**
  1. **Dosage**
     Loading dose: an initial slow IV bolus of 5 g (10 ml, ie 2 ampoules of 49.3% $MgSO_4$ solution) magnesium sulphate diluted in 50 ml of normal saline, administered over 10–15 minutes by syringe pump
     Maintenance dose: IV infusion of magnesium sulphate at rate of 2 g/h (50 ml, ie 10 ampoules of 49.3% $MgSO_4$ diluted with normal saline to 120 ml infused at rate of 5 ml/h) till 24 hours after delivery

Note: The drug should only be given if these criteria are satisfied: (1) The patellar reflex is present: **most important**; and (2) Respiratory rate is not depressed, ie rate is >16/min.

  2. **Side effects**: flushing, nausea, epigastric discomfort
  3. **Clinical signs of magnesium toxicity**: diminished deep tendon reflexes, muscle weakness manifesting as ptosis, slurred speech and respiratory difficulty, and oliguria/anuria
  4. **Management of magnesium toxicity**:
     a. Administer 10 ml (1 ampoule) calcium chloride IV over 3 minutes
     b. Stop $MgSO_4$ infusion if
        (1) Patellar reflexes are absent
        (2) Respirations <16/minute
        (3) SpO_2 <90% in spite of supplemental oxygen
        (4) Anuria (or oliguria persisting beyond 2 hours)
     c. If oliguric, do serum magnesium levels and stop infusion if level >3 mmol/l

- **Diazepam (Valium®)**: the second choice anticonvulsant, which is indicated if magnesium sulphate therapy is contraindicated or magnesium toxicity is evident.

1. **Dosage**: 10 mg slowly IV over 2 minutes; can be repeated to a total of 20 mg

Note: 5 mg dose is too low for pregnancy.

2. **Infusion**: 1 mg/min.
3. **Management of recurrent convulsions**:
   a. Repeat $MgSO_4$ 2.5–5.0 g IV
   b. Diazepam 10 mg IV
   c. If there is no response, or the patient has a prolonged period of obtundation after only being given $MgSO_4$, then the possibility of intracranial haemorrhage exists, and a head CT scan should be sought at an appropriate juncture
   d. Consider consulting Anaesthesia regarding thiopentone infusion

Drug therapy for hypertension

Women with blood pressures >110 mm Hg diastolic or >170 mm Hg systolic risk arterial damage and should be treated. The aim of therapy is smooth reduction of blood pressure over 20–30 minutes, to a level of 90–100 mm Hg diastolic or 140–150 mm Hg systolic. Too rapid or too great a reduction in blood pressure may have adverse effects on both the mother and baby.

Note: Antihypertensive therapy **should not be given** before IV fluid administration. Due to vasoconstriction, eclamptics usually have a low intravascular volume which may predispose to renal shut-down and precipitous falls in BP when antihypertensive therapy is commenced.

- **Hydralazine (Apresoline®)**
  Dosage: 5 mg IV or PO bolus and repeated in doses of 5–10 mg IV or PO every 20 minutes prn, or
- **Labetalol (Trandate®/Normadyne®)**: see notes below
  Dosage: 20 mg over 5 minutes, followed by increasing doses of 20–80 mg by IV bolus q 10 min till the desired effect is achieved, or to a maximum cumulative dose of 300 mg

Note:
1. Avoid felodipine or nifedipine if magnesium sulphate is being used for control of convulsions since a synergistic hypotensive effect may be seen.
2. If there is no response to hydralazine or the patient is unconscious, the drug of choice is labetalol. Experience suggests a smoother control of BP and there is published evidence suggesting that it may be of benefit to the foetus by accelerating lung maturity.

References/further reading

1. Schwab, R. Preeclampsia/eclampsia: Establishing the diagnosis and providing prompt, effective treatment. *Emerg Med Rep.* November 25, 1996:237–244.

55 Ectopic pregnancy

Irwani Ibrahim

CAVEATS

- Any sexually active woman presenting with abdominal pain and vaginal bleeding with or without amenorrhoea has an ectopic pregnancy until proven otherwise.
- Diagnosis is easily missed unless suspected. Hence consider ectopic pregnancy in all females of childbearing age.
- Absence of cervical motion tenderness does not exclude ectopic pregnancy.

> ☛ **Special Tips for GPs**
> - Ectopic pregnancy must be suspected in all females of childbearing age presenting with abdominal pain.
> - Most presentations are atypical (Table 1).
> - History of tubal ligation does not exclude an ectopic pregnancy.
> - Urine pregnancy test is a simple tool that can be used but beware of its limitations.

MANAGEMENT

Urine HCG

- Most urine human chorionic gonadotrophin (HCG) kits have almost 100% specificity but sensitivities vary (generally still around 90%).
- All females of childbearing age with abdominal pain should have a urine pregnancy test done to exclude ectopic pregnancy. In one study, the percentage of potentially missed cases drops from 40% if based on history alone, to 3% if urine HCG is negative, to 2% if serum HCG is negative, and to 1% if ultrasound is negative.
- Urine pregnancy test becomes positive 4th to 5th week after conception and serum HCG becomes positive from 3rd to 4th week post conception.
- Different urine pregnancy test kits give different sensitivities. Some can detect as low as 10 IU/l, eg the Abbott Test Pack Plus detects urine HCG of 25 IU/l.
- **False positive results** can be due to trophoblastic diseases (hydatidiform moles or choriocarcinoma), HCG producing pituitary tumours as well as drugs such as anticonvulsants and phenothiazines.

- **False negative results** occur if urine specimen is too dilute (the best specimen is the first morning specimen) and in patients who are on diuretics.
- In a recent article, a HCG-based urine pregnancy test is sensitive to 90% only if conducted on the first day of missed period, as 10% of women may not have implanted yet. Sensitivity rises to 97% if conducted within 1 week after the first day of missed period.

Unstable patient

- The patient must be managed in the critical care area.
- Maintain airway and give supplemental high-flow oxygen.
- Monitoring: ECG, vital signs q 5 min, pulse oximetry.
- Establish 2 large bore intravenous lines.
- Fluid challenge of 1 litre crystalloid. Reassess parameters.

Table 1: Risk factors and presentations of ectopic pregnancy

Risk factors	*Presentations*
Previous ectopic tubal surgery History of infertility Invitro fertilization Increased age Smoking History of pelvic inflammatory disease Intrauterine contraceptive device	Usually around 8 weeks of amenorrhoea. The **spectrum** of clinical symptoms ranges from pelvic pain and vaginal bleeding indistinguishable from spontaneous abortion, ovarian accident or pelvic inflammatory disease to catastrophic intraabdominal haemorrhage. They may present with syncope. **Typical presentation**: Sudden onset of unilateral severe abdominal pain accompanied by collapse and fresh vaginal bleeding. Commonest presenting symptom is abdominal pain with or without vaginal bleeding. **Atypical presentation**: Chronic recurrent lower abdominal pain combined with irregular vaginal bleeding, gastrointestinal symptoms (vomiting and diarrhoea), and urinary symptoms such as dysuria or shoulder tip pain.

- Labs (mandatory):
  1. FBC
  2. Urea/electrolytes/creatinine
  3. GXM 2–4 units
  4. Urine HCG
  5. DIVC screen
- Insert urinary catheter to monitor urinary output.
- Inform Obstetrics and Gynaecology Registrar.

Stable

- Keep patient NBM.
- Put patient in a monitored bed.
- Monitor vital signs every 5–10 minutes.
- Establish at least 1 large bore peripheral line (14/16G).
- Administer crystalloids at maintenance rate.
- Labs:
  1. Mandatory: GXM 4 units
  2. Optional: FBC, urea/electrolytes/creatinine
- Insert urinary catheter to monitor urine output.
- Inform Obstetrics and Gynaecology Registrar who may arrange for immediate ultrasound scan.

References/further reading

1. Carson SA, Buster JE. Ectopic pregnancy. *N Engl J Med*. 1993;329(16):1174–1181.
2. Ankum WM. Diagnosing suspected ectopic pregnancy: Hcg monitoring and transvaginal ultrasound lead the way. *BMJ*. 2000;321:1235–1236.
3. Wong E, Ooi SBS. Ectopic pregnancy: A diagnostic challenge in the emergency department. *Eur J Emerg Med*. 2000;7(3):189–194.
4. Brennan, DF. Ectopic Pregnancy Part 1:Clinical and laboratory diagnosis. *Acad Emerg Med. 1995;*2(12):1081–1089.
5. Wilox AJ, Baird DD, Dunson D, et al. Natural limits of pregnancy testing in relation to the expected menstrual period. *JAMA*. 2001;286(14):1759–1761.

56 Electrical and lightning injuries

Peter Manning • Chong Chew Lan

CAVEATS

- Low-voltage injuries (<1,000 volts) are less frequently serious than high-voltage injuries. As voltage increases, the likelihood of extensive burns increases.
- Resistance varies from tissue to tissue, with bones being the most resistant.
- The longer the duration of contact, the more severe the injury.
- Dry skin takes 3,000 volts to induce VF, whereas wet skin only requires household current (220–240 volts).
- Alternating current (AC) is more dangerous than direct current (DC), causing flexor muscle tetanic contractions 'freezing' the victim to the point of electrical contact.
- Direct current will cause a single muscle contraction that can throw the victim from his/her current location; lightning does the same.
- Pathway: once skin is breached, current passes through the least resistant tissues (nerves, vessels, muscles) with damage being inversely proportional to the cross-sectional diameter of the affected tissue.
- True electrical-conduction injuries are more like crush injuries than thermal in that the total amount of damage is often not apparent.
- **Good fluid management** is **essential** to avoid acute renal failure.

Note: Fluid replacement cannot be calculated based on the Wallace Rule of 9 as in thermal burns.

- Never forget to address possible **associated injuries**:
  1. Cervical spine injuries
  2. Toxic inhalations
  3. Falls with fractures/dislocations
  4. Thermal burn care with possible inhalation injury
  5. Foetal injury during pregnancy

> **☛ Special Tips for GPs**
> - Ensure electricity supply is switched off before approaching victim, if called to scene first.

TYPES OF ELECTRICAL INJURY

- **True electrical injuries** occur when current actually passes through the body to the ground.

Table 1: Complications of electrical and lightning injuries

Body system affected	*Shared complications*	*Unique features*
CVS	Ventricular dysrhythmias, low BP (fluid loss), High BP (catecholamine release), myocardial ischaemia.	Myocardial infarction is rare and tends to be a late finding in both types of injury.
Neurologic	LOC, altered mental state, convulsions, aphasia, amnesia, peripheral neuropathy.	Respiratory centre paralysis, ICH, cerebral oedema and infarction, parkinsonism are features of lightning injury. Neuralgias are a late feature.
Skin	Electrothermal contact burns, non-contact arc and 'flash' burns, secondary thermal burns of varying depth (clothing ignition and heating of metal jewellery).	Scars and contractures are late features.
Vascular	Thrombosis, coagulation necrosis, intravascular necrosis, intravascular haemolysis, delayed vessel rupture, compartment syndrome.	Disseminated intravascular coagulation in lightning injuries.
Respiratory	Respiratory arrest, aspiration pneumonia, pulmonary contusion.	Pulmonary infarction and pneumonia are late features.
Renal/metabolic	Myoglobinuria, haemoglobinuria, metabolic acidosis, hypokalaemia, hypocalcaemia, hyperglycaemia.	Renal failure is uncommon.
GI tract	Gastric atony and intestinal ileus, bowel perforation, intramural oesophageal haemorrhage, hepatic and pancreatic necrosis, GI bleeding.	

Muscular	Compartment syndrome, clostridial myositis and myonecrosis.	
Skeletal	Secondary blunt trauma common in both types including vertebral compression fractures (from falls), long bone fractures (from victim being flung or violent muscle contractions), large joint dislocations; aseptic necrosis, periosteal burn, osteomyelitis.	
Eye	Corneal burns, intraocular haemorrhage or thrombosis, uveitis, retinal detachment, orbital fracture.	Late injuries are delayed cataracts, macular degeneration and optic atrophy.
Ear	Hearing loss (temporary), tinnitus, haemotympanum, CSF rhinorrhoea.	Tympanic membrane rupture is rare.
Oral burns	Delayed labial artery haemorrhage (from child biting electrical cord) with subsequent scarring and facial deformity, delayed speech development, impaired mandibular/dentition development.	These injuries are almost always seen in electrical injuries only.
Foetal	Spontaneous abortion, foetal death, oligohydramnios, intrauterine growth retardation, hyperbilirubinaemia.	
Psychiatric	Hysteria, anxiety, sleep disturbance, depression, storm phobia, cognitive dysfunction.	These features tend to be more common in lightning injuries.

- **Flash burns**:
  1. Current does not involve internal body.
  2. Wounds are characterized by central blanching with surrounding erythema; these are simple thermal burns and are treated as such.
- **Flame burns**:
  1. Caused by ignition of clothing and are **not** considered true electrical injuries.
  2. Managed as thermal burns once electrical injury is excluded.
- **Lightning injury**: see Table 1 for details of complications.
  1. High-voltage (in the millions) direct current.
  2. Cardiac injury results in asystole: treated via ACLS protocols with delayed recovery possible.
  3. Skin around entry site may have a spidery or pine tree appearance.

MANAGEMENT

Supportive measures

- Patients with altered mental state or cardiac dysrhythmias should be managed in the critical care area.
- Maintain airway with cervical spine immobilization.
- Monitoring: ECG, vital signs q 5–15 min, pulse oximetry.
- Establish peripheral IV access (2 lines if patient haemodynamically unstable).
- **Labs**: FBC, urea/electrolytes/creatinine, DIVC screen, urinalysis including myoglobin, cardiac screen, creatinine kinase, ABGs and COHb levels in associated inhalation injury and GXM if injury warrants it.
- ECG in all electrical injuries.
- IV crystalloid at a rate to maintain peripheral perfusion and urine output of 1–1.5 ml/kg/h.
- **X-rays**: C spine; then as indicated by injuries, CXR in associated inhalation injury.
- **Pain management**:
  1. Pethidine® 50–75 mg IM or 25 mg IV, **or**,
  2. Diclofenac sodium (Voltaren®) 50–75 mg IM.
- Insert Foley catheter.
- Consider alkalinization of urine to prevent renal tubular necrosis if myoglobin is demonstrated in the urine.
  Dosage: IV sodium bicarbonate 1 mmol/kg/body weight over 2 hours (1 ml of 8.4% sodium bicarbonate = 1 mmol).
- Consider placement of Ryle's tube if paralytic ileus suspected.
- Administer ATT 0.5 ml IM according to standard protocols.

- Consider need for **fasciotomy** and consult Hand Surgery or Orthopaedics in the case of:
  1. Muscle tightness
  2. Sensory loss
  3. Circulatory compromise
  4. Rapid tissue swelling
- In case of cardiac arrest, follow standard ACLS protocols except that prolonged resuscitative efforts should be made since recovery from prolonged asystole is possible.

Special situations

- **Paediatric considerations**
  1. **Oral commissure burns** are almost exclusively found in children and can involve considerable morbidity.
  2. Fatalities are rare since the electrical circuit is completed locally in the mouth.
  3. There is **local sloughing of tissue** on the 7th to 10th days and this may lead to brisk bleeding.
  4. **Admit** all such burns on the day of presentation.
- **Obstetric considerations**
  1. Foetal injury depends on the flow of current through the mother's body.
  2. Significant foetal injury (death or IUGR) may occur following even minor degrees of electrical shock to the mother, especially in cases of oligohydramnios.
  3. Obtain O&G consultation in all cases of electrical injuries during pregnancy and keep in view foetal monitoring.

Disposition

- **Admission criteria**
  1. All patients with high-voltage injury (>1,000 volts).
  2. All patients with specific organ system involvement.
  3. All patients with suspected neurovascular compromise to the extremities.
  4. All patients with oral commissure burns.
  5. Deep hand burns.
- **Discharge criteria**
  1. Patients without evidence of burns.
  2. Patients with minor injuries with appropriate referral to an outpatient setting.

References/further reading

1. Tintinalli JE, Kelen GD, Stapczynski JS, et al, eds. *Emergency Medicine: A Comprehensive Study Guide*. 5th ed. New York: McGraw-Hill; 2000:1292–1301.

57 ENT Emergencies

Peng Li Lee

☛ Special Tips for GPs

- Suspect **FB nose** in a child who presents with foul smelling nasal discharge.
- Enquire about history of **FB ingestion** in patients who present with chest pain not suggestive of angina.
- Do **not** use **syringing technique** to remove **organic FB** (eg pea, sponge, tissue paper) in the ear as it may swell up rendering removal difficult, and there may also be danger of tympanic membrane perforation.
- Suspect **epiglottitis** in a sick patient with severe sore throat, muffled voice and an absence of significant findings from examination of the oral cavity.

BELL'S PALSY

- The most common cause of facial paralysis worldwide.
- A diagnosis of exclusion.
- **Role of Emergency Physician** is to
  1. Exclude other causes of facial paralysis.
  2. Begin appropriate treatment.
  3. Protect eye.
  4. Arrange appropriate follow-up.
- **Clinical features**
  1. Sudden onset: a partial paralysis of gradual onset is likely to have an underlying aetiology.
  2. Unilateral paralysis/weakness of one side of the entire face: pay particular attention to sparing of the upper third (orbicularis and frontalis) of face, which is indicative of upper motor neurore lesion.
  3. Other symptoms include drooling, tearing from eye, altered taste, pain behind ear.
  4. Association with recent URTI/viral syndrome.
- **Differential diagnosis** of Bell's Palsy may be considered in relationship to the course of the 7th nerve
  1. Intracranial: meningioma, acoustic neuroma
  2. Intratemporal: acute/chronic ear disease, herpes zoster, temporal bone fracture or tumour

3. Extratemporal: parotid malignancy, facial laceration

A careful history and ENT/parotid gland/neurological examination should be able to differentiate the above causes

- **Management**
  1. **Steroids**
     a. Still debatable and literature does not have sufficiently large number of patients to prove conclusively its benefit. However, as there are minimal side effects associated with steroid therapy in Bell's palsy, the general consensus is to start steroids as soon as possible
     b. Dosage: 1 mg/kg for 7 days
     c. Contraindicated in diabetes, PUD, hepatic dysfunction
  2. **Acyclovir (zovirax)**
     a. Recent evidence supports HSV as the presumed cause in >70% of cases. However, acyclovir is not useful in late presentations.
     b. Dosage: 800 mg 5 times per day for 10 days
  3. **Eye Care**
     a. Artificial tears and eyeglasses/shields/taping of eyelids at night to decrease risk of corneal drying and ulceration
  4. **Referrals**
     a. Neurology: atypical presentation of Bell's palsy or other neurologic signs found
     b. ENT: all typical Bell's palsy
     c. EYE: unexplained ocular pain or abnormal eye findings

EPISTAXIS

- Priorities are to:
  1. Assess and **stabilize** the haemodynamic status
  2. **Identify the site** and cause of bleed
  3. **Stop the bleed**
- Most nose bleeds come from ruptured blood vessels on the nasal septum. Absence of anterior bleeding site, presence of bilateral nose bleed or blood draining down oropharynx is suggestive of a posterior source.
- **Differential diagnosis**: blood dyscrasias, local vascular malformation, eg hereditary telangiectasia, nasal tumour.
- Institute **stabilization** efforts upon arrival at ED:
  1. Pinch the nostril between a finger and the thumb for at least 10 minutes.
  2. Apply ice packs to the bridge of nose.
  3. Sit patient up and hold a bowl into which the blood can drip. Swallowing, which may displace the accumulating clot, must be discouraged.
  4. If patient is unstable haemodynamically:
     a. Transfer patient to critical care area.
     b. Establish peripheral IV line and administer crystalloids at a rate sufficient to maintain perfusion.

c. Take blood for GXM, FBC, urea/electrolytes/creatinine, coagulation profile.
d. Monitoring: ECG, vital signs q 5–15 min, pulse oximetry.

- Proceed **to identify the source of bleed** (good illumination with headlight required).
  1. Remove clotted blood with Tilley's forceps or sucker.
  2. As each part of nasal septum comes into view, it may be sprayed with cophenylcaine (constricts the blood vessels and anaesthetizes the mucosa).
- **Upon cessation of haemorrhage**:
  1. Bleeding points seen may be cauterized with a bead of silver nitrate on a stick (avoid cauterizing both sides of nasal septum due to small risk of septal perforation) or packed with gauze soaked in adrenaline 1:10,000 for 15–30 min.
  2. If no further bleeding after a short period of observation, patient may be discharged with bed rest advice and an early ENT clinic review.
  3. **If bleeding persists**, anterior nasal packing is required:
     a. Inform ENT MO.
     b. Options: Merocel (# 8–10 cm for adult) lubricated with tetracycline ointment, BIPP (bismuth subnitrate and iodoform paste) using a Tilley's nasal dressing forceps.
     c. Patient is admitted for observation and oral antibiotics.
  4. **If bleeding persists despite the presence of an effective anterior nasal pack**, posterior nasal packing is required.
     a. Inform ENT MO.
     b. Reassess haemodynamic stability: monitor vital signs, take blood for FBC, coagulation profile, GXM, urea/electrolytes/creatinine.
     c. A Foley catheter (# 12) is inserted via the nostril (choose the side from which more bleeding is suspected) until the tip is seen in the oral pharynx.
     d. Inflate the balloon with 8 ml of water and withdraw the Foley catheter until the balloon sits snugly at the postnasal space, at which point, further inflate the Foley catheter with another 8 ml of water.
     e. Secure the catheter at the nose with an umbilical clamp and guard the ala from the pressure of the catheter.
     Tip: Cut the proximal end of the Foley catheter and thread the clamp through the catheter to act as a cushion for the ala.
- **Disposition**: admit the patient for observation and oral antibiotics **after** ENT consultation. **Always refer to ENT MO** to review if:
  1. Epistaxis is prolonged.
  2. Repeat visit.
  3. Recurrent epistaxis.
  4. Patient is elderly.

FRACTURE OF NASAL BONE

- **Caused** by direct trauma to the nose.
- **Clinical features:**
  1. Distorted shape of nose.
  2. Soft tissue swelling.
  3. Tenderness of nasal bone.
- **Important to exclude**
  1. Injuries to other parts of the facial skeleton.
  2. **Septal haematoma** (bluish swelling on both sides of the nasal septum visible from the front of the nose): if present **urgent ENT referral** is required for haematoma aspiration/I&D, in order to prevent the development of septal ischaemia or abscess, which may lead to necrosis, collapse and deformity of the cartilaginous structure of the nose.
- Nasal **x-ray** is done more for medicolegal reasons. It does not affect the clinical management.
- Need for **M&R** should be assessed 5–7 days postinjury, when the soft tissue swelling has subsided; M&R is usually done within 7–10 days of the injury before the nasal bones become firmly set.

FOREIGN BODY: EAR

- Generally FB can be removed using microforceps or a blunt hook (under otoscopy) or syringing.
- In a uncooperative child, removal under GA is advised.
  1. Insect FB: kill it with a few drops of 1% lignocaine or olive oil before removal with microforceps
  2. Organic FB (eg pea/tissue paper/sponge): **do not** use syringing technique as they may swell up, rendering removal difficult.
- If FB removal is deemed difficult under otoscopy, refer to the ENT clinic (during office hours) where microscope is available
- One attempt by ED staff is recommended, failing which the patient should be referred to the ENT clinic.

FOREIGN BODY: NOSE

- Usually occurs in a child, presenting with unilateral, foul smelling nasal discharge.
- There is the danger of inhalation and obstruction of respiratory tract during removal, especially if the patient is supine during the removal attempt. **Tip**: secure child in papoose restrainer held vertically against assistant's legs for removal attempt.
- If irregular shape FB, use small alligator forceps for removal.
- If round or smooth FB, use a blunt hook (eg jobson horn) to engage posterior end of FB before removing it.

- Nasal cophenylcaine spray may be used to aid removal of FB by causing mucosal shrinkage.
- One attempt at removal by ED staff is recommended, failing which, the ENT MO should be informed for KIV removal of FB under GA.

FOREIGN BODY: THROAT

- Ask about nature of FB: fish bone, chicken bone, etc.
- Ask for exact site of pain: pain over lower part of neck or chest may suggest oesophageal FB which is not easily visualized clinically and radiologically (lateral neck XR).
- Enquire about presence of haemoptysis or haemetemesis.
- Inspect tonsillar region carefully. Options are
  1. Indirect laryngoscopy (IDL).
  2. Direct pharyngolaryngoscopy using laryngoscope with patient supine after throat has been sprayed with cophenylcaine: the advantage of this technique is that an FB can be removed easily with Magill's forceps. It allows a quick look and this should only be done for children as they are often uncooperative. For an adult, it is better to use IDL or fibreoptic nasopharyngoscopy to visualize, and Nagashima forceps or bronchoscopy to remove.
  3. However, there is a small risk of FB aspiration and dislodgement of FB into pharyngeal wall.
  4. Fibreoptic nasopharyngoscopy.
  5. Inspect closely for FBs at the tonsillar poles, base of tongue, vallecular region and pyriform fossae.
- If no FB can be seen, proceed with lateral (soft tissue) x-ray of the neck.
- If x-ray shows FB, inform ENT MO.
- Paediatric FB throat: Attempt visualization with tongue depression; if FB cannot be seen, refer to ENT MO.
- If **x-ray and IDL** are **negative** for FB **and patient is comfortable**, reassure and treat symptomatically with lozenges and gargle. Oral antibiotic (eg amoxicillin) may be considered if ulcer or abrasion is seen. Refer to ENT clinic in 1–2 days for review. The discharge advice should be to return immediately if there is dyspnoea, fever, chest pain or haemetemesis.
- If **x-ray and IDL** are **negative** for FB but **patient is still symptomatic**, inform ENT MO for review and KIV barium swallow (especially for lower neck pain and chest pain) or rigid oesophagoscopy.
- See Figure 1 for the algorithm showing the management of FB throat.

HEARING LOSS: SUDDEN, SENSORINEURAL

- A medical emergency

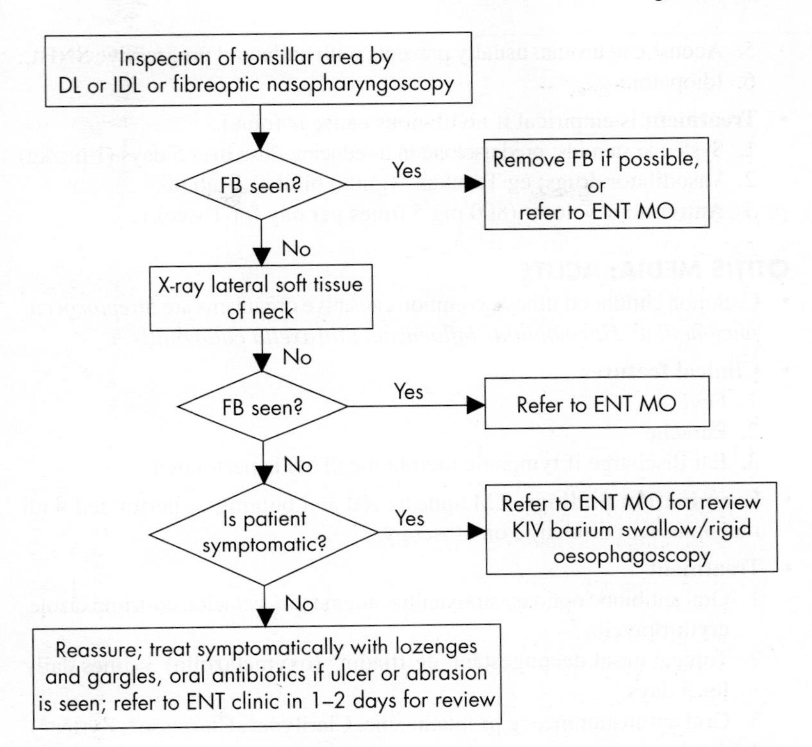

Figure 1: A practical algorithm showing the management of FB throat

- Differentiate from:
  1. Bilateral progressive sensorineural hearing loss (SNHL): presbyacusis is a common cause.
  2. Unilateral progressive SNHL: Ménière's disease and acoustic neuroma.
- **Clinical features**
  1. Usually unilateral.
  2. Weber test: lateralized towards unaffected ear.
  3. Rinne test may be positive (in a partially deaf ear: Air conduction is still better than bone conduction in SNHL) or falsely negative (in a totally deaf ear: bone conducted sound from deaf ear will be heard by intact cochlear on the unaffected side).
- **Causes**
  1. Trauma to head or ear: traumatic tears to intralabyrinthine membrane (perilymph fistula).
  2. Viral infection, eg mumps, measles, varicella.
  3. Vascular: sudden impairment of cochlear blood flow.
  4. Syphilis.

5. Acoustic neuroma: usually presents with unilateral progressive SNHL.
6. Idiopathic.

- **Treatment** is empirical if no obvious cause is found.
  1. Systemic steroids: prednisolone in a reducing dose over 5 days (1 mg/kg)
  2. Vasodilator drugs: eg Tanakan® (ginko biloba) 1 tab tds
  3. Antiviral: acyclovir (800 mg 5 times per day for 1 week)

OTITIS MEDIA: ACUTE

- Common childhood illness: common causative organisms are *Streptococcus pneumoniae*, *Haemophilus influenzae*, *Moraxella catarrhalis*
- **Clinical features**
  1. Fever
  2. Earache
  3. Ear discharge if tympanic membrane (TM) is perforated.
- **Examination findings**: TM appears red and bulging or perforated with mucopurulent discharge on otoscopy.
- **Treatment**
  1. Oral antibiotic options: amoxicillin, augmentin, cefaclor, co-trimoxazole, erythromycin.
  2. Topical nasal decongestant, eg Iliadin® (oxymetazolin) 3 times daily for 5 days.
  3. Oral antihistamine, eg promethazine, Clarityne®, Clarinase®, Zyrtec®).
  4. Analgesia.
  5. Antibiotic ear drops are indicated only if TM is ruptured (this differs from the treatment of traumatic rupture of tympanic membrane).
- Refer to ENT clinic for follow-up.

OTITIS MEDIA: CHRONIC

- COM refers to a chronic non-healing TM perforation, usually associated with a conductive hearing loss.
- Patient often presents with an acute superinfection with mucopurulent discharge; otalgia is unusual.
- Treat with topical antibiotic and refer to ENT clinic for aural toilet.

Note: Oral antibiotic is only indicated if concurrent pharyngitis/sinusitis is suspected.

- Patient should be advised on ear hygiene, ie to keep ear dry with ear plugs or putty made with hand cream and cotton wool.

OTITIS EXTERNA: ACUTE

- **Presents** with itching, ear pain and ear discharge.
- **Clinically** there may be diffuse inflammation or a furuncle.

- **Treatment** is with topical antibiotic (with steroid combination), eg otosporin or sofradex 2 drops tds and analgesia.
  1. Oral antibiotic is indicated **only** when there is a **systemic illness with fever and lymphadenitis**.
  2. Refer to ENT for follow-up.
- **Suspect 'malignant' otitis externa** if pain is excessive of clinical signs, especially in elderly/diabetics.
  1. Requires admission for IV antibiotic.
  2. Risk of spread of infection to base of skull and adjacent soft tissues.

PERITONSILLAR ABSCESS (QUINSY)

- **Presents** with typical picture of tonsillitis but
  1. Is almost always unilateral
  2. Associated with increasing difficulty in swallowing (dysphagia)
  3. Associated with painful swallowing (odynophagia)
  4. Trismus
- **Clinical examination**: involved tonsil is often obscured by swollen soft palate and uvula is displaced contralaterally.
- **Treatment**: I&D under LA; refer to ENT MO.

SINUSITIS

- **Classically divided into**:
  1. Acute: symptoms lasting <3 weeks.
  2. Subacute: symptoms lasting between 3 weeks to 3 months.
  3. Chronic: symptoms lasting >3 months.
- **Commonly presents with**:
  1. A persistent cold.
  2. Nasal congestion.
  3. Purulent discharge.
  4. Facial pain with headache.
- **Clinical findings**
  1. Purulent secretions in the middle meatus may be seen using a nasal speculum and a direct light.

     Tip: purulent secretions may be seen better if the nasal mucosa is first decongested with cophenylcaine nasal spray).
  2. Facial tenderness on palpation.
- **X-rays**
  1. Uncomplicated sinusitis is often a clinical diagnosis and imaging is not mandatory.
  2. Plain sinus films have a high (40%) false negative. Rate radiographic signs of infection: air-fluid level in affected sinus on paranasal sinus x-ray.

- Exclude **complications**: intracranial extension of infection, osteomyelitis and orbital cellulitis in children.
- **Goal of treatment** in uncomplicated sinusitis is:
  1. To relieve obstruction of the sinus ostia.
  2. Avoid antihistamines as they thicken secretions.
     a. **Nasal decongestant**: oxymetazoline (Iliadin®) nose drops
     Dosage: Adult 0.05%; Paediatric 0.025%; Infants 0.01% for 3–5 days
     b. **Systemic decongestant:** pseudoephedrine (Sudafed®)
     c. **Antibiotics**: empiric coverage for *H. influenzae* and *Strep pneumoniae*; in addition *Moraxella catarrhalis* in children
     Dosage: for a minimum of 10–14 days

	Augmentin	**Bactrim**
Adult	625 mg bd	2 tab bd
Child: 2–6 yrs	5 ml bd	
Child: 7–12 yrs	10 ml bd (228 mg/5 ml)	

If patient is allergic to penincillin, alternative antibiotics are cephalosporins or azithromycin.

- Refer to ENT clinic for follow-up.

TONSILLITIS: ACUTE

- Patient presents with sore throat and fever.
- **Clinical examination**: tonsils are injected, swollen and may show purulent exudates.
- **Differentials** to consider: diphtheria, infectious mononucleosis.
- **Treat** with antibiotic (penicillin is the antibiotic of choice), gargles, lozenges and antipyretic.
- Consider admission for IV antibiotics/hydration if
  1. Tonsillitis is prolonged.
  2. Patient has had prolonged fever.
  3. Patient has difficulty swallowing.
  4. Patient is clinically dehydrated.
- Patient can be discharged with oral antibiotics for 10 days with a referral for review by the GP if non-recurrent. Refer to ENT clinic if there are recurrent episodes over several years or multiple episodes per year.

TYMPANIC MEMBRANE: ACUTE, TRAUMATIC PERFORATION

- Usually caused by a slap or punch to the side of the head.
- **Clinical features**
  1. Unilateral otalgia.
  2. Possible hearing loss.
  3. Perforation of tympanic membrane seen on otoscopy (often blood-stained).

- **Management**
  1. Broad spectrum oral antibiotics, eg amoxicillin.
  2. Analgesics.
  3. **Do not** prescribe ear drops.
  4. Inform patient of the need to:
     a. **Prevent** water getting into the ear canal.
     b. **Not** use ear plugs or cotton balls, etc.
- **Disposition**
  1. If there is **hearing loss**, refer patient to ENT clinic on **next** working day for documentation of hearing loss.
  2. If there is **no hearing loss**, refer patient to ENT clinic within a week.

References/further reading

1. Ludman H. *ABC of Otolaryngology.* 4th ed. London: BMJ; 1997.

58 Geriatric emergencies

Chong Chew Lan • Shirley Ooi

CAVEATS

- Vague complaints of, eg malaise or decreased functional ability may indicate serious illness.
- Abnormalities in cognitive status are easily missed unless a formal assessment is performed in the ED. Cognitive status is evaluated through a 2-step process:
  1. Orientation to time, place and person.
  2. 3-item recall after 1 minute.

  If these are abnormal, a formal mental status instrument, the Abbreviated Mental Test (AMT), can be used to assess the patient's cognitive abilities.
- **Factors** that **affect diagnosis** and **treatment** of geriatric patients:
  1. **Under-reporting of signs and symptoms** by the patient and dismissal of symptoms as due to **old age** by patient, caregiver as well as physician.
  2. **Atypical** or attenuated **manifestation** of serious illness in elderly makes diagnosis difficult. Be prepared to perform further diagnostic tests even with initial non-specific findings.
  3. Presence/accumulation of **multiple coexisting chronic disorders** may mask clinical presentation of new disease.
  4. **Polypharmacy** lowers compliance and may cause adverse effects due to drug interaction. Evaluate all medications to exclude this as a cause of symptoms for every elderly.
  5. Avoid polypharmacy and prescription of drugs which may affect the elderly's cognitive, renal or hepatic function, balance, bowel and urinary function adversely.
- Age alone is not a contraindication for diagnostic and therapeutic interventions.

☛ Special Tips for GPs

- Do not dismiss complaints of functional decline as due to 'old age'.
- Vague complaints may indicate serious illness or depression.
- Beware of atypical presentation of AMI in the elderly. Have low threshold for doing ECG and for admission.
- Fever may be absent in sepsis in the elderly.

SPECIFIC CONDITIONS AND THEIR MANAGEMENT

Altered mental state (AMS)

- AMS manifests itself in the form of a decreased level of consciousness, an altered content of consciousness, or a combination.
- Look for these **4 features of delirium**:
  1. Acute onset or fluctuating course
  2. Inattention
  3. Disorganized thinking
  4. Altered level of consciousness

  The diagnosis of delirium requires the presence of features 1 and 2, and either 3 or 4. After making the diagnosis, focus on finding the underlying cause.
- Elderly patients with acute changes in their mental state should be assumed to have an **organic aetiology**.
- **Myoclonus** and **asterixis** when present are **pathognomonic** for delirium.
- AMS may be the sole presenting feature of **myocardial infarction**, **pneumonia**, **GI haemorrhage**, **sepsis** or **pulmonary embolism**.
- **Medications** are the most common cause of AMS in the elderly.
- The elderly patient with delirium should be admitted to hospital for further workup and treatment.
- Some patients who have subacute or chronic cognitive impairment (dementia) may be discharged, provided prompt medical follow-up and safe home environment with reliable caregiver are assured.

Functional decline

- Functional decline may be defined as a **recent or progressive** difficulty in performing the activities of daily living.
- There are 2 errors that the Emergency Physician can make with regard to functional decline:
  1. To miss it.
  2. To dismiss it as part of 'normal ageing'.
- Assume that functional decline is a symptom of **new medical illness** or established **chronic diseases** that are **decompensating**.
- The best way in assessing functional decline is the patient history and corroborating history from a caregiver who is in a position to comment objectively on new or worsening functional impairment.

Trauma and falls

- When faced with an injured elderly patient, look beyond the injuries and consider the **cause** of the **fall**. Common medical causes of falls are CVA/TIA, giddiness, postural hypotension and syncope.

Table 1: Atypical presentation of AMI in the elderly

1. SOB
2. Acute confusion
3. Syncopal attacks
4. Strokes
5. Giddiness, vertigo, faintness
6. Palpitations
7. Vomiting
8. Peripheral gangrene, increased claudication
9. Renal failure
10. Pulmonary embolism
11. Restlessness
12. Sweating
13. Weakness
14. Abdominal pain
15. Burning sensation or indigestion in 20%

- If there is suspicion of medical cause for a fall, it may be appropriate to admit the patient to a medical discipline.
- Also consider the impact the injury has on the patient's functional status and ability to care for himself or herself. A priority is to prevent further injury.

Acute myocardial infarction

- Although the elderly may present with the classical symptoms of AMI, it is **common** for them to present **atypically** (Table 1). Those older than 85, in fact, are unlikely to present with classic chest pain. About 60% of those >85 years old with AMI do not have chest pain. Atypical AMI is associated with greater mortality.
- **Dyspnoea** is the **commonest presenting complaint** of **AMI** in the elderly.
- Acute CVA and AMI are much more likely to present together in the elderly. Hence, ECG should be done in every case of CVA in the elderly.
- As AMI may present in a myriad of ways, it is a good practice to do ECG in elderly patients presenting with seemingly unrelated complaints.
- Therapy should be based on physiologic age, functional status, known risks and benefits, and the patient's wishes, if known.
- Thrombolytic therapy and anticoagulation can be well tolerated by the elderly patient with AMI, with a significant reduction in death and disability. The small but significant risk of haemorrhage and other complications should be discussed with the patient.

Acute abdominal pain

- The elderly patient with acute abdominal pain is a great challenge to the Emergency Physician.
- The rate of required admission and subsequent surgery is very high in elderly patients with acute abdominal pain.
- Pain perception and the physical examination may be altered in older patients, creating diagnostic difficulties. Abdominal guarding or muscular rigidity may be lacking in the face of serious intraabdominal pathology with peritoneal irritation. This well-recognized phenomenon is partially attributed to the relatively thin abdominal musculature in elderly patients.
- In the elderly patient with **appendicitis**, anorexia, leukocytosis or the classic migration pattern of pain may be lacking. However, the right lower quadrant tenderness is generally present.
- Note also that although less than 10% of all appendicitis patients are elderly, 50% of deaths occur in this age group. Suspect appendicitis in any patient who presents with abdominal pain. If the cause of the abdominal pain is unclear, tell the patient to have a follow-up examination within 12–24 hours.
- Half the elderly patients with **perforated peptic ulcer** do not report sudden onset of pain. The pain may be generalized or in the lower quadrant. Epigastric rigidity and presence of free air on plain radiography are absent in a large percentage of these patients.
- **Large bowel obstruction** may be present despite the patient's complaint of diarrhoea. Colonic pseudoobstruction should be suspected in patients appearing to have large bowel obstruction who have non-tender abdomen or a cavernous rectal vault.
- **Acute mesenteric ischaemia** must always be suspected in any elderly patient with abdominal pain out of proportion to physical signs. This is particularly so if there is underlying cardiovascular disease, hypotension, peripheral vascular disease, atrial fibrillation or with associated symptoms of chronic ischaemic bowel such as weight loss, post-prandial abdominal pain, diarrhoea and malabsorption. These patients must undergo angiography before 'hard evidence' of mesenteric infarction develops. Refer to *Pain, Abdominal*.
- A **ruptured abdominal aortic aneurysm** must be considered in any elderly patient with acute abdominal or back pain. A pulsatile mass will often not be detectable on examination. Syncope may be the primary complaint.
- Suspect **cholecystitis** in any elderly patient who presents with abdominal pain or signs of sepsis.

Infections

- An ageing immune system, when accompanied by chronic conditions such as diabetes, dementia, malnutrition, cardiovascular disease, chronic lung disease, cancer and alcohol abuse, places the older individual at greater risk of serious infection and secondary complications.
- The **chief presenting complaint** with infection may be anorexia, excess fatigue, unexplained weight loss, new incontinence, falls or mental confusion. Fever and leukocytosis may be absent in sepsis in the elderly. The neutrophil count is usually increased.
- Infections in the independent, community dwelling individual differ from those residing in nursing homes and those who have been recently hospitalized. **Respiratory tract infections** are most common among community living elderly and include influenza, bronchitis and pneumonia. **UTI** follows next in frequency and then **intraabdominal infections**, including cholecystitis, diverticulitis and appendicitis. In contrast, 70–80% of infections in nursing home residents can be accounted for by the acronym **pus: pneumonia, urinary traet** and **soft tissue infections**.
- Whether to treat any elderly patient infection as an outpatient or an inpatient often can be a difficult decision. Consider the patient's clinical status, comorbid conditions, functional status, social support and availability of timely, appropriate support.
- In general, lower the threshold for admission in the elderly with suspected infections as their likelihood for decompensation is very high.

References/further reading

1. Sanders AB. *Emergency Care of the Elder Person*. St Louis, MO: Beverly Cracom Publications; 1996.
2. Kingsley A. Relevance of aging issues in the emergency department. In: Yoshikawa TT, Norman DC, eds. *Acute Emergencies and Critical Care of the Geriatric Patient*. New York: M Dekker; 2000:1–9.
3. Fernandez-Frackelton M. Abdominal pain in elderly patients. *Foresight*. 2001 Oct;52:1–7.

59 Heart failure

Quek Lit Sin • Shirley Ooi

CAVEATS

- Acute heart failure can be placed into 3 clinical groups:
  1. Acute cardiogenic pulmonary oedema (refer to *Pulmonary Oedema, Cardiogenic*)
  2. Cardiogenic shock (refer to *Shock/Hypoperfusion States*)
  3. Acute decompensation of chronic left heart failure which is the focus of this chapter.
- Exclude **renal failure** as a cause of fluid overload before diagnosis of heart failure.
- Heart failure may present as **non-specific complaints**:
  1. Weakness
  2. Lightheadedness
  3. Abdominal pain
  4. Malaise
  5. Wheezing
  6. Nausea
- Always look for precipitating causes of heart failure (Table 1).
- The cardiac conditions combined with asthma or symptoms of chronic obstructive airway disease are difficult clinical challenges and will require a multidisciplinary approach.
- Patients with coexisting insulin-dependent diabetes mellitus have a significantly increased mortality rate.

Table 1: Precipitating causes of heart failure

Cardiac	*Non-cardiac*
Myocardial ischaemia or infarction	Pulmonary embolism
Dysrhythmias	Superimposed systemic infection
Valvular heart disease	Systemic illness, eg severe hypertension, severe anaemia, thyrotoxicosis, heavy alcohol consumption
Non-compliance with therapeutic regimen including failure to restrict fluid intake	Drugs: cocaine, amphetamines, excess use of bronchodilators, 1st-generation calcium antagonist, beta-blockers, NSAIDs
Bacterial endocarditis	Pregnancy

☛ **Special Tips for GPs**

- Always look for a cause of heart failure in patients especially if they have been stable and on medication for a long time. Coronary events or renal impairment must be identified.
- Patient in severe heart failure may present with wheezing. This is **cardiac asthma** and will require aggressive management in the ED before it deteriorates to pulmonary oedema. Ventolin nebulization will not make the patient improve symptomatically.
- Elderly patients have altered autonomic regulation and are sensitive to the side effects of the drugs used in the therapy for heart failure. Special precaution is necessary to tailor the therapy.

MANAGEMENT

- Manage patient in a monitored area: vital signs, pulse oximeter, continuous ECG monitoring.
- Maintain airway.
- Administer supplemental oxygen, initially 100% non-rebreather face mask to maintain SpO_2 >95%.
- Obtain IV access and obtain bloods for FBC, urea/electrolytes/creatinine, cardiac enzymes and serum cardiac markers.
- To reduce venous return, patient can be seated upright with legs hanging over the bed.
- Do **ECG** to diagnose concomitant cardiac ischaemia, prior MI, cardiac dysrhythmias, chronic hypertension, and other causes of left ventricular hypertrophy.
- Order **CXR**. Look for cardiomegaly and upper lobe diversion. Classic radiographic progression is often not found as there is a radiographic lag from the onset of symptoms (about 12 hours after the onset of symptoms). In addition, radiographic findings frequently persist for several days despite clinical recovery.
- Give **diuretics**, eg IV frusemide 40–60 mg if patient is haemodynamically stable.
- A **nitrodisc** 5–10 mg can be given to the patient to relieve the symptoms of pulmonary congestion.
- In severe cases, **IV infusion of GTN** will lower the left ventricular end-diastolic volume and pressure rapidly with prompt resolution of symptoms.

- Monitor urine output to assess response to therapy.

Disposition

- To date, there have not been any prospective studies done to evaluate the admission criteria for patients presenting to the ED with heart failure.
- **Discharge** if patient:
  1. Has no chest pain or concomitant illness.
  2. Responds to diuretics given at the ED (comfortable at rest on room air, SpO_2 on room air ≥95%).
  3. Show no radiographic evidence of chronic heart failure.
- Discharge with the following and refer patient for follow-up at the cardiology outpatient clinics:
  1. Loop diuretics, eg Lasix® 40 OM, and potassium supplements, eg span K 1.2 mg OM if patient is not on diuretics before and urea/electrolytes/creatinine are normal.
  2. Increase dose of loop diuretics if patient is already on diuretics.
  3. If patient has **concurrent hypertension**, besides loop diuretics, angiotension converting enzyme inhibitor, eg captopril 6.25–12.5 mg tds or hydralazine 25 mg tds may be given.
  4. Dietary advice to decrease salt intake and fluid restriction.
- **Admit** if patient has:
  1. Symptomatic dysrhythmias:
     a. syncope or presyncope
     b. cardiac arrest
     c. multiple discharges of implantable defibrillator
  2. New MI or ischaemia.
  3. Rapid onset of new symptoms of heart failure.
  4. Decompensation of chronic heart failure.
  5. Precipitating factors identified which are not easily reversible on an outpatient basis.
  6. Anasarca or significant oedema.
  7. Lack of home support.
  8. Hypotension.

References/further reading

1. Goldman L, Braunwald E, eds. *Primary Cardiology*. Philadelphia: WB Saunders Company; 1998:310–329.
2. American College of Cardiology/American Heart Association Task Force Report: Guidelines for the evaluation and management of heart failure. *J Am Coll Cardiol*. 1995;26:1376–1398.
3. Cole K. Congestive heart failure. In: Frank LR, Jobe KA, eds. *Admission and Discharge Decisions in Emergency Medicine*. Philadelphia: Hanley & Belfus; 2002:32–33.

60 Hepatic encephalopathy, acute

Malcolm Mahadevan • Lee Yin Mei • Lim Seng Gee

DEFINITION

Hepatic encephalopathy is defined as a syndrome of altered mental state and reversible neuropsychiatric state complicating liver disease.

CLASSIFICATION

There are two classifications each with widely differing aetiologies, clinical presentations, physical findings, and management principles:

- Encephalopathy associated with acute liver failure.
- Encephalopathy associated with liver cirrhosis and portal hypertension.

> ☛ **Special Tips for GPs**
> - Avoid narcotics, tranquillizers and sedatives that are metabolized in the liver.
> - Be aware that not all hepatic encephalopathies arise in patients with chronic liver cirrhosis: acute hepatic failure can arise from ingestion of toxins, recreational drug use, and hepatitis A, B and E.

Encephalopathy associated with acute liver failure

- A medical emergency that requires prompt recognition and treatment as the patient may deteriorate into a coma and require a liver transplant.
- Typically the patient is previously well with **no history of liver disease**.
- Symptoms are vague and non-specific, ie malaise and fatigue with nausea; jaundice and encephalopathy follow, and may progress rapidly to coma.
- **History**: care should be taken in the history to exclude the following:
  1. Overdose of paracetamol.
  2. Ingestion of toxins such as fenfluramin.
  3. Use of recreational drugs such as cocaine and Ecstasy.
  4. IV drug use.
  5. A recent travel history in an attempt to exclude hepatitis A and E.
  6. A history of recent sexual exposure significant for possible hepatitis B.
- The **physical examination** should show no signs of chronic liver disease, focal neurology or a high fever. Such findings should prompt the search for an alternative cause for encephalopathy.

- **Grades of encephalopathy**:
  - **I** Trivial lack of awareness, anxiety, euphoria or short attention span.
  - **II** Lethargy or apathy with minimal disorientation for time or place. Patient may show subtle personality change or inappropriate behaviour.
  - **III** Stupor and confusion.
  - **IV** Coma.
- **Management**:
  1. Patient should be managed in the critical care area of the ED.
  2. Airway maintenance and oxygenation: if patient is comatose or has airway compromise, perform endotracheal intubation.
  3. Monitoring: ECG, vital signs q 5–15 min, pulse oximetry.
  4. Establish peripheral IV line.
  5. IV fluids: normal saline infusion at a rate sufficient to maintain peripheral perfusion is best performed with haemodynamic monitoring.
- **Drug therapy:** IV mannitol 20%: 1 g/kg body weight.
- **Investigations**:
  1. Stat capillary blood sugar.
  2. FBC, urea/electrolytes/creatinine, coagulation profile, liver function tests
  3. Serum toxicology (where relevant).
  4. Screen for hepatitis A, B, C, D and E (anti-HAV IgM, HbsAg, anti-HBS, anti-HCV, anti-delta, anti-HBE).
  5. Urgent head CT scan to detect cerebral oedema.
- **Disposition**: consult Gastroenterology and admit to ICU.

Encephalopathy associated with liver cirrhosis and portal hypertension

- The patient **has established liver disease** and has a disturbance of consciousness that develops over a short period of time and fluctuates in severity, or may be a more chronic phenomenon.
- The current classification consists of 3 categories: episodic, persistent or minimal. Encephalopathy in cirrhosis is caused by portosystemic shunting and altered amino acid metabolism with ammonia playing a strong role as well as other neuro-transmitters.
- **History**: the recognition of a history of established cirrhosis or liver disease is important.
- **Precipitating events** that tip patients with chronic liver disease into hepatic encephalopathy include the following:
  - **H** Haemorrhage from the GI tract, eg from varices or erosions
  - **E** Electrolyte imbalance (hypokalaemia, alkalosis as seen in diuretic use, and vomiting and diarrhoea), hypoglycaemia
  - **P** Protein intake (excessive)
  - **A** Azotemia from volume contraction, diuretics
  - **T** Tranquillizers, other sedatives

I Infection, eg spontaneous bacterial peritonitis, UTI or pneumonia, also surgery
C Constipation

- The **physical examination**:
  1. May show signs of chronic liver disease, eg spider naevi, gynaecomastia, liver palms, leuchonychia and a hepatic flap.
  2. May show enlargement of the liver or spleen as well as ascites.
  3. Should include a rectal examination for melaena.
- **Management**:
  1. Patient should be managed in the critical care area of the ED.
  2. Airway maintenance and oxygenation: if patient is comatose or has airway compromise, perform endotracheal intubation.
  3. Monitoring: ECG, vital signs q 5–15 min, pulse oximetry.
  4. Establish peripheral IV line.
  5. IV fluids: normal saline infusion at a rate sufficient to maintain peripheral perfusion is best performed with haemodynamic monitoring.
- **Investigations**: these are targeted to confirm the **diagnosis** of **encephalopathy** complicating cirrhosis as well as to look for the **precipitating cause**:
  1. Stat capillary blood sugar.
  2. FBC, urea/electrolytes/creatinine, ammonia, coagulation profile, liver function tests.
  3. Blood cultures and urinalysis as indicated.
  4. CXR.
- **Drug therapy**:
  1. IV dextrose 50% 40 ml for hypoglycaemia, and IV thiamine 100 mg if patient has alcoholic cirrhosis.
  2. IV naloxone 2 mg if patient has significant obtundation.
  3. IV flumazenil 0.5 mg repeated after 5 min (shown in small controlled trials to improve the grade of encephalopathy).
- **Reversal of encephalopathy**:
  1. **Lactulose** 30 ml PO or a lactulose enema: produces an osmotic diarrhoea altering intestinal flora that decreases ammonia production.
  2. **Oral antibiotics**: randomized controlled trials show no clinical benefits.
  3. **Protection of GI mucosa**: omeprazole 20–40 mg IV slowly over 5 min.
- **Disposition**: consult Gastroenterology with a view to admit to a HD unit (or ICU if intubated).

References/further reading

1. Sherlock S, Dooley J. *Diseases of the Liver and Biliary System*. 10th ed. Oxford: Blackwell Science; 1997.
2. Ferenci P, Lockwood A, Mullen K, et al. Hepatic encephalopathy: Definition, nomenclature, diagnosis and qualification. Final report at the 11th World Congress of Gastroenterology, Vienna, 1998.

61 Hepatobiliary emergencies

Kenneth Mak

The acute problems originating from the hepatobiliary system that present to the emergency physician are usually complications of biliary stone disease. These present as follows.

BILIARY COLIC

- The most common presentation of patients with biliary stone disease.
- Can present in any patient from teens onwards, although it is most often seen in obese women between the ages of 30 and 50 years.
- Pain is centred in the right upper quadrant or epigastrium.
- Pain usually starts acutely and may radiate to the inferior angle of the right scapula.
- Pain is colicky without pain-free intervals between exacerbations (unlike ureteric colic in which pain-free intervals are commonly reported).
- Pain may be triggered by the recent ingestion of food and, in particular, a fatty or large meal.
- Associated features are a sensation of upper abdominal distension or 'bloating', nausea and vomiting.

Caveats

- Always look for symptoms of **obstructive jaundice** since this suggests the presence of **biliary ductal stone** rather than gallstone disease *per se*.
- The presence of pain plus fever suggests **acute cholecystitis** has occurred.
- The presence of pain plus fever and obstructive jaundice suggests **cholangitis**.

ACUTE CHOLECYSTITIS

- Patients often present with an initial visceral pain whose character is like biliary colic. The pain may change over time and evolve into a relatively constant parietal pain which is sharply localized to the right hypochondrium. The pain worsens over time and is exacerbated by movement.
- There is often a background of repeated episodes of upper abdominal pain resembling biliary colic, worsening progressively in terms of severity or frequency.
- Associated features are fever with or without chills, loss of appetite, nausea and vomiting.
- On examination, there may be localized guarding in the right hypochondrium.

- A tender, globular mass palpable below the right costal margin that descends with respiration may represent either an inflammatory mass formed by omentum wrapping itself around an inflamed gallbladder, or an empyema of the gallbladder.
- **Murphy's sign** is present when the patient complains of pain and catches his breath while being palpated in the right hypochondrium; this is due to the gallbladder coming in contact with the tips of the examiner's fingers during inspiration.

Caveats

- **Tenderness** in the **right hypochondrium** is not pathognomonic for **cholecystitis**; this sign is also present in **cholangitis**.
- Classically, there are **no** signs of **obstructive jaundice**.
- Always look for features of **dehydration** or **haemodynamic lability** in patients with acute cholecystitis. These patients are predisposed to volume depletion due to vomiting and anorexia and may further be in shock due to septicaemia.

CHOLANGITIS

- The classic scenario is **Charcot's triad** (right upper abdominal pain, fever and obstructive jaundice).
- There may be a history of previously asymptomatic gallstones which were managed conservatively, or of previous biliary surgery. One local study found that only 35.7% of patients with cholangitis presented with the complete Charcot's triad but most patients (95.7%) had upper abdominal pain as the chief complaint.

Caveats

- As with cholecystitis, always look for features of **dehydration** or **haemodynamic lability** in patients with cholangitis. These patients are predisposed to volume depletion due to vomiting and anorexia and may further be in shock due to septicaemia.

Differential diagnosis

- One must consider hepatic pathologies such as **hepatitis** and **liver abscess**, exacerbation of **ulcer dyspepsia**, **acute peptic ulcer perforation**, **ureteric colic**, **pancreatitis**, **diverticulitis** as well as **right basal pneumonia**.

MANAGEMENT

Stable patient

- This group of patients should be managed in the intermediate acuity care area of the ED.

☛ **Special Tips for GPs**

- The analgesic of choice for biliary colic is an opioid agonist (Pethidine® or Tramal®) administered in *small* doses via the IV route.
- The common practice of giving antispasmodics such as Buscopan® to patients with biliary colic-like symptoms has no evidence-based support.
- NSAIDs, while effective analgesics, are generally not used to treat the pain of biliary colic until peptic ulcer disease has been excluded as a differential diagnosis.

- **Keep patient fasted** while undergoing investigations and treatment.
- **Labs**: the diagnosis of biliary colic is clinical. Any investigations that are to be performed in the acute setting is generally aimed at excluding the complications associated with biliary colic (ie cholangitis or cholelithiasis) as well as the other differential diagnoses.
- **FBC**: a polymorphonuclear leucocytosis is consistent with a bacterial infection (cholangitis or cholecystitis).
- **Liver function tests**:
  1. These tests are normal in biliary colic.
  2. There is typically a cholestatic picture in cholangitis, ie elevated conjugated bilirubin **and** elevation of the cholestatic hepatic ductal enzymes (ALP/GGT), out of proportion to any associated rise in the intracellular hepatic enzymes (AST/ALT).
  3. There is generally no cholestasis in acute cholecystitis.
- **Urea/electrolytes/creatinine**: to detect electrolyte abnormalities and renal dysfunction secondary to vomiting and volume depletion.
- **PT and PTT**: to be performed in the presence of jaundice to detect coagulopathy.
- **Serum amylase**: to exclude coexisting acute pancreatitis.
- **Urinalysis**: to exclude the possibility of urolithiasis and pyelonephritis.
- **ECG**: to exclude myocardial ischaemia.
- **Erect chest x-ray**: to exclude basilar pneumonia and subdiaphragmatic air.
- **KUB**: to detect intraabdominal calcifications, free air, or air-fluid levels.

Unstable patient (haemodynamic lability or presumed septic)

- This group of patients should be managed in the critical care area of the ED.

- **Early** consultation with a surgeon depending on local practice.
- **Monitoring**: vital signs q 10–15 min, ECG, pulse oximetry.
- Administer **supplemental oxygen**.
- **Provide adequate vascular access** with large bore (14/16G) IV cannulae for fluid resuscitation.
- **Labs**: as above.
- Draw first **blood cultures** in ED (from 2 sites and minimum 10 ml blood per bottle).
- **Administer IV antibiotics**: a cephalosporin such as ceftriaxone or cefuroxime to cover gram-negative organisms, and metronidazole 500 mg IV, particularly in the setting of previous biliary surgery.

Note: (1) If patient is allergic to penicillin, ciprofloxacin is an alternative. (2) Avoid use of nephrotoxic antibiotics such as gentamicin, given the predisposition to renal dysfunction in patients who are dehydrated and jaundiced.

- **Consider inotropic support** for those patients who do not respond to an initial adequate fluid challenge.
- **Keep patient fasted** and insert a **nasogastric tube** for gastric decompression and symptomatic relief.
- Insert a **urinary catheter** to monitor urine output.
- **Provide analgesia**: small doses of opioid agonist via IV route titrated to response. Avoid antispasmodics and NSAIDs (see comments in *Special Tips for GPs*).

Disposition

- Patients with **biliary colic** only and without features of jaundice and sepsis may be discharged to early surgical outpatient follow-up assuming the pain has been controlled by analgesia.
- Patients with acute **cholecystitis or cholangitis** should be admitted for further management. Consider high dependency or ICU placement for the unstable patient by liaison with the consulting surgical team.

References/further reading

1. Chew RK, et al. Acute cholangitis in Singapore. *Ann Acad Med Singapore*. 1986;15(2):172–175.
2. Riviello RJ, Bradley WJ. Presentation and management of acute biliary tract disorders in the emergency department: Optimizing assessment and treatment of cholelithiasis and cholecystitis. *Emerg Med Rep*. 2002;23(17):203–210.

62 Hyperosmolar hyperglycaemic state (HHS)

Also known as Hyperosmolar Hyperglycaemic Non-ketotic state (HHNK)

Peter Manning • Chong Chew Lan • Shirley Ooi • Sim Tiong Beng

CAVEATS

- The history of this condition runs to days rather than the hours associated with *diabetic ketoacidosis*.
- The fluid losses tend, therefore, to be significantly greater than those of DKA.
- Some patients with HHS are exquisitely sensitive to insulin.
- HHS is associated with high mortality and needs to be identified early.
- **HHS diagnostic criteria**:
  1. Blood glucose >33 mmol/l
  2. Arterial pH >7.3, bicarbonate >15 mmol/l
  3. Absence of severe ketonaemia or ketonuria
  4. Serum total osmolality >330 mOsm/kg H_2O, or, effective serum osmolality (2 × Na^+ + glucose level + urea) >320 mOsm/kg H_2O
- Exclude other causes of obtundation such as meningitis if serum osmolality is not sufficiently high for the obtundation to be attributed to HHS.

> **☛ Special Tips for GPs**
> - Consider the diagnosis of HHS in an elderly patient with abnormalities in vital signs or mental state, or with complaints of weakness, anorexia or fatigue.
> - HHS may be unexpectedly found in patients who present with concurrent medical insults such as acute CVA, severe burns, MI, infection, pancreatitis or drugs (eg diuretics, beta-blockers, glucocorticoids, neuroleptics, phenytoin and calcium channel blockers). Hence check the bedside glucose level in an elderly patient fairly liberally to avoid missing HHS or DKA.
> - Put up a normal saline infusion before sending the patient by ambulance to hospital.

MANAGEMENT

Supportive measures

- Patient must be managed in a monitored area.
- Administer supplemental high-flow oxygen.
- Monitoring: ECG, pulse oximetry, vital signs q 15–30 min, blood levels of glucose and potassium q 1–2 h.
- Circulatory support: the average fluid deficit in HHNK is 6–10 litres. One-half of the estimated water deficit will need to be replaced during the first 12 hours.
- Labs: FBC, urea/electrolytes/creatinine/calcium/magnesium/phosphate, serum osmolality, ABGs, urinalysis.
- ECG, CXR to look for a cause of the HHNK state.
- Urinary catheter to monitor urine output.

Specific measures

- **IV volume replacement**:
  1. If the patient shows significant tissue hypoperfusion, use **normal saline** as a rapid bolus till perfusion improves and BP stabilizes. Administer at least 1 litre normal saline in the first hour; another over the next 2 hours. Then switch to 1 litre **0.45% NS** over the next 4 hours.
  2. If the patient is **hypertensive** or has significant hypernatraemia (>155 mmol/l), use **0.45% NS** and change to IV D_5W when the serum glucose level reaches 16 mmol/l.
- **Potassium replacement**: total body potassium depletion in HHNK states is usually greater than that in DKA. Establish that there is urine output first, then replace as follows:
  1. Serum K^+ <3.3 mmol/l give 20–40 mEq KCl in the first hour.
  2. Serum K^+ 3.3–4.9 mmol/l give 10–20 mEq K^+ per litre of IV fluid (can be given as 2/3 KCl and 1/3 $KHPO_4$; phosphate replacement is indicated when serum phosphate <0.3 mmol/l).
  3. Serum K^+ >5.0 mmol/l, withhold K^+ but check serum potassium every 1–2 hours.
- **Insulin administration:** bolus not needed since these patients can be exquisitely sensitive to insulin. Administer an infusion of regular insulin at 0.1 units/kg body weight/h. Adjust insulin infusion to keep blood glucose at 14–16 mmol/l, until serum osmolality ≤315 mOsm/l and patient is mentally alert.

Note: Venous blood glucose level should be checked every 1–2 hours as it will be 'HHH' using a bedside glucometer.

Guidelines

- The **serum osmolality** can be calculated by the following equation: $(2 \times Na^+)$ + glucose + urea mOsm. (Normal = approximately 280–290 mOsm.)
- The **osmolal gap** is determined by using the above formula and then comparing it with the lab result measured by the molal freezing point depression method. The difference should be about 10; if higher, some other osmotically active particles are in the serum, eg an alcohol or IVP dye.

Disposition

- Obtain General Medicine or Endocrine consultation; keep in view admission to HD bed. After the initial volume replacement, most patients do not require ICU beds.

References/further reading

1. Wyatt JP, Illingworth RN, Clancy MJ, et al, eds. *Oxford Handbook of Accident and Emergency Medicine*. Oxford: Oxford University Press; 1999:152–153.
2. Singapore Ministry of Health Clinical Guidelines on Diabetes Mellitus. 1999.
3. Graffeo GS. Hyperosmolar hyperglycemic non ketotic syndrome. In: Tintinalli JE, Kelen GD, Stapczynski JS, et al, eds. *Emergency Medicine: A Comprehensive Study Guide*. 5th ed. New York: McGraw-Hill; 2000:1340–1343.
4. Rosen P, Barkin R. *Emergency Medicine: Concepts & Clinical Practice*. 2nd ed. St. Louis: Mosby Year Book; 1992:2180–2187.
5. American Diabetes Association Position Statement. Hyperglycemic crises in patients with diabetes mellitus. *Diabetes Care*. 2003:26:S109–117.
6. Kitabchi AE, Umpierrez GE, Murphy MB, et al. Management of hyperglycemic crises in patients with diabetes (technical review). *Diabetes Care*. 2001;24(1):131–153.

63 Hypertensive crises

Benjamin Leong • Peter Manning

DEFINITIONS

- **Hypertension**: defined as BP levels of 140/90 mm Hg or higher, although it should be recognized that BP levels are a continuous variable. Table 1 shows the classification based on the seventh report of the Joint National Committee (JNC VII) on Prevention, Detection, Evaluation and Treatment of High Blood Pressure.
- **Hypertensive crisis**: a critical elevation in the BP with markedly elevated diastolic BP. No absolute BP level defines a hypertensive crisis, but diastolic BP in the range of 120–130 mm Hg may be used as a guide. Hypertensive crises include hypertensive emergencies and urgencies.
  1. **Hypertensive emergency**: when elevated BP is associated with acute or ongoing end-organ dysfunction or damage.
  2. **Hypertensive urgency**: when elevated BP is associated with imminent end-organ dysfunction or damage. Severe hypertension in an otherwise relatively asymptomatic patient does not constitute a hypertensive emergency and is at most described as urgency.
- The patient may present in several different ways. There are **hypertensive emergencies** such as:
  1. Hypertensive encephalopathy: to be differentiated from stroke/subarachnoid haemorrhage
  2. Hypertensive left ventricular failure (acute pulmonary oedema)
  3. Acute aortic dissection
  4. Acute myocardial infarction/acute coronary syndrome (ACS)
  5. Haemorrhagic or ischaemic stroke/subarachnoid haemorrhage
  6. Acute renal failure
  7. Eclampsia/preeclampsia (refer to *Eclampsia*)
  8. Phaeochromocytoma crises
  9. Recreational drugs (eg ecstasy)

Table 1: JNC VII classification of BP for adults aged 18 years or older

BP (mm Hg)	*Systolic*	*Diastolic*
Normal	<120	<80
Prehypertension	120–139	80–89
Hypertension		
Stage 1	140–159	90–99
Stage 2	≥160	≤100

- There are **hypertensive urgencies** such as:
  1. Elevated BP with retinal change (without associated end-organ damage)
  2. Chronic renal failure
  3. Preeclampsia

CAVEATS

- If the BP measured by a monitoring device is too high (or too low), repeat using a *manual* measurement, with a cuff of appropriate size.
- Hypertensive crises occur mostly in patients known to have hypertension, though some can present *de novo*, with no previous history. **Secondary causes of hypertension** are also more often found in patients with hypertensive crises but by themselves are still uncommon.
- The terms **accelerated hypertension**, **malignant hypertension**, and **accelerated-malignant hypertension** were used to describe severe hypertension with associated retinal changes according to the Keith-Wagener-Barker grading. While it was previously found that grades 3 (haemorrhages, cotton wool patches, arteriosclerosis) and 4 (papilloedema) were associated with poorer outcomes, recent authors have found no difference based simply on these fundoscopic findings. The terms 'hypertensive emergencies' or 'hypertensive urgencies' are preferred now.
- **Hypertensive encephalopathy** is now believed to be rare and often the patient's altered mental state is found to be secondary to a **stroke** (refer to *Stroke*). Making the distinction is important as lowering the BP acutely in a patient with stroke may be hazardous. In the former the BP is raised often significantly, whereas in a stroke it is often only mildly raised. Head CT scan also assists in differentiating the two.
- **Hypertensive left ventricular failure** (commonly labelled as acute pulmonary oedema) occurs when the severe hypertension results in acute LV failure from excessive afterload causing decompensation. Refer to *Pulmonary Oedema, Cardiogenic*.
- **Hypertension with aortic dissection** needs to be considered when the patient presents with acute chest pain, or AMI (when the dissection affects the coronary arteries) or a new aortic regurgitation murmur is detected. The classical history of tearing pain radiating to the back may not be present. Refer to *Aortic Dissection*.
- **Hypertension with AMI/ACS** occurs when the severe hypertension leads to increased ventricular wall tension and myocardial oxygen demands. A BP of >180/110 mm Hg is a contraindication to thrombolysis.
- **Preeclampsia and eclampsia** need to be considered in pregnant women after 20 weeks amenorrhoea. Refer to *Eclampsia*.
- **Never treat the patient on a single BP measurement alone**: when measuring BP, ensure the patient is comfortable and use an appropriate sized cuff.

- **Over-zealous correction of BP** may be dangerous and may result in CVA or AMI. In the vast majority of severely hypertensive patients, BP may be reduced with oral medications and long-term control of BP is probably the most important factor in influencing prognosis. Avoid sublingual calcium channel blockers: the absorption is unpredictable and BP may drop too fast.

> ☛ **Special Tips for GPs**
> - Good BP control of patients known to have hypertension helps to reduce the number of cases presenting with hypertensive emergency or urgency.
> - The use of sublingual nifedipine, though popular in the past, lowers BP imprecisely and has been found to be associated with serious adverse events. It is now an unacceptable practice.

MANAGEMENT

The aims are to stabilize the patient, identify true hypertensive emergencies and manage them appropriately.

Manage the patient in a monitored area (critical or intermediate)

- Administer supplemental low-flow oxygen.
- Monitoring: ECG, pulse oximetry, vital signs q 5–10 min.

Is the BP reading correct?

- Repeat using a manual sphygmomanometer.
- Check for correct cuff size.
- Check the other arm.
- Recheck later if the patient is otherwise asymptomatic.

Is it a hypertensive emergency or urgency?

- Look for evidence of **end-organ damage**.
- **Clinical examination should include the following**:
  1. Fundoscopy for haemorrhages, exudates, papilloedema.
  2. Neurological examination for altered mental states, focal deficits.
  3. Cardiovascular examination for left ventricular failure, new aortic regurgitation murmurs, evidence of aortic dissection.
- **Bedside investigations**: ECG, urine dipstick for haematuria and proteinuria, urine pregnancy test in females who may be pregnant.

- **Lab investigations**: FBC, urea/electrolytes/creatinine, cardiac enzyme screen, troponin T.
- **Radiology**:
  1. Chest x-ray for left ventricular failure, widened mediastinum.
  2. Head CT scan if altered mental state.
  3. CT thorax if aortic dissection is suspected.

Does the BP need to be lowered acutely? If so, how?

- The optimal rate of BP lowering has not been established.
- If **hypertensive emergency** is diagnosed, the goal is generally to lower MAP (Diastolic BP + 1/3 Pulse Pressure) within a few hours to 20–25% below presenting level, or DBP to no less than 100–110 mm Hg, then towards 160/100 mm Hg over the next 2–6 h.
- For patients presenting with a stroke syndrome, if a head CT scan can be done promptly it may be advisable to resist lowering the BP acutely until an intracerebral bleed can be demonstrated. Refer to *Stroke* for details.
- **Drug therapy**
  1. **Sodium nitroprusside**: suitable for all hypertensive emergencies except predelivery eclampsia. Limited by toxic metabolite thiocyanate especially after prolonged use (24–48 h), which may lead to cyanide or thiocyanate toxicity, manifesting as lactic acidosis, altered mental state and clinical deterioration. Needs to be protected from light. Very powerful drug that should be used only when close monitoring facilities are available.
     Dosage: IV infusion starting at 0.25 μg/kg/min titrated to response. The average effective dose is 3 μg/kg/min, with a range of 0.25 to 10 μg/kg/min (maximal dose for 10 min only).
  2. **Labetalol hydrochloride**: use primarily, or in the case of treatment failure with nitroprusside. Useful for patients with IHD in reducing myocardial oxygen demand and tachycardia. Also effective in aortic dissection by reducing force of systolic ejection and shear stress. **Contraindicated** in patients with asthma, COLD, CCF, bradycardia and AV block. While useful for phaeochromocytoma, low doses may result in paradoxical hypertension because the beta-blocking effect is stronger than the alpha-blocking effect.
     Dosage: Give IV 25–50 mg bolus, followed by 25–50 mg every 5–10 min to a maximum of 300 mg (effect lasts about 50 min), or by an infusion at a rate of 0.5–2.0 mg/min.
  3. **Nitroglycerine**: the drug of choice for moderate hypertension complicating unstable angina. Complicated by headache and vomiting, and thus may be of limited value in patients with hypertensive encephalopathy.
     Dosage: IV infusion at 5–100 μg/min, titrated to response.

4. **Propranolol**: may be used in conjunction with nitroprusside for thoracic aortic dissection. Use in conjunction with phentolamine for catecholamine crises.
   Dosage: Give IV 1 mg boluses and titrate.
5. **Esmolol**: short-acting beta-blocker. Useful in aortic dissection.
   Dosage: Give IV 250–500 μg/kg/min for 1 min, then 50–100 μg/kg/min for 4 min; may repeat sequence.
6. **Phentolamine**: an alpha-blocking agent, used in conjunction with IV propanolol for catecholamine crises.
   Dosage: Give IV 5–15 mg.
7. **Hydralazine**: the treatment of choice in predelivery eclampsia.
   Dosage: Give IV 5–10 mg boluses q 15 min and titrate.

- If **hypertensive urgency** is diagnosed, the goal generally is to lower BP gradually over a period of 24–48 hours to a target DBP of 100–110 mm Hg. Medications are given orally. Patient's own medications may be given, if compliance was poor.
- **Drug therapy**
  1. **Felodipine**
     a. Give PO 2.5 mg age >65 yo
     b. Give PO 5.0 mg age <65 yo, then 5.0 mg bd
  2. **Captopril**: Give PO 25.0 mg stat, then bd or tds

Disposition

- **Hypertensive emergency**: patients should be admitted to an ICU in consultation with General Medicine and the respective subspecialties involved.
- **Hypertensive urgency**: can be discharged **if** response is prompt and BP acceptable after 4 hours of monitoring; **but** follow-up must be arranged within 48 hours. In patients with newly diagnosed hypertension where the cause is uncertain, admit to General Medicine for evaluation and exclusion of secondary causes of hypertension.

References/further reading

1. The Seventh Report of the Joint National Committee on Prevention, Detection, Evaluation, and Treatment of High Blood Pressure, *JAMA* 2003;289(19):2560–2572..
2. Crawford MH, DiMarco JP, eds. *Cardiology*. London: Mosby International Limited; 2001.
3. Wyatt JP, Illingworth RN, Clancy MJ, et al, eds. *Oxford Handbook of Accident and Emergency Medicine*. Oxford: Oxford University Press; 1999:90.
4. Bales A. Hypertensive crisis: How to tell if it's an emergency or an urgency. *Postgrad Med.* 1999;105(5):119–126,130.
5. Cherney D, Straus S. Management of patients with hypertensive urgencies and emergencies: A systematic review of the literature. *J Gen Intern Med.* 2002;17(12):937–945.

64 Hyperthermia

Francis Lee

CAVEATS

- The **classic triad** for heat stroke is:
  1. Rectal temperature >41°C
  2. Altered mental state
  3. Hot dry skin

  This is an advanced stage of the condition and should be used with caution. If followed too rigidly, one may miss many cases of early heat stroke.
- There is no clinical marker for heat stroke and many of the symptoms and signs are non-specific. Diagnosis, therefore, requires a high index of suspicion. Altered mental state, acute behavioural change and syncope with a history of exposure to a high ambient temperature should alert one to the diagnosis of heat stroke.
- Many would associate high ambient temperature with the outdoors. It is important to note that prolonged activity or incarceration in an enclosed space without proper ventilation or air-conditioning (nursing homes, sauna, boiler room) is a significant risk factor for heat stroke.
- **Heat exhaustion** is a precursor of heat stroke and has the following features:
  1. Anxiety, irritability and fatigue
  2. Thirst, polydipsia
  3. Hyperventilation, carpopedal spasm
  4. Nausea, vomiting
  5. Raised rectal temperature
  6. Mild liver enzymes abnormalities
  7. Raised creatinine kinase levels
- There is no clear distinction between heat exhaustion and heat stroke and the two conditions share some common features, making diagnosis difficult. As a general guide, patients with **heat exhaustion** usually have **no history of altered mental state**.

RISK FACTORS FOR HEAT STROKE

- Several factors may predispose a person to heat stroke:
  1. Lack of acclimatization and poor physical fitness
  2. Obesity
  3. Extremes of age
  4. Concurrent diseases such as ischaemic heart disease, diabetes mellitus, skin disorders, infectious disease
  5. States of dehydration such as alcohol use, diarrhoea, vomiting
  6. Drugs such as anticholinergics, antihistamines, diuretics, beta-blockers

7. Recreational drugs such as amphetamines, cocaine
8. Preceding pyrexia
9. Previous history of heat injuries

DIFFERENTIAL DIAGNOSIS

- Many conditions producing altered mental state with pyrexia mimic heat stroke:
  1. Intracranial infections such as meningitis, encephalitis
  2. Infections such as typhoid, malaria
  3. Malignant hyperthermia, neuroleptic malignant syndrome
  4. Neurologic disorders such as stroke, epilepsy
  5. Metabolic conditions such as thyroid storm

☛ Special Tips for GPs

- Call ambulance for transport to the ED.
- Institute early cooling by undressing patient as much as possible and sponging or spraying with water to wet the skin. A fan directed at the victim will aid cooling by evaporation.
- Hydration is important. Oral fluids could be given if patient is alert and able to tolerate it. Establishment of an IV drip would be ideal.

MANAGEMENT

- The **initial steps** in the **management of heat stroke** are:
  1. Transfer patient to resuscitation or critical care area of the ED.
  2. Secure ABCs.
  3. Provide supplemental oxygen.
  4. Set up large bore IV in both cubital fossae and infuse cool fluids.
  5. Set up cardiac and vital signs monitoring.
  6. Assess rectal temperature.
- **Cooling** of the patient must be carried out next:
  1. Remove all clothing
  2. Use a body cooling unit (evaporative cooling method) or sponge and spray with cold water and fan patient
  3. Cooling should be carried out until rectal temperature reaches 38.5°C
- **ECG** to look for cardiovascular problems. In acute heat disorders, tachycardia is almost always present. Other features may include non-specific ST and T changes and conduction abnormalities. ECG may indicate any preexisting cardiovascular disorders.
- **CXR** to look for evidence of pulmonary oedema or ARDS. Pulmonary infarctions have been described in heat stroke.

- **Stat capillary blood glucose** to look for hypoglycaemia so that treatment can be instituted. However, hyperglycaemia may be seen in heat stroke and does not necessarily indicate the presence of diabetes mellitus.
- **Blood investigations**:
  1. FBC: leukocytosis is common without infection. Thrombocytopaenia may be seen.
  2. Electrolytes: sodium and potassium levels may be elevated, normal or low, depending on many factors. Hypomagnesaemia and hypocalcaemia may occur.
  3. Muscle enzymes are commonly raised.
  4. Liver function test: abnormalities of hepatic enzymes are almost always present.
  5. ABG may indicate alkalosis from hyperventilation or metabolic acidosis from tissue injury and hypoxia.
  6. Coagulation profile may indicate the onset of coagulopathy
- **Urine dipstick** to look for blood and myoglobin. Alternatively, a sample may be sent to the lab to measure urine myoglobin.
- During cooling, shivering may occur, countering efforts in lowering the body temperature. This can be controlled with IV diazepam 5 mg or IV chlorpromazine 25–50 mg.
- Insert a nasogastric tube to manage acute gastric distension.
- Give IV cimetidine 400 mg stat to prevent acute gastritis.
- Patient must be catheterized to measure urine output.
- **Precautions**
  1. The mechanism for heat stroke does not involve a shift in the 'physiological thermostat' and therefore **antipyretics** are **not helpful**. Aspirin must be avoided as it may cause coagulation problems while the use of paracetamol may aggravate hepatic injury.
  2. **Alcohol cannot be used** for cooling despite a higher specific heat for vapourization because skin absorption may cause progressive drowsiness and obtundation.
  3. **Hypotension must be corrected** before effective cooling can be carried out.
  4. Beware of **rebound pulmonary oedema** when vasoconstriction occurs after the heat stroke is controlled.
- **Disposition**
  1. Admit all heat strokes.
  2. Recovered heat exhaustion without end-organ damage can be observed in the ED and then discharged.

References/further reading

1. Weiner KS, Khogali M. A physiological body-cooling unit for heatstroke. *Lancet.* 1980;1:507.
2. Gaffin SL, Gardner JW, Flinn SD. Cooling methods for heatstroke victims. *Ann Intern Med* 2000;132(8):678.

65 Hypoglycaemia

Benjamin Leong

DEFINITION

Hypoglycaemia may be defined as a low blood glucose level, usually of less than 3.0 mmol/l in a venous reading, accompanied by typical symptoms and signs, which are relieved upon correction of the low blood glucose.

CAVEATS

- Always check a stat capillary blood sugar on any patient presenting with altered mental state or seizures.
- Capillary blood sugar readings read lower than venous readings and may be artificially low in the presence of hypotension, hypothermia and oedema; hence always confirm the presence of hypoglycaemia with a venous sample to the lab.

Causes

- Up to half of the cases are diabetic patients on treatment with insulin or sulphonylureas.
- **Causes of hypoglycaemia** in a **healthy-appearing patient**
  1. Medications/drugs
     a. Alcohol
     b. Salicylates
     c. Non-selective beta-blockers (which attenuate the adrenergic response to stress)
     d. Factitious hypoglycaemia or overdose with insulin or oral hypoglycaemic agents
  2. Intense exercise
  3. Insulinoma
- **Causes of hypoglycaemia** in an **ill-appearing patient**
  1. Sepsis and shock
  2. Infection: malaria, especially with Quinine or Quinidine treatment
  3. Starvation, anorexia nervosa
  4. Liver failure
  5. Cardiac failure (diffuse liver dysfunction)
  6. Renal failure (impaired gluconeogenesis)
  7. Endocrine
     a. Hypothalamus-pituitary-adrenal axis insufficiency in cortisol and growth hormone
     b. Insulin antibodies

8. Non-islet cell tumour, eg sarcoma, mesothelioma
9. Congenital liver problems including defects of carbohydrate, amino acid and fatty acid metabolism

Clinical features

Hypoglycaemia may present with a **wide spectrum of neurological manifestations**. The following are common patterns of presentation:

- Neurogenic/autonomic (BSL approx 2.8–3.0 mmol/l): sympathetic overdrive state with diaphoresis, tachycardia, jitteriness, and pallor
- Neuroglycopenia (BSL <2.5–2.8 mmol/l)
  1. Behavioural disturbances such as irritability, confusion, and aggression
  2. Decreased conscious level
  3. Seizures
  4. Focal neurological deficits

☛ **Special Tips for GPs**

- **Prevention** is better than cure.
- **Good education** of patients and their caregivers on oral hypoglycaemic agents, insulin and appropriate meal and snack plans.
- **Avoid long-acting sulphonylureas, especially glibenclamide and chlorpropamide, in patients who are elderly, or who have liver, renal or cardiac impairment.**
- **Close monitoring** of patients' blood glucose, including self-blood glucose monitoring, will help to reduce the incidence of hypoglycaemia in the diabetic population.
- Encourage **medication safety at home**.
  1. Keep drugs locked out of reach of children.
  2. Discourage the practice of taking medication out of their original blister packs and filling them into recycled containers to prevent confusion.
  3. Label packages clearly.
- **Check the capillary blood glucose** of all patients presenting with altered mental state. Early treatment of hypoglycaemia reduces morbidity and mortality.

MANAGEMENT

- **Manage the patient in a monitored area**
  1. Monitoring: ECG, pulse oximetry, vital signs.
  2. Administer supplemental low-flow oxygen.
  3. Check the capillary blood glucose for all patients presenting with altered mental state.
- **History and examination**
  1. Check for diabetes mellitus, medication history, recent change in drug doses, recent and chronic illnesses.
  2. If patient is unconscious, obtain history from family or caregiver, and look for clues like medicine packages, Medik Awas cards, or other medication alert cards.
- **Investigation**
  1. **Venous blood glucose**, urea/electrolytes/creatinine, liver function tests, FBC.
  2. If patient is not diabetic, take **1–2 extra plain tubes of blood on ice** for serum insulin, C-peptides and cortisol prior to giving treatment to help the inpatient management team in the subsequent endocrine evaluation of the patient.
  3. **Do not wait for final lab results before instituting treatment**.
- **Treatment** depends on the conscious level and cooperation of the patient
  1. **Conscious and cooperative patient**
     a. **Oral therapy** is preferred.
     b. Give a **carbohydrate rich drink** (eg Glucolin, Lucozade, Ensure, Isocal, Milo, Horlicks) and feed the patient. Note that 1 can of Ensure has 250 calories, cf 1 pint of D_5W, which has 100 calories.
  2. **Unconscious or uncooperative patient**
     a. If **IV access is available**, give **IV dextrose 50% 40–50 ml**. Remember to flush with normal saline as the hypertonic solution can cause thrombophlebitis.
     b. If **IV access is unavailable** or if the patient is very uncooperative, **IM** or **SC glucagon 1 mg** may be given. Note that IM or SC glucagon takes a few minutes longer to work than IV dextrose. It is also not suitable for use in hypoglycaemia secondary to sulphonylureas or liver failure.
  3. If chronic alcoholism is suspected, give **IV thiamine 100 mg**.
  4. If adrenal insufficiency is suspected, give **IV hydrocortisone 100–200 mg**.
  5. If there are associated injuries, give **tetanus prophylaxis**.
- **Monitoring**
  1. Check the **capillary blood glucose** 15 min later, then every 30 min for the first 2 hours, and hourly thereafter. Prolonged monitoring is required in the case of a sulphonylurea overdose with Glibenclamide or Chlorpropamide.

2. **Consider repeat doses** if there is poor response to therapy, or a **continuous infusion of dextrose 5% or 10%** if there is a likelihood for a continued fall in the blood glucose level.
3. The majority of patients should recover in **20–30 minutes**.
4. If there is a **persistent altered mental state** despite the resolution of hypoglycaemia, other pathology must be considered, and a CT scan of the brain may be indicated.

- **Disposition**
  1. The disposition of the patient depends on several factors, which include the following:
     a. the **aetiology** of the hypoglycaemia, including the causal agent
     b. the **severity** of the neurological deficit and its response to treatment
     c. the **response** of the blood glucose levels and need for continuous replacement
     d. the presence of **comorbidities**, such as head injury
     e. the **social circumstances**, such as the availability of a responsible caregiver, or suicidal patients
  2. In general, most patients should be admitted under the care of Endocrinology or General Medicine or other subspecialty depending on etiology and comorbidities as appropriate. All cases of hypoglycaemia due to sulphonylureas must be admitted because of the relatively long half-life of the agent.
  3. In conditions which result in a strong tendency to hypoglycaemia (eg massive overdose of OHGA, acute liver failure, severe sepsis), consider admission to a HD ward or ICU.
  4. If the cause of hypoglycaemia has been clearly recognized and reversed (such as a diabetic who missed a meal after injecting insulin) with good clinical recovery, the patient may be discharged home under the care of a responsible caregiver.

References/further reading

1. Wyatt JP, Illingworth RN, Clancy MJ, et al, eds. *Oxford Handbook of Accident and Emergency Medicine*. Oxford: Oxford University Press; 1999.
2. Tintinalli JE, Kelen GD, Stapczynski JS, et al, eds. *Emergency Medicine: A Comprehensive Study Guide*. 5th ed. New York: McGraw-Hill; 2000.
3. Service JF: Classification of hypoglycemic disorders. *Endocrinol Metab Clin North Am.* 1999;28:501–517.
4. Service JF: Hypoglycemic disorders. *N Engl J Med.* 1995;332:1144–1152.

66 Intestinal obstruction

Irwani Ibrahim

CAVEATS

- Classical presentation includes abdominal pain, distension, vomiting and constipation. However, vomiting may be delayed in low obstruction and distention may be minimal in high bowel obstruction.
- Intestinal obstruction can be divided into **mechanical** (Table 1) and **non-mechanical obstruction (ileus)** (Table 2).
- Always **examine** the **hernia orifices** and perform a **rectal examination**. Impacted faeces would indicate a pseudoobstruction instead.
- Once diagnosis is made, determine if there is evidence of **strangulation** (Table 3) since bowel gangrene follows quickly.

Table 1: Causes of mechanical obstruction
Adhesions from previous surgery
Hernias
Tumours
Volvulus
Gallstones
Intussusception
Inflammatory bowel disease, namely Crohns' disease

Table 2: Causes of ileus
Postoperative
Hypokalaemia
Uraemia
Pseudoobstruction

Table 3: Evidence of strangulation
Febrile
Shock
Persistent pain despite decompression
Peritonism on examination and shock
In case of strangulation by external hernia, the lump is tense, tender, irreducible, has no expansile cough impulse and there is recent increase in size

☛ **Special Tips for GPs**

- Small frequent amounts of stools, which may be termed 'diarrhoea' by the patient, may be 'spurious diarrhoea' and does not exclude the diagnosis of intestinal obstruction.

MANAGEMENT

- Maintain airway and give supplemental oxygen .
- Establish peripheral IV line and infuse crystalloid 500 ml over 1–2 hours.
- Labs: FBC, GXM 2–4 units, urea/electrolytes/creatinine.
- Keep nil by mouth.
- Insert nasogastric tube and allow passive/free drainage to decompress stomach.
- Do **AXR (erect and supine)** to look for dilated bowel loops and multiple fluid levels.
- Supine AXRs give us more information than erect AXRs (eg the likely level of obstruction). If you have to do only one film, do a supine one.
- Consider ECG especially in the elderly.
- Insert urinary catheter to monitor urine output.
- If there is evidence of strangulation or peritonitis, immediate consultation with General Surgery registrar should be made.
- IV Rocephin® 1 g and IV metronidazole 500 mg should be given if there is evidence of bowel sepsis.

References/further reading

1. Winslet MC. Intestinal obstruction. In: Russell RCG, Williams NS, Bulstrode CJK, eds. *Bailey & Love's Short Practice of Surgery*. 23rd ed. London: Arnold Hodder Headline Group; 2000:1058–1075.
2. Wyatt JP, Illingworth RN, Clancy MJ, et al, eds. *Oxford Handbook of Accident and Emergency Medicine*. Oxford: Oxford University Press; 1999:528–529.

67 Ischaemic bowel

JP Travers • Irwani Ibrahim

CAVEATS

- Ischaemic bowel needs to be excluded in patients who are at risk, who present with sudden onset of abdominal pain, out of proportion to examination findings.
- Following occlusion, gangrene and perforation of the bowel follows rapidly.
- Early diagnosis is difficult when physical signs are minimal.
- **Risk factors** include:
  1. Age >50 years
  2. Valvular heart disease
  3. Chronic congestive cardiac failure
  4. Peripheral vascular disease
  5. Recent myocardial infarction
  6. Dysrhythmias, especially atrial fibrillation which predisposes to embolization
  7. Hypovolaemia
  8. Hypotension

Note: However, ischaemic bowel can occur without these classic risk factors and in the young. It should be suspected in all patients with peritoneal signs, when the pain seems out of proportion to the physical findings, and the patient looks too sick to be accounted for by a benign process, and especially if patient has metabolic acidosis as well.

> ☛ **Special Tips for GPs**
> - Do not dismiss abdominal pain as benign in high-risk patients.

MANAGEMENT

- Manage patient in at least monitored bed since these patients are prone to extensive peritonitis, shock and metabolic acidosis.
- Maintain airway and give supplemental **high-flow oxygen**.
- Establish at least 1 wide intravenous line and infuse crystalloid at maintenance rate, unless in shock.
- **Labs**:
  1. FBC
  2. Urea/electrolytes/creatinine

3. **ABG**, the most important lab test, to look for a metabolic acidosis which cannot be explained by other pathologies
4. Coagulation screen
5. GXM 2–4 units

- **AXR** may reveal dilated and/or thickened bowel loops or intramural gas. Most specific is free intraperitoneal air indicating perforation of gangrenous bowel.
- ECG may show dysrhythmias. AF is common.
- Consider inserting nasogastric tube and commencing antibiotics (eg an IV cephalosporin and metronidazole 500 mg).
- Insert urinary catheter to monitor urine output.
- Immediate consultation with the General Surgery Registrar.

References/further reading

1. Wyatt JP, Illingworth RN, Clancy MJ, et al, eds. *Oxford Handbook of Accident and Emergency Medicine*. Oxford: Oxford University Press; 1999.
2. Mann CV, Russell RCG. *Bailey & Love's Short Practice of Surgery*. 21st ed. London: Chapman and Hall; 1991.

68 Malaria

Chong Chew Lan

Caveats

- Classically, patients may present with paroxysms of high spiking **fever every 48 hours** (*Plasmodium vivax, P. ovale*) or **72 hours** (*P. malariae*). Infection with *P. falciparum* may not manifest these paroxysms.
- Consider malaria in all patients with fever, especially army recruits, foreign workers and patients with recent travel history to India, South America, Africa or South East Asia.
- Chemoprophylaxis may not prevent malaria as a result of drug resistance and inadequate dosages.
- **Clinical features** are **highly variable** and include the following:
  1. Malaise
  2. Vomiting
  3. Diarrhoea
  4. Haemolytic anaemia
  5. Jaundice
  6. Splenomegaly
  7. Headache
  8. Cerebral oedema
  9. Heart failure
  10. Pulmonary oedema
  11. Shock
  12. Renal failure
  13. Hypoglycaemia
- **Deterioration** can be **rapid**, particularly with ***P. falciparum*** infection.
- Look out for **hypoglycaemia** as both malaria and quinine may cause hypoglycaemia.
- Always be on the look out for **complications** of malaria as follows:
  1. Superimposed gram-negative sepsis
  2. Malarial respiratory distress or pulmonary oedema
  3. Cerebral malaria
  4. Shock
  5. Anaemia
  6. Acidosis
- **Mefloquine** is **not recommended** in patients with neuropsychiatric or cardiac conduction defects.

MANAGEMENT

- Send **blood for thin and thick film** examination for malaria in any ill patient who has been to a malarious area.
- If parasites are not visualized, repeated smears should be taken at least twice daily for 3 days to exclude malaria.
- **Admit** all patients with malaria.

☛ **Special Tips for GPs**

- Treat with **quinine** or **mefloquine**, when malaria is diagnosed, or, **chloroquine if vivax** is positively identified, before sending the patient to the ED as the patient may deteriorate very quickly.
- Check bedside glucose level at the clinic and treat hypoglycaemia if necessary.
- **Simple preventive measures against malaria in adults include:**
  1. Advising patients to avoid mosquito bites by utilizing repellant, eg 30% DEET, nets, appropriate clothing and avoidance of dusk and dawn bare exposure.
  2. If patients are going to a malarious area, start **chemoprophylaxis** 1 week before travel and continue for 4 weeks after returning. Give:
     a. mefloquine 250 mg weekly **or**
     b. doxycycline 100 mg OM **or**
     c. maloprim 1 tab weekly

- The **parasite count**, which is related to prognosis, and infecting species should be identified.
- **Labs**:
  1. FBC (anaemia, low or normal TW, thrombocytopaenia)
  2. Urea/electrolytes/creatinine (renal failure)
  3. Liver function test (jaundice)
  4. Blood glucose (*P. falciparum* infection or treatment with quinine)
  5. Urine for haemoglobinuria (blackwater fever)
- For ***P. vivax, P. ovale, P. malariae*** and **mild chloroquine sensitive *P. falciparum* infections (<0.1% parasite count)**:
  1. Adult: **Chloroquine phosphate** 1 g stat (chloroquine base 600 mg) 500 mg 6 h later, then 500 mg per day for the next 2 days
  2. Child: **Chloroquine phosphate** 10 mg/kg base to maximum of 600 mg load then 5 mg/kg base in 6 h, and 5 mg/kg base per day for 2 days

  This is followed by **primaquine phosphate** (ensure normal G6PD status) 26.3 mg load (15 mg base) per day for 14 days upon completion of chloroquine therapy for *P. ovale* and *P. vivax* infections. Give 0.3 mg/kg base for 14 days in children.

Note: Primaquine therapy is for eradication of extraerythrocytic stage and prevents relapses.

- For **uncomplicated, moderate (>0.1% but <5%) chloroquine sensitive *P. falciparum***, give oral **quinine sulfate** 600–650 mg (8.3–10 mg/kg for children) tds for 7 days and **doxycycline** 100 mg bd for 7 days. **Doxycycline is contraindicated in children <8 years old**. In this case, extend quinine sulphate therapy to 10 days. Fansidar (pyrimethamine-sulfadoxine), mefloquine and artemisinin (qinghaosu) have also been used.
- **For complicated (cerebral malaria, renal failure, Hb <7g/dL, ARDS, hypoglycaemia and DIVC)** or **severe (>5%) *P. falciparum* infection**, admit to ICU for close monitoring of BP, urine output, cardiac rhythm and blood sugar level:
  1. Give **IV quinine dihydrochloride** 20 mg/kg over 4 h, then 10 mg/kg over 8 h q 8 hourly for 72 h.
  2. Switch to oral regime when possible or counts <1% to finish 7 days of therapy. Monitor parasitemia every 6 hours. If treatment is effective, expect about 75% decrease in parasite level after 48 hours of treatment. If parasitemia >10–15%, consider exchange transfusion. Steroids are harmful in cerebral malaria.

References/further reading

1. White NJ. Current concepts: The treatment of malaria. *NEJM.* 1996;335:800–806.
2. Warrell DA, Gilles HM. *Essential Malariology*. London: Arnold; 2002.

69 Meningitis

Francis Lee

CAVEATS

- Meningitis **typically presents** with fever, headache and meningeal signs such as neck stiffness. This may be accompanied by nausea, vomiting, irritability and lethargy. Photophobia may be present.
- One must be aware of **atypical presentations**. Infants with meningitis tend to present with non-specific symptoms like irritability, vomiting and poor feeding. Children and the elderly may have no meningeal signs and the latter may present with altered mental states.
- In the management of patient with meningitis, one should consider the possibility of **meningococcaemia**, especially if the patient has a purpuric rash. This fulminant infection runs a rapid course with associated high mortality. Healthcare personnel who have contact with such a patient may require **antibiotic prophylaxis, ie 1 dose of ciprofloxacin 500 mg**.

> ☛ **Special Tips for GPs**
> - If **meningococcaemia** is suspected, **IV crystalline penicillin 4 mega units** can be given stat if there is delay in getting the patient to the hospital by ambulance.
> - Chemoprophylaxis to be considered for office staff – **ciprofloxacin 500mg × 1 dose**.

MANAGEMENT

- Transfer the patient to a monitored area of the department. Those with unstable parameters or altered mental state should be managed in the critical care area.
- Secure the airway and give supplemental oxygen.
- Establish an IV line and do blood investigations such as FBC and urea/electrolytes/creatinine. DIVC screen should be done if meningococcaemia is suspected.
- Monitoring: BP, pulse rate, respiration rate, temperature, SpO_2 and conscious level.
- Do blood culture/urine culture.
- Lumbar puncture may be performed in the ED (after visualization of optic discs for evidence of raised ICP). Send CSF specimens for:

Table 1: Empirical antibiotic regime for bacterial meningitis

Group	Suspected organisms	Empiric therapy
Elderly Alcoholic Debilitated	*Streptococcus pneumoniae* *Neisseria meningitidis* *Haemophilus influenzae* *Listeria monocytogenes*	IV ceftriaxone 2 g 12 h **and** IV ampicillin 50 mg/kg body weight 6 h
HIV-positive Immunocompromised	*Streptococcus pneumoniae* *Neisseria meningitidis* *Haemophilus influenzae* *Listeria monocytogenes* *Cryptococcus neoformans* *Toxoplasma gondii* *Staphylococcus aureus*	IV ampicillin 50 mg/kg body weight 6 h
Indwelling CNS devices (V-P Shunt)	Coagulase +ve *Staphylococcus aureus* *Streptococcus pneumoniae* *Neisseria meningitidis* *Haemophilus influenzae* *Enterobactericae*	IV ceftriaxone 2 g 12 h **or** IV vancomycin 1 g 12 h
Nosocomial (postneurosurgical) Penetrating CNS trauma	*Staphylococcus aureus* *Streptococcus pneumoniae* *Pseudomonas aeruginosa* *Neisseria meningitidis* *Haemophilus influenzae*	IV ceftazidime 2 g 8–12 h
Meningococcaemia	*Neisseria meningitidis*	IV penicillin G 400,000 units/kg/d (Up to 24 mega units/day) **or** IV ampicillin 2 g 4–6 h **or** IV ceftriaxone 2 g 12 h

Table 2: CSF picture in bacterial and viral meningitis

	Normal	Bacterial meningitis	Viral meningitis
Colour	Clear	Cloudy	Clear
Opening pressure	<18 cm H_2O	>20 cm H_2O	<18 cm H_2O
WBC count	0	200–10,000/mm^3	25–1,000/mm^3
Glucose	>40 mg/dl	<40 mg/dl	>40 mg/dl
Protein	<40 mg/dl	100–500 mg/dl	50–100 mg/dl

1. Tube 1: cell count and cytospin for cell and differential count.
2. Tube 2: protein, glucose.
3. Tube 3: microbiology (gram stain, C&S, AFB smear, TB culture, Indian ink, fungal culture).
4. Tube 4: crytococcal antigen, bacterial antigens, ie *Strep pneumoniae*, *N. meningitidis*, *H. influenzae B*, *Group B streptococcus*.
5. Tube 5: virology studies if viral meningitis is suspected

- Start **IV antibiotics** therapy early (Table 1). If delay in definitive diagnosis is expected, this should be administered prior to lumbar puncture.
- Prescribe antipyretics and antiemetics accordingly.
- The use of corticosteroids in meningitis is controversial. Most studies that show benefits of steroids have been done on children. Many experts feel that the paediatric experience could be extrapolated to adults. The recommended dose is 0.15 mg/kg of dexamethasone.
- All patients with meningitis should be admitted for further management and investigation.

CEREBROSPINAL FLUID

- There is no absolute necessity to routinely perform a **head CT scan** prior to a lumbar puncture. This is **indicated only** when there is **raised intracranial pressure** and suspected mass lesion:
  1. Head injury
  2. Brain tumour
  3. Brain abscess
  4. Neurological deficits
  5. HIV positive patients
- The **CSF picture** depends on aetiology. See Table 2.
- **Cryptococcal meningitis** shares similar CSF picture to that of bacterial meningitis except for a lower white count. Definitive diagnosis depends on a positive Indian ink and cryptococcal antigen results.
- **Tuberculosis meningitis** also produces CSF changes similar to viral meningitis. Definitive diagnosis depends on AFB stain and AFB culture.

References/further reading

1 Walsh-Kelly C, Nelson D, Smith D, et al. Clinical predictors of bacterial versus aseptic meningitis in childhood. *Ann Emerg Med.* 1992;21:910–914.
2. Graham T, Moran G. Meningitis update: Pearls, pitfalls, guidelines, and controversies. *Emerg Med Rep.* 1995;16(22).
3. Lipton JD, Schafermeyer RW. Evolving concepts in paediatric bacterial meningitis. Part 1: Pathophysiology and diagnosis. *Ann Emerg Med.* 1993;22:1062–1615.

70 Myocardial infarction, acute

Shirley Ooi

CAVEATS

- 2–4% of all cases of MI are inappropriately discharged home. The majority of these cases involve young patients with unsuspected AMI, and, elderly patients with atypical presentations (refer to *Geriatric Emergencies*). Hence, AMI should be excluded in older patients as well as diabetic patients presenting with unexplained cardiac, respiratory and neurologic symptoms.
- Factors leading to the **missed diagnosis of MI** cited in successful litigation include:
  1. Failure to order study (ECG or serum marker)
  2. Diagnosis not considered
  3. Inappropriate discharge from ED
  4. Incorrect interpretation of tests (ECG or serum marker)
  5. Over-reliance of negative studies (both ECG and a single *negative* serum marker)
- Characteristics of the **atypical AMI presentation** include:
  1. Personality traits (masculinity, calmness, independence, low anxiety)
  2. Behaviour pattern (low rates of physician presentation for past medical issues, the stoic patient, the patient with denial)
  3. Higher pain thresholds (both non-cardiac and cardiac pain issues)
  4. Major depression or psychosis
  5. Demented patient or other factors reducing effective communication
  6. Physician and patient misinterpretation of symptoms and signs resulting from AMI
  7. Sensory, motor and autonomic neuropathy
  8. Impaired CNS recognition of the ischaemia
- The following are **anginal equivalent complaints**, **syndromes and presentations**:
  1. Anginal equivalent complaints: dyspnoea, nausea/vomiting, diaphoresis, weakness/dizziness, cough, syncope.
  2. Anginal equivalent syndromes: delirium, confusion, CVA.
  3. Anginal equivalent presentations and findings: cardiac arrest, new-onset dysrhythmia, new-onset congestive cardiac failure, unexplained bronchospasm, unexplained tachycardia, peripheral oedema.
- The following are **risk management tips** for patients with possible MI:
  1. Age and female gender should not rule out the diagnosis of ischaemia or infarction.
  2. History of heart disease is a critical factor. For the patient with a known history of angina or MI who presents with a potentially new ischaemic

event, risk factors have limited diagnostic significance since the presence of cardiovascular disease is a known fact.
3. The following are risk factors relevant in patients with chest pain: family history, diabetes mellitus, hypertension, hyperlipidaemia, smoking and a history of cocaine use.
4. Consider implementing a policy of old ECG retrieval as a normal departmental routine in any patient with a potential cardiac-related presentation.
5. Chest pain in the presence of a new left bundle branch block should be considered an AMI. All new LBBB with consistent chest pain should be considered for thrombolysis therapy.
6. Resting chest pain in a patient with known heart disease should be considered an ominous finding.

☛ **Special Tips for GPs**

- Patients with AMI may present atypically clinically and from ECGs.
- Beware of the atypical presentation of AMI in the elderly, diabetic and the young with risk factors.
- Once AMI is diagnosed, do not send the patient to the ED by his own transport! Call for the ambulance.
- Give aspirin 300 mg immediately before sending the patient to the hospital.

MANAGEMENT

Refer to *Pain, Chest, Acute* for general management.

- Oxygen by mask, vital signs monitoring.
- Oral **aspirin** 300 mg stat.
- **S/L GTN** 1 tab stat and repeat ECG after 5 minutes (to exclude ECG changes due to coronary spasm).
- Do right-sided ECG in inferior MI to exclude concomitant right ventricular infarct.
- IV plug and blood tests, ie FBC, urea/electrolytes/creatinine, cardiac enzymes, troponin T, PT/PTT, and GXM 2U PCT. Avoid arterial punctures.
- IV **morphine** 2–5 mg slow bolus. Repeat at 10 min intervals until pain relief is achieved.
- Consider IV metoclopramide 10 mg as antiemetic.
- **IV GTN** 20–200 μg/min, especially in:
  1. Continuing ischaemic chest pain
  2. Left ventricular failure, or
  3. Hypertension

Increase by increments of 5–10 μg/min at 5–10 min intervals until chest pain resolves or mean arterial pressure decreases by 10%. Discontinue if hypotensive. Caution in inferior MI as patient may have concomitant right ventricular infract, in which case nitrates are contraindicated.

- Consider **myocardial salvage therapy**, ie procedural coronary intervention (PCI) versus thrombolysis (PCI is the preferred strategy when available). See Table 1 for the value and limitations of the two reperfusion strategies.

Table 1: The reperfusion dichotomy in AMI, illustrating the advantages and disadvantages of the two reperfusion strategies

	Thrombolysis	*Procedural coronary intervention*
Advantages	Rapid administration Widely available Convenient	Better clinical efficacy, ie superior vessel patency, TIMI grade 3 flow rates and reduced occlusion rates Less haemorrhage Early definition of coronary anatomy allows tailored therapy and more efficient risk stratification
Disadvantages	Patency ceiling, ie infarct-related artery, is restored in only 60–85% of patients, with a normal TIMI grade 3 epicardial coronary flow in only 45–60% of patients Less clinical efficacy, ie optimal reperfusion is not achieved in >50% of patients, and re-occlusion of infarct vessel occurs in 5–15% at week 1 and 20–30% by 3 months Haemorrhagic risk	Delay limits efficacy Less widely available Requires expertise

- Consider whether patient is a candidate for **thrombolytic therapy** by reviewing criteria **for** thrombolysis:
  1. Typical chest pain of AMI
  2. ST segment elevation of at least 1 mm in at least 2 inferior ECG leads **or** elevation of at least 2 mm in at least 2 contiguous anterior leads
  3. Less than 12 hours from onset of chest pain
  4. Less than 75 years of age
- If patient satisfies criteria for consideration for **thrombolysis**, review list of **contraindications**:
  1. Suspected aortic dissection
  2. Previous stroke
  3. Known intracranial neoplasm
  4. Recent head trauma
  5. Other intracranial pathology
  6. Severe hypertension (BP >180/110)
  7. Acute peptic ulcer (not merely vague history of 'gastric')
  8. Acute internal bleeding
  9. Recent (<1 month) internal bleeding
  10. Major surgery (<1 month) recently
  11. Current use of anticoagulants
  12. Known bleeding diathesis
  13. Prolonged CPR (>5 minutes)
  14. Previous administration of thrombolytics
  15. Pregnancy
  16. Diabetic retinopathy
  17. Hypotension (SBP <90 mm Hg)
  18. ECG shows LBBB
  19. Any other medical problem which may preclude use of thrombolytics

  If the answer to **any** of the above is 'yes', do not administer thrombolytics. Discuss the case with cardiologist on-call first.
- If there are no contraindications, consider **choice of thrombolytics,** ie Streptokinase (SK) versus recombinant tissue plasminogen activator (rtPA):

  SK
  1. The most commonly used and cost-effective choice
  2. The better choice when the risk for intracranial haemorrhage is the highest (eg the elderly) because usage of rtPA results in increased likelihood of intracranial haemorrhage

  rtPA
  1. Can be used in either gender
  2. Less than 50 years of age
  3. Anterior AMI
  4. Less than 12 hours from onset of chest pain
- Take verbal consent from patient and relatives. Inform them of the benefits and risks of thrombolytic therapy.

- **Adverse effects of thrombolytic therapy** include:
  1. Risk of intracranial bleeding (1%) is higher when
     a. Patient's age is >65
     b. Low body weight of <70 kg
     c. Hypertension on presentation
     d. rtPA is used, compared to SK
  2. **SK allergy** occurs in approximately 5% of patients treated for the first time, especially those with a recent *Streptococcus* infection, and 0.2% of patients experience a serious anaphylactic reaction.
  3. **Hypotension** during IV SK infusion (15%), but this responds to decreasing the rate of infusion and volume expansion.
- **Dosage of thrombolytic therapy**

SK	rtPA
1. IV SK 1.5 mega units in 100 ml normal saline over 1 hour	1. 100 mg rtPA is dissolved in 100 ml sterile water
	2. Administer 15 mg IV bolus
	3. Administer IV infusion of 0.75 mg/kg over 30 minutes (not to exceed 50 mg)
	4. Followed by IV infusion of 0.5 mg/kg over 60 minutes (not to exceed 35 mg)

- If patient is in **shock**, always look for precipitating causes:
  1. Do a gentle rectal examination to look for **GI bleed**.
  2. Is patient **bradycardic**? Treat according to ACLS guidelines.
  3. Is patient **tachycardic**? Treat according to ACLS guidelines.
  4. Is patient having **right ventricular infarct**?
     a. Do right-sided leads in presence of ST elevation in II, III and aVF as in inferior AMI (Figure 1a). Look for at least 1mm ST elevation in V4R, V5R and V6R (Figure 1b).
     b. If so, give fluid challenge of 100–200 ml NS over 5–10 min and assess response.
     c. This can be repeated if patient does not become breathless and there are no clinical signs of pulmonary oedema.
     d. Start inotropes (IV dobutamine/dopamine 5–20 μg/kg/min) if BP remains low despite 500 ml of IV fluid.
  5. Is patient in **cardiogenic shock** because of **mechanical complications**, eg papillary muscle dysfunction or rupture, septal rupture or cardiac tamponade from free wall rupture?
     a. Call cardiologist and cardiothoracic surgeon.
     b. Meanwhile, start inotropic support, eg IV dobutamine/dopamine 5–20 μg/kg/min.
     c. Catheterize patient to measure urine output.

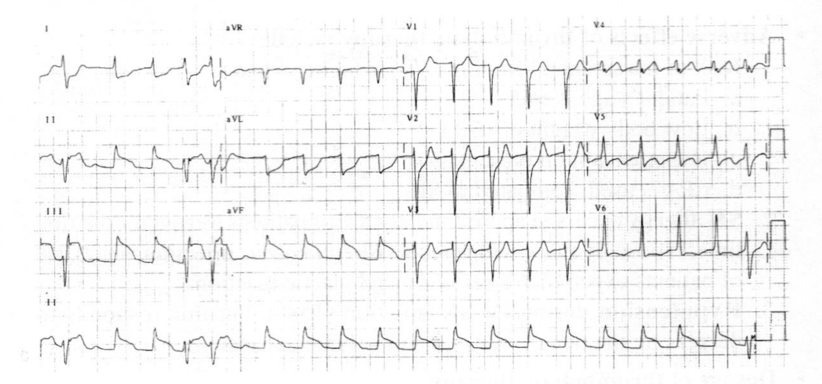

Figure 1a: ECG showing hyperacute phase of inferoposterior ST elevation MI

Note: ST elevations concave upwards, tall widened T waves in the inferior leads (leads II, III, aVF). There are reciprocal ST depression changes seen in leads I and aVL. The posterior MI changes are shown by ST depression in leads V_{2-3}

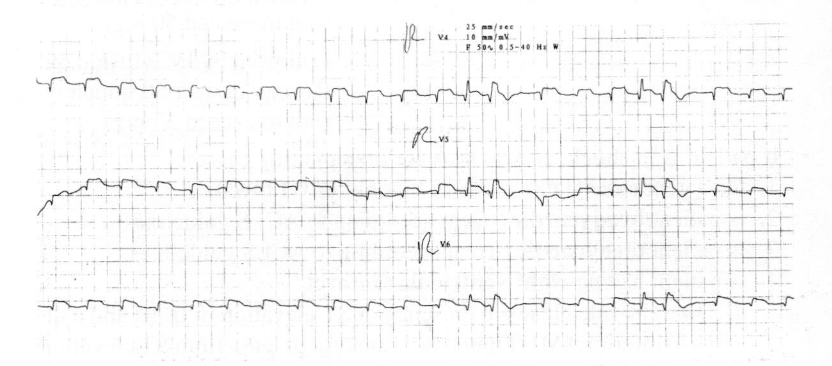

Figure 1b: Right-sided leads in the same patient

Right ventricular infarct is indicated by ST elevation in V_{4R} to V_{6R}. Nitrates are contraindicated in this patient.

References/further reading

1. Brady WJ, Jr. Missing the diagnosis of acute MI: Challenging presentations, electrocardiographic pearls, and outcome-effective management strategies. *Emerg Med Rep*. 1997; 18(10):91–102.
2. McPherson JA, Gibson RS. Reperfusion therapy for acute myocardial infarction. *Emerg Med Clin North Am*. 2001;19(2):433–449.

71 Near drowning

Francis Lee

DEFINITIONS

Drowning syndromes range from minimal aspiration of water with good survival to severe pulmonary injury with death. Several terminologies have been used to describe these events:

- **Drowning**: a process whereby air-breathing animals succumb on submersion in a liquid.
- **Near drowning**: submersion with temporary survival.
- **Submersion incident**: a more neutral term used to describe a person who is adversely affected by being submersed in water.

CAVEATS

- **Immediate rescue** (<5 min) and **early on-site resuscitation** is key to patient survival.
- An important part of the assessment is to look for a **cause** (eg trauma, suicide, poisoning, sea creature sting).
- **Hypothermia** is a potential complication, especially in the younger age group.

> ☛ **Special Tips for GPs**
> - In-water resuscitation is difficult to perform and potentially endangers the life of the rescuer.
> - Attempts to drain water using various techniques, such as the Heimlich manoeuvre, are controversial.

INITIAL PREHOSPITAL MANAGEMENT

- Immediate rescue from water
- Assessment of ABCs
- Initiate CPR if necessary
- Provide oxygen
- Establish intravenous access (if equipment is available)

MANAGEMENT

- The management of near drowning focuses on securing ABCs and correction of hypoxia.

- The distinction between **fresh water** (surfactant loss from washout) and **salt water** (surfactant loss by denaturation) **drowning** or between **wet** and **dry** (asphyxiation due to laryngospasm precipitated by initial water entry into the larynx) **drowning** is useful to help us understand possible pathophysiologic mechanisms of morbidity and mortality but does not affect the way a patient is managed in the ED.
- **Lung drainage procedure**, eg Heimlich manoeuvre, is controversial. These are **not** recommended because their effectiveness is not concretely proven, the execution of the manoeuvres could potentially cause more harm than good to the victim and distracts the care provider from more urgent goals of resuscitation.
- **Antibiotics and steroids** have **no proven benefit** in near-drowning victims.
- **Diuretics** are of **no help** in non-cardiogenic pulmonary oedema.

Initial hospital management

- Transfer patient to a high acuity area of the department.
- **Primary survey**:
  1. Check ABCs. Consider intubation if airway is not secured.
  2. C-spine must always be stabilized and neck movements avoided.
  3. Give 100% oxygen. Assist ventilation if breathing is inadequate.
  4. Providing PEEP will often improve oxygenation.
  5. Resuscitative actions: start CPR if patient is in a collapsed state.
  6. Establish IV line and draw blood for FBC, urea/electrolytes/creatinine, and ABG.
  7. Put patient on full monitoring: ECG, parameters and pulse oximetry.
  8. **Chest x-ray** to assess severity of aspiration.
  9. Keep patient warm at all times.
  10. Treat **hypothermia** (in the tropics, hypothermia is uncommon and if it occurs, it is usually mild: 32–35°C):
      a. All wet clothing should be removed and patient dried.
      b. Provide adequate insulation (wrap patient in clean dry blanket or aluminium foil).
      c. Apply external warming if necessary (warming blanket).
      d. All fluids for the patient should be warmed.
- **Secondary survey**:
  1. Do a head-to-toe examination for possible causes or effects of the near-drowning incident.
  2. Pay special attention to the following:
      a. Altered sensorium after resuscitation: possible alcohol and drug use.
      b. Head injury: look for signs on the scalp and face.
      c. Cervical spine injury may be the cause or effect of near drowning.
      d. Epilepsy: abrasions and injury to tongue is a clue.
      e. Cardiac dysrhythmias: ECG assessment and monitoring is important.

   f. Diving injuries: eg decompression illness (DCI) or cerebral arterial gas embolism (CAGE).
3. Perform serial GCS assessment.

Disposition

- **Generally all** near-drowning victims should be **admitted**.
- Those who look well should be managed in an observation ward for at least 12 hours and subsequently be **discharged** if:
  1. Patient looks well and alert.
  2. No abnormal vital signs.
  3. Normal chest x-ray.
  4. Reliable guardian or caregiver at home.
- A patient should be admitted to **ICU** if:
  1. Patient is intubated.
  2. Continued altered mental state.
  3. Unstable parameters despite resuscitation.

Prognosis

- Patients with the following factors have a poor prognosis:
  1. Children <3 years old.
  2. Estimated submersion time >5 min.
  3. No resuscitation provided within 10 min of rescue.
  4. Presenting at the ED in coma or collapsed state.
  5. Delayed respiratory gasp only 20 min after rescue.

References/further reading

1. Newman A. Submersion incidents. In: Auerbach P, ed. *Wilderness Medicine*. 4th ed. St. Louis: Mosby; 2001:1340.
2. Modell JH. *Pathophysiology and treatment of drowning and near drowning*. Springfield, Illinois: Thomas; 1971.
3. Orlowski JP. Prognostic factors in drowning and near-drowning. *J Am Coll Emerg Phys*. 1979;8:176.
4. Pearn J. The management of near drowning. *BMJ*. 1985;292:1447–1452.

72 Oncology emergencies

Shirley Ooi

CAVEATS

- Patients with malignancies are prone to emergencies either arising from their treatment or related to their malignancy.
- There are some **important principles** to follow when managing them in the ED:
  1. If need be, the managing physician should be notified early.
  2. As these patients have been 'through the system' on numerous occasions, a direct assessment with early senior clinician involvement, early symptom management, eg pain control and early decision-making, are all desirable.
  3. It is useful to find out the extent of the malignancy, the patient's response to treatment, what the prognosis is and the objectives of treatment so as to decide on palliative care versus active treatment. This is especially important if the patient presents in a critical condition and a decision must be made as to whether active resuscitation should be carried out.
- The **4 most common and life-threatening oncologic emergencies** are:
  1. Neutropenic sepsis
  2. Thrombocytopaenia
  3. Hypercalcaemia
  4. Cord compression
- Reduction of mortality from neutropenic sepsis is dependent on the speed of administration of IV antibiotics.

> ☛ **Special Tips for GPs**
> - Do not attempt to treat oncology patients presenting with a fever by administering antibiotics in the office. Refer immediately to the ED, especially if the fever is >38°C.
> - Suspect **hypercalcaemia** in all oncology patients who are generally unwell.
> - Think of **bony metastases** with a possibility of **cord compression** in all oncology patients presenting with back pain. Do not dismiss it as being due to 'arthritis'.

Table 1: A guide to the occurrence of neutropenia postchemotherapy

Drugs	*When neutropenia is expected to start*	*Expected duration of neutropenia*
Taxane Camptothecin	Days 7–10	3 days
Anthracyclines, eg adriamycin Alkylating agents, eg cyclophosphamide	Days 12–14	5–7 days
Mitomycin C	Week 3	1 week

NEUTROPENIC FEVER/SEPSIS

- This is an emergency and is the most common fatal side effect of chemotherapy!
- **Definition of neutropenia:** absolute neutrophil count (ANC) <1,000.

Management

- The occurrence of postchemotherapy neutropenia depends on the drugs given. See Table 1 for a guide to the occurrence of neutropenia.
- All patients undergoing chemotherapy/radiotherapy with fever (T >38°C) should ideally be managed in the **intermediate care area** with high prioritization given to them.
- Do the following **investigations for all patients undergoing chemotherapy/radiotherapy presenting with a fever**:
  1. FBC
  2. Urea/electrolytes/creatinine
  3. Liver function test
  4. CXR
- If **neutropenic**, perform **septic workup**. Do
  1. Blood cultures (aerobic and anaerobic) × 2 (one from each arm)
  2. Urine C&S, and
  3. Culture any purulent drainage
- Administer **IV antibiotics immediately** (after blood cultures drawn) before admission:
  1. IV **ceftazidime** (Fortum®) 1–2 g stat, and,
  2. IV **gentamicin** 2 mg/kg body weight stat
- If patient is more ill, give:
  1. IV ceftazidime (Fortum®) 2 g, and
  2. IV amikacin 7.5 mg/kg body weight stat

Note: If the patient is allergic to penicillin, an appropriate initial antibiotic combination would be IV **ciprofloxacin** and **gentamicin**. In the presence of possible infection with gram-positive organisms such as cutaneous infections, **cloxacillin** should be initiated.

- **Disposition**: admit to Oncology ward (isolation room).

Note:
1. No IM injections, urinary catheters or rectal examinations unless critical to management.
2. For patients on chemotherapy/radiotherapy with fever but who are not neutropenic, there is no need to do blood cultures and IV antibiotics at the ED level.

If a patient on chemotherapy is having a non-neutropenic fever, unless the patient's primary care physician is consulted, it is better to admit such a patient especially if the expected duration of the neutropenia is not over yet.

THROMBOCYTOPAENIA

There is a significant chance of central nervous system bleeding if platelet count is <20,000.

Management

- GXM random platelets 6 units.
- **Precautions**:
  1. Avoid IM injections
  2. Avoid NSAIDs
  3. Enforce complete bed rest
- **Disposition**: admit to Oncology general ward.

HYPERCALCAEMIA OF MALIGNANCY

Definition: elevated serum ionized calcium.

Diagnostic considerations

- This is a common problem and difficult to diagnose as symptoms and signs are non-specific including:
  1. aches and pains
  2. lethargy
  3. weakness
  4. nausea/vomiting
  5. dehydration
  6. polyuria
  7. polydipsia
  8. constipation
  9. confusion
  10. obtundation
  11. seizures
  12. coma

- Suspect hypercalcaemia in all cancer patients who do not feel well, or who are unusually depressed especially in cancers associated with hypercalcaemia, eg squamous cell carcinoma, breast, lymphomas, myelomas, clear cell.
- If untreated, it can be life-threatening!

Investigations

- Serum ionized calcium, urea/electrolytes/creatinine.

Management

- Aggressive hydration with IV normal saline; may need up to 3–4 litres in first 24 hours in severe cases to correct dehydration and to improve urine output and excretion of calcium (100–250 ml/h).
- Save diuretics only for impending fluid overload as premature use may worsen the hypercalcaemia.

CORD COMPRESSION

- This complication usually signifies advanced malignancy and a limited survival.
- The ability to walk and remain independent contributes immensely to the quality of life of an oncology patient. Hence, cord compression is a **true emergency**, as the prognosis for regaining function is at least in part related to early diagnosis and institution of treatment.

Presenting signs and symptoms

- Back pain (localized or radicular) in >95%.
- Localized tenderness on palpation.
- Other physical signs (eg weakness, sensory changes, or decreased reflexes) are late. Do not wait for them to appear!

Management

- Do **plain x-rays of spine** (85% sensitivity) to look for:
  1. Vertebral collapse (87% sensitivity)
  2. Pedicle destruction (31%)
  3. Lytic destruction (7%)
- **Practical approaches**:
  1. Back pain and no neurological deficit
     a. Do plain x-rays. If normal, perform non-urgent bone scan
     b. If abnormal, perform early MRI/myelogram
  2. Back pain with neurological deficit: administer **steroids** first in patients with known history of cancer (pathology established)
     a. As soon as cord compression is confirmed or strongly suggested **or**
     b. Collapsed vertebrae **or**

c. Absence of pedicles are noted on plain x-rays
   Dosage: IV dexamethasone 12–16 mg in 50 ml normal saline infusion immediately, followed by 4 mg q 6 h
d. Contact oncologist immediately

Note: In the absence of a known diagnosis of cancer, **do not start steroids**, but contact oncologist for further advice.

MASSIVE PLEURAL EFFUSION CAUSING RESPIRATORY COMPROMISE

- Presents with breathlessness, classical clinical signs of 'stony dullness', impaired vocal resonance, reduced breath sounds on auscultation, and a 'white out' hemithorax on chest x-ray. Tracheal and mediastinal deviation may be present.
- Check for previous chest imaging for comparison.

Management

- Prop up patient and administer supplemental oxygen to maintain >95% if possible.
- Monitor patient.
- Insert chest tube size 28–32 F on the affected side.

PERICARDIAL EFFUSION CAUSING ACUTE BREATHLESSNESS

- Pericardial effusions are particularly common in lung cancers, but can occur with other malignancies such as lymphoma, due to pericardial metastases.
- Recognition of this condition may be difficult but it should be suspected on **clinical** grounds in the presence of:
  1. Sinus tachycardia
  2. Small voltages on ECG
  3. Clear breath sounds
  4. Elevated jugular venous pressure (Kussmaul's sign)
  5. Palpable pulsus paradoxus (drop in systolic BP of >10 mm Hg on inspiration)
- **Diagnosis** is **confirmed** on transthoracic echocardiography.

Management

- In the presence of hypotension, urgent drainage is necessary. Refer to Cardiology for pericardiocentesis, which is temporary (definitive pericardial window should be performed eventually).

SUSPECTED MASSIVE PULMONARY EMBOLISM

- Patients with malignancy are at increased risk of deep venous thrombosis and pulmonary embolism due to factors including immobility and hypercoagulability. Refer to *Pulmonary Embolism.*

- Early recognition and proper management will lead to a better outcome.

Management

- Immediate Oncology/General Medicine consultation. Keep in view urgent spiral CT scan with IV contrast.

Acknowledgements

The author is grateful to the Oncology Department of the National University Hospital, Singapore, for sharing with us their protocol in the care of oncological emergency patients.

References/further reading

1. Edwards R. The oncological patient in the emergency department. In Fulde GWO, ed. *Emergency Medicine: The Principles of Practice.* 3rd ed. Sydney: MacLennan & Petty; 1998:383–386.

73 Pancreatitis, acute

Kenneth Mak • Peter Manning

DEFINITIONS

- An acute inflammatory process of the pancreas, with variable involvement of other regional tissues or remote organ systems.
- Classically, it is characterized by the presence of abdominal pain and associated with the presence of hyperamylasaemia.

CAVEATS

- Classically, acute pancreatitis is associated with high levels of **serum amylase** (the threshold value with high specificity being above 1,000 U/L or at least 4 times the normal range). This, however, is not always present.
- Patients with **acute exacerbations of chronic pancreatitis** often **present 'subthreshold' elevations of serum amylase** due to a reduced volume of functioning pancreatic tissue.
- **Raised amylase** levels may also be seen in **practically any acute abdominal pathology** but these do not classically reach threshold values.
- See Table 1 for the differential diagnosis of pancreatitis.

> ☛ **Special Tips for GPs**
>
> - Beware atypical presentations: the pain is often in the central abdomen or epigastrium, but not always so. When associated with other pathologies, eg common bile duct (CBD) stone and/or cholangitis, patients may also report symptoms related to the associated pathology, eg biliary colic from a CBD stone. When pancreatitis affects the pancreatic body and tail, pain may also be in the left hypochondrium rather than central. **Acute pancreatitis must therefore always be considered a possible diagnosis in any patient presenting with upper abdominal pain.**

GOALS OF MANAGEMENT

When a diagnosis of acute pancreatitis is made, the emergency physician should consider the following key questions:

Table 1: Differential diagnosis of pancreatitis

Site of pathology	*Examples*
Abdominal	Perforated peptic ulcer Acute exacerbation of peptic ulcer dyspepsia Biliary colic Cholangitis Ischaemic bowel Abdominal aortic aneurysm Abdominal aortic dissection
Supradiaphragmatic	Basal pneumonia Acute coronary syndrome

- **What is the cause of pancreatitis?** An attempt should be made to try and determine a possible cause of the pancreatitis from the clinical history. In the local setting, the most commonly defined cause is gallstone disease and patients may give a history of previous biliary colic or fat dyspepsia. Chronic alcohol consumption is also a major cause and the abdominal pain may present after a bout of heavy alcohol consumption. A list of the possible causes of pancreatitis is given in Table 2. There is no need to investigate further beyond a good clinical history in the ED to define the aetiology of the pancreatitis.
- **How severe is the pancreatitis?** Look for clues which will give an indication of the severity of the pancreatitis. This includes the following:
  1. **Signs of excessive fluid loss** ('third space losses') and **compromised end-organ perfusion**

Table 2: Possible causes of pancreatitis

Metabolic	*Vascular*
Alcohol	Postcardiopulmonary bypass
Hyperlipoproteinaemia	Polyarteritis nodosa and other vasculitic disorders
Hypercalcaemia	Atheroembolism
Genetic	
Drugs	
Scorpion Venom	*Infection*
	Mumps
Mechanical	Coxsackie B
Cholelithiasis	CMV
Postoperative	Cryptococcus
Pancreas divisum	
Posttraumatic	
ERCP	
Pancreatic tumour	

   a. Clinical dehydration
   b. Confusion
   c. Ascites
   d. Haemoconcentration (haematocrit elevated more than 10%)
   e. Raised urea/creatinine
   f. Metabolic acidosis
2. **Signs of organ failure**
   a. Coagulopathy (DIC screen positive)
   b. Renal failure (raised creatinine, metabolic acidosis, hyperkalaemia)
   c. Respiratory distress and hypoxia (lowered PaO_2 and SaO_2)
3. **Signs of sepsis**
   a. Local septic complications (eg pancreatic abscesses or infected pancreatic necrosis) do not occur early. Typically, these are complications which occur after the first week of disease. They should only be considered to be present if the patient presents with >1 week duration of disease, with signs of sepsis (high fevers and raised TWC).
   b. If high fever is present in a patient presenting early with pancreatitis, consider a non-pancreatic cause of sepsis. The most common cause is cholangitis secondary to biliary obstruction. Look for a cholestatic picture in the LFT results.
4. **Other signs of severe pancreatitis**
   a. Abdominal ecchymosis. This may be in the flanks (**Grey-Turner's sign**) or in the periumbilical area (**Cullen's sign**).
   b. Signs of hypocalcaemia, eg carpopedal spasm and tetany.
   c. Blood glucose >10 mmol/l.

MANAGEMENT PROTOCOL

- In all patients with acute pancreatitis:
  1. Keep patient fasted.
  2. Start IV saline drip. In the absence of dehydration, this can be at a maintenance rate of about 2.5–3 litres/day.
  3. Give supplemental oxygen by mask.
  4. If patient has vomiting (due to gastroparesis), insert a nasogastric tube for gastric decompression.
  5. Give parenteral analgesia. Opiates like Pethidine® are not strictly contraindicated and give the best pain relief. Avoid NSAIDs in patients with dehydration or organ compromise due to the risk of nephrotoxicity.
  6. In patients with history of peptic ulcer disease, give prophylactic acid suppressive therapy. Acid reduction, however, does not affect the severity or disease course of pancreatitis.
  7. Perform a **serum amylase** determination.
  8. Perform a **chest x-ray**. This will allow baseline evaluation of the lung fields for respiratory compromise and exclude other differential diagnoses, eg basal pneumonia or perforated viscus.

9. In patients with cardiac risk factors, perform an **ECG** and cardiac enzymes to exclude atypical angina/AMI.
10. In patients with signs of cholangitis (high fever, raised TWC and cholestatic LFTs), start **IV antibiotics after an initial blood culture**. Use a third-generation cephalosporin, eg cefuroxime or ceftriaxone, together with metronidazole. In patients with penicillin sensitivity, substitute the cephalosporin with ciprofloxacin. Avoid gentamicin due to potential nephrotoxicity.

Note: There is no need to give antibiotics in uncomplicated pancreatitis.

11. Start input/output charting to allow assessment of overall fluid losses.
12. It is not necessary to always perform all the relevant lab investigations in the ED to fully prognosticate the severity of the pancreatitis. In the absence of any clinical signs of severe pancreatitis, most of these tests can be performed in the ward after admission.
13. **Mild** cases of acute pancreatitis can either be admitted to the General Surgery service or to the Gastroenterology service. Try to get a ward (HD) bed for the patient if possible.

- In patients with signs of **severe pancreatitis**:
  1. Carry out the measures listed above.
  2. Monitor the patient in either the critical or intermediate case areas of the ED.
  3. If respiratory failure is present, intubate and ventilate patient.
  4. Carry out the following series of laboratory tests:
     a. FBC
     b. Urea/electrolytes/creatinine including calcium
     c. Liver function tests
     d. ABG
     e. Blood culture
  5. Start prophylactic systemic antibiotics. The choice of antibiotics is as above.
  6. There is no overall evidence-based benefit for the use of other medications like somatostatin or octreotide.
  7. When any of the features of acute pancreatitis is present, or if pancreatitis is diagnosed in an elderly patient (above the age of 70 years), contact the attending General Surgeon to review the patient urgently in the ED. Such patients are better admitted under the surgical service for possible surgical intervention in case of potential complicating infected pancreatic necrosis or pancreatic abscesses.
  8. Patients with severe pancreatitis should as a minimum be admitted to high dependency care. Patients with any feature of organ failure must be admitted to the SICU for definitive care.

References/further reading

1. Bradley EL 3rd. A clinically based classification system for acute pancreatitis. Summary of the International Symposium on Acute Pancreatitis, Atlanta, GA, September 11 through 13, 1992. *Arch Surg*. 1993;128(5):586–590. Review.
2. Vissers RJ, Abu-Laban RB, McHugh DF. Amylase and lipase in the emergency department evaluation of acute pancreatitis. *J Emerg Med*. 1999;17(6):1027–1037. Review.
3. Toouli J, Brooke-Smith M, Bassi C, et al. Guidelines for the management of acute pancreatitis. *J Gastroenterol Hepatol*. 2002;17 Suppl:S15–39.
4. Ratschko M, Fenner T, Lankisch PG. The role of antibiotic prophylaxis in the treatment of acute pancreatitis. *Gastroenterol Clin North Am*. 1999;28(3):641–659, ix–x. Review.
5. Bassi C, Falconi M, Sartori N, et al. The role of surgery in the major early complications of severe acute pancreatitis. *Eur J Gastroenterol Hepatol*. 1997;9(2):131–136. Review.

74 Pelvic inflammatory disease (PID)

John Yam Pei Yuan

CAVEATS

- Consider ectopic pregnancy and PID in any pregnancy-capable female patient with lower abdominal pain.
- **Criteria for the clinical diagnosis of acute PID**: the **classic triad** of lower abdominal pain/tenderness, cervical motion tenderness and bilateral adnexal tenderness detected on either vaginal or rectal examination is present in most cases. Other symptoms include vaginal discharge, vaginal bleeding and dyspareunia. Fever >38°C, nausea and vomiting may be present. On speculum examination, a purulent discharge is seen in about 95% of women with PID. If an adnexal mass is palpated and a tubo-ovarian abscess is suspected, pelvic ultrasonography should be performed.
- **Predisposing factors**:
  1. Multiple sexual partners
  2. Young age at sexual debut
  3. History of sexually transmitted diseases
  4. Recent instrumentation to lower genital tract (eg D&C, hysterosalpingography)
  5. Recent abortion, miscarriage or delivery
  6. Foreign body (eg IUCD)
  7. Frequent douching
  8. Smoking
- **Classical presentation** is that of subacute lower abdominal pain that is dull in nature and usually bilateral. Unilateral lower abdominal pain and adnexal tenderness is probably not PID. On the other hand, bear in mind other possible diagnoses in the face of bilateral lower abdominal pain and adnexal tenderness (eg ectopic pregnancy, tubo-ovarian abscess, adnexal torsion).
- Generally, women with appendicitis have been symptomatic for a shorter period of time and have more pronounced gastrointestinal symptoms. They are clinically more unwell, with signs localizing to the right iliac fossa.
- It is mandatory to **exclude a pregnancy**. Other investigations: FBC, urine dipstick.

MANAGEMENT

- Manage in intermediate acuity care area.
- Take high vaginal swabs for culture/sensitivity, endocervical swabs for *Chlamydia* and *Gonococcus*.

> ☛ **Special Tips for GPs**
>
> - Admit following O&G consultation if the following apply: toxic patient, poor response to outpatient treatment, pregnancy, presence of vomiting, surgical emergency causing the pain cannot be excluded, suspected tubo-ovarian abscess, immunodeficiency, poor likelihood of outpatient follow-up.

- Establish IV access and take blood for FBC, urea/electrolytes/creatinine.
- IV rehydration should be initiated if needed and pain should be controlled.
- Consideration should be given to removal of an IUCD, if present.
- In acute PID, consider **admission** for **IV antibiotics**:
  1. second or third generation cephalosporin (eg **ceftriaxone** 250 mg IM)
  2. **Tetracycline** 500 mg PO qd for 10–14 days or **doxycycline** 100 mg PO for 10–14 days (substitute **erythromycin** 500 mg PO qd for 10–14 days if patient is allergic to tetracycline)
  3. Consider **metronidazole** (IV or oral) for up to 14 days
- If the patient is discharged, complete discharge instructions should be given, with the following advice: close follow-up in the next 48–72 hours, abstention from sexual intercourse for two weeks and treatment of sexual partners.
- Patient should also be counselled (1) to avoid sexual contact until patient and partner have completed treatment, and (2) about condom use.
- Patients should be encouraged to be tested for syphilis, hepatitis and the human immunodeficiency virus (HIV).

Acknowledgement

The author is grateful to Associate Professor Arijit Biswas, Head, Division of Feto-Maternal Medicine, Department of Obstetrics and Gynaecology, National University Hospital, Singapore, for his assistance in the preparation of this chapter.

References/further reading

1. Moors A, Bevan CD, Thomas EJ. Pelvic inflammatory disease. In: Shaw RW, Soutter WP, Stanton SL, eds. *Gynaecology*. London: Churchill-Livingstone; 1997:813–825.

75 Peptic ulcer disease/dyspepsia

Andrea Rajnakova • Lim Seng Gee

CAVEATS

- Most patients will not present to the ED with peptic ulcer disease since it can only be diagnosed either endoscopically or radiologically. Most would present with upper abdominal pain/discomfort.
- **Dyspepsia** should be reserved for those who present with chronic upper abdominal pain/discomfort.
- All patients suffering from dyspepsia over the age of 40 years must be fully investigated for gastric malignancy.
- Duodenal ulcers usually occur in people aged 30 to 50 years and gastric ulcers in people aged 60+ years.
- *Helicobacter pylori* (*H. pylori*) is responsible for >95% of duodenal ulcers and 70–80% of gastric ulcers.
- The second most important cause of peptic ulcers is NSAIDs, which account for most cases of *H. pylori*-negative ulcers.
- Rare causes of peptic ulcers include pathological hypersecretory conditions such as gastrinoma (Zollinger-Ellison syndrome).
- Alcohol has not been found to be associated with peptic ulcers. However, ulcers are more common in people who have cirrhosis of the liver, a disease linked to heavy alcohol consumption.

☛ Special Tips for GPs

- *H. pylori* and NSAIDs cause over 90% of peptic ulcers.
- All people >40 years with **dyspepsia** should be **investigated endoscopically** to rule out gastric malignancy.
- All patients with **dyspepsia** and **alarm features**, such as weight loss, anaemia, dysphagia, palpable abdominal mass should be referred to a gastroenterologist for endoscopy.
- Always enquire about the **complications** of ulcer such as bleeding (weakness and melaena) and vomiting (pyloric obstruction). These are emergencies which need urgent hospital referral.
- Surgery is rarely necessary and only if complications such as recurrent severe bleeding, perforation or obstruction develop.

SYMPTOMS

- The patient with an uncomplicated peptic ulcer usually presents with abdominal pain or discomfort. Poor appetite, burping, nausea, vomiting may also be present.
- Alarm features include: weight loss, haematemesis or melaena, anaemia, dysphagia, palpable abdominal mass.
- It is not possible on the basis of history alone to differentiate between gastric and duodenal ulcers, although gastric ulcer patients tend to be older and are more likely to complain of weight loss.
- The pain is typically situated in the epigastrium, but may occur in the lower chest or right or left hypochondrium, and be localized to a very small area (pointing sign).
- The pain tends to occur when the patient is hungry, 1 to 3 hours after meals, to wake the patient in the night, to be relieved by food, antacids, vomiting, and also to be characterized by remission and exacerbations. Ulcer pain may radiate to the back.
- The diagnosis of peptic ulcer cannot be established or excluded based on history alone. Typical ulcerlike pains may occur in patients with non-ulcer dyspepsia. On the other hand, asymptomatic ulcers are more common in patients taking NSAIDs.
- Asymptomatic ulcers may present with bleeding. Patients may be unaware that they have a bleeding ulcer and may feel tired and weak due to anaemia. If the bleeding is heavy, haematemesis and melaena will be present.

MANAGEMENT

The **aims** of management of upper abdominal discomfort are to:

- Make a provisional diagnosis (refer to *Pain, Abdominal*)
- Relieve the symptoms
- Decide on who to admit
- Decide on who to refer for specialist consultation

Symptom management

- After **excluding life-threatening causes,** eg AMI, aortic dissection, ruptured abdominal aortic aneurysm and other important causes such as perforated peptic ulcer, pancreatitis, the patient should be given symptomatic relief.
- Give mist **magnesium trisilicate (MMT)/aluminium hydroxide** 40–80 ml and an **anti-spasmodic**, eg IV or IM hyoscine-N-butylbromide (Buscopan®) 40 mg or oral H_2-blockers.

Note: Statistically, peptic ulcer disease represents 10–15% of abdominal pain which will respond to MMT.

There is **no role for IV H_2-blockers or proton pump inhibitors**. The only evidence is that it is effective for those with bleeding peptic ulcers.

- Discharge the patient with MMT or Buscopan® for dyspeptic patients while waiting for a definitive diagnosis to be made at the Gastroenterology Specialist Outpatient Clinic (SOC).
- For patients with acute abdominal pain/discomfort, no further treatment is indicated.
- There is no role for *H. pylori* eradication for PUD and non-ulcer dyspepsia in the ED.

DISPOSITION

Indications for admission

- Bleeding: haematemesis, melaena. Admit to Gastroenterology or General Surgery depending on your hospital policy.
- Perforation: admit to General Surgery
- Narrowing and obstruction: difficult to diagnose in ED, but patient presents with vomiting or signs of IO. Admit to General Surgery.
- Non-responsive to treatment at the ED only if they have severe symptoms: admit to Gastroenterology
- Abdominal pain with fever and jaundice: admit to Gastroenterology.

Indications for referral to Gastroenterology (SOC)

- Recent onset of new symptoms in patients >40 years old.
- Presence of alarm features: weight loss, loss of appetite, haematemesis, melaena, anaemia, dysphagia, palpable abdominal mass.
- Persistence of symptoms despite a trial of empirical treatment (H_2-antagonists).

Note: **Single episode of abdominal pain/discomfort** (without any alarm features) **should not be referred to SOC** since this complaint is very common and is usually self-limiting and non-specific.

Discharge advice

Always remember to discharge patients with advice to return to the ED immediately if there is fever, lower abdominal pain, persistent diarrhoea or vomiting. Remember **upper abdominal pain** may be an **early symptom of acute appendicitis**.

References/further reading

1. Chan FKL, To KF, Wu JCY, et al. Eradication of *Helicobacter pylori* and risk of peptic ulcers in patients starting long-term treatment with non-steroidal anti-inflammatory drugs: A randomized trial. *Lancet.* 2002;359:9–13.

2. Hawkey CJ, Karrasch JA, Szczepanski L, et al. Omeprazole compared with misoprostol for ulcers associated with non-steroidal anti-inflammatory drugs. Omnium study. *NEMJ*. 1998;338:727–734.
3. Yeoh KG, Kang JY. Peptic ulcer disease. In: Guan R, Kang JY, Ng HS, et al, eds. *Management of Common Gastrointestinal Problems*. Singapore: Habas MediMedia Asia Pte Ltd; 2000;31–46.
4. Graham DY, Rakel RE, Fendrick AM, et al. Recognizing peptic ulcer disease: Keys to clinical and laboratory diagnosis. *Postgrad Med*. 1999;105(3):113–133.
5. Lahaie RG, Gaudreau C. *Helicobacter pylori* antibiotic resistance: trends over time. *Can J Gastroenterology*. 2000;14(10):895–899.
6. Manes G, Balzano A, Iaquinto G, et al. Accuracy of the stool antigen test in the diagnosis of *Helicobacter pylori* infection before treatment and in patients on omeprazole therapy. *Aliment Pharmacol Ther*. 2001;15(1):73–79.

76 Perianal conditions

Charles Bih-Shiou Tsang

CAVEATS

- Bleeding from the anal canal is usually fresh and bright red. Blood mixed with stool suggests a more proximal aetiology.
- **Pain and bleeding** with bowel movements occur in **anal fissures**. Bleeding from **piles** is usually **painless**.
- Deep seated anal abscesses can present with constant chronic anal pain and few physical signs. An endoanal ultrasound evaluation by a colorectal surgeon is required.
- Recurrent perianal abscesses in the same area suggests an underlying fistula-in-ano.

> ☛ **Special Tips for GPs**
> - Do not attribute rectal bleeding in a middle-aged or elderly patient solely to bleeding piles. Refer to a colorectal surgeon to exclude lesions in the more proximal gastrointestinal tract.
> - Never assume that rectal bleeding with bowel movements in a patient is due to piles without performing a digital rectal examination and anoscopy. If bleeding persists despite conservative treatment, always exclude a more proximal aetiology, eg barium enema, colonoscopy.

HAEMORRHOIDS

- **Clinical features**
  1. Bright red rectal bleeding usually after passage of stool.
  2. Bleeding can be variable in quantity but is usually self-limiting.
  3. Prolapsing mass requiring digital reduction.
  4. Painful and prolapsing mass with a bluish hue represents thrombosis and are usually not reducible.
  5. **First-degree piles** do not appear at the anus after defecation. Main symptom is bleeding after defecation.
  6. **Second-degree piles** protrude through the anus on defecation but spontaneously reduce.
  7. **Third-degree piles** remain outside the anus unless pushed back manually.
  8. **Fourth-degree piles** cannot be pushed back inside the anus.

- **Acute management**
  1. **Bleeding first- and second-degree piles**
     a. Provide reassurance.
     b. Perform rectal examination and anoscopy to exclude a proximal aetiology.
     c. Discharge with a 6-week course of bulking agents eg 1 satchet of ispaghula husk twice daily (Fybogel®, Metamucil®, Mucilin®), or micronized flavonoids (Daflon 500®) in a dose of 3 tabs bd for 3 days, then 2 tabs bd for 2 weeks.
  2. **Bleeding third-degree piles with mild thrombosis**
     a. Lie patient prone with an ice pack placed in the buttock cleft to reduce oedema.
     b. Administer parenteral analgesia, eg NSAIDs or opioid agonist.
     c. Attempt digital reduction with generous amount of lubricant.
     d. If successful, discharge with analgesics, bulking agents and flavonoid agents.
     e. If unsuccessful, admit the patient for further management.

PERIANAL HAEMATOMA

- **Clinical features**
  1. Due to rupture of blood vessels of the external haemorrhoidal venous complex.
  2. On examination there is an exquisitely tender and bluish discrete pea-shaped lump.
  3. The pain usually peaks within the first 2 days and settles by the 5th day.
- **Acute management**
  1. In the first 2 days, I&D in the ED:
     a. Prepare perianal skin with betadine (ask about allergy first).
     b. Infiltrate around haematoma with 1% lignocaine solution 5 ml using 22G needle.
     c. Make a small radial incision towards the anus and evacuate haematoma by expressing it.
     d. Apply direct pressure to stop any oozing.
     e. Insert a small ribbon pack.
     f. Discharge with analgesics, and, bulking agents to prevent constipation or straining.
     g. The ribbon pack can be removed the next day by the patient after a sitz bath (2 tablespoons of salt in a tub of warm water).
     h. Refer to colorectal surgeon for outpatient follow-up.
  2. After 2 days, provide reassurance and discharge with analgesics and bulking agents.

ANAL FISSURES

- **Clinical features**
  1. Present with bright red rectal bleeding with bowel movements.

2. Severe pain differentiates this condition from piles.
3. Common aggravating causes are poor fluid intake and a fibre-deficient diet.
4. Rectal examination reveals an acute linear tear posteriorly or anteriorly when gently effacing the anal verge. Digital rectal examination **may not be possible** due to severe anal pain and spasm.

- **Acute management**: if the pain is so severe as to preclude a proper rectal examination, admit the patient for examination under anaesthesia. Most acute fissures heal spontaneously with proper bowel regulation. However, if symptoms persist beyond 8 weeks, the fissure may not heal without surgical intervention. Signs of chronicity include the appearance of a boat-shaped ulcer with white anal sphincter fibres seen at the base. There is often a skin tag (aka sentinel pile) at the distal margin of the fissure and a hypertrophic anal papilla at the apex. The **mainstay of treatment** is **conservative** consisting of:
  1. A 6-week course of bulking agents, eg 1 sachet of ispaghula husk twice a day (Fybogel®, Metamucil®, Mucilin®) and 2 litres of oral fluids a day.
  2. Topical analgesia: lignocaine jelly 2% applied around the anus before a bowel movement to help ease the pain; this can be followed by a sitz bath (see above for directions).
  3. GTN paste can be useful for 'chemical sphincterotomy'.
  4. Note that stool softeners, eg Agarol® lactulose, are seldom necessary, and the resultant diarrhoea may aggravate the fissure.
  5. Arrange for outpatient follow-up with a colorectal surgeon.

ANORECTAL SEPSIS

- **Classification**: Park's classification categorizes anorectal sepsis in relation to the anal sphincter complex. Most abscesses arise from anal glands that are present within and around the anal sphincters and may be submucous, perianal, intersphincteric, ischiorectal or supralevator in location.
- Persistent drainage from an abscess that has been drained previously (2 months or more) suggests the presence of a fistula.
- **Clinical features**
  1. **A classic abscess** presents as a red, warm and tender swelling, which may already be pointing or draining pus.
  2. **Differential diagnosis of a perianal abscess from an ischiorectal abscess**: look at the relationship of the abscess to the pigmented perianal skin. Abscess within pigmented skin means **perianal abscess**, whereas abscess lying more laterally outside the pigmented skin means **ischiorectal**.
  3. A small deep-seated abscess may present with few external signs other than pain and tenderness during a rectal examination. Typically, this patient has received several courses of antibiotics or analgesics from his/her own doctor. Hence, chronic perianal pain should be referred to a colorectal surgeon for the exclusion of a deep abscess.

4. Persistent discharging sinuses or swelling for more than 2 months after the drainage of an abscess suggests an **anal fistula**. Rectal examination often reveals an indurated subcutaneous cord running radially from the external opening towards the anus. This cord is the fistula track.

- **Acute management**
  1. **Acute abscess**:
     a. Incision and drainage in ED under conscious sedation and local anaesthesia: a linear incision over the most fluctuant part of the abscess is then converted into a cruciate incision and the edges are trimmed to deroof the abscess.
     b. After expression of all pus, lightly pack with ribbon gauze for haemostasis (can be removed the next day after a sitz bath).
     c. Prescribe analgesics for 1–2 days with referral for review by colorectal surgeon within a week. If pain or fever persists, advise the patient to return to ED earlier as the abscess may have been incompletely drained.
     d. **Criteria for admission**: (1) **diabetics with perianal abscess** for surgical drainage and control of blood sugar levels, (2) suspicion of **necrotizing fasciitis** (tender induration with crepitus around the abscess).
  2. **Recurrent perianal abscesses or suspected underlying anal fistula**: admit for drainage by a colorectal surgeon.
  3. **Ischiorectal abscess**: admit for drainage by a colorectal surgeon.

PROLAPSED RECTUM

- **Clinical features**
  1. **'True' prolapse** is seen in infants and elderly females but is uncommon. The entire thickness of the rectal wall is intussuscepted out through the anus. The 'pinch' test reveals a double layer or 'a sleeve within a sleeve'.
  2. **'Pseudo' prolapse** is a prolapsed haemorrhoid or rectal mucosal prolapse and is common. The 'pinch' test fails to reveal another layer of rectal wall beneath. The mucosal prolapse is often associated with a history of chronic straining. The resultant mucus seepage may also cause pruritis.

- **Acute management**
  1. **'True' prolapse**: gentle digital reduction, bowel regulation in adults to avoid straining, and an early referral to paediatrician (infants) or colorectal surgeon (adults). If reduction is not possible, then it is deemed to be incarcerated and is a surgical emergency.
  2. **'Pseudo' prolapse of rectal mucosa**: prescribe a course of bulking agents (see above) and advise adequate fluid intake to avoid straining during defaecation. Refer to colorectal surgeon for definitive management (rubber band ligation).

POSTHAEMORRHOIDECTOMY BLEEDING

- **Clinical features**: fewer than 5% of such patients may present with secondary haemorrhage 7–10 days postsurgery; this may occur after a difficult bowel movement with straining. The bleeding is usually self-limiting and minor. However, in a small percentage, it can be sufficient to cause hypovolaemic shock.

- **Acute management**
  1. If severe, resuscitate with rapid fluid replacement via large-bore IV cannulae; GXM bood if necessary.
  2. Prepare to inspect the anal canal, identify the bleeding point and secure haemostasis.
     a. Prepare proper lighting, proctoscope, suction equipment, 20 ml of adrenaline solution diluted 1:10,000 in a syringe with a long spinal needle 23G.
     b. With the patient in the left lateral position, apply generous amounts of lignocaine jelly to the anus prior to the insertion of the proctoscope; evacuate the clots and slowly withdraw the proctoscope to visualize the anal canal, in particular the haemorroidectomy wound.
     c. Identify the bleeding point and inject the adrenaline solution.
     d. Insert an adrenaline pack and leave in situ for minor persistent oozing.
  3. Arrange an immediate colorectal consultation in the ED if you cannot control the bleeding. In the interim a size 18 F Foley catheter can be inserted into the anus and the balloon filled with 30 ml water and traction applied with the catheter being taped to the thigh. The balloon creates a tamponade effect on the haemorrhoidectomy wound.
  4. In minor cases of bleeding that has already stopped:
     a. Discharge patient with a course of metronidazole 400 mg tds for a week and a course of micronized flavonoids, eg Daflon®, (see p. 344 for dosage).
     b. Arrange early follow-up with patient's surgeon.

References/further reading

1. Misra MC, Parshad R. Randomized clinical trial of micronized flavonoids in the early control of bleeding from acute internal haemorrhoids. *Br J Surg*. 2000;87(7):868–872.
2. Ho YH, Tan M, Seow-Choen F. Micronized purified flavonidic fraction compared favorably with rubber band ligation and fiber alone in the management of bleeding hemorrhoids: randomized controlled trial. *Dis Colon Rectum*. 2000;43(1):66–69.
3. Eu KW, Seow-Choen F, Goh HS. Comparison of emergency and elective haemorrhoidectomy. *Br J Surg*. 1994;81(2):308–310.
4. Keighley M. Haemorrhoidal disease. In: Keighley MRB, ed. *Surgery of the Anus, Rectum and Colon*. London: W.B. Saunders; 1993:304–305.
5. Sorgi MB, Sardinas C. Anal fissure. In: Wexner SD, ed. *Clinical Decision Making in Colorectal Surgery*. Tokyo: Igaku-Shoin Medical Publishers, Inc; 1995:123–126.
6. Grace, R. Anorectal sepsis. In: Dudley CH, Russell RCG, eds. *Atlas of General Surgery*. Kent: Butterworth & Co; 1986:614–621.
7. Goldberg S. Rectal Prolapse and Rectoanal Intussusception in Clinical Decision Making. In: Wexner SD, ed. *Clinical Decision Making in Colorectal Surgery*. Tokyo: Igaku-Shoin Medical Publishers, Inc; 1995.
8. Ho YH, Tan M, Seow-Choen F, et al. Prospective randomized controlled trial of a micronized flavonidic fraction to reduce bleeding after haemorrhoidectomy. *Br J Surg*. 1995;82(8):1034–1035.

77 Pneumonia, community acquired (CAP)

Malcolm Mahadevan

CAVEATS

- **Defined** as acute infection of the pulmonary parenchyma.
- To be **diagnosed** if:
  1. Infiltrate on CXR consistent with pneumonia
  2. Altered breath sounds and/or localized crepitation
  3. Patient must not be a hospitalized patient or resident of a long term facility 14 days before onset of symptoms.
- Several **symptoms** of lower respiratory tract infection (≥2) may be present:
  1. Fever/hypothermia
  2. Rigors, sweats
  3. New cough with/without sputum
  4. Chest pain
  5. Dyspnoea
- **Non-specific symptoms** also include:
  1. Fatigue
  2. Myalgia
  3. Abdominal pain
  4. Anorexia
  5. Headache
- Pneumonia is the most common cause of death from an infective cause in Singapore. The most **common bacterial pathogens include**:
  1. *Strep pneumoniae* (65%)
  2. *Haemophilus influenzae* (appoximately 10%)
  3. Atypicals: mycoplasma and legionella (appoximately 10%)
  4. *Staph aureus* (2%) and gram-negatives (1%) are rare (5–10% may be due to multiple infections)
- The **risk factors** for **mortality** include:
  1. Old age
  2. Alcoholism
  3. Active malignancy
  4. Neurological disease
  5. Heart failure
  6. Diabetes mellitus

  Previous pneumonia, pneumonia due to gram-negatives and aspiration pneumonia are adverse risk factors for death.

☛ **Special Tips for GPs**

- Penicillin resistant (40%) multiple drug resistant *Strep pneumoniae* is becoming common in Singapore.
- The incidence and virulence of gram-negative CAP is much higher in Singapore: *Burkholderia pseudomallei* and *Klebsiella pneumoniae* accounts for about 25% of severe CAP in Singapore and is associated with >50% mortality.
- Tuberculosis accounts for 15–20% of CAP in Singapore and should be considered in all patients, especially the elderly.
- HIV patients normally present with *Pneumocystis carinii* pneumonia (disproportionate hypoxaemia with mild CXR abnormalities) or PTB (extensive).
- CAP can only be diagnosed with confidence on a chest radiograph.

MANAGEMENT

- **Risk stratification**: Figure 1 shows risk stratification based on a prediction rule that stratifies patients into 5 classes. It has been validated in a large number of patients in the US.
- **Scoring system**: Table 1 shows the prediction model for the identification of patient risk for persons with community acquired pneumonia.
  1. A **risk score** (total point score) for a given patient is obtained by summing the patient age in years (age –10 for females) and the points for each applicable patient characteristic (Tables 1 and 2).
  2. Oxygen saturation <90% also was considered abnormal.
  3. This model may be used to help guide the initial decision on site of care (Table 3); however, its use may not be appropriate for all patients with this illness and therefore should be applied in conjunction with physician judgement.
- **Treatment**: see Table 4.

References/further reading

1. Lim TK. Emerging pathogens for pneumonia in Singapore. *Ann Acad Med S'pore.* 1997;26:651–658.
2. Fine MJ, Auble TE, Yealy DM, et al. A prediction rule to identify low risk patients with community acquired pneumonia. *N Eng J Med.* 1997;336:243–250.
3. Koh TH, Lui RVTP. Increasing antimicrobial resistance in clinical isolates of *Strep pneumoniae*. *Ann Acad Med S'pore.* 1997;26:604–608.
4. Lee KH, Hui KP, Lim TK. Severe community acquired pneumonia in Singapore. *S'pore Med J.* 1996;37:374-377.
5. Singapore Ministry of Health Clinical Practice Guidelines 1/2000. Use of antibiotics in community acquired pneumonia. 1/2000:27–38. From www.gov.sg/moh/pub/cpg/cpg.htm.

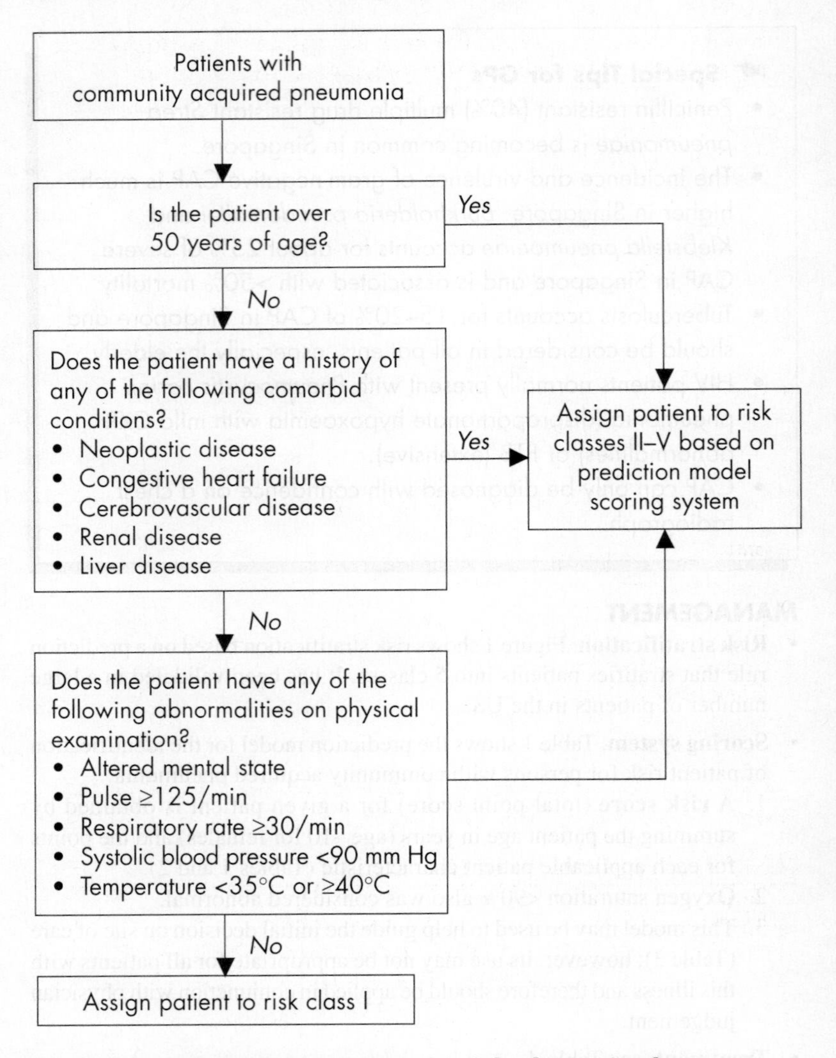

Figure 1: Identifying patients in risk class I in the derivation of the prediction rule

Source: Reproduced with permission from Fine MJ, et al[2] Figure 1, p. 246.

Table 1: Scoring system for identification of patient risk for persons with community acquired pneumonia

Patient characteristic	*Points assigned*[1]
Demographic factors	
• Age: Males	Age (in yr)
Females	Age (in yr) −10
• Nursing home resident	+10
*Comorbid illnesses**	
• Neoplastic disease	+30
• Liver disease	+20
• Congestive heart failure	+10
• Cerebrovascular disease	+10
• Renal disease	+10
*Physical examination findings**	
• Altered mental state	+20
• Respiratory rate ≥30/min	+20
• Systolic blood pressure <90 mm Hg	+20
• Temperature <35°C or ≥40°C	+15
• Pulse ≥125/min	+10
Laboratory findings	
• pH <7.35	+30
• BUN >10.7 mmol/l	+20
• Sodium <130 mEq/l	+20
• Glucose >13.9 mmol/l	+10
• Haematocrit <30%	+10
• PO_2 <60 mm Hg	+10
• Pleural effusion	+10

Source: Reproduced with permission from Fine MJ, et al,[2] Table 2 p. 247.

Table 2: Stratification of risk score

Risk	*Risk class*	*Based on*
	I	Absence of features marked with asterisks in Table 1 and age ≤50 years
Low	II	≤70 total points
	III	71–90 total points
Moderate	IV	91–130 total points
High	V	>130 total points

Source: Adapted from Fine MJ, et al,[2] Table 3, p. 248 with permission.

Table 3: Risk class mortality for CAP points

Risk class	*Points*	*Mortality (%)*	*Recommendations for site of care*
I	0	0.1	Outpatient
II	≤ 70	0.6	
III	71–90	2.8	
IV	91–130	8.2	Inpatient
V	>130	29.2	

Source: Adapted from Fine MJ, et al;[2] Table 3, p. 248 with permission.

Table 4: Empirical antibiotics for initial treatment of CAP

	Class: Outpatient (oral)	Antibiotics	Dosage
Class I	*Category I*		
	Macrolide	Erythromycin	500 mg 6 h × 7–10 days
		Erythromycin ES	800 mg bd × 7–10 days
		Clarithromycin	250 mg bd × 7–10 days
		Azithromycin	500 mg × 3 days
	or		
	Tetracycline	Doxycycline	200 mg om × 7–10 days
Class II	*Category II*		
	Macrolide	(as above)	
	or		
	2nd generation cephalosporin	Cefuroxime	500 bd × 7–10 days
	or		
	Penicillin ±lactamase inhibitor	Amoxicillin-clavulanic acid	375 mg tds × 7–10 days
		Ampicillin-sulbactam	750 mg bd × 7–10 days
	Class: Inpatient (IV±oral)	*Antibiotics*	*Dosage*
Class III	*Category III (general ward)*		
	Penicillin (high dose)	≥10 million U per day ±oral macrolide	6 h IV
	or		
	3rd generation cephalosporin	Ceftriazone ±oral macrolide	1 g bd IV
	or		
	Penicillin ±lactamase inhibitor	Amoxicillin-clavulanic acid	375 mg tds IV
	or		
	'respiratory quinolones'	Levofloxacin	
		Gatifloxacin	
		Moxifloxacin	

Source: Table from Singapore Ministry of Health Clinical Practice Guidelines:[5] Use of antibiotics in community acquired pneumonia. Reproduced

78 Pneumothorax

Francis Lee

CAVEATS

- The management of pneumothorax is dependent on the size, clinical state of patient and whether the lung is diseased or normal.
- **Tension pneumothorax** is a medical emergency that requires a clinical diagnosis and treatment before CXR. Tracheal displacement is a **late** development in tension pneumothorax.
- It is important to give appropriate advice to all patients discharged from a health facility.

☛ Special Tips for GPs

- Pneumothorax must be considered in all patients presenting with acute shortness of breath or a young Marfanoid patient with sudden onset of unilateral chest pain.
- Suspect **tension pneumothorax** in patients with severe dyspnoea, tachycardia, signs of impaired peripheral perfusion, diminished breath sounds in one hemithorax and raised jugular veins. Do immediate needle decompression by inserting a 14G IV venula into the 2nd intercostal space mid-clavicular line and remove the metal stylet before sending the patient by ambulance to hospital. If not, patient will die! For further details, refer to *Trauma, Chest*.

CLASSIFICATION OF SPONTANEOUS PNEUMOTHORAX

- Spontaneous pneumothorax has no antecedent traumatic or iatrogenic cause.
- This can be further divided into:
  1. **Primary**: where there is no underlying lung abnormalities or underlying disease that predisposes to pneumothorax.
  2. **Secondary**: where the underlying lung is diseased (eg COLD, pneumonia).

INITIAL MANAGEMENT

- A patient with suspected pneumothorax and unstable vital signs must be managed in the resuscitation area. Other patients with pneumothorax can be managed in the intermediate care area.

- Measure vital signs and monitor patient for ECG, vital signs and pulse oximetry.
- Administer 100% oxygen.

Investigation

- The main investigation is the chest x-ray.
- The **size of the pneumothorax** is determined by the distance from the lung apex to the ipsilateral cupola (apex of the lung) at the parietal surface: (1) Small pneumothorax <3 cm, and (2) large pneumothorax ≥3 cm.

MANAGEMENT

- Management depends on the following factors:
  1. Stability of patient
  2. Size of pneumothorax
  3. Type of pneumothorax

Small primary pneumothorax (stable patient)

- Observe patient in the ED for 3 h.
- Thereafter the patient may be discharged if:
  1. The patient is clinically stable.
  2. A repeat CXR does not show enlargement of pneumothorax.
- Give pneumothorax advice (see p. 355).
- Give follow-up appointment with a respiratory specialist.

Large primary pneumothorax (stable patient)

- Drain the pneumothorax with a 20–24 F chest tube
- Connect the chest tube to a Heimlich valve or underwater seal.
- Admit patient for observation.

Unstable patient with large pneumothorax

- If the patient has tachypnoea and/or tachycardia only, the pneumothorax should be drained expediently with a 24–28 F chest tube.
- If the patient is hypotensive,
  1. The patient should be considered to have tension pneumothorax.
  2. Needle thoracostomy using 14G IV venula should be performed stat in 2nd intercostal space mid-clavicular line.
  3. Thereafter, a 24–28 F chest tube should be inserted.
- Patient must be admitted.

Patient with secondary pneumothorax

- All patients should be admitted for management and observation as there is a risk of delayed expansion of lung.

- Those with a large pneumothorax should have a chest tube inserted prior to admission.
- Unstable patients should be treated as above.

PNEUMOTHORAX ADVICE

- Pneumothorax advice should be given to all patients discharged from the ED, regardless of whether the lungs have expanded or not.
- **Absolute contraindications**, even after complete resolution of pneumothorax include:
  1. Mountain climbing
  2. Deep sea diving
- **Relative contraindications**, for a period of 1 month after complete resolution of pneumothorax (demonstrated clinically and on x-rays) include:
  1. Air travel
  2. Strenuous activity (eg pushing and pulling heavy weights)

References/further reading

1. Management of spontaneous pneumothorax. An American College of Chest Physician Delphi Consensus Statement. *Chest*. 2001;199:590–602.

79 Poisoning, benzodiazepine

Suresh Pillai

CAVEATS

- Death from benzodiazepine overdose is generally rare unless it is combined with other sedative agents, ethanol or barbiturates.
- General supportive treatment measures are usually all that is required with special emphasis on airway, breathing and ventilation.
- The use of **benzodiazepine antagonists** like flumazenil in overdose is controversial. Do not give IV flumazenil to patients who are benzodiazepine dependent and to patients with concomitant ingestion of tricyclic antidepressants, or an unspecified mixed overdose.
- If there is associated head trauma then this must be evaluated separately with a head CT scan even though the major contribution to a patient's altered mental state may be due to benzodiazepines.

> ☛ **Special Tips for GPs**
> - All patients should be referred to the ED if there is any suspicion of a benzodiazepine overdose even though they may only exhibit mild drowsiness initially.

PATHOPHYSIOLOGY

- Benzodiazepines cause a generalized depression of spinal reflexes as well as inhibit the reticular activating system resulting in lethargy, slurred speech, ataxia, hyporreflexia, drowsiness, stupor, coma or even respiratory arrest.
- The **pupils** in patients with benzodiazepine overdose are usually **non-specific** and are generally not pin point as in pure opiate overdoses.
- Hypotension and cardiopulmonary arrest are possible after rapid IV injection of diazepam.
- The **half-lives** of benzodiazepine vary widely from 2–5 hours for midazolam, 5–30 hours for chlordiazepoxide and 50–100 hours for flurazepam.

MANAGEMENT

Supportive Measures

- Patients having altered mental state with impaired gag reflex and respiratory depression, haemodynamic instability or are comatose should be managed in the critical care area.

- The airway should be maintained and if necessary the patient intubated and ventilated if indicated. Otherwise the patient should be on 100% O_2 via a non-rebreather mask.
- The patient should be placed on vital signs, cardiac and pulse oximetry monitoring q 15 min.
- Maintain a peripheral IV infusion line.
- Take blood for FBC, urea/electrolytes/creatinine. Perform bedside blood glucose estimation.
- **Serum benzodiazepine** levels are **not necessary** during the acute management of overdoses but qualitative urine or blood-screening methods, if available, can be performed in cases where the diagnosis is in doubt.
- Induced emesis is not recommended in benzodiazepine overdose because of CNS depression.
- Administer **activated charcoal** if the time of ingestion is within 4 hours. **Gastric lavage** is limited to large ingestions or mixed ingestions within one hour. However, the airway must be protected and the patient intubated, if necessary, during gastric lavage or activated charcoal administration.

Antidotal therapy

- **IV flumazenil** in a dose of 0.2 mg given over 30 seconds can be given depending on the response and repeated till 0.5 mg is administered. As its effects are generally short-lived, repeat doses may be required. However, the **contraindications** in using it are:
  1. If there is **concomitant tricyclic antidepressant overdose** where reversal of benzodiazepine effects may precipitate status epilepticus induced by the former.
  2. Flumazenil can precipitate an acute withdrawal reaction, manifested by seizures and autonomic instability, in patients who may be **addicted** to **benzodiazepines**.
- If the history is not accurate, then the administration of IV thiamine, IV 50% dextrose and IV naloxone should be considered in patients presenting with altered mental state. IV naloxone should not be used routinely unless there are signs suggestive of opioid overdose (refer to *Poisoning, General Principles*).

Disposition

- All patients with benzodiazepine overdose should be admitted to the General Medical Ward and if necessary to the High Dependency Unit or the Intensive Care Unit especially if ventilatory support is required.

References/further reading

1. Bose GM. Benzodiazepines. In: Tintinalli JE, Ruiz E, Krome RL, eds. *Emergency Medicine: A Comprehensive Study Guide*. 3rd ed. New York: McGraw-Hill; 1992:624–625.
2. Sporer KA. Benzodiazepines. In: Olson KR, ed. *Poisoning and Drug Overdose*. 2nd ed. East Norwalk, Conn.: Appleton and Lange; 1994:97–99.
3. Amrein R, Leishman B, Bentzinger C, et al. Flumazenil in benzodiazepine antagonism: Actions and clinical use in intoxications and anaesthiosology. *Med Toxicol.* 1987;2:411.
4. Hojer J, Baehrendtz S, Gustafsson L. Benzodiazepine poisoning: Experience of 702 admissions to an intensive care unit during a 14 year period. *J Intern Med.* 1989;226:117.
5. Boccuzzi-Chmura L, Robertson DC. Flumazenil (romazicon) and the patient with benzodiazepine overdose: Risks versus benefits. *J Emerg Nurs.* 1996;22(4):330–333. Review.

80 Poisoning, carbon monoxide

Peter Manning

CAVEATS

- Carbon monoxide (CO) is a respiratory asphyxiant which binds preferentially to haemoglobin (HgB) and myoglobin, subsequently reducing the oxygen-carrying capacity of blood.
- **Half-life** in the body is **5–6 hours**.
- Carbon monoxide has an affinity for HgB 250 times that of oxygen; it shifts the oxyhaemoglobin dissociation curve to the left, impairing release of oxygen to the tissues.
- It binds to and inactivates myoglobin (cardiac myoglobin 3 times more than skeletal myoglobin). During hypoxaemia, cardiac myoglobin takes up CO even more avidly, resulting in myocardial necrosis and depressed myocardial function.
- Causes diffuse demyelination of the brain, with autopsy findings of cerebral oedema, necrosis of superficial white matter, globus pallidus, cerebrum and hippocampus. Delayed neuropsychiatric sequlae occur in up to 40% of cases following apparent recovery.
- CO poisoning is difficult to diagnose since there are **few pathognomonic signs and symptoms**. Mild symptoms are non-specific, eg headache, nausea and vomiting, dizziness. Several members of the same family may present at the same time, seemingly indicating a flu-like illness.

> ☛ **Special Tips for GPs**
> - Always consider CO toxicity in patients presenting with altered mental state who were found in a confined space or who were involved in a fire or explosion some hours before.
> - Remember: the classic cherry red appearance described in most texts is an autopsy finding. Cyanosis is more common in a living survivor.

METABOLISM

- Carbon monoxide (exhaust gas, house gas) is a colourless, odourless and tasteless gas.
- Absorption is by inhalation without further metabolism; widespread distribution by blood, with elimination via the lungs by exhalation.

- Binds to cytochrome oxidase system: competes with oxygen for binding sites on cytochrome A_3.
- **Sources**:
  1. Endogenous: CO is a normal degradation product of haemoglobin and other haem-containing compounds:
     a. The carboxyhaemoglobin (COHb) level is <5% in non-smokers and <10% in smokers.
     b. In pregnant women the COHb level can be up to 2–5%.
     c. In normal infants the COHb level can be 4–5%.
     d. In haemolytic anaemia the level can rise as high as 6%.
  2. **Exogenous**:
     a. Cigarette smoke: smoke at tip of cigarette contains 2½ times as much CO as the inhaled portion.
     b. Smokers often have COHb levels of 4–10%.
     c. Fires: smoke from a major fire contains up to 10% CO (100 times the concentration needed to produce a lethal COHb level).
     d. Car exhausts contain up to 8% CO: rear seat passengers are affected more due to closer proximity to exhaust system.
     e. Methylene chloride in paint removers, aerosols and fumigants is readily absorbed through skin and is slowly metabolized to CO. Note that the half-life of COHb due to methylene chloride exposure is twice that of inhaled CO.

ACUTE EXPOSURE

- **CNS**: headache, peripheral neuropathy, altered mental state, coma, seizure, cerebral oedema, behavioural and personality changes, ataxia, memory impairment.
- **Respiratory**: dyspnoea and hyperpnoea, bronchopneumonia and non-cardiogenic pulmonary oedema.
- **Cardiovascular**: angina, ST-segment changes, tachycardia, ventricular dysrhythmias, hypotension, myocardial infarction, heart block, CCF and cardiac arrest.
- **Renal**: oliguria from acute renal failure, proteinuria, myoglobinuria and haematuria.
- **Haematological**: carboxyhaemoglobinaemia, tissue hypoxia, polycythaemia, haemolytic anaemia, DIVC, leukocytosis.
- **Skin:** cyanosis is more common than the often quoted cherry red discolouration; bullae.
- **Ophthalmologic**: flame-shaped retinal haemorrhages, decreased visual acuity, cortical blindness, papilloedema, scotomas.
- **Musculoskeletal**: rhabomyolysis, myonecrosis, compartment syndrome.

Note: ABG will typically reveal a normal PaO_2 because PaO_2 is a measurement of the dissolved oxygen in arterial blood, not the amount of oxygen bound to Hb. Many blood gas analyzers calculate the percentage of oxygen saturation based on the PaO_2. The calculated oxygen saturation will be falsely high when compared to those directly measured by oximetry. This 'saturation gap' is characteristic of CO poisoning.

- **Potential sequelae**: delayed neuropsychiatric sequelae (3 weeks to 3 months after exposure) occur in up to 40% of cases after apparent recovery:
  1. Headache/dizziness
  2. Memory deficits
  3. Personality alterations
  4. Parkinsonism

ED MANAGEMENT

Consists of **supportive measures** and **supplemental oxygen therapy**.

- **ABCs**
  1. Evaluate and support airway.
  2. Perform orotracheal intubation if ventilation/oxygenation are compromised.
  3. Administer 100% supplemental oxygen via tight-fitting face mask.

Note: The serum elimination half-life of COHb when breathing room air is 520 min, compared to 80 min when breathing 100% oxygen. Oxygen therapy should not be discontinued until the patient is symptomatic and the COHb level is <10%.

  4. Monitoring: ECG (showing sinus tachycardia and ST-segment changes), vital signs q 15 min, pulse oximetry.
  5. Consider use of sodium bicarbonate by IV infusion in the face of significant metabolic acidosis (arterial pH <7.1).

- **Lab tests:**
  1. Routine: FBC, glucose, urea/electrolytes/creatinine, ABG with COHb level, 12-lead ECG.
  2. Optional: CXR (for severe inhalation injury, pulmonary aspiration, bronchopneumonia or pulmonary oedema)

- **Antidote therapy**: A study by Weaver et al (2002) shows that 3 hyperbaric oxygen treatments within a 24-hour period appeared to reduce the risk of cognitive sequelae 6 weeks and 12 weeks after acute CO poisoning. The benefit of hyperbaric oxygen is the prevention of damage caused by CO exposure rather than the removal of CO.

DISPOSITION AND FOLLOW UP

- Refer for **hyperbaric oxygen therapy** the following patients by contacting your local hyperbaric oxygen source, military or civilian, according to local protocols:
  1. All patients with syncope, neurological abnormalities, and cardiac abnormalities with elevated levels of COHb.

2. All patients with COHb levels >25%.
3. Pregnant patients with COHb levels >10% .
4. Myocardial ischaemia.
5. Worsening symptoms despite oxygen therapy.
6. Symptoms persisting after 4 h of 100% O_2 therapy (including abnormal psychometric testing and tachycardia).
7. Neonate.

Note: With **hyperbaric oxygen therapy**, the elimination **half-life** of **CO** is reduced to **23 min**, though outside of a military setting, it is very unlikely that you would be able to implement this therapy sufficiently promptly to achieve this reduction in half-life.

- Admit to General Medicine patients with COHb levels <20%, administer high-flow oxygen at 15 l/min via a tight-fitting mask for at least 4 h till the COHb level has dropped to normal.
- Asymptomatic patients with COHb level <10% are unlikely to develop complications and may be discharged from the ED with advice to seek medical care promptly if any of the following symptoms develop:
  1. Difficulty breathing or shortness of breath.
  2. Chest pain or tightness.
  3. Difficulties with coordination of limbs.
  4. Memory difficulties.
  5. Prolonged headache or dizziness.
- Discharged patients should be referred for psychiatric review with a view to possible carbon monoxide neuropsychiatric screening battery (CONSB) to detect subtle deteriorations.
- The patient should be told to refrain from smoking for 72 hours.

References/further reading

1. Scheinkstel CD, et al. Hyperbaric or normobaric oxygen for acute carbon monoxide poisoning: A randomized controlled clinical trial. *Med J Aust*. 1999;170:203–210.
2. Gosselin RE, Smith RP, Hodge HC. *Clinical Toxicology of Commercial Products*. 5th ed. Baltimore: Williams and Wilkins; 1984.
3. Weaver LK, Hopkins RO, Chan KJ, et al. Hyperbaric oxygen for acute carbon monoxide poisoning. *N Engl J Med*. 2002;347(14):1057–1066.

81 Poisoning, cyclic antidepressants

Peter Manning • Suresh Pillai

CAVEATS

- Commonly prescribed cyclic antidepressants are imipramine, trimipramine, desipramine, amitriptyline, doxepin, maprotiline and amoxapine.
- Heterocyclics are highly protein-bound (92% at physiological pH); forced diuresis, dialysis and haemoperfusion have no role in the management of OD.
- The mainstay of treatment is the administration of **sodium bicarbonate** because it alters binding of the drug to the myocardial sodium channels, and may also increase protein binding of the drug, thus rendering it pharmacologically less active.
- **Drugs to avoid**:
  1. Type IA (eg quinidine, procainamide) and IC (eg flecainide) antidysrhythmics, which can worsen the 'quinidine-like' toxicity on the myocardium.
  2. Beta-blockers and calcium channel blockers which may exacerbate hypotension.
  3. Phenytoin may increase the incidence of ventricular dysrhythmias and its use is controversial.
  4. Flumazenil (Anexate®) carries the risk of precipitating fits.
  5. Physostigmine has the risk of cardiac toxicity and asystole.

☛ Special Tips for GPs

- Do not induce emesis or administer activated charcoal if patient appears drowsy because they can rapidly lose consciousness necessitating airway protection.
- Do not administer flumazenil to reverse a concomitant benzodiazepine OD as this may precipitate fits induced by the cyclic antidepressants.
- Widened QRS complexes >100 msec on ECG indicates serious intoxication.
- IV **sodium bicarbonate therapy** administered in the hospital is the mainstay of therapy and is effective for TCA-induced hypotension and dysrhythmias.

CLINICAL PATHOPHYSIOLOGY

Cardiac effects

- Anticholinergic activity that can induce tachycardia.
- Quinidine-like activity (sodium and potassium channel blockade) that can induce intraventricular and atrioventricular blocks. Bundle branch and fascicular blocks are usually preceded by a widening QRS complex. See Figure 1a. A **coexistent sinus tachycardia may simulate ventricular tachycardia.**
- Hypotension due to peripheral alpha-adrenergic blockade.
- Pulmonary oedema.

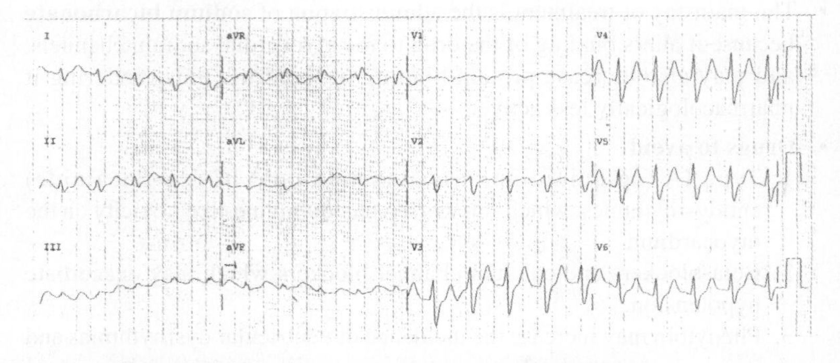

Figure 1a: ECG showing widened QRS complexes in a patient with cyclic antidepressant overdose

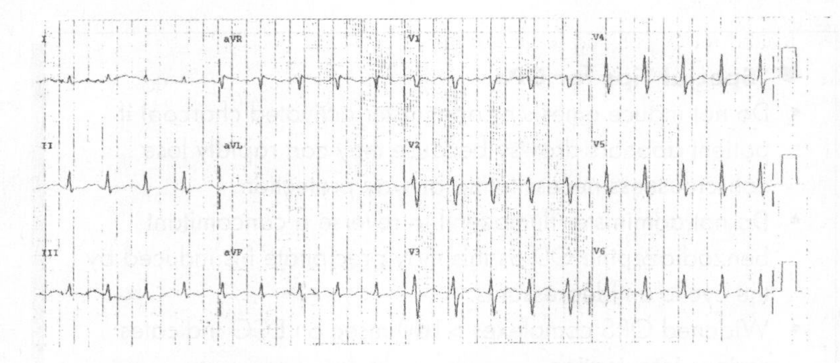

Figure 1b: ECG of patient in Figure 1a showing normalization of width of QRS complexes posttreatment

CNS effects

- Confusion, agitation and hallucinations before the patient rapidly succumbs to coma.
- Seizures are common and usually single; status epilepticus is more likely to occur with amoxapine or maprotiline.
- Physical findings may include:
  1. Clonus
  2. Choreoathetosis
  3. Myoclonic jerks
  4. Increased muscle tone
  5. Hyperreflexia
  6. Extensor plantar responses

Anticholinergic effects (may or may not occur; their absence does not exclude toxicity)

- Flushing
- Dry mouth/skin
- Dilated pupils
- Fever
- Absent bowel sounds
- Urinary retention
- Blurred vision from paralysis of accommodation

Other effects

- Skin blisters
- Rhabdomyolysis and renal failure
- Pneumonia
- ARDS

Signs that indicate a serious overdose

- Ventricular dysrhythmias
- Bradycardia and AV blocks
- Intraventricular conduction defects with a QRS complex >100 msec
- Fits
- Hypotension
- Pulmonary oedema
- Cardiac arrest

MANAGEMENT

Supportive measures

- Patient must be managed in a monitored area with resuscitation equipment, including defibrillator, immediately available.
- Maintain airway; intubate patient if depressed level of consciousness is noted or if gag reflex is absent.
- Administer supplemental high-flow oxygen by non-rebreather reservoir mask.
- Monitoring: ECG, VS q 5–15 min, pulse oximetry.
- Establish peripheral IV line.
- IV fluid of choice is normal saline.
- **Labs**: FBC, urea/electrolytes/creatinine, blood drug screen (send drug screen tube to ward with patient if mixed OD suspected).

Note: Do not ask for plasma antidepressant level; it adds nothing to the management.

- ABGs to monitor blood pH as therapy continues.
- CXR for pulmonary oedema, aspiration pneumonia, ARDS.
- Place urinary catheter to monitor urine output/fluid status.
- Perform gastric lavage if indicated and send first effluent specimen to ward with patient.

Drug therapy

- **Activated charcoal**: dosage = 1 g/kg body weight. Administer via orogastric tube.
- Alkalinization of the blood to a pH of 7.45 to 7.50. This is best achieved by a combination of **hyperventilation** and **sodium bicarbonate** administration:
    1. If intubated, mechanical ventilation at respiratory rate of 20/min is adequate for most adults.
    2. Dosage of **sodium bicarbonate** = 1–2 mmol/kg body weight in slow IV boluses, ie over 20–30 minutes.
    3. Bicarbonate therapy is indicated if the QRS is at least 100 msec wide.

SPECIFIC CLINICAL SITUATIONS

Note: Sodium bicarbonate is the most effective therapy for improving hypotension and abolishing dysrhythmias.

Dysrhythmias unresponsive to sodium bicarbonate

- **Lignocaine** may abolish ventricular dysrhythmias. Dosage: IV bolus of 1.0–1.5 mg/kg, then an infusion of 1–4 mg/min.

- **Magnesium sulphate** may be used to treat torsades de pointes. Dosage: IV bolus of 1–2 g over 60 seconds, then an infusion of 1–2 g/h.
- **Synchronized cardioversion** may be used for the treatment of supraventricular tachydysrhythmias.
- **Emergency pacing** (transcutaneous pacing in ED followed, if necessary, by transvenous pacing in ICU) is indicated for severe bradydysrhythmias and AV blocks.

Hypotension

- First approach is the use of **normal saline** and **alkalinization**.
- Poor or no response: attempt **drug therapy**.
- Noradrenaline or high-dose dopamine: both are more effective early in toxicity.
  Dosage: **noradrenaline**: infusion **only** of 0.5–1.0 μg/min and titrated to effect
  dopamine: infusion **only** of 10–20 μg/kg/min and titrated to effect
- Failure of above measures necessitates consideration of an intraaortic balloon pump.

Control of fits resistant to use of sodium bicarbonate

This is important since ensuing lactic acidosis can worsen cardiac toxicity by lowering protein binding and making more active drug available to the susceptible tissues.

- **Diazepam**: Dosage: 2–5 mg IV bolus, repeated q 5 min to a total of 20 mg, **or**,
- **Lorazepam**: Dosage: 0.1 mg/kg IV bolus to a total of 8 mg.
- **Phenobarbital**:
  Dosage: IV 100 mg/min to a total of 10 mg/kg or fits are controlled, if ineffective, give
  IV 50 mg/min to a total of (including previous dose) 20 mg/kg or fits are controlled,
  IV 50 mg/min to a total of (including previous dose) 30 mg/kg or fits are controlled.
- **Paralysis/general anaesthesia**: obtain consultation from Anaesthesia.

DISPOSITION

- Obtain consultation from General Medicine; keep in view admission to a HD/ICU setting for monitoring. Significant deterioration of such cases has been known to occur several hours or days after the initial ingestion.

References/further reading

1. Callaham M. Cyclic antidepressant overdose. In: Tintinalli JE, Ruiz E, Krome RL, eds. *Emergency Medicine: A Comprehensive Study Guide*. 3rd ed. New York: McGraw-Hill; 1992:551–554.
2. Benowitz NL. Cyclic antidepressants. In: Olson KR, ed. *Poisoning and Drug Overdose*. 2nd ed. East Norwalk, Conn.: Appleton and Lange; 1994:147–150.
3. Callaham M. Cyclic antidepressant toxicity. In Rosen P, Baker F, Braen R, et al, eds. *Emergency Medicine: Concepts and Clinical Practice*. 2nd ed. St Louis: Mosby; 1987:2087–2098.
4. Frommer DA, Kullig KW, Marx JA, et al. Tricyclic antidepressant overdose: A review. *JAMA* 1987;257:521–526.
5. Brown TCK, Barker GA, Dunlop ME, et al. The use of sodium bicarbonate in the treatment of tricyclic antidepressant induced arrhythmias. *Anesth Intensive Care*. 1973;1:203–210.
6. Wedin GP, Oderda GM, Klein'Schwartz W. Relative toxicity of cyclic antidepressants. *Ann Emerg Med*. 1986;15:797–804.
7. Sasyniuk BI, Jhamandas V. Mechanism of reversal of toxic effects of amitriptylline on cardiac Purkinje fibres by sodium bicarbonate. *Ann Emerg Med*. 1986;15:1052–1059.

82 Poisoning, organophosphates

Peter Manning • Suresh Pillai

CAVEATS

- The active agent in most pesticides and insecticides is **parathion**, which binds irreversibly with cholinesterase to form a diethylphosphate bond.
- **Atropine** is a physiologic antimuscarinic antidote that acts by competitively blocking the muscarinic effects of acetylcholine.
- Atropine has no effect on the nicotinic receptors at myoneural junctions in skeletal muscle, ie it will not reverse paralysis.
- **Pralidoxime** is a biochemical antidote that reactivates the cholinesterase that has undergone the process of phosphorylation by the organophosphate; however, the pralidoxime must be administered within 24–36 hours after exposure, otherwise the cholinesterase molecule may be irrevocably bound and new cholinesterase will then take weeks to regenerate.
- **Classic presentation**: a patient with vomiting and diarrhoea, diaphoresis, breath smelling strongly of insecticide and small pupils. Beware erroneous diagnosis of gastroenteritis.

> ### ☛ Special Tips for GPs
>
> - Refer all patients with suspected organophosphate poisoning to hospital even if they are asymptomatic.
> - Be aware that vomiting, diarrhoea and hypotension can occur and can be misdiagnosed as severe GE. Look for the DUMBELS signs and symptoms (see next section).
> - Ensure that the implicated receptacle containing the insecticide is brought along with the patient to the hospital.

PATHOPHYSIOLOGY

- Organophosphates inhibit acetylcholinesterase, which results in excess acetylcholine accumulating at the myoneural junctions and synapses.
- Excess acetylcholine initially excites, then paralyzes, neurotransmission at the motor endplate and stimulates nicotinic and muscarinic sites:
  1. **Muscarinic** effects: the mnemonic **DUMBELS** is useful to remember since these signs and symptoms develop **first**, 12–24 hours after ingestion:

D Diarrhoea
U Urination
M Miosis (absent in 10% of cases)
B Bronchorrhoea/Bronchospasm/Bradycardia
E Emesis
L Lacrimation
S Salivation and hypotension

2. **Nicotinic** effects
   a. Diaphoresis, hypoventilation and tachycardia
   b. Muscle fasciculations, cramps and weakness leading to flaccid muscle paralysis
3. **CNS** effects
   a. Anxiety and insomnia
   b. Respiratory depression
   c. Convulsions and coma

MANAGEMENT

Supportive measures

- Ensure all staff are wearing protective equipment since percutaneous absorption and inhalation in the course of care may cause toxicity.
- Patient must be managed in the critical care area with resuscitation equipment immediately available.
- Start detoxification by removing patient's clothes and washing skin thoroughly (ED staff should take appropriate precautions: see *Poisoning, General Principles*).
- Maintain airway patency; perform orotracheal intubation if patient is obtunded, apnoeic or has no gag reflex. Frequent suctioning may be required due to bronchorrhoea.
- Administer supplemental high-flow oxygen via non-rebreather reservoir mask.
- Perform gastric lavage if indicated, especially within a few hours in early ingestions.
- Monitoring: ECG, vital signs q 5–15 min, pulse oximetry.
- Establish peripheral IV line.
- IV fluids: crystalloids to replace fluids lost by vomiting and diarrhoea.
- Labs: FBC, urea/electrolytes/creatinine, plasma cholinesterase gastric and serum toxicology specimens to accompany patient to ward.

Drug therapy

- **Activated charcoal** via gastric lavage tube.
  Dosage: 1 g/kg body weight

- **Atropine**: first drug to be given in the treatment of symptomatic poisoning.
  1. Its major use is in the reduction of bronchorrhoea /bronchospasm.
  2. Large doses may be needed to control airway secretions.

  Dosage: Adult: 2 mg IV q 10–15 min prn; the dosage may be doubled q 10 min until secretions have been controlled **or** signs of atropinization are obvious (flushed and dry skin, tachycardia, mydriasis and dry mouth).
  Children: 0.05 mg/kg body weight q 15 min prn; the dosage can be doubled q 10 minutes until secretions are controlled

- **Pralidoxime (2-PAM®, Protopam®)**
  1. Pralidoxime should be given with atropine to every symptomatic patient.
  2. Effects will be apparent within 30 minutes and include disappearance of convulsions and fasciculations, improvement in muscle power and recovery of consciousness.
  3. The administration of pralidoxime usually necessitates reduction in the amount of atropine given and may unmask atropine toxicity.

  Dosage: Adult: 1 gm IV over 15–30 min; can be repeated in 1–2 hours prn
  Children: 25–50 mg/kg/body weight IV over 15–30 min; can be repeated in 1–2 hours

Note: In very severe cases with bradycardia/hypotension and respiratory arrest, half the dosage of **pralidoxime** can be given IV over 1 min.

- **Diazepam (Valium®)**: used to reduce anxiety and restlessness and to control convulsions.

  Dosage: 5–10 mg IV for anxiety/restlessness.

Note: Doses up to 10–20 mg IV may be needed for the control of convulsions.

Disposition

- Obtain General Medicine consultation on HD/ICU admission.
- For cases of subclinical poisoning treatment is not necessary, **but** the patient should be admitted for observation for at least 24 hours to ensure that delayed toxicity does not develop.

References/further reading

1. Tafuri J, Roberts J. Organophosphate and carbamate poisoning. In: Tintinalli JE, Ruiz E, Krome RL, eds. *Emergency Medicine: A Comprehensive Study Guide*. 3rd ed. New York: McGraw-Hill; 1992:609–613.
2. Woo OF. Organophosphates – Cyclic antidepressants. In: Olson KR, ed. *Poisoning and Drug Overdose*. 2nd ed. East Norwalk, Conn.: Appleton and Lange; 1994:240–243.
3. Kurtz PH. Pralidoxime in the treatment of carbamate intoxication. *Am J Emerg Med.* 1990;8:68.
4. Dikart WL, Kiestra SH, Sangster B. The use of atropine and oximes in organophosphate intoxication: A modified approach. *J Toxicol Clin Toxicol.* 1988;26:199–208.
5. Lotti M. Treatment of acute organophosphate poisoning. *Med J Aust.* 1991;154:51–55.
6. Wang EIC, Braid PR. Oxime reactivation of diethylphosphoryl human serum cholinesterase. *J Biol Chem.* 1967;242:2683–2687.

83 Poisoning, paracetamol

Peter Manning • Shirley Ooi • Benjamin Leong

CAVEATS

- Commonest form of drug overdose locally, where a single ingestion of 7.5 g (15 tablets) is used empirically as a threshold for possible toxicity.
- **Toxicity** has been shown to occur with ingested doses >150 mg/kg body weight or **7.5 g (15 tablets)** in an average-sized adult.
- Toxicity may occur at lower doses in patients with hepatic enzyme induction, eg patients taking anticonvulsants, or anorexic patients who may have preexisting glutathione depletion. In such cases, use the high-risk treatment line on the Rumack-Matthew nomogram (Figure 1) rather than the normal treatment line.
- Use of the Rumack-Matthew nomogram is useful in determining the need for N-acetylcysteine (Parvolex®) therapy following a single, acute ingestion **only** (see management section).
- **N-acetylcysteine (NAC)** is most effective if given within 8 hours of the ingestion, though it may also be used up to 24 hours after ingestion, if the history suggests a significant overdose and the serum paracetamol level is not available.
- A guiding philosophy in managing paracetamol poisoning is **'if in doubt, treat with N-acetylcysteine'**.

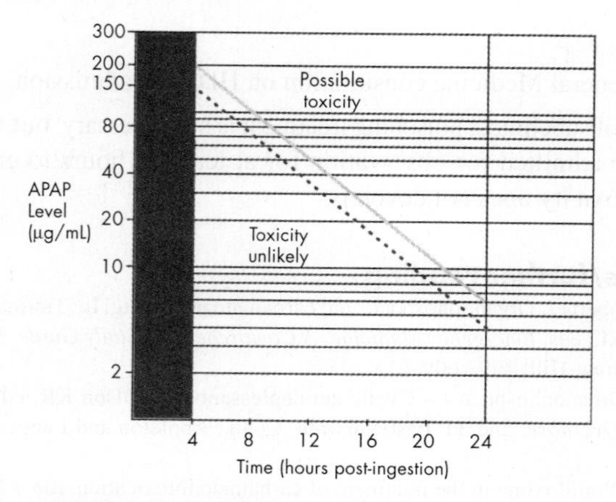

Figure 1: Rumack-Matthew nomogram

Figure reproduced with permission of the McGraw-Hill Companies, from Tintinalli JE, Kelen GD, Stapczynski JS, eds. *Emergency Medicine: A Comprehensive Study Guide*. New York: McGraw-Hill; 2000:1128, Fig. 165-4.

☛ **Special Tips for GPs**

- Patients with paracetamol overdose often look well in the initial stages except for nausea and vomiting.
- If there is any doubt as to the accuracy of history or the amount ingested, patients should be referred to the ED for further evaluation.
- Do not induce emesis before sending patient to the ED.

STAGES OF PARACETAMOL TOXICITY

- **Stage I (up to 24 hours)**: symptoms are vague with abdominal pain, loss of appetite, nausea and vomiting. Examination will probably reveal pallor and sweating.
- **Stage II (24 to 48 hours)**: the vague symptoms of Stage I have diminished though examination may reveal an enlarged and tender liver. Labs will reveal mild elevations of serum bilirubin and liver enzymes and prothrombin time (PT). Renal function tests may also be abnormal.
- **Stage III (72 to 96 hours)**: vague symptoms may persist. Examination reveals obvious clinical jaundice. Liver function tests are at their highest level of abnormality. Hepatic and, rarely, renal failure may occur during this stage, and occasionally death.
- **Stage IV (4 days to 2 weeks)**: if such a patient presents late or has not been treated earlier in the disease, then hepatotoxicity induced by paracetamol may progress to hepatic failure, coma and possibly death.

MANAGEMENT

Supportive measures

- Patient should be managed in the intermediate care area, although transfer to the critical care area is mandatory if there is significant derangement of vital signs or depressed mental state.

Note: Depressed mental state should trigger the search for concomitant drug ingestion since obtundation is unusual in isolated paracetamol poisoning.

- Maintain airway; perform orotracheal intubation if patient is significantly obtunded or the gag reflex is absent (anticipating gastric lavage or the administration of activated charcoal, or both).
- Administer supplemental oxygen if SpO_2 is decreased.
- Monitoring: ECG, vital signs q 15 min, pulse oximetry.
- Establish peripheral IV line.
- Perform gastric lavage if patient presents within 1 hour of ingestion and collect first effluent for toxicology specimen.

Note: Send to ward/unit with patient. Current evidence does **not** support gastric lavage unless the patient has ingested a potentially toxic dose of paracetamol, and has presented within the first hour. Some authors even suggest that lavage may be omitted if activated charcoal was given.

- **Labs**
  1. FBC, urea/electrolytes/creatinine, liver function tests, prothrombin time.

Note: Plasma ALT >5,000 IU/l is highly suggestive of hepatotoxicity due to paracetamol since such levels are seldom seen in viral hepatitis. From an EBM standpoint **only** serum paracetamol level is required to be drawn in patients with paracetamol overdose who show no signs of hepatotoxicity.

  2. Serum paracetamol level (**mandatory**).
  3. If the initial level is in the toxic range when plotted on the Rumack-Matthew nomogram (Figure 1), then NAC therapy should be initiated immediately.
  4. A more precise judgement is based on the level taken 4 hours postingestion for those cases where NAC therapy is not indicated earlier (see next section).

Drug therapy

- Activated charcoal: administer via the gastric lavage tube.
  Dosage: 1 g/kg body weight (50 g for the average Asian).

Note: Activated charcoal is only useful within the first hour of ingestion **and** multidose charcoal therapy is no longer considered useful.

- **N-acetylcysteine (Parvolex®)**, administer if:
  1. The 4-hour serum paracetamol level lies in the toxic range on the Rumack-Matthew nomogram (see Figure 1).
  2. The initial serum paracetamol level (drawn earlier than 4 hours post ingestion) is already in the toxic range.
  3. The history is sufficiently convincing of a significant overdose, ie 15 tablets or 7.5 g. **Do not** wait for a serum paracetamol level to return, though a specimen should still be sent from the ED to enable appropriate monitoring of the paracetamol level on the ward.
  4. The liver function tests show evidence of hepatotoxicity. NAC therapy should be given in patients with hepatic failure until recovery or death.

PARVOLEX® (N-ACETYLCYSTEINE) IV INFUSION

Dosage in adults (Table 1)

- Initial dosage: 150 mg/kg IV over **15 min**, followed by continuous infusion (50 mg/kg in 500 ml of 5% dextrose in **4 h**), followed by continuous infusion (100 mg/kg in 1 litre 5% dextrose over **16 h**).
- Total dosage: 300 mg/kg in 20 h.

Table 1: Treatment with Parvolex®

Patient's body weight (kg)	Volume of Parvolex® (ml) Initial 150 mg/kg in 200 ml of 5% dextrose in 15 min	Second 50 mg/kg in 500 ml of 5% dextrose in 4 h	Third 100 mg/kg in 1 l of 5% dextrose in 16 h	Total Parvolex (ml)
50	37.5	12.5	25	75
60	45.0	15.0	30	90
70	52.5	17.5	35	105
80	60.0	20.0	40	120
90	67.5	22.5	45	135
x	0.75x	0.25x	0.5x	1.5x

Mechanism of action of N-acetylcysteine (Parvolex®)

- Normal usage of paracetamol in appropriate dosages results in the conversion of the paracetamol by the cytochrome P-450 system to a toxic metabolite, which is detoxified by glutathione in the liver.
- Excess amounts of paracetamol, eg acute, large overdose, depletes glutathione stores and the toxic metabolite causes centrilobular hepatic necrosis.
- While the action of N-acetylcysteine (Parvolex®) is complex and multifactorial, it can be said to act as a glutathione substitute.

Adverse effects of Parvolex® (seen most commonly in the first hour of treatment)

- Nausea, flushing, urticaria and pruritus are the commonest (true anaphylactic reaction is rare). Treatment is to stop infusion for 15 minutes and restart the infusion at the slowest rate (100 mg/kg in 1 litre 5% dextrose over 16 h).

References/further reading

1. Jones AL, Volens G. Management of self poisoning. *BMJ.* 1999;319:1414–1417.
2. Vale JA, American Academy of Clinical Toxicology, European Association of Poison Centres and Clinical Toxicologists. Position statement: Gastric lavage. *J Toxicol Clin Toxicol.* 1997;35(7):711–719.
3. Bateman DN. Gastric decontamination: A view for the millenium. *J Accid Emerg Med.* 1999;16(2):84–86.
4. Zed PJ, Krenzelok EP. Treatment of acetaminophen overdose. *Am J Health Syst Pharm.* 1999;56(11):1081–1091.
5. Chyka PA, Seger D, American Academy of Clinical Toxicology, European Association of Poison Centres and Clinical Toxicologists. Position statement: Single-dose activated charcoal. *J Toxicol Clin Toxicol.* 1997;35(7):721–741.
6. Hung O, Nelson LS. Acetaminophen. In: Tintinalli JE, Kelen GD, Stapczynski JS, eds. *Emergency Medicine: A Comprehensive Study Guide*. 5th ed. New York: McGraw-Hill; 2000:1125–1132.

84 Poisoning, salicylates

Suresh Pillai • Peter Manning

CAVEATS

- Sources include aspirin, Peptobismol, sports liniments, Oil of Wintergreen and traditional Chinese medicines.
- **Mild toxicity** is manifested by:
  1. Hyperpnoea with respiratory alkalosis (due to stimulation of the respiratory centre).
  2. Ototoxicity as the prominent symptom (especially tinnitus).
- **Moderate toxicity** is manifested by:
  1. Vomiting generally starting 3–6 hours postingestion.
  2. Severe hyperpnoea, hyperthermia, dehydration, abdominal pain and diaphoresis.
- **Severe toxicity** is manifested by:
  1. CNS alterations with signs of stimulation initially, followed soon after by depression, leading to convulsions and coma.
  2. Non-cardiogenic pulmonary oedema, dysrhythmias, haemorrhage and acute renal failure.
- Due to its limitation and deceptive utility, the use of the Done nomogram is not recommended. Instead, the patient's clinical condition and early course, rather than the nomogram, should guide clinical therapy.
- **Serum salicylate estimations**:
  1. The first level should be drawn approximately 2 hours postingestion, with a repeat test drawn at 6 hours. Subsequently, serial levels should be monitored until the salicylate level is declining.
  2. Significant toxicity can develop very rapidly in acute overdosage even before the 6-hour test is drawn.
  3. A salicylate level of <30 mg % (non-toxic range) drawn less than 6 hours postingestion **does not** rule out impending toxicity.
- **Urine alkalinization** is indicated for those patients with a rising and toxic salicylate level (>30 mg %):
  1. Salicylate is an acid whose renal excretion is increased by ionization.
  2. The kidney reabsorbs only unionized salicylate; since salicylate is an acid it ionizes in alkaline urine.
  3. If urine pH is increased to pH 8 the urinary excretion of salicylate increases 10–20 fold.
- **Haemodialysis** is the most effective means of lowering the serum salicylate level. Indications are:

1. Serum salicylate level >100 mg/dL
2. Severe acid base imbalance, ie pH 6.5–6.8
3. Severe cardiac toxicity, eg ARDS
4. Renal or pulmonary failure
5. Neurologic signs or symptoms, eg psychosis, confusion, convulsions or coma
6. Rising serum salicylate levels despite urinary alkalinization and multidose activated charcoal therapy

☛ **Special Tips for GPs**

- Patients with severe salicylate toxicity may appear well initially. Always refer suspected cases to the ED for evaluation.
- Look out for the early signs of salicylate toxicity like tinnitus, vertigo or hearing loss.
- Be aware that ingestion of small amounts of concentrated salicylates like methylsalicylate liniments or Oil of Wintergreen can be lethal especially in a child.

MANAGEMENT

Supportive measures

- Patients with altered mental states or derangement of vital signs should be managed in the critical care area.
- Maintain airway; intubate if gag reflex is absent (in anticipation of gastric lavage) or patient is hypoxaemic.
- Administer 100% O_2 via non-rebreather reservoir mask.
- Monitoring: ECG, vital signs q 5–15 min, pulse oximetry.
- Perform gastric lavage even beyond 1 hour as salicyclates delay gastric emptying.
- Establish peripheral IV line.
- Administer IV crystalloids at a rate sufficient to maintain peripheral perfusion.
- **Labs**
  1. Serum salicylate level stat and at 2 hours postingestion
  2. ABG to determine the presence, type and degree of acid base derangement
  3. FBC, urea/electrolytes/creatinine, PT

Drug therapy

- Activated charcoal via lavage tube or PO
  Dosage: 1 g/kg body weight (or 50 g for the average adult locally)
- Sodium bicarbonate
  Dosage: bolus 1–2 mmol/kg 8.4% $NaHCO_3$
  Infusion: 150 mmol $NaHCO_3$ (150 ml of 8.4% solution) in 850 ml D_5W. Start at 1.5 to 2 times maintenance fluid rate; titrate flow rate against urine pH of 7.5–8.0

Note: Monitor serum potassium level (either via lab tests or by T wave morphology on ECG monitor).

Contraindications to bicarbonate therapy

- Salicylate-induced non-cardiogenic pulmonary oedema as it may aggravate fluid overload.
- Concomitant oral bicarbonate therapy as this will increase salicylate absorption.
- Patient is already on acetazolamide as this will worsen systemic acidosis, thereby increasing CNS levels of salicylate.

Disposition

- For severe toxicity or those patients with rising serum salicylate levels, obtain General Medicine consultation in anticipation of admission to ICU/HD.
- Cases of mild toxicity can be managed by admission to a general ward.

References/further reading

1. Gaudreault P, Temple AR, Lovejoy F. The relative severity of acute versus chronic salicylate poisoning in children. A clinical comparison. *Paediatrics.* 1982;70:566.
2. Prescott LF, Balali-Mood M, Critchley JH, et al. Diuresis or urinary alkalinization for salicylate poisoning. *Br Med J.* 1982;285:1383.
3. Snodgrass W, Rumack BH, Petereson RG, et al. Salicylate toxicity following therapeutic doses in young children. *Clin Toxicol.* 1981;18:247.
4. Thisted B, Krantz T, Strom J, et al. Acute salicylate self-poisoning in 177 consecutive patients treated in ICU. *Acta Anaesthesiol Scand.* 1987;31:312.
5. Walters JSW, Woodring JH, Stelling CB, et al. Salicylate induced pulmonary edema. *Radiology.* 1983;146:289.

85 Pulmonary embolism

Shirley Ooi

CAVEATS

- Thrombotic pulmonary embolism (PE) is not an isolated disease of the chest but a complication of venous thrombosis. Deep venous thrombosis (DVT) and PE are therefore parts of the same process, venous thromboembolism.
- Leg DVT is found in 70% of patients with PE. Conversely, PE occurs in 50% of patients with proximal DVT of the legs (involving popliteal and/or more proximal veins), and is less likely when the thrombus is confined to the calf veins.
- As PE is preceded by DVT, the **factors predisposing** to the two conditions are the same and broadly fit Virchow's triad of venous stasis, injury to the vein wall and enhanced coagulability of the blood (Table 1).

Table 1: Some common risk factors for venous thromboembolic disease

Flow stasis	Prolonged immobilization including long journeys, stroke Major trauma or surgery within 4 weeks Congestive heart failure Obesity Advanced age Spinal cord injuries Shock syndromes
Endothelial damage	Local trauma Surgery of legs and pelvis Vasculitis Burns Electric shock Infection Previous history of thromboembolism
Coagulation abnormalities	Polycythaemia Platelet abnormalities Oral contraceptive drugs with high oestrogen content Malignant neoplasia Deficiency of antithrombin III, protein C or S

Note: In **surgical series**, the risk of venous thromboembolism rises rapidly with age, length of anaesthesia, and the presence of previous venous thromboembolism or cancer. The incidence is highest in those undergoing emergency surgery following trauma (eg for hip fractures) and pelvic surgery. In **medical series**, venous thromboembolism is frequent in cardiorespiratory disorders (eg congestive heart failure, irreversible airways disease), with leg immobility (caused by stroke and other neurological disease), and by cancer.

Table 2: Clinical forms of pulmonary embolism

Pulmonary embolism	*History*	*Vascular obstruction*	*Presentation*
Acute minor	Short, sudden onset	<50%	Dyspnoea with or without pleuritic pain and haemoptysis
Acute massive	Short, sudden onset	>50%	Right heart strain with or without haemodynamic instability and syncope
Subacute massive	Several weeks	>50%	Dyspnoea with right heart strain

Source: Table adapted with permission from Riedel et al,[1] Table 3.

Notes:

1. Massive PE without hypoxaemia is so rare that if the arterial oxygen tension (PaO_2) is normal, an alternative diagnosis should be considered.
2. Although PE impairs the elimination of carbon dioxide, hypercapnia is rare.
3. A patient with massive PE is obviously dyspnoeic but **not orthopnoeic**.
4. The third and least common presentation, ie subacute massive PE, mimics heart failure or indolent pneumonia, especially in the elderly.

Note: The identification of risk factors not only aids in clinical diagnosis of venous thromboembolism, but also guides decisions about prophylactic measures and repeat testing in borderline cases.

- **Case fatality rate** is less than 5% in treated patients who are haemodynamically stable at presentation but approximately 20% in those with persistent hypotension.
- **PE** can be **classified** into 3 main types as shown in Table 2.
- Nearly all patients with PE will have **one or more** of the following **clinical features**:
  1. Dyspnoea of sudden onset
  2. Tachypnoea (>20 breaths/minute)
  3. Chest pain (pleuritic or substernal).

Note: If the clinician remembers these 3 features, the possibility of PE will rarely be overlooked. When these clinical features are associated with ECG signs of right ventricular strain and/or radiologic signs of plump hilum, pulmonary infarction or oligaemia, the likelihood of PE is high. It is further strengthened in the presence of risk factors for venous thromboembolism and arterial hypoxaemia with hypocapnia. On the contrary, the absence of all these 3 clinical features virtually excludes the diagnosis of PE.

- Table 3 shows the **estimation of the pretest clinical likelihood of PE**.

Table 3: Estimation of the (pretest) clinical likelihood of pulmonary embolism

High (>85% likely)	Otherwise unexplained sudden onset of dyspnoea, tachypnoea, or chest pain and at least 2 of the following: *Significant risk factor present* (immobility, leg fracture, major surgery) Fainting with new signs of right ventricular overload in ECG Signs of possible leg DVT (unilateral pain, tenderness, erythema, warmth, or swelling) Radiographic signs of infarction, plump hilum, or oligaemia
Intermediate (15–85% likely)	Neither high nor low clinical likelihood
Low (<15% likely)	Absence of sudden onset of dyspnoea and tachypnoea and chest pain Dyspnoea, tachypnoea, or chest pain present but explainable by another condition *Risk factors absent* Radiographic abnormality explainable by another condition Adequate anticoagulation (INR>2 or aPPT >1.5 times control) during the previous week

Source: Table reproduced with permission from Riedel et al,[1] Table 4.

Note: In patients with low pretest probability for PE, if **D-dimer ELISA assay** tested is found to be negative, PE can be confidently excluded. In contrast, if D-dimer is found to be positive in patients with low pretest probability for PE, the patient should be reevaluated. A negative D-dimer test cannot be used to confidently exclude a PE in intermediate or high risk patients.

MANAGEMENT

Massive PE with signs of haemodynamic instability

- Monitor vital signs at critical care area.
- Give **oxygen** via non-rebreather mask or intubate if unable to maintain oxygenation.

Note: Intubation may cause the haemodynamic situation to deteriorate further by impeding venous return.

- Set up 2 **large bore IV lines** and send blood for investigations. Start fluid resuscitation.

Special Tips for GPs

- Remember that PE is one of the 6 life-threatening causes of chest pain!
- Clinical features of PE are deceivingly non-specific, but PE is highly unlikely in the absence of all of the following: dyspnoea, tachypnoea and chest pain.
- When an ECG is done for chest pain and T wave inversion is seen in lead III, look for the presence of $S_1Q_3T_3$ and the other associated ECG features of PE.

Note: When thrombolytic treatment is considered, the antecubital route should be preferred and the insertion of arterial lines avoided.

- If BP is still low despite fluid resuscitations, start **inotropes**.

Note: Inotropes may do no more than precipitate dysrhythmias when the cardiac output is reduced, the dilated right ventricle is hypoxic and already near maximal stimulation from the high concentration of endogenous catecholamines. The judicious use of IV noradrenaline titrated against a moderate increase in BP might be beneficial.

- Give **pain relief**.

Note: Opiates should be used with caution in the hypotensive patient.

- Contact Cardiothoracic Registrar-on-call for admission to CT ICU.

General emergency investigations

- **ECG** findings in PE:
  1. ECG changes are usually non-specific.
  2. Non-specific ST depression and T wave inversion are the most common findings.
  3. In minor PE, there is no haemodynamic stress and thus the only finding is sinus tachycardia.
  4. In acute or subacute massive PE, evidence of **right heart strain** may be seen. They are:
     a. Rightward shift of QRS axis
     b. Transient right bundle branch block
     c. T wave inversion in leads V_{1-3}
     d. P pulmonale
     e. Classical $S_1Q_3T_3$ (only present in 12%)
  5. Normal ECG in 6%.
  6. The main value of ECG is in excluding other potential diagnoses, such as myocardial infarction or pericarditis. Refer to Figure 1 for ECG of PE.

- **Arterial blood gas**: the characteristic changes are a **reduced PaO_2 and a $PaCO_2$ that is normal or reduced** because of hyperventilation. The PaO_2 is almost never normal in massive PE but can be normal in minor PE, mainly due to hyperventilation. In such cases the widening of the alveolo-arterial PO_2 gradient ($AaPO_2$>20 mm Hg) may be more sensitive than PaO_2 alone. (For more details, refer to *Acid Base Emergencies* and *Useful Formulae*.) Both hypoxaemia and a wide $AaPO_2$ may obviously be due to many other causes. Blood gases, therefore, may heighten the suspicion of PE, but are of insufficient discriminant value to permit proof or exclusion of PE. Note FiO_2 at time of blood sampling.
- FBC.
- Urea/electrolytes/creatinine.
- **DIVC screen**: D-dimer assay has a sensitivity of 85–94% for diagnosing pulmonary embolism. However, its specificity is only 67–68%. A normal D-dimer ELISA test result is useful in excluding PE in patients with a low pretest probability of PE or a non-diagnostic lung scan.
- GXM 4-6U packed cells.
- **Chest x-ray**: findings in PE:
  1. In general, CXR is not specific or diagnostic in PE, but comparison with previous films may be helpful.
  2. The **findings** may show the following:
     a. Normal (~40%).

Note: A normal film is compatible with all types of acute PE. In fact, a normal film in a patient with severe acute dyspnoea without wheezing is very suspicious of PE.

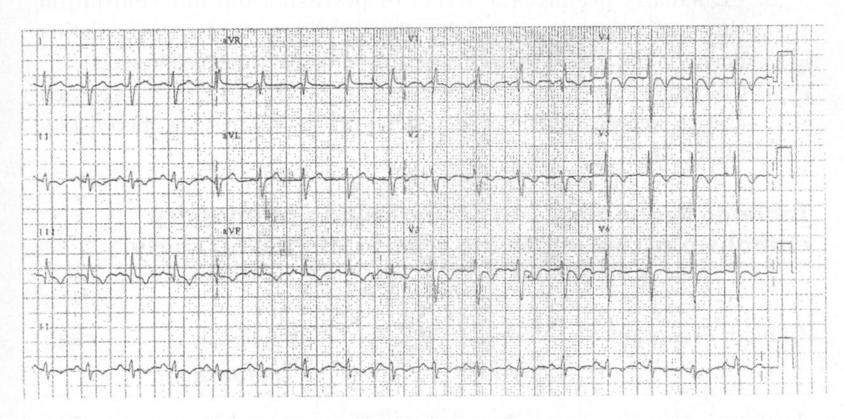

Figure 1: ECG of a 71-year-old man who presented with right-sided chest discomfort, dyspnoea and coughing

Spiral CT scan confirmed pulmonary embolism. Note the following ECG changes: sinus tachycardia, $S_1Q_3T_3$, right axis deviation, RBBB, T inversion in V_{1-5} and P pulmonale.

b. Evidence of pulmonary infarction: peripheral opacities, sometimes wedge shaped with apex pointing towards the hilum or semicircular with its base on the pleural surface (**Hampton's hump**).
c. Focal pulmonary oligaemia in parts of the lung affected by emboli (**Westermark sign**) but this is difficult given the type of film usually available in the acute situation.
d. Atelectasis.
e. Small pleural effusions.
f. Raised diaphragm.

Note: Features d, e and f have low specificity for PE.

g. Localized infiltrate.
h. Consolidation.
i. 'Plump' pulmonary arteries in massive PE.

3. The CXR is especially valuable in excluding other conditions mimicking PE (pneumothorax, pneumonia, left heart failure, tumour, rib fracture, massive pleural effusion, lobar collapse), but PE may coexist with other cardiopulmonary processes.

Definitive investigations

- **Lung scintigraphy**
  1. A normal perfusion scan essentially excludes the diagnosis of a clinically relevant recent PE because occlusive PE of all types produces a defect of perfusion.
  2. However, many conditions other than PE, such as tumours, consolidation, left heart failure, bullous lesions, lung fibrosis, and obstructive airways disease, can also produce perfusion defects.
  3. PE usually produces a defect of perfusion but not ventilation ('mismatch') while most of the other conditions produce a ventilation defect in the same area as the perfusion defect (matched defects).
  4. The probability that perfusion defects are caused by PE can be assessed as high, intermediate or low depending on the type of scans abnormality (Table 4).

Table 4: Probability (%) of underlying pulmonary embolism according to the criteria of PIOPED study

	Scan probability			
Clinical likelihood	*Normal/ very low*	*Non-diagnostic*		*High*
		Low	*Intermediate*	
Low	2	4	16	56
Intermediate	6	16	28	88
High	0	40	66	96

Source: Table reproduced with permission from Riedel et al,[1] Table 5.

- **Computed tomography (CT, spiral or electron beam)**
  1. This is emerging as a non-invasive testing modality to complement or replace the standard lung scintigraphy.
  2. Its **advantages** include the following:
     a. Faster
     b. Less complex
     c. Less operator dependent than conventional pulmonary angiography
     d. Has about the same frequency of technically insufficient examinations (about 5%) as pulmonary angiography compared to 70% non-diagnostic scintigrams
     e. Better interobserver agreement in the interpretation of CT than for scintigraphy
     f. Imaging of lung parenchyma and great vessels is possible (eg pulmonary mass, pneumonia, emphysema, pleural effusion, mediastinal adenopathy) and diagnosis can be made if PE is absent. Hence, CT helps in diagnosing alternative causes of dyspnoea. CT can also detect right ventricular dilatation, thus indicating severe, potentially fatal PE
  3. CT has over **90% specificity and sensitivity** in diagnosing PE in the main, lobar and segmental pulmonary arteries but smaller, subsegmental emboli can be overlooked. When CT is used to evaluate patients with a non-diagnostic lung scan, the sensitivity is lower. CT has greater sensitivity and specificity for PE than lung scintigraphy.
  4. Currently, because of significant sources of false negative and false positive examinations, CT cannot yet be regarded as a new 'gold standard' to replace angiography. However, because of its small number of non-diagnostic results and a potentially greater out-of-hours availability, spiral CT may replace scintigraphy as the primary test in patients with suspected PE.
- **Pulmonary angiography**
  1. This remains the '**gold standard**'.
  2. The **indications** are as follows: (1) if cardiovascular collapse and hypotension are present, and (2) when other investigations are inconclusive.
  3. The **disadvantages** include: (1) its limited availability, and (2) small (<0.3%) but definite risk of mortality.
  4. The relative **contraindications** include: (1) pregnancy, (2) significant bleeding risk, (3) renal insufficiency, and (4) known right heart thrombus.
- **Echocardiography**: in **critically ill patients** suspected of having massive PE, particularly those with cardiovascular collapse, **echocardiography** can be rapidly performed at the **bedside** to exclude other diseases or to establish the diagnosis by finding clots in the central pulmonary arteries or the right heart. When evidence of right heart strain without clots is present on echo, spiral CT or pulmonary angiography should follow.

Suspected PE

- Start IV heparin 5,000U bolus or SC fraxiparine 0.4 ml for weight <50 kg, 0.5 ml for weight 50–65 kg, 0.6 ml for weight >65 kg.
- Investigate.
- Contact General Medical or Respiratory Medical Registrar.
- Admit patient to Respiratory Medicine.

References/further reading

1. Riedel M. Acute pulmonary embolism 1: Pathophysiology, clinical presentation, and diagnosis. *Heart.* 2001;85:229–240.
2. Riedal M. Acute pulmonary embolism 2: Treatment. *Heart.* 2001;85:351–360.
3. Kline JA, Israel EG. Diagnostic accuracy of a bedside D-dimer assay and alveolar dead-space measurement for rapid exclusion of pulmonary embolism: A multi-center study. *JAMA.* 2001:285:761–768.
4. Ginsberg JS, Wells PS, Kearon C, et al. Sensitivity and specificity of a rapid whole-blood assay for D-dimer in the diagnosis of pulmonary embolism. *Ann Intern Med.* 1998;129:1006–1011.
5. Lim TK. Non-invasive tests for acute pulmonary embolism: What are the real advances? *Singapore Med J.* 2001;42(10):446–449.
6. Brown MD, Rowe BH, Reeves M. The accuracy of the enzyme-linked immunosorbent assay D-dimer test in the diagnosis of pulmonary embolism: A meta-analysis. *Ann Emerg Med.* 2002;40(2):133–144.

86 Pulmonary oedema, cardiogenic

Francis Lee • Shirley Ooi

CAVEATS

The following aspects of cardiogenic pulmonary oedema are to be noted:

- The main pathogenic mechanism is sympathetic overdrive with central distribution of blood volume resulting in elevated left ventricular enddiastolic volume and pressure.
- As there is no volume overload *per se*, management with the use of vasodilators should be the mainstay of pharmacological therapy compared to the use of diuretics.
- The end point of pulmonary oedema treatment is dictated by the resolution of sympathetic overdrive, as suggested by the normalization of pulse rate, restoration of warm dry extremities and comfort of patient.
- The BP will serve as a guide to therapy rather than an end point in itself.
- CPAP mask is effective but requires an alert and cooperative patient. Its utility in pulmonary oedema is perhaps limited.

DIAGNOSIS OF PULMONARY OEDEMA

- The **diagnosis** is made clinically, supported by the following features:
  1. Severe respiratory distress, with inability to maintain a supine posture
  2. Cold clammy extremities
  3. Thready pulse
  4. SpO_2 (many severe patients have saturation typically around 80–90%), due to true hypoxia compounded by peripheral vasoconstriction affecting the sensor
- Clinical features that signal **impending respiratory failure** are as follows:
  1. Altered mental state, eg confusion, obtundation of sensorium
  2. Poor and incoordinated respiratory effort
  3. Progressive desaturation, as shown on pulse oximetry
  4. If rapid blood gas analysis is available
     a. PaO_2 <50 mm Hg, $PaCO_2$ >50 mm Hg
     b. Normalization of $PaCO_2$
- As deterioration can occur fairly quickly, a clinical judgement for more aggressive intervention should be made without the need for blood gas sampling. A **low threshold for intubation and mechanical ventilation** should be instituted as it may be life saving.

☛ **Special Tips for GPs**

- Sit patient with pulmonary oedema upright and give supplemental oxygen.
- Set up an IV line and give IV frusemide 40–80 mg bolus.
- Give SL GTN or nitroglycerine spray if available.
- If time permits, do a 12-lead ECG.
- Send patient to the hospital by ambulance.

MANAGEMENT

- Patient must be treated in the critical care area.
- Full monitoring. Defibrillator attached.
- ABC assessed, with a view to intubate if signs of impending respiratory failure is present.
- 100% oxygen is administered by non-rebreather reservoir mask.
- Establish peripheral IV access.
- Do a 12-lead ECG to exclude the presence of an inferior/right ventricular infarction (which contraindicates the use of nitrates).
- Blood is taken for standard investigations, FBC, urea/electrolytes/creatinine, cardiac enzymes and troponin T.
- ABG is taken as a baseline.
- Portable CXR is done.
- Patient is catheterized to measure urine output.

PHARMACOLOGICAL TREATMENT

- **Drugs of choice**
  1. **Nitroglycerine**: 10–200 μg/min. Start with 10 μg/min, slowly stepping up at 5 μg every 5 min.
     Titrate to response and BP effects. No invasive monitoring is required. Fall in BP can be rapid when high doses are used. Patient must be on continuous BP monitoring. Infusion should be slowed down when MAP reaches 90 mm Hg.
  2. **Nitroprusside**: 0.25–10 μg/kg/min. Start at lowest dose and titrate to response.
     Very powerful vasodilator. Invasive monitoring is usually needed. Care should be taken to prevent precipitous drop in BP.
  3. **Hydralazine**: IV 10 mg every 30 min.
     Powerful vasodilator. Once given, effects could last for a while. Care should be taken to monitor patients, especially when combined with other agents.

- **Other drugs**
  1. **Frusemide**: 40–80 mg IV bolus.
     Effective but variance in onset of effects from 20 min to 2 h. Effects not titratable. Effects are not physiological. Higher doses may be needed in patients with renal failure.
  2. **Morphine**: 0.1 mg/kg. Given in incremental boluses of 1 mg. Some regimes start with IV morphine 3–5 mg.
     Comparatively, a weaker venodilator than other available agents. Not easily titratable. Also decreases respiratory drive. Care should be taken to avoid large intravenous bolus dose as this may cause apnoea.

- **Oral agents**: these can be given in situations where IV access is delayed or not possible. They can also be added to other drugs in combination therapy of acute pulmonary oedema.
  1. **Glyceryl trinitrate**: 0.5–1.5 mg could be given SL stat. Comes in tablet form or aerosol spray.
     Effects similar to the IV form but not as pronounced.
  2. **Captopril**: SL captopril 6.25 mg or 12.5 mg.
     Dosage depends on BP and whether it is used alone or in combination with other agents. Effects are not easily titratable.

- **Combination regimes**
  1. **IV GTN plus frusemide**: frusemide is given as a stat dose while IV GTN is given as a titratable infusion. Doses of IV GTN infusion should be smaller.
  2. **IV GTN plus captopril**: SL captopril is given as a stat dose. IV GTN is given as above.
  3. **Frusemide plus morphine**: traditional combination.

HYPERTENSION IN PULMONARY OEDEMA

- It is often difficult to tell whether hypertension is the cause of pulmonary oedema as almost all patients have a sympathetic response that will cause BP to rise.
- Features that will lend support to hypertension as a primary cause include:
  1. History of severe uncontrolled hypertension
  2. Florid fundal changes, Grade III or Grade IV retinopathy

- If evidence points towards a hypertensive crisis as a cause for pulmonary oedema, the management of such cases should involve the use of vasodilators with the aim of reducing the BP quickly but safely.

HYPOTENSION IN PULMONARY OEDEMA

- Hypotension is indicative of severe heart failure with poor cardiac output (Killip Class IV). The management of pulmonary oedema with hypotension poses a big challenge to any emergency physician.

- IV **dobutamine** (5–20 μg/kg/min) or IV **dopamine** (5–20 μg/kg/min) may be added to the treatment regime for pulmonary oedema to help maintain the BP at least 90 mm Hg SBP. In such situations, agents used for managing pulmonary oedema must be in IV form, of rapid action and effectively titratable.
- Patient may have to be **intubated early** as most of the drugs used in the treatment of pulmonary oedema will cause further decrease in BP. Avoid induction agents which have a negative inotropic effect such as thiopentone.
- IV **etomidate** is a good choice as it is cardiovascularly stable.

CPAP IN PULMONARY OEDEMA

CPAP (continuous positive airway pressure) ventilation may be useful in patients who are unresponsive to supplemental oxygen. It helps to prevent alveolar collapse and improve gas exchange. The starting pressure is 5–10 cm H_2O and should be adjusted with care to prevent decrease in cardiac output and BP. The patient must be conscious, cooperative and have a good breathing effort for this to work.

DISPOSITION

- Admit all patients with the following to the **CCU**:
  1. Intubated patients
  2. Concomitant acute coronary syndrome
- Admit patients requiring CPAP to the High Dependency Unit
- Admit the rest of the patients to the Cardiology general ward.

References/further reading

1. Weir EK, Reeves JT, eds. *Pulmonary Edema.* American Heart Association Monograph Series. Armonk, New York: Reeven Futura Pub Co.; 1998.
2. Rezakovic DE, Alpert JS, eds. *Nitrate Therapy and Nitrate Tolerance: Current Concepts and Controversies.* Basel: Karger Publishing; 1993.
3. Alexander R, Fuster V, O'Rourke R, et al. *Hurst's The Heart.* 10th ed. New York: McGraw-Hill Professional; 2000.

87 Renal emergencies

Peter Manning

HYPERKALAEMIA

Caveats

- The severity of hyperkalaemia is related to the plasma potassium level but there is considerable interpatient and intrapatient variability. The rapidity of the development of hyperkalaemia would have a significant bearing on the clinical severity. **Do not** wait for the potassium level to come back from the lab if either clinical state or ECG suggests hyperkalaemia; rather, treat empirically.
- Clinical manifestations can be protean. ECG changes when present are useful but may be difficult to interpret and may even be absent in some patients with severe hyperkalaemia. Metabolic acidosis and hypocalcaemia can worsen the severity of hyperkalaemia.
- In the appropriate clinical setting (eg chronic renal failure, diabetic with nephropathy, etc.) with ECG changes consistent with severe hyperkalaemia (see Figure 1), it would be appropriate to consider empiric therapy if the serum potassium result is anticipated to be unavailable rapidly.
- Serum potassium level greater than 5.5 mmol/l is considered hyperkalaemia. Pseudohyperkalaemia is most commonly due to extravascular haemolysis. Other causes include severe thrombocytosis and leucocytosis.
- **Severity of hyperkalaemia** is as follows:

  Mild: potassium level <6.0 mmol/l and ECG may be normal or show only peaked T waves.

  Moderate: potassium level 6.0–7.0 mmol/l and ECG may show peaked T waves.

  Severe: potassium level 7.0–8.0 mmol/l and ECG shows flattening of the P wave & QRS widening; 8.0–9.0 reveals fusion of QRS with T wave (sine wave) that leads to A-V dissociation, ventricular dysrhythmias and death.

Four-step management of hyperkalaemia

Step 1: Stabilization of membrane potential

- Administer **calcium chloride** or **gluconate** 10%: 10 to 20 ml IV over 3–10 min, to a maximum of 20 ml. Onset: 1–2 min. Repeat same dose if no improvement. Duration: 30–60 min.

Note: **IV calcium** should be **used only** when there is ECG evidence of severe hyperkalaemia, significant neuromuscular weakness or serum potassium >7.0 mmol/l. Use absolute caution in patients on digoxin as it can bring about severe digitalis toxicity. Ensure IV line is working well because extravasation of calcium into the subcutaneous tissue can cause skin necrosis.

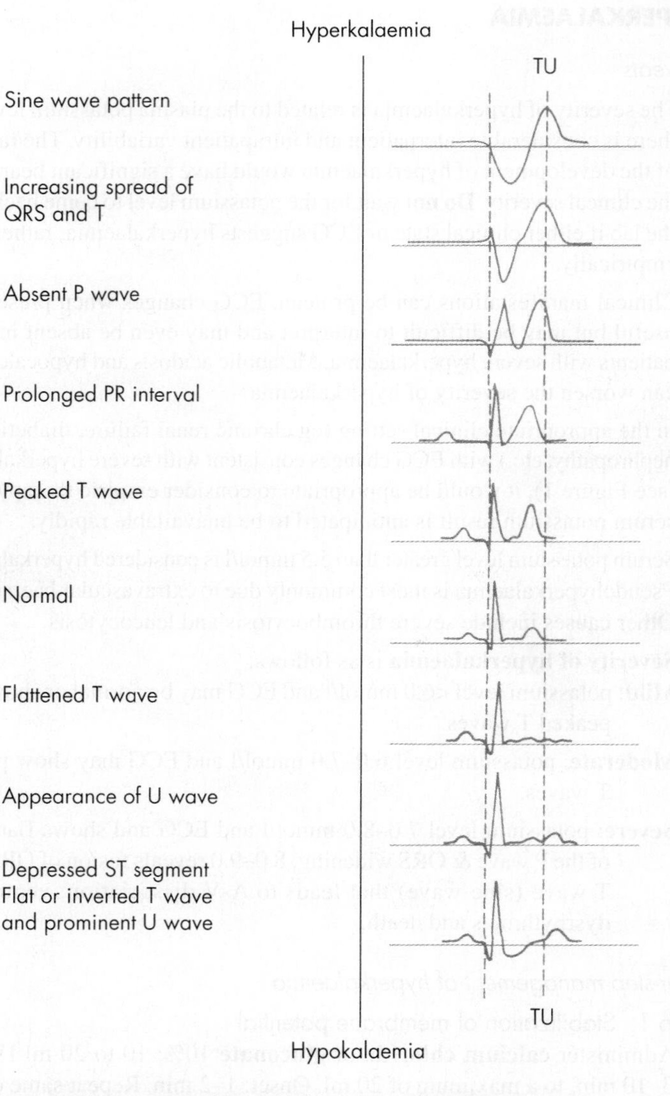

Figure 1: Electrocardiographic manifestations of hypokalaemia and hyperkalaemia

Source: Reproduced with permission from Zull DN.[2]

Step 2: Shift ECF potassium into the ICF

- Administer **dextrose/insulin**: 40–50 ml $D_{50}W$ IV over 5–10 min and 10 units regular insulin as separate bolus. Onset: 30 min, duration: 4–6 h. Recommended over sodium bicarbonate therapy.
- Administer **sodium bicarbonate** 1 mEq/kg body weight IV as a bolus over 5 min in patients with moderate to severe metabolic acidosis; repeat in 30 min in patients with severe metabolic acidosis. Onset: 5 min, duration: 1–2 h.

Note: Most useful in the severely acidotic patient (may have no effect in non-acidotic patient). It should be used with caution in CRF patients since it may lead to fluid overload and provoke hypocalcaemic tetany or fits due to acute alkalosis.

- Administer **salbutamol**: add 5 mg salbutamol to 3–4 ml saline and nebulize over 10 min. Onset: 30 min, duration: 2 h. Salbutamol should be used with caution in patients with known or suspected ischaemic heart disease.

Step 3: Remove potassium from the body

- **Resonium A:** 15 g PO 4–6 hourly. Onset: 1–2 h, duration: 2 h. Caution in patients with significant constipation or ileus.
- **Haemodialysis** (contact Renal Medicine first): onset: minutes, duration: 4 h.

Step 4: Prevent further potassium increase

- Review all medications: eg Span K, ACE inhibitors, beta-blockers.
- Dietary review and advice.

Note: Steps 3a and 4 usually suffice for stable mild to moderate hyperkalaemia. However, repeat a serum potassium level to ensure there is no continued increase in potassium and improvement in the serum potassium level.

CRF with fluid overload and not on dialysis

- Patient to be managed in the critical care area.*
- Place patient in upright position.*
- Administer supplemental high-flow oxygen.*
- Monitoring: ECG, vital signs q 5–10 min, pulse oximetry.*
- Preserve one upper-limb vessel for future arterio-venous access (no blood taking or drip setting).
- Draw blood for FBC, urea/electrolytes/creatinine, and ABG; also cardiac enzymes if cardiac ischaemia suspected.
- Drug therapy
  1. **morphine** 2.5–5 mg IV (if there is severe pulmonary oedema)
  2. **GTN** 0.5 mg SL or nitroderm 5–10 mg patch or IV 10–200 µg/min.

3. **felodipine** 2.5 mg PO if BP is high
4. **frusemide** 120–240 mg IV

- Consider dialysis if there is severe fluid overload, hyperkalaemia, metabolic acidosis or the patient is not responding to above measures (contact Renal physician on call).

CRF with fluid overload without accessible peripheral venous access

- Asterisked steps 1–4 noted in previous section.
- Drug therapy
  1. **morphine** 5–10 mg IM
  2. **GTN** 0.5 mg SL or **nitroderm** 5–10 mg patch
  3. **felodipine** 2.5 mg PO if BP is high
  4. **frusemide** 120–240 mg PO

SEVERE METABOLIC ACIDOSIS

Caveats

- Patients often present with non-specific symptoms with its clinical effects being overshadowed by the signs and symptoms of the underlying disorder.
- Metabolic acidosis should be suspected in any patient with hyperventilation, altered mental state and haemodynamic instability.

Management

- **Supportive Measures**
  1. Patient should be managed in the critical care area.
  2. Ascertain airway patency and manage accordingly.
  3. Monitoring: ECG, vital signs q 5–10 min.
  4. Establish peripheral IV access with normal saline at 'keep open' rate.
  5. **Labs**: FBC, urea/electrolytes/creatinine, stat capillary blood glucose, ABG, serum osmolality, urinalysis, ECG.
  6. **X-rays**: no specific role in acid base states. However, a **KUB** may be useful to identify an ingested substance, eg iron tablets, or a GI problem causing or complicating the acid base imbalance, eg bowel obstruction or ischaemic bowel.

Decision Priorities

- Once the lab values are available, and assuming they are accurate, 3 steps are followed in the **evaluation** for an **acidotic state**. Refer to *Acid Base Emergencies* and *Useful Formulae* for more details.
  1. Determine primary and secondary acid base abnormalities.
  2. Calculate osmolal gap to detect presence of low molecular weight osmotically active substances (refer to *Useful Formulae*).
  3. Review the potassium level in relation to the abnormal pH (refer to *Useful Formulae*).

Specific therapy

- Bicarbonate therapy is reserved for severe organic acidoses or those not easily reversed. The goal is to raise the arterial pH above 7.2. No need to correct if pH is 7.2 or greater unless there is some life-threatening problem that needs to be addressed. No perfect formula exists but the following is useful: **Dose of $NaHCO_3$ [mEq] = (desired [HCO_3^-] − measured [HCO_3^-]) × 50% body weight in kg**. One half this dose is given initially with the remainder depending on repeat laboratory evaluation. **Do not** aim to correct bicarbonate to normal levels.

  Dosage: Bolus therapy is recommended only for those with severe acidosis or when there is haemodynamic compromise. Patients with less life-threatening acidosis may be treated with IV bicarbonate infusion. Add 100–150 mEq $NaHCO_3^-$ (2–3 ampoules of 8.4% $NaHCO_3^-$) to 1 litre D_5W and run over 1–2 hours with repeated ABGs as a guide to therapy.

  Potential complications of therapy are hypernatraemia, hyperosmolality, volume overload, hypokalaemia and posttreatment alkalosis.

INDICATIONS FOR DIALYSIS

- Severe pulmonary oedema
- Severe uncontrollable hypertension from severe fluid overload not responding to diuretics
- Hyperkalaemia
- Severe metabolic acidosis
- Some poisoning, eg methanol, ethylene glycol, salicylates (severe)
- Uraemia, including pericarditis and encephalopathy

PROBLEMS ASSOCIATED WITH DIALYSIS

Haemodialysis

A. Vascular access-related complications

- **Bleeding**
  1. Apply pressure but **do not** occlude/thrombose the vessel with excess pressure.
  2. Document presence of a thrill following procedure.
  3. Continued bleeding mandates consultation with Dialysis Access Team and Renal Medicine.
- **Loss of thrill in shunt:** immediate consultation with Dialysis Access Team and Renal Medicine: **Do not** forcefully manipulate vessel.
- **Infection**
  1. While classic signs are common, patient may present with fever only.
  2. Draw FBC and first blood culture; administer first dose of antibiotics, eg IV ceftazidime 1–2 g.

3. Admit to Renal Medicine; inform Renal physician on call if overtly septic.

B. Non-vascular access-related complications

- **Hypotension**
  1. Posthaemodialysis hypotension may be due to reduction in circulating intravascular volume in a patient whose compensatory mechanisms are inadequate. Check with patient how much fluid was removed during haemodialysis session.
  2. Similar problem may be seen in patients on peritoneal dialysis. Again, check with patient how much negative balance was achieved with the peritoneal dialysis session.
  3. Most cases respond to observation postdialysis, but may require IV fluids.
  4. However, consider and exclude:
     a. Occult haemorrhage: do PR to detect GIT bleeding
     b. Acute AMI/dysrhythmias or cardiac tamponade
     c. Life-threatening hyperkalaemia: treat empirically if there are severe changes of hyperkalaemia
     d. Infection
     e. Pulmonary or air embolism and acute haemolysis in haemodialysis

- **Dyspnoea**
  1. Most commonly due to volume overload; consider sudden cardiac failure, pericardial tamponade, pleural effusion, severe acidosis, severe anaemia (from acute and chronic blood loss) and sepsis.
  2. Exclude acute MI; others include pulmonary or air embolism and acute haemolysis in haemodialysis.

- **Chest pain**
  1. Commonly ischaemic in origin with underlying IHD exacerbated by the transient hypotension and hypoxaemia associated with the dialysis process. Also consider pulmonary embolism, acute haemolysis and air embolism in haemodialysis.
  2. Management: ECG, monitoring, cardiac enzymes.
  3. Conduct appropriate consultations with Renal Medicine and/or Cardiology.
  4. Consider non-ischaemic causes of chest pain including pericarditis, lung/pleural diseases, reflux oesophagitis, gastritis or peptic ulcer disease.

- **Neurologic dysfunction**
  1. Exclude electrolyte abnormalities, infection, major intracranial catastrophes.
  2. Management:
     a. Draw stat capillary blood sugar, urea/electrolytes/creatinine, ABG
     b. Monitoring: ECG, vital signs q 5–15 min, pulse oximetry

   c. Search for new focal neurological abnormalities and perform head CT scan
3. Fits: treat as per normal. Consult Renal Medicine on call and/or Neurology.

Peritoneal Dialysis

Dialysis access-related complications:

- **Peritonitis**
  1. Cloudy effluent, non-specific abdominal pain, malaise, fever and chills in mild to moderate cases.
  2. Vomiting, severe pain, shock and classic signs of peritonitis in more severe cases.
  3. Management
     a. Draw FBC, urea/electrolytes/creatinine and first blood culture
     b. Administer first dose of antibiotics, eg IV ceftazidime 1–2 g.
  4. Inform Renal Medicine on call regarding admission.
- **Leaking catheter**: admit and inform Renal Medicine on call of admission.
- **Hypotension**: see p. 396.
- **Acute abdomen**
  1. Due to serious intraabdominal condition whose presentation mimics peritonitis.
  2. Obtain combined Renal Medicine on call and General Surgery consultations.

Note: CAPD patients are at risk for abdominal/inguinal herniae due to chronically elevated intraabdominal pressures, and intestinal obstruction secondary to adhesions.

- **Infection of tunnel/catheter exit site**
  1. Often difficult to detect clinically.
  2. Consult with Renal Medicine.

References/further reading

1. Wilson RF. Fluid and electrolyte problems. In: Tintinalli JE, Ruiz E, Krome RL, eds. *Emergency Medicine: A Comprehensive Study Guide*. 3rd ed. New York: McGraw-Hill; 1992:72–74.
2. Zull DN. Disorders of potassium metabolism. In: Wolfson AB, ed. Endocrine and metabolic emergencies. *Emerg Med Clinics N Am*. 1989;7(4):783.

88 Respiratory failure, acute

Chong Chew Lan

DEFINITIONS

- Type I: PaO_2 ≤60 mm Hg (8 kPa)
- Type II: $PaCO_2$ ≥55 mm Hg (7 kPa) with/without poor oxygenation

CAVEATS

- Patients with **type II failure alone** may look **deceptively 'comfortable'**, ie, they are often not tachypneoic. A hypercarbic patient is drowsy while a hypoxic patient is often agitated, and, sometimes violent. They will need repeated ABG for monitoring of $PaCO_2$ or end tidal CO_2 monitoring.
- SaO_2 of 91% corresponds to PaO_2 of 60 mm Hg in general but this is affected by pH, temperature and 2,3 DPG level.
- **Do not treat the high $PaCO_2$** level in patients with chronic compensated type II respiratory failure, ie they have **normal pH (pH >7.35)**.
- Always give as much oxygen as is necessary to correct hypoxia (SaO_2>90% but not >95%).
- Use pulse oximetry to titrate oxygenation (SaO_2) and ABG to evaluate ventilation (CO_2 and pH).
- If CO_2 is climbing due to the loss of hypoxic drive, the patient needs ventilatory support in terms of **biphasic positive airway pressure (BIPAP)** or **intermittent positive pressure ventilation (IPPV)**.
- **Common causes** include:
  1. Pulmonary oedema
  2. Pneumonia
  3. Pulmonary embolism
  4. Severe asthma/COLD
  5. Chest trauma
  6. Drowning
  7. Aspiration
  8. Acute respiratory distress syndrome
  9. Pulmonary metastasis

Note: For a hyperventilating patient with normal chest findings on physical examination, refer to *Hyperventilation*.

- Seriously consider the diagnosis of **pulmonary embolism** in a hypoxic patient with normal CXR. Refer to *Pulmonary Embolism*.
- Patients who have **aspirated** may have delayed CXR changes.
- **Oxygen therapy**: see Table 1.

Table 1: Devices used for oxygen delivery

Device	*Features*	*Advantages*	*Disadvantages*	*Indications*
Nasal prongs	1. Low flow (1–6 l/min) 2. FiO_2 0.24–0.40 (approx. 3–4%/l) 3. FiO_2 delivered is variable	1. Simple to use 2. Does not interfere with talking or eating 3. Better compliance	1. Imprecise FiO_2 2. Maximum FiO_2 <40%	1. Less hypoxic patients 2. Patients with history of retaining CO_2
Simple mask	1. Low flow (5–10 l/min) 2. FiO_2 0.35–0.50 (approx. 3–4%/l)	1. Provides higher FiO_2 than nasal prongs	1. Less comfortable, hot and confining 2. Interferes with talking and eating 3. May cause CO_2 rebreathing if flow is set too low 4. Variable delivered FiO_2	1. Moderately hypoxic patients not known to have COLD
Venturi mask	1. Provides high flow of up to 60 l/min 2. FiO_2 0.24–0.50	1. More precise FiO_2 2. Maximum FiO_2 50%	1. Needs 2 settings and higher risk of errors in application* 2. Poorer compliance 3. CO_2 rebreathing possible if flow rate inadequate 4. Difficult to talk and eat	1. Controlled oxygen therapy, eg for Type II failure from COLD
Non-rebreathing mask	1. Low flow (6–15 l/min) 2. FiO_2 0.50–0.80	1. Maximum FiO_2 80%	1. Poorer compliance 2. Obstructs access to mouth 3. Claustrophobic	1. High FiO_2 necessary to correct hypoxia

* Correct application for Venturi masks:

1. Decide on the FiO_2 desired (24–30%: use green diluter on mask; 35–50%: use white diluter).
2. Set oxygen to appropriate flow rate for FiO_2 desired.
3. Set the size of the Venturi aperture on the face mask to the desired FiO_2.

> **☛ Special Tips for GPs**
> - Give supplemental oxygen to all patients who are dyspnoeic till arrival of the ambulance even if they do not look cyanosed.

MANAGEMENT

- Manage these patients in the resuscitation room.
- Give high-flow O_2 via face mask and continuously monitor heart, respiratory rate and oxygen saturation. Reduce the FiO_2 according to pulse oximetry and/or frequent blood gas monitoring after improvement in patients with COLD. The target O_2 saturation for patients with COLD is 90–92% but not >92%. Watch these patients carefully as there is a risk of worsening CO_2 retention and narcosis.
- Clinical signs of worsening CO_2 retention and respiratory acidosis are not reliable. ABG examination is needed.
- **All** patients with **COLD need ABG examination** after O_2 titration and initial medical treatment with repeated nebulizations of bronchodilators.
- Take a quick history and perform a targeted examination to determine the underlying cause of the respiratory failure.
- Treat the underlying cause.
- If the patient does not improve with supplemental oxygen and treatment of the underlying cause, consider mechanical support of ventilation.
- In severe hypoxic or **type I acute respiratory failure**, consider **CPAP (non-invasive)** or **PEEP (intubate patient)**.
- In severe hypercapnic or **type II acute respiratory failure**, consider **IPPV** either non-invasively or post-intubation.
- Consider **BIPAP** for COLD patients with CO_2 retention and **pH between 7.26** and **7.32**. Patients with **pH <7.26** usually require **intubation** and mechanical ventilation.
- **Do not give sodium bicarbonate to patients with low pH due to CO_2 retention!** This will exacerbate the respiratory acidosis.

References/further reading

1. Respiratory failure. In: Kumar P, Clark M, eds. *Clinical Medicine*. 4th ed. Edinburgh: WB Saunders; 1998:849–851.
2. Lim TK. Acute breathlessness and acute respiratory failure. In: Lee KH, Wong J, Tan CC, eds. *Survival Guide to Acute Medicine*. Singapore: Singapore University Press; 1998:4–6.

89 Sepsis/septic shock

Irwani Ibrahim

DEFINITIONS

- **Infection**: microbial phenomenon characterized by an inflammatory response to the presence of microorganisms or the invasion of normally sterile host tissue by those organisms.
- **Bacteraemia**: the presence of viable bacteria in the blood.
- **Systemic inflammatory response syndrome (SIRS)**: the systemic inflammatory response to a variety of severe clinical insults. The response is manifested by ≥2 of the following conditions:
  1. Temperature >38°C or <36°C
  2. Heart rate >90 beats per minute
  3. Respiratory rate >20 breaths per minute or $PaCO_2$ <32 mm Hg
  4. White blood cell count >12,000/mm^3, <4,000/mm^3, or >10% immature (band) forms
- **Sepsis**: the systemic response to infection, manifested by ≥2 of the following conditions as a result of infection.
  1. Temperature >38°C or <36°C;
  2. Heart rate >90 beats per minute;
  3. Respiratory rate >20 breaths per minute or $PaCO_2$ <32 mm Hg
  4. White blood cell count >12,000/mm^3, <4,000/mm^3, or >10% immature (band) forms.
- **Severe sepsis**: sepsis associated with organ dysfunction, hypoperfusion, or hypotension. Hypoperfusion and perfusion abnormalities may include, but are not limited to, lactic acidosis, oliguria, or an acute alteration in mental state.
- **Septic shock**: sepsis-induced hypotension despite adequate fluid resuscitation along with the presence of perfusion abnormalities that may include, but are not limited to, lactic acidosis, oliguria, or an acute alteration in mental state. Patients who are receiving inotropic or vasopressor agents may not be hypotensive at the time perfusion abnormalities are measured.
- **Sepsis-induced hypotension**: a SBP <90 mm Hg or a reduction of ≥40 mm Hg from baseline in the absence of other causes for hypotension.
- **Multiple organ dysfunction syndrome (MODS)**: presence of altered organ function in an acutely ill patient such that homeostasis cannot be maintained without intervention.

CAVEATS

- In the **elderly**, the **very young** or **immunocompromised**, the clinical presentation may be atypical and non-specific with no fever or localizable source of infection (refer to *Geriatric Emergencies*).
- **Symptoms** of sepsis include fever, chills and constitutional symptoms of fatigue, malaise, anxiety or confusion. These symptoms are not pathognomonic for infection and may be seen in a wide variety of non-infectious inflammatory conditions. They may be absent in serious infections especially in the elderly.
- Vital signs abnormalities such as tachypnoea, tachycardia and increased pulse pressure may suggest sepsis even if fever is absent.

Note: In the early stages of sepsis, cardiac output is well maintained or increased, resulting in warm skin and extremities. As sepsis progresses, patient starts to show signs of poor distal perfusion, eg cool skin and extremities. Hence, late septic shock without a fever is indistinguishable from other types of shock and a high index of suspicion is required. It is often a diagnosis by exclusion.

- The most frequent **sites of infection** are the lungs, abdomen and the urinary tract (Table 1).

Table 1: Predisposing factors for gram-negative and gram-positive bacteraemia

Gram-negative bacteraemia	*Gram-positive bacteraemia*
Diabetes mellitus	Vascular catheters
Lymphoproliferative disease	Indwelling mechanical devices
Cirrhosis of the liver	Burns
Burns	Intravenous drug injections
Chemotherapy	

☛ **Special Tips for GPs**

- If delay to the nearest hospital is anticipated, start IV fluid resuscitation immediately.
- In patient with signs of meningococcaemia, start IV crystalline penicillin 4 mega units immediately as patient can deteriorate rapidly within a few hours.

MANAGEMENT

- Patient must be managed in the resuscitation area.
- Monitoring: ECG, vital signs q 5 min, pulse oximetry.

- Maintain airway, give supplemental high-flow oxygen. Endotracheal intubation should be considered if airway is not secured or ventilation and oxygenation are inadequate.
- Establish 2 large bore IV lines and aggressively correct the hypotension with fluid resuscitation (eg rapid fluid administration of at least 1–2 litres crystalloid). Consider inserting central venous line.
- Labs:
  1. Capillary blood sugar
  2. FBC
  3. Blood culture (2 different sites)
  4. DIVC screen
  5. Urea/electrolytes/creatinine
  6. ABG
  7. Urine culture
- Chest x-ray to look for consolidation and signs of ARDS.
- Consider ECG.
- Insert urinary catheter to monitor urine output.
- All patients should receive **empiric antimicrobial therapy** as soon as possible. The route of administration should be intravenous.

Note: Table 2 is only a guide. The spectrum of bacteria and their sensitivities vary in different hospitals.

Table 2: A guide to choices of antibiotics

Suspected infection	*Suggested antibiotics*
Immunocompetent without obvious source	Third-generation cephalosporin (eg IV ceftriaxone 1 g) or quinolones (eg, ciprofloxacin 200 mg)
Immunocompromised without obvious source	Antipseudomonal beta-lactamase susceptible penicillin (eg IV ceftazidime 1 g) or quinolones plus aminoglycoside (eg gentamicin 80 mg)
Gram-positive	IV cefazolin 2 g. Consider IV vancomycin 1 g if there is history of intravenous drug abuse or indwelling catheter or penicillin allergy
Anaerobic source (intraabdominal, biliary, female genital tract, aspiration pneumonia)	IV metronidazole 500 mg Add ceftriaxone 1 g and IV gentamicin 80 mg to cover for gram-negative bacteria in these infections

- **Inotropic vasoactive agents support** may be needed if there is no response to fluid challenge. Noradrenaline is the agent of choice in septic shock, started at 1 μg/kg/min. Alternatively, dopamine can be used (dosage at 5–20 μg/kg/min). Successful fluid resuscitation is indicated by stabilization of mentation, BP, respiration, pulse rate, skin perfusion and good urine output.
- The use of corticosteroids in septic shock is still controversial. However it plays a primary role if adrenal insufficiency is suspected or documented.
- Consult the Intensive Care team for transfer to their care.

References/further reading

1. Jui J. Septic Shock. In: Tintinalli JE, Kelen GD, Stapczynski JS, et al, eds. *Emergency Medicine: A Comprehensive Study Guide*. 5th ed. New York: McGraw-Hill; 2000:229–239.
2. Astiz ME, Rackow EC. Septic shock. *The Lancet*. 1998;351(9114):1501–1505.
3. Bone RC, Balk RA, Cerra FB, et al. Definitions for sepsis and organ failure and guidelines for the use of innovative therapies in sepsis. The ACCP/SCCM Consensus Conference Committee. *Chest.* 1992; 101:1664–1673.
4. Rivers E, Nguyen B, Havstad S, et al. Early goal-directed therapy in the treatment of severe sepsis and septic shock. *N Engl J Med.* 2001;345(19):1368–1377.
5. Annane D, et al. Effect of treatment with low doses of hydrocortisone and fludrocortisone on mortality in patients with septic shock. *JAMA*. 2002;288:862–871.
6. Bernard GR, Vincent JL, Laterre PF, et al. Efficacy and safety of recombinant human activated protein C for severe sepsis. *N Engl J Med.* 2001;344(10):699–709.

90 Spinal cord injury

Peng Li Lee • Shirley Ooi

MECHANISMS OF INJURY

- Penetrating injury.
- Blunt trauma with disruption of vertebral column causing transection or compression of neural elements.
- Primary vascular damage to spinal cord, eg compression by extradural haematoma.

CAVEATS

- **Spinal cord injury** should be suspected and cervical immobilization maintained from the time of injury in the following:
  1. Unconscious trauma patient
  2. Survivors of high velocity accident
  3. Presence of associated injuries:
     a. Significant head or facial trauma: 4–20% incidence of associated cervical injury
     b. Scapular contusion: may suggest flexion-rotation of thoracic spine
     c. Seat belt injuries: may be associated with thoracic and lumbar injuries
     d. Injury to feet/ankle from a fall from height: may be associated with compression injury to lumbar spine
- Be on the lookout for **signs of spinal cord injury**:
  1. Vital signs: **neurogenic shock** (hypotension with bradycardia).

Note: Although neurogenic shock should be considered in trauma patients with hypotension in the absence of tachycardia, hypovolaemia from blood loss must still be excluded first as patient may not mount the tachycardic response, eg patients on beta-blockers.

  2. On **inspection**:
     a. Diaphragmatic breathing
     b. Flexed posture of upper limbs suggests a high cervical cord injury
     c. Spontaneous muscle fasciculations
     d. Priapism
  3. On **testing**:
     a. **Myotomic pattern of power loss:** see Table 1
     b. **Dermatomic pattern of sensory loss:** see Figure 1
     c. **Complete spinal cord lesion**: complete loss of motor power and sensation distal to the site of spinal cord injury. Differential diagnosis is spinal shock (usually less than 24 h). Look for **sacral sparing** (prognosticate for functional recovery):
     Intact perianal sensation.

Table 1: Nerve function

Nerve root	*Motor/function*	*Sensory*	*Reflex*
C4	Diaphragm/ventilation	Suprasternal notch	
C5	Deltoid/shoulder shrug	Below clavicle	Biceps
C6	Biceps/elbow flexion, wrist extension	Thumb	Biceps
C7	Triceps/elbow extension	Middle finger	Triceps
C8	Flexor digitorum/finger flexion	Little finger	
T1	Interossei/spread fingers	Medial forearm	
T4	Intercostal/ventilation	Nipples	
T8		Xiphoid	
T10	Abdominal musculature	Umbilicus	
T12		Pubic symphysis	
L1/L2	Iliopsoas/hip flexion	Upper thigh	
L3	Quadriceps/knee extension	Medial thigh	Patellar
L4	Quadriceps/knee extension	Big toe	Patellar
L5	Extensor hallucis longus/ great toe dorsiflexion	Middle toe	
S1	Gastrocnemius and soleus/ ankle plantarflexion	Little toe	Achilles
S2/S3/S4	Anal sphincter/bowel and bladder	Perianal area	Bulbocavernosus

Source: Reproduced with permission of the McGraw-Hill Companies, from Scaletta TA and Schaider JJ. *Emergent Management of Trauma*. Boston: McGraw-Hill; 2001: Table 10.1.[3]

Intact rectal sphincter tone.
Slight flexor toe movement.
Presence of bulbocavernosus reflex: external anal sphincter contraction felt with a gloved finger when the glans penis/clitoris is squeezed or the in-situ Foley's catheter is gently tugged.

d. **Incomplete cord lesions**: classify into 3 main types.

(1) **Central cord syndrome** (Figure 2), commonly seen in degenerative arthritis of cervical spine.
Disproportionately greater loss of motor power in upper limbs than lower limbs.
There is varying degrees of sensory loss.
Fibres controlling voluntary bowel and bladder function are centrally located and often affected, although 'sacral sparing' is usually present.
Mechanism: hyperextension, eg typically a forward fall onto the face in an elderly person.

(2) **Brown sequard syndrome** (Figure 3)
Ipsilateral motor paralysis.

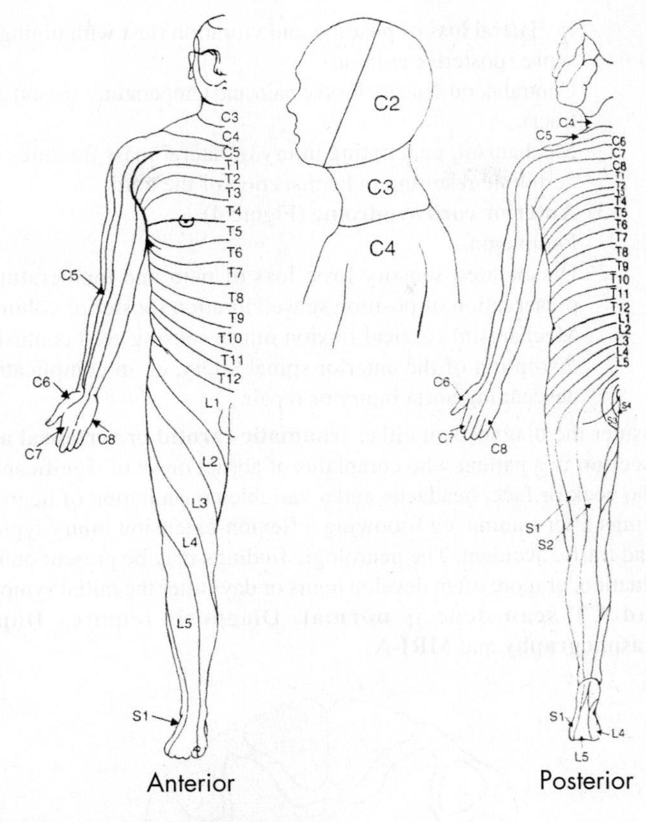

Figure 1: Sensory function
Reproduced with permission from Scaletta and Schaider, Figure 10-11[3]

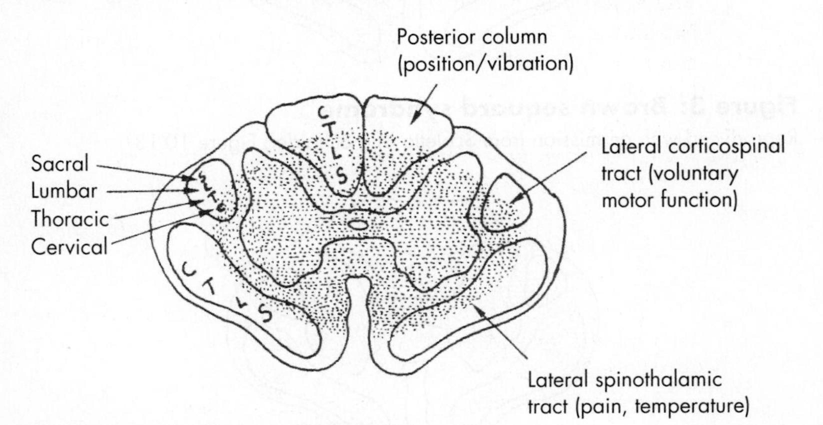

Figure 2: Central cord syndrome
Reproduced with permission from Scaletta and Schaider, Figure 10-12[3]

Ipsilateral loss of position and vibration (test with tuning fork) sense (posterior column).
Contralateral sensory loss of pain and temperature (spinothalamic tract).
Mechanism: penetrating injury or lateral mass fractures of the vertebrae resulting in hemisection of the cord.

(3) **Anterior cord syndrome** (Figure 4)
Paraplegia.
Dissociated sensory loss: loss of pain and temperature but preservation of position sense/vibration (posterior column).
Mechanism: cervical flexion injury causing cord contusion or disruption of the anterior spinal artery, eg in complication of descending aorta injury or repair.

- Consider the diagnosis of either **traumatic carotid** or **vertebral artery dissection** in a patient who complains of abrupt onset of significant pain in the neck or face, headache and a variable constellation of neurologic findings after trauma, eg following a flexion-extension injury typical of a road traffic accident. The neurologic findings may be present on initial evaluation, or more often develop hours or days after the initial symptoms. **Head CT scan** done is **normal**. Diagnosis requires **Doppler ultrasonography** and **MRI-A**.

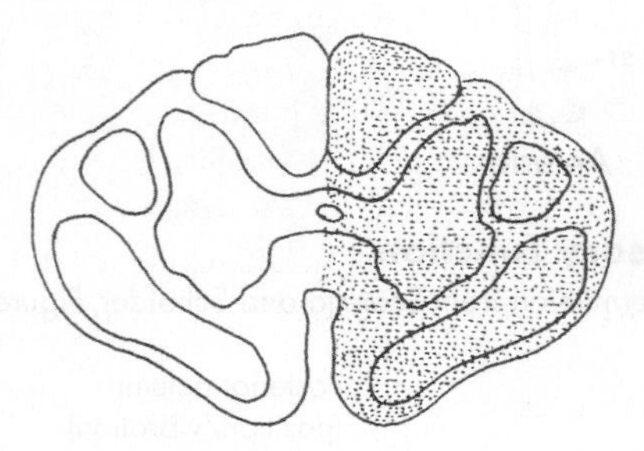

Figure 3: Brown sequard syndrome
Reproduced with permission from Scaletta and Schaider, Figure 10-13[3]

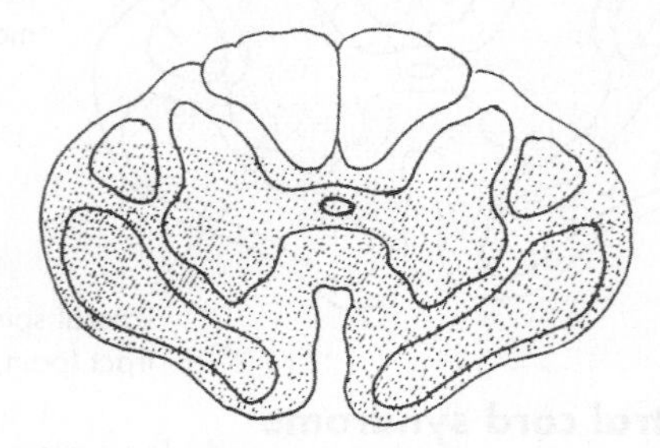

Figure 4: Anterior cord syndrome
Reproduced with permission from Scaletta and Schaider, Figure 10-14[3]

☛ **Special Tips for GPs**
- Always immobilize the neck of all trauma patients from the time of injury till transfer to the ED.
- A whiplash injury or neck sprain is often not very painful immediately. However, patient should be warned that the neck stiffness may worsen over the next few days and to return to the ED should he/she develop neurological signs or symptoms.

MANAGEMENT

- Attend to life-threatening injuries first while minimizing movement of the spinal column.
- Immobilize the spine in neutral position.
- Document neurological deficits.
- **Radiological investigations**:
  1. C-spine x-ray: mandatory AP/lateral view (patient's shoulders may have to be pulled down during lateral view to ensure adequate visualization of C7/T1 junction). Consider:
     a. Swimmer's view if C7/T1 junction not seen on lateral view.
     b. Open mouth odontoid view if C1/2 injury suspected, when there is upper cervical/occipital pain.
  2. Thoracic and lumbar spine x-ray: AP/lateral views.
  3. CT scan is indicated in the following:
     a. Good visualization of the lower C-spine not obtained on x-ray.
     b. Suspicious abnormality seen on x-ray.
  4. MRI:
     a. Provides the most accurate data in the presence of neurological deficits.
     b. Limitation is its availability in the urgent setting.
- **IV fluids:**
  1. Avoid overzealous fluid administration as it may precipitate pulmonary oedema.
  2. Insert urinary catheter to monitor urinary output.
  3. For neurogenic shock, consider vasopressors if the BP does not improve after fluid challenge.
- Consider **IV methylprednisolone:**
  1. Indications:
     a. Proven non-penetrating spinal cord injury.
     b. Within 8 h postinjury.
  2. Dosage: 30 mg/kg over 15 min followed by 5.4 mg/kg/h for the next 23 h

3. Contraindications
   a. Paediatric: <13 years old
   b. Pregnancy
   c. Mild injury limited to cauda equina/nerve root
   d. Presence of abdominal trauma
   e. Major life-threatening morbidity

- **Disposition**: refer to Orthopaedic surgeon and/or Neurosurgeon depending on local practice.

References/further reading

1. Spine and spinal cord trauma. In: Committee on Trauma of the American College of Surgeons. *Advanced Trauma Life Support for Doctors Student Course Manual*. 6th ed. Chicago: American College of Surgeons; 1997:215–230.
2. John AM, Hockberger RS, Walls RM, et al. *Rosen's Emergency Medicine*. 5th ed. St. Louis: Mosby; 2002.
3. All pictures and tables in this chapter were reproduced with permission of the McGraw-Hill Companies, from Scaletta TA and Schaider JJ, *Emergent Management of Trauma*. Boston: McGraw-Hill; 2001.
4. Stahmer SA, Raps EC, Mines DI. Carotid and vertebral artery dissection. In: Neurologic emergencies. *Em Med Clin North Am* 1997;15:677–698.
5. Chong CL, SBS Ooi. Neck pain after minor neck trauma – is it always neck sprain? *Eur J Em Med* 2000;7:147–149.

91 Stroke

Peng Li Lee • Shirley Ooi

DIAGNOSIS

- Acute stroke is characterized by the sudden onset of focal neurological deficits, usually referable to a brain vascular territory. Common clinical presentations include hemiparesis, hemisensory loss, facial weakness, dysarthria, aphasia and visual disturbance, occurring alone or in combination.
- **Strokes** are **classified** as:
  1. **Ischaemic** strokes (IS, 70–90%, higher incidence in Caucasians). Common aetiologies include large artery atherothrombosis, cardioembolism and small vessel disease (lacunar strokes).
  2. **Haemorrhagic** strokes, which are **intracerebral haemorrhage** (ICH, 10–30%, higher incidence in non-Caucasian ethnic groups) and **subarachnoid haemorrhage** (SAH, about 2%).

CAVEATS

- Although the diagnosis of stroke is often straightforward, some common 'stroke mimics' should be considered (Table 1). Always perform a **capillary (finger-stix) glucose level to exclude hypoglycaemia**.
- Stroke is recognized as a time-sensitive emergency, especially with the more common use of intravenous rt-PA (alteplase) treatment for acute ischaemic stroke within 3 h of symptom onset. Patients with suspected stroke should be transported by ambulance to the nearest ED to expedite triage and management.
- Neurological deficits associated with headache, nausea, vomiting, decreased conscious level and grossly elevated BP are more likely to occur in **haemorrhagic strokes**.
- Treatment of hypertension in acute stroke is often controversial and should be approached cautiously (see the following discussion).

Table 1: Differential diagnosis of stroke

Hypoglycaemia/hyperglycaemia
Postepileptic (Todd's) paralysis
Complicated migraine
Hypertensive encephalopathy
Head trauma (epidural/subdural haematoma)
Brain tumour/abscess
Meningitis/encephalitis
Aortic dissection
Bell's palsy
Functional (psychiatric) conditions

☛ **Special Tips for GPs**

- Stroke patients who are **potential candidates for thrombolysis** (Figure 1) should be transferred to the ED by ambulance without delay, given the narrow time window for this treatment.
- Most patients with suspected stroke should also be assessed emergently at the ED for timely management. Home visit and outpatient assessment are not advisable except for patients who present with mild non-disabling symptoms which are non-progressive and had already lasted for more than 48 hours.
- The GP can play an important role in educating at-risk patients (eg those with hypertension, diabetes mellitus, hypercholesterolaemia, cardiac disease, smoking, and history of stroke or transient ischaemic attack [TIA]) and their families to recognize common stroke symptoms, thus facilitating early presentation when stroke occurs.
- Always check the **capillary blood sugar level** to exclude hypoglycaemia.
- **Bell's palsy** is often confused with stroke. Although Bell's palsy (isolated lower motor neuron-type facial nerve palsy) usually presents with complete paralysis of the entire half of the face **without** sparing the forehead muscles, clear distinction from stroke is sometimes difficult in cases of partial facial weakness, and neurology referral is warranted.
- Patients who present with a recent **TIA** (acute neurological deficits attributed to a cerebrovascular aetiology with complete remission within 24 hours of symptom onset) are at high risk of suffering from ischaemic stroke early in the post-TIA period. They require urgent referral to a neurologist or a stroke clinic. If a same-day neurology appointment is not available, an antiplatelet agent (eg aspirin 150–300 mg stat, followed by 75–100 mg daily) may be commenced if not contraindicated. Patients with recurrent TIAs or crescendo TIAs should be urgently referred to the ED.

MANAGEMENT

The management of a suspected stroke patient in the ED include:

- Maintenance of optimal physiological status, including oxygenation, hydration and satisfactory blood glucose level. All patients should initially be put on nil-by-mouth, and started on maintenance IV isotonic saline. Fever should be investigated for infective sources and controlled with antipyretic agents. BP management is discussed below.
- Definitive diagnosis of stroke and the stroke subtype (IS, ICH or SAH). This requires a head CT scan that should be performed on all patients with suspected stroke within 24 hours of admission.
- An **emergent head CT scan** to be performed in the ED is indicated in:
  1. IS patients who are candidates for thrombolytic or anticoagulant therapies, eg present within 3 hours of symptom onset, atrial fibrillation.
  2. Suspected ICH, eg grossly elevated BP, headache, vomiting, possibly drowsiness, low platelet count, impaired clotting profile, anticoagulant use or addiction of stimulant drugs.
  3. Suspected SAH, eg worse headache in life, meningism or loss of consciousness. Refer to *Subarachnoid Haemorrhage (SAH)*.
  4. Patients at risk of early deterioration, eg severe cortical stroke with hemiplegia, forced eye deviation, and aphasia or hemineglect; suspected stroke in the posterior fossa.

  Results of the head CT scan in these groups of patients will assist in starting appropriate medical therapy, timely neurosurgical consultation and early prognostication.

Management of hypertension in acute stroke

Haemorrhagic stroke

- Acute reduction of BP may reduce rebleeding and haematoma expansion.
- However, aggressive BP control may exacerbate ischaemia in the regions immediately adjacent to the haematoma.
- Goals of BP management in patients with acute haemorrhagic stroke:

SBP <180 mm Hg DBP <105 mm Hg	Usually do not require treatment in ED. More aggressive treatment may be considered after admission.
SBP 180–220 mm Hg DBP 105–120 mm Hg	Transdermal nitroglycerin 5–10 mg, or IV labetalol, esmolol, enalapril or diltiazem in small titrated doses.
SBP >220 mm Hg DBP >120 mm Hg	IV nitroglycerin 0.6–6 mg/h.

Ischaemic stroke

- No data show a benefit of routine aggressive BP control in acute ischaemic stroke.

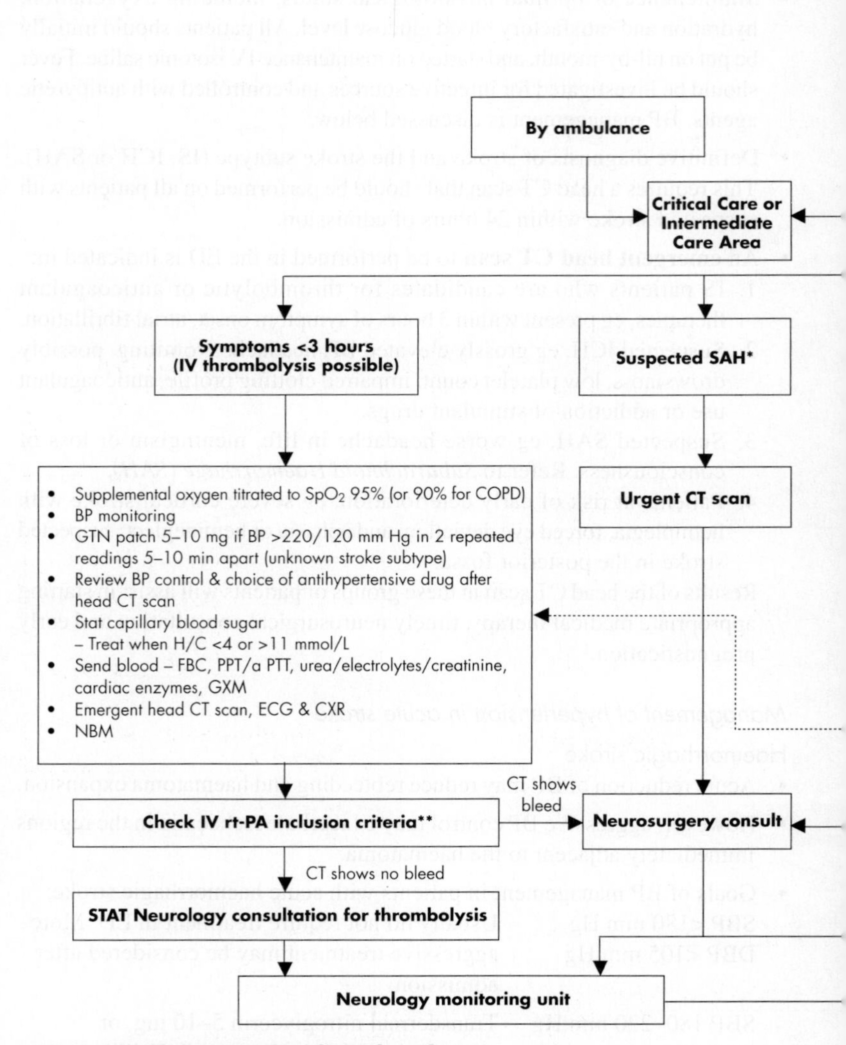

Figure 1: The ED stroke clinical pathway

* Suspected SAH:

1. Any 2 of the 3 clinical features:
   - Headache
   - LOC
   - Meningism

   Neurological deficit may/may be present
2. Isolated headache that is severe, of sudden onset, and the 1st episode of such pain.

** Inclusion criteria for IV rt-PA:

1. Age 18–80 years (upper age limit may differ according to institution/physician)
2. Acute stroke <3 h (time of assessment – time of onset). Most conservative estimate taken, ie time of onset = time patient last seen to be well
3. Measurable deficit in motor, visual, or language domain.

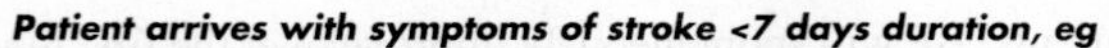

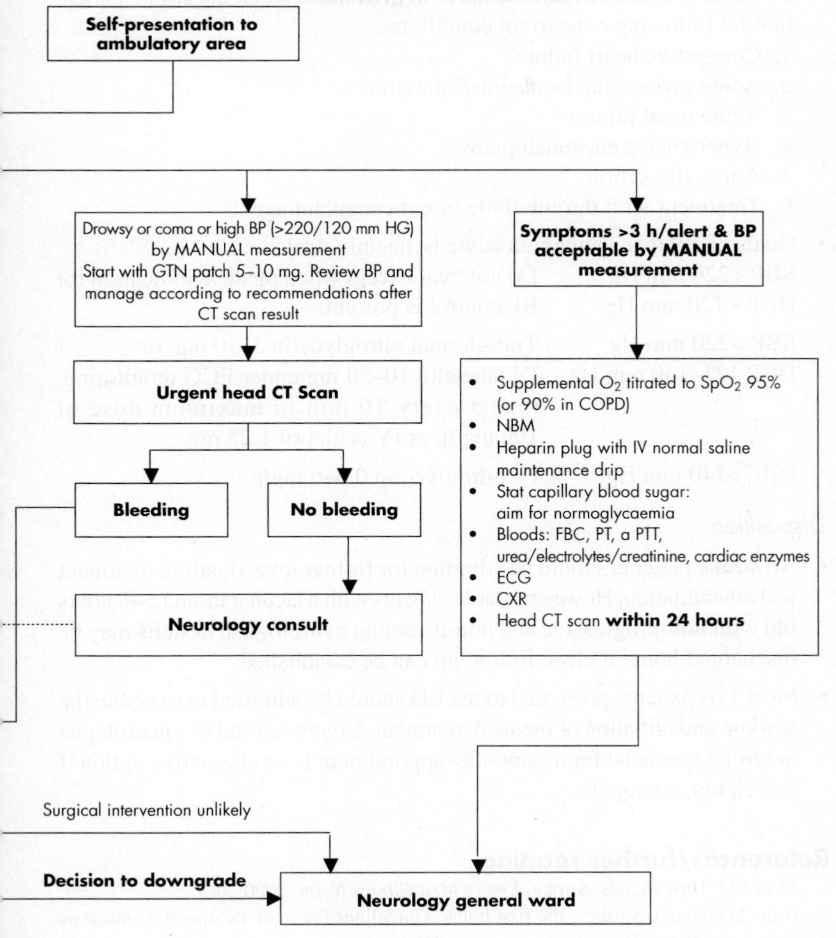

Patient arrives with symptoms of stroke <7 days duration, eg
✓ weakness on one side of the body
✓ incoordination of limbs on one side
✓ slurring of speech
✓ vertiginous giddiness with slurring of speech
✓ numbness on one side of the body
✓ inability to express one's thought, or to understand others
✓ blindness affecting part or all of visual field in one or both eyes
✓ double vision or weakness of face and/or limbs
Self-presentation to ambulatory area
Drowsy or coma or high BP (>220/120 mm HG) by MANUAL measurement
Start with GTN patch 5–10 mg. Review BP and manage according to recommendations after CT scan result
Symptoms >3 h/alert & BP acceptable by MANUAL measurement
Urgent head CT Scan
Bleeding
No bleeding
Neurology consult
Supplemental O_2 titrated to SpO_2 95% (or 90% in COPD)
NBM
Heparin plug with IV normal saline maintenance drip
Stat capillary blood sugar: aim for normoglycaemia
Bloods: FBC, PT, a PTT, urea/electrolytes/creatinine, cardiac enzymes
ECG
CXR
Head CT scan within 24 hours
Surgical intervention unlikely
Decision to downgrade
Neurology general ward

- Most patients' BP will spontaneously improve over the first few hours and return to baseline over the first few days after stroke onset.
- Most neurologists regard significant BP lowering may be harmful by decreasing collateral perfusion in the ischaemic penumbra, resulting in infarct extension.
- **BP control is indicated on a more urgent basis** when the stroke patient has the following concurrent conditions:
  1. Congestive heart failure
  2. Acute myocardial ischaemia/infarction
  3. Acute renal failure
  4. Hypertensive encephalopathy
  5. Aortic dissection
  6. Treatment with thrombolytic or anticoagulant agents
- Goals of BP management in acute ischaemic stroke

SBP <220 mm Hg DBP <120 mm Hg	Do not treat **except** when medical indication for BP control is present.
SBP >220 mm Hg DBP 121–140 mm Hg	Transdermal nitroglycerin 5–10 mg, or IV labetalol 10–20 mg under ECG monitoring, repeat every 10 min to maximum dose of 100 mg/h, or IV enalapril 1.25 mg.
DBP >140 mm Hg	IV nitroglycerin 0.6–6 mg/h.

Disposition

- All stroke patients should be admitted for further investigation, treatment and rehabilitation. However, stable patients with a lacunar infarct >48 hours old with non-progressive and non-disabling neurological deficits may be discharged home if close follow-up can be established.
- Most TIA patients presented to the ED should be admitted to expedite the workup and initiation of medical treatment. Urgent referral to a neurologist or stroke specialist for a same-day appointment is an alternative option if this can be arranged.

References/further reading

1. Shah SM, Huff JS, eds. Stroke. *Emerg Med Clinics N Am.* 2000;20(3).
2. Brott TG (chair). Stroke – the first hours. Guidelines for acute treatment. Consensus Statement, National Stroke Association. 2000.
3. Adams Jr HP (chair). Guidelines for the early management of patients with ischemic stroke. A scientific statement from the Stroke Council of the American Stroke Association. *Stroke.* 2003;34:1056–1083.
4. Broderick JP, Adams HP Jr., Barsan W. Guidelines for the management of spontaneous intracerebral hemorrhage. A statement for healthcare professionals from a special writing group of the Stroke Council, American Stroke Association. *Stroke.* 1999;30:905–915.

92 Subarachnoid haemorrhage (SAH)

Seet Chong Meng • Peter Manning • Shirley Ooi

CAVEATS

- SAH increases in age until it plateaus after age 60 years, with a peak incidence from 40–60 year old.
- The **speed of the onset** of the headache (**sudden**, like a **thunder-clap**) is a more useful guide than the severity of the headache.
- On presentation, 50% of patients are alert, 30% are lethargic and the remaining 20% are stuporous or comatose.
- Neck stiffness may take 2–3 hours to develop.
- Fundoscopic examination reveals preretinal haemorrhage in up to 20% of patients.
- Non-focal neurological symptoms and signs are common, eg nausea, vomiting, fever, syncope, confusion, migraine-like headache, or coma.
- Patients with **posterior cerebral artery communicating aneurysms** may present with an ipsilateral dilated pupil, or deviated gaze from third cranial nerve palsy.
- Patients with **middle cerebral artery aneurysms** may have contralateral hemiparesis secondary to haemorrhage in the temporal lobe or Sylvian fissure.
- Nystagmus and ataxia may be present when haemorrhage occurs into the **posterior fossa** (10% of berry aneurysms).

Note: Most (90%) spontaneous cerebral aneurysms can be found in the anterior circulation which includes the anterior and posterior communicating arteries and the middle cerebral artery.

- On presentation, 20–50% of patients report a severe headache with days to weeks before presentation. This is known as a **warning** or **sentinel**, **headache**, thought to be secondary to fleeting haemorrhage from an aneurysmal sac and subsequent thrombosis.
- Contrary to patients with aneurysmal SAH, patients with haemorrhage secondary to **arteriovenous malformations** (AVMs) are more likely to present with seizures, cerebral bruits, dysphasia and ischaemic events.
- **Do not** diagnose migraine if the first episode of headache occurs after the age of 50 years.
- SAH is most commonly due to bleeding from a saccular (berry) aneurysm or AVM (3–6%), but may occur with trauma as well. The history will often differentiate the two but, occasionally, the haemorrhage will precede a

traumatic incident. Careful history-taking is essential. Rare causes are mycotic, oncotic and flow related aneurysms.

- Various ECG changes, eg peaked or symmetrically inverted T waves, U waves, prolongation of the QRS complex, prolonged QT interval and dysrhythmias, may occur in association with SAH and confuse the physician into pursuing a cardiac diagnosis.
- See Table 1 on Hunt and Hess Classification of SAH for the signs and survival rate.

Table 1: Hunt and Hess classification of subarachnoid haemorrhage

Grade	*Signs*	*Survival (%)*
1	Normal mental state Mild headache No neurologic deficits No meningeal signs	70
2	Moderate-to-severe headache Cranial nerve palsy	60
3	Drowsy, confused Mild focal neurologic deficit	50
4	Stupor Hemiparesis, early vegetative posturing	40
5	Coma Decerebrate posturing	10

☛ **Special Tips for GPs**

- The initial misdiagnosis rate for SAH is 20–50%.
- Absence of headache makes the diagnosis of SAH unlikely.
- Characterized by abrupt onset of symptoms (usually headache and vomiting) and rapid progression of neurological deficits.
- The initial BP is usually high.
- Patient suspected of having SAH should be referred to the ED by ambulance.

MANAGEMENT

Supportive measures

- Patient must be managed in the critical care area.
- Intubation and resuscitation equipment must be immediately available.
- Ensure patent airway.
- Provide supplemental high-flow oxygen via reservoir mask.
- Elevate head of bed to 30 degrees.
- Monitoring: ECG, vital signs q 10–15 min, pulse oximetry.
- Establish peripheral IV line at 'keep open' rate.
- Labs: FBC, urea/electrolytes/creatinine, PT/aPTT, GXM 2 units.
- ECG, CXR (watch out for neurogenic pulmonary oedema)
- Look out for acute complications (0–48 hours after initial haemorrhage). These include:
    1. **Rebleeding**: this is the most significant acute complication after spontaneous SAH. The risk of rebleeding is 4% on the first day after spontaneous SAH and increases 1.5% with each additional day for the next 13 days. Mortality is 80% with rebleeding.
    2. **Cerebral salt wasting** causing hyponatremia.
    3. **Acute hydrocephalus** (15%).
    4. **Seizures** (6%).
    5. **Neurogenic cardiac disease** (10%).
    6. **Neurogenic pulmonary oedema**: this can occur minutes to hours after the initial haemorrhage.

Specific measures

- Non-opioid analgesia, eg IM diclofenac, may be given for relief of the headache.
- Antiemetics: IM prochlorperazine 12.5 mg or IM metoclopramide 10 mg.
- Nitroglycerin by IV infusion if diastolic BP >130 mm Hg by manual measurement. Start at 10 μg/min and titrate to response but **avoid** lowering diastolic BP lower than 100 mm Hg in order to maintain cerebral perfusion.
- Organize head CT scan (without contrast) **coincidental with consultation** with Neurology or Neurosurgery, consistent with institutional practice.

Note:

1. A CT scan does not detect all SAHs. Its sensitivity for detecting SAH is only 93%. The sensitivity of CT decreases with time. It is most sensitive within the first 12 hours and dramatically decreases after 2–7 days.
2. An LP is essential in workup of SAH when the initial CT scan is negative. The presence of xanthochromia in a fresh CSF specimen is pathognomonic for SAH.

Disposition

- Admit all SAH patients under Neurology or Neurosurgery depending on institutional practice.

References/further reading

1. Fontanarosa P. Subarachnoid Haemorrhage. In: Harwood-Nuss AL, Linden CH, Luten RC, eds. *The Clinical Practice of Emergency Medicine.* 2nd ed. Philadelphia: Lippencott-Raven; 1996.
2. Gallagher EJ. Headache. In: Harwood-Nuss AL, Linden CH, Luten RC, eds. *The Clinical Practice of Emergency Medicine.* 2nd ed. Philadelphia: Lippencott-Raven; 1996.
3. Lipinski CA, Benz AG. Subarachnoid haemorrhage. In: Frank LR, Jobe KA, eds. *Admission and Discharge Decision in Emergency Medicine*. Philadelphia: Hanley & Belfus; 2002:152–136.
4. Hunt WE, Hess RM. Surgical risk as related to the time of intervention in the repair of intracranial aneurysms. *J Neurosurg.* 1968;28:14–20.

93 Temporal arteritis

Seet Chong Meng • Shirley Ooi • Peter Manning

DEFINITION

Temporal arteritis is a granulomatous inflammation of one or more branches of the external carotid artery.

DIAGNOSIS

According to the American College of Rheumotology, the diagnosis of temporal arteritis requires the presence of 3 of the following criteria:

- Age >50 years
- New onset of localized headache
- Temporal artery tenderness of decreased pulse
- ESR ≥55 mm/h
- Positive histology on biopsy

CAVEATS

- Suspect temporal arteritis in a **woman, usually over 50 years of age**, presenting with a severe throbbing, burning, and unilateral temporal headache. Often, the headache has been present for several months. Associated symptoms may include malaise, anorexia, weight loss, jaw/tongue claudication, amaurosis, muscle aches, TIA, neuropathy and stroke.
- **Sudden, painless, monocular loss of vision** (due to vascular occlusion of the ophthalmic or posterior ciliary artery with infarction of the optic nerve or retina) is the **most serious complication** since visual loss is usually permanent.
- There is increased incidence of temporal arteritis with **polymyalgia rheumatica**.

☛ **Special Tips for GPs**

- Treat temporal arteritis with **prednisolone** 30–60 mg (1 mg/kg) PO stat once diagnosis is suspected before sending patient to the hospital as delay in diagnosis and treatment can result in permanent blindness.

MANAGEMENT

Supportive measures

- Patient can be managed in the intermediate care area.
- Measure and record the visual acuity.
- Labs: FBC, ESR.

Specific measures

- Start therapy immediately if history and physical examination are suspicious and ESR is elevated.
- Prednisolone 30–60 mg (1 mg/kg) PO stat.
- Analgesia, eg diclofenac IM.

Disposition

- Admit under Neurology following appropriate consultation.

References/further reading

1. Levine SM, Hellmann DB. Giant cell arteritis. *Curr Opin Rheumatol*. 2002;14(1): 3–10. Review.
2. Field AG, Wang E. Evaluation of the patient with nontraumatic headache: An evidence based approach. In: Fontanarosa PB, ed. Evidence based emergency testing: Evaluation and diagnostic testing. *Emerg Med Clin North Am* 1999;17(1):139.

94 Tetanus

Suresh Pillai

CAVEATS

- A high index of suspicion must be maintained in order to pick up patients presenting with tetanus.
- Wound debridement as well as management in an ICU is mandatory for all suspected cases of tetanus.

> ☛ **Special Tips for GPs**
>
> - Apart from ensuring adequate tetanus prophylaxis in all patients with tetanus prone wounds, a high index of suspicion must be maintained for patients presenting with either localized or generalized muscular rigidity with or without a tetanus susceptible wound.
> - All suspected cases should be immediately referred to the ED for further management.

PATHOPHYSIOLOGY

- Tetanus is caused by the introduction of exotoxin liberated by *Clostridium tetani*, an anaerobic gram-positive rod, into a wound. *Clostridium tetani* is usually introduced into a wound in the spore-forming, non-invasive state, but can germinate into a toxin-producing, vegetative form if tissue is compromised and tissue oxygen tension is reduced.
- Tetanus originates in puncture wounds, lacerations, crush injuries as well as in parenteral drug abusers when anaerobic conditions facilitate the germination of spores.
- The clinical signs and symptoms arise because of the transport of exotoxin to the CNS, where it blocks the transmission at the inhibitory interneurones leading to unopposed muscle spasm.

CLINICAL PRESENTATION

- The incubation period can vary from 3–21 days from the onset of infection.
- The signs of generalized tetanus include painful stiffening of the jaw and trunk muscles.
- The typical features of tetanus, including risus sardonicus, dysphagia, opisthotonus, flexing of the arms, clenching of fists, abdominal muscle

rigidity and extension of the lower limbs, are caused by intermittent tonic contractions of the involved muscle groups.

- Fractures of the spine or long bones may arise from convulsive spasms of skeletal muscles as well as from seizures.
- Consciousness is usually not lost unless laryngospasm or spasm of the respiratory muscles develop.
- Autonomic instability resulting in fever, diaphoresis, tachycardia and hypertension are commonly present as well.

MANAGEMENT

- Management is best achieved in quiet isolation in an ICU environment.
- The mainstay of therapy includes neuromuscular paralysis, orotracheal intubation and ventilation. Tracheostomy is often indicated for prolonged ventilatory care.
- Wound debridement is essential to minimize further progression of the disease.
- A single intramuscular dose of Human Tetanus Immune Globulin at 3,000–5,000 IU should be administered.
- A complete course of Intramuscular Anti-Tetanus Toxoid (ATT) 0.5 ml should be initiated once the patient recovers from the acute phase, then at 6 weeks and subsequently at 6 months.
- Intravenous penicillin G 10 million IU/day in divided doses should be initiated. Alternative antibiotics include IV metronidazole 500 mg q 6 h or IV doxycycline 100 mg q 12 h. If the patient is allergic to penicillin, IV erythromycin 2 g/day or tetracycline 2 g/day can be substituted.
- Muscle relaxation with IV diazepam 10 mg q 1–3 h/prn is essential to control reflex painful muscle spasms.
- Prolonged neuromuscular blockade can be achieved with IV atracurium or pancuronium.
- Autonomic instability should be controlled with appropriate medications. Consult an Intensivist.

References/further reading

1. Carden DL. Tetanus. In: Tintinalli JE, Ruiz E, Krome RL, eds. *Emergency Medicine: A Comprehensive Study Guide*. 3rd ed. New York: McGraw-Hill; 1992:525–526.
2. Applegate CN, Fox PT. Neurologic emergencies in internal medicine. In: Dunagan WC, Ridner ML, eds. *Manual of Medical Therapeutics*. 26th ed. St. Louis, Missouri: Little Brown and Co.; 1989:480–481.
3. CDC. Diphtheria, tetanus and pertussis: Recommendations for vaccine use and other preventive measures. Recommendations of the Advisory Committee on Immunization Practices (ACIP). *MMWR*. 1991;40(RR-10):1–28.

95 Thyrotoxic crisis

Malcolm Mahadevan

CAVEATS

- Thyrotoxic crisis is defined as a sudden severe life-threatening exacerbation of hyperthyroidism associated with multiple organ decompensation.
- Suspect the existence of **thyroid storm** in any **known case of hyperthyroidism developing a fever**.
- Thyroid storm is fatal if untreated: mortality rate is 20–50%.
- Avoid aspirin-based antipyretics: they release free T4 and free T3 from protein-bound sites.
- **Clinical presentation**:
  1. **Fever** as indicator of underlying sepsis or a consequence of thyroid storm.
  2. **Tachycardia out of proportion to fever** classically persists during sleep.
  3. **Accentuated thyrotoxic symptoms and signs** such as weight loss, tremors.
  4. **Multiorgan dysfunction**:
     a. CNS dysfunction: altered mental state with mental confusion, delirium, agitation, stupor, coma
     b. GI dysfunction: abdominal pain, diarrhoea and vomiting may simulate a surgical abdomen; jaundice may occur with liver dysfunction
     c. CVS dysfunction: systolic hyper- or hypotension, heart failure, rapid atrial fibrillation/flutter
  5. Recent history of thyroid disease requiring treatment, precipitating event, eg sepsis, recent surgery, iodinated CT contrast.
  6. Trauma patient with increasing pulse and BP.
  7. Volume depletion from fever, increased metabolism, diarrhoea.
- Beware atypical presentation especially in the elderly where a high index of suspicion is essential. They may only present with weakness, heart failure or atrial fibrillation, and goitre may not be evident.

☛ Special Tips for GPs

- Thyroid storm often must be recognized and treated based on clinical grounds because laboratory confirmation of the disease cannot be obtained in a timely manner.

- **Physical examination findings**:
  1. Hyperpyrexia is an indicator of underlying sepsis or a consequence of thyroid storm.
  2. Systolic hyper- or hypotension, heart failure, rapid atrial fibrillation/flutter.
  3. Tachycardia out of proportion to fever.
  4. Altered mental state (**mandatory** diagnostic criterion) delirium, agitation, stupor, coma.
  5. Volume depletion from fever, increased metabolism, diarrhoea.
  6. Stigmata of hyperthyroidism is goitre, tremors, lid lag/retraction, myopathy.

MANAGEMENT

Supportive measures

- Patient must be managed in the critical care area due to the life-threatening nature of this disease entity.
- Administer supplemental high-flow oxygen by non-rebreather reservoir mask.
- Monitoring: ECG, vital signs q 10–15 min, pulse oximetry.
- Establish peripheral IV line.
- IV fluids: dextrose-saline by slow infusion with appropriate electrolytes and vitamins; **correct volume depletion cautiously** to avoid precipitating or worsening heart failure; however, immense fluid losses may require replacement of 3–5 litres/day.
- Labs:
  1. FBC
  2. Urea/electrolytes/creatinine
  3. Liver panel
  4. Thyroid screen to include TSH, free T4. Send blood tube to ward with patient.
  5. CXR for evidence of heart failure and infection
  6. ECG to determine presence of ischaemia, infarction or dysrhythmia
  7. Urinalysis by dipstick reagent; and C&S if sepsis suspected
- Correct precipitating factors, eg sepsis, AMI.
- Administer paracetamol, tepid sponging or other cooling techniques to relieve fever.

Drug therapy

- **Beta-blockers**: crucial even in the presence of high cardiac output heart failure.
  1. Give ultra-short acting IV **esmolol**; test dose 250 μg/kg followed by infusion of 50 μg/min if available, or

2. Give IV **propranolol** 1 mg q 5 min until severe tachycardia is controlled. If patient is able to tolerate orally, then **propranolol 60 mg PO q 4 h** or **80 mg PO q 8 h** can be given.

Note: Treat other cardiovascular complications with conventional means, eg digoxin, diuretics.

- **PTU** (propylthiouracil) blocks iodination as well as the conversion of T4 to T3.

  Dosage: 400–600 mg stat PO or via Ryle's tube, followed by 200–300 mg q 4 h.

Note: Per rectal PTU can be given if patient NBM. Dissolve in a paediatric Fleet enema and give through a Nelaton catheter.

- **Iodine** solution inhibits the release of thyroid hormone; **must** give 1–2 hours post-PTU therapy.

  Dosage: Lugol's iodine 5 drops PO or via Ryle's tube q 8 h.

Note: If NBM, give IV sodium iodide 1 g/500 ml saline q 12 h.

- **Dexamethasone**: 2 mg IV to provide glucocorticoid support; also blocks conversion of free T4 to free T3.

Disposition

- Consult with Endocrine/General Medicine regarding anticipated admission to MICU.

References/further reading

1. Smallridge RC. Metabolic and anatomic thyroid emergencies: A review. *Crit Care Med.* 1992;20:276–291.
2. Burch HB, Wartofsky L. Life-threatening thyrotoxicosis: Thyroid storm. *Endocrinol Metab Clin North Am.* 1993;22(2):263–277.

96 Trauma, abdominal

Peng Li Lee • Shirley Ooi

CAVEATS

- Intraabdominal trauma is a significant cause of preventable deaths.
- Emergency care personnel should have a high index of suspicion for its presence, and investigate and manage accordingly.
- All penetrating injuries below (between) the nipple line should also be suspected of entering the abdominal cavity.
- Patients should always be log-rolled to examine the back and flanks to complete the abdominal examination in trauma cases.
- All multiple trauma patients with hypotension are presumed to have intraabdominal injury until proven otherwise.
- Clinical examination of the abdomen may be compromised in the following setting:
  1. Change in sensorium: alcoholic intoxication, use of illicit drugs, head injury.
  2. Change in sensation: injury to spinal cord.
  3. Distracting injury to adjacent structures: lower ribs, pelvis, lumbar spine.
- Resuscitation and stabilization of patient takes precedence over investigations.

> ☛ **Special Tips for GPs**
>
> - In alert patients, the most reliable signs indicating abdominal injury are tenderness on abdominal palpation, guarding or rebound. However, the lack of such signs does not reliably exclude significant intraabdominal injury.
> - For those with significant mechanism of injury but who present with minimal abdominal findings initially, refer to ED for further evaluation.
> - For those who present to the clinic with early signs of shock, start an IV infusion of crystalloid and call the ambulance for transfer to hospital.

MANAGEMENT

- Patient should be managed in the critical care area.
- Physical examination and resuscitation should proceed simultaneously.

- **Principles of ATLS** should be followed with priorities given to:
  1. Airway: establish and maintain airway.
  2. Breathing: high-flow O_2 for the conscious and spontaneously breathing. The unconscious may require endotracheal intubation with mechanical ventilation.
  3. Circulation: establish 2 large (14/16G) cannulae for venous access. In hypotensive patients, fluid should be infused rapidly. Start with normal saline (up to 2 litres) and followed by blood products (start Group O emergency blood if available in the ED).
- Send blood for GXM, FBC, urea/electrolytes/creatinine.
- **Targeted examination** should include:
  1. Chest wall: bruise, fractured ribs, penetrating injury
  2. Abdomen: external injuries, eg bruising and signs of peritonism, eg tenderness, guarding and absent bowel sounds
  3. Pelvis: tenderness and instability suggesting fracture
  4. External genitalia and rectum: bleeding or haematoma
  5. Neurological status
- Insert nasogastric tube and urinary catheter unless there is suspicion of urethral injury based on physical examination.
- Mandatory trauma series x-rays are indicated as time permits: CXR, pelvic XR, C-spine (C-spine x-rays may not be indicated in selected cases where the neck may be cleared clinically. Refer to *Cervical Spine Clearance*).
- Abdominal stab wounds with implements in-situ should not be removed until the patient is in the operating room.
- Refer and consult General Surgeon early.

Indications for immediate laparotomy

- Evisceration, stab wounds with implement in-situ and gunshot wounds traversing the abdominal cavity.
- Any penetrating injury to the abdomen with haemodynamic instability or peritoneal irritation.
- Obvious or strongly suspected intraabdominal injury with shock or difficulty in stabilizing the haemodynamics.
- Obvious signs of peritoneal irritation.
- Rectal exam reveals fresh blood.
- Persistent fresh blood aspirated from nasogastric tube if oropharyngeal injuries have been excluded as a cause for bleeding.
- X-ray evidence of pneumoperitoneum or diaphragmatic rupture.

Investigations

- In the absence of the above indications for immediate laparotomy, Figure 1 shows the mode of investigations to be considered depending on the stability of the patient.

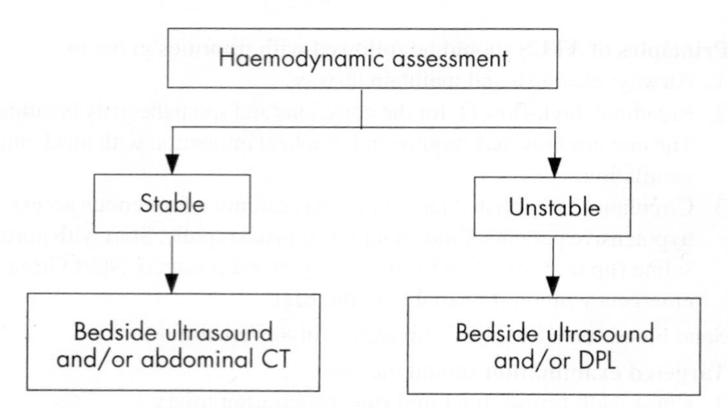

Figure 1: Mode of investigations in a suspected abdominal trauma patient

- Patient going to CT scan room must have **continuous monitoring** of vital signs and must be accompanied by a doctor.
- **CT scan abdomen**:
  1. Indications:
     a. Blunt trauma with stable haemodynamics and with no indication for urgent laparotomy.
     b. Further assessment for pelvic fracture, retroperitoneal, diaphragmatic and urogenital injuries.
  2. Sensitivity is consistently reported as greater than 90%.
  3. With the advent of CT, diagnostic peritoneal lavage (DPL) is uncommonly done in stable patients due to its invasive nature.
  4. **Advantages**
     a. Able to precisely locate intraabdominal lesions preoperatively.
     b Able to evaluate retroperitoneum.
     c. Able to identify injuries that can be managed non-operatively.
     d. Not invasive.
  5. **Disadvantages**
     a. Expensive.
     b. Time required to perform the study.
     c. Need to transport patient to the radiology suite.
     d. Use of contrast materials needed.
- **Diagnostic peritoneal lavage** performed by surgical team:
  1. **Indications**:
     a. Any unstable patient with suspicion of abdominal trauma or where clinical exam is difficult or equivocal.
     b. Unexplained hypotension in multiple trauma.
     c. Patient sustaining blunt trauma requiring immediate operation for extraabdominal injuries.
     d. Stable patients with suspicion of intestinal injury: 'delayed' DPL may be performed.

2. **Contraindications**: the first is an absolute contraindication but the rest are relative contraindications.
   a. Absolute indications for laparotomy already exist.
   b. Previous abdominal surgery or infections.
   c. Gravid uterus.
   d. Morbid obesity.
   e. Coagulopathy.
3. Prerequisite: decompress bladder and stomach with urinary catheter and nasogastric tube respectively.
4. Open technique with an infraumbilical incision. Alternatively, the percutaneous method using the Seldinger technique is also acceptable.
5. Indicators of a positive DPL:
   a. Frank blood (>5 ml) or obvious bowel contents aspirated
   b. Lavage fluid seen to exit from chest drain or urinary catheter
   c. Effluent RBC >100,000 per mm^3
      WBC >500 per mm^3
      Gram stain positive for bacteria
6. DPL is exceptionally sensitive.
7. **Advantages**:
   a. DPL can promptly reveal or exclude the presence of intraperitoneal haemorrhage in a haemodynamically unstable patient with multiple injuries.
   b. DPL is especially valuable in the discovery of potentially lethal bowel perforations when patients are poor candidates for serial clinical observations.
8. **Disadvantages**:
   a. There is morbidity, although low, associated with DPL. They include: (1) wound complications, including haematoma and infections (0.3%); (2) intraperitoneal injury; (3) technical failure whereby insertion of a catheter through an abdominal wall haematoma can create a haemoperitoneum to produce a false positive result.
   b. False negative rate (2%) results from failure to recover lavage fluids, early hollow visceral injury, diaphragmatic injuries and injuries due to retroperitoneal structures (eg pancreas and duodenum).

- **Focused assessment using sonography in trauma (FAST)**:
  1. Increasingly being used as an adjunct in the bedside assessment of abdominal trauma. The indications are the same as for DPL.
  2. It is especially useful in situations where DPL is relatively contraindicated, eg obesity, previous laparotomy or coagulopathy, and patient is too unstable for transfer to CT scan room.
  3. Its accuracy is operator as well as equipment dependent. The amount of free fluid may be quantified based on ultrasound, which gives an idea of the degree of intraabdominal haemorrhage. It is sensitive in detecting as little as 100 ml and more typically 500 ml of peritoneal fluid from 60–95%.

4. Four quadrants are looked at to detect free fluid:
   a. Subxiphoid: Pericardium
   b. RUQ: Morrison's pouch (potential space between liver and kidney)
   c. LUQ: Splenorenal recess and between the spleen and diaphragm
   d. Pelvis: The pouch of Douglous
5. **Advantages**:
   a. Portable instrument that can be brought to the bedside.
   b. Examinations can be done quickly in <5 min. Hence it helps emergency physicians to rapidly answer whether haemoperitoneum, free pericardial fluid and free pleural fluid are present.
   c. FAST can be used for serial examinations.
   d. Unlike CT scanning, it is not a potential radiation hazard and does not require administration of contrast agents.
6. **Disadvantages**:
   a. FAST does not image solid parenchymal damage, the retroperitoneum, diaphragmatic defects or bowel injury well.
   b. It is technically compromised by the uncooperative, agitated patient, as well as by obesity, substantial bowel gas and subcutaneous air.
   c. Indeterminate studies require follow-up attempts or alternative diagnostic tests.
   d. It is less sensitive and more operator dependent than DPL in revealing haemoperitoneum and cannot distinguish blood from ascites.
   e. FAST will not detect the presence of solid parenchymal damage if free intraperitoneal blood is absent as in subcapsular splenic injury.
7. For the haemodynamically stable blunt trauma patient with positive FAST examination results, further evaluation with CT scan may be warranted before admission to General Surgery.

Investigations: penetrating trauma

- In the absence of the above indications for immediate laparotomy, the following mode of investigations are considered depending on the stability of the patient:
  1. Stab wound: explore wound in ED. No penetration of fascia: home. Penetration of fascia: involve surgeon.
  2. Gunshot wound: establish trajectory by examining the entrance/exit wounds or using x-rays if exit wound missing. If trajectory traverses peritoneal cavity, will require immediate laparotomy. If trajectory is tangential, involve surgeon.

References/further reading

1. Marx JA. Abdominal trauma. In Marx JA, Hockberger RS, Walls RM, eds. *Emergency Medicine: Concepts and Practice*. 5th ed. St. Louis: Mosby Year Book; 2002:415–436.
2. Committee on Trauma of the American College of Surgeons. *Advanced Trauma Life Support for Doctors Manual*. 6th ed. Chicago: American College of Surgeons; 1997:157–175.
3. Ma OJ. Abdominal trauma. In: Cline DM, Ma OJ, Tintinalli JE. *Emergency Medicine: A Comprehensive Study Guide. Companion Handbook*. 5th ed. New York: McGraw-Hill; 2000:855–859.

97 Trauma, chest

Francis Lee • Shirley Ooi

CAVEATS

- Management of chest trauma follows standard ATLS protocol:
  1. Securing the ABCs is the priority.
  2. Give immediate management for detected lesions.
  3. Early involvement of the hospital trauma team according to institutional practice is important.
- During primary survey, the clinician should detect the following potentially **life-threatening** but salvageable conditions:
  1. Airway obstruction (eg due to laryngeal injury or posterior/fracture dislocation of sternoclavicular joint)
  2. Tension pneumothorax (sucking chest wound)
  3. Open pneumothorax
  4. Flail chest
  5. Massive haemothorax
  6. Pericardial tamponade

> ☛ **Special Tips for GPs**
>
> - Always consider the diagnosis of **tension pneumothorax** in a patient with signs of simple pneumothorax, haemodynamic instability, severe respiratory distress and neck vein distension.
> - Immediately perform needle thoracostomy, preferably with a large bore 14/16G IV venula at the 2nd intercostal space, midclavicular line.
> - A delay in performing this procedure will cause the patient to die! A wrong diagnosis will at most cause patient to have chest tube insertion but will not kill a patient!
> - In a patient with **open pneumothorax**, cover the wound with any sterile dressing taped only on 3 sides leaving 1 side free so as to act as a flutter-valve effect. Do not tape on all sides as it may create a tension pneumothorax!
> - Splinting a **flail chest** segment is controversial. However, in the process of transfer, it may be considered for pain relief.

INITIAL MANAGEMENT

- Transfer patient to critical care or resuscitation area of the ED.

- Activate in-house Trauma Team according to institutional protocol.
- Assess patient according to ATLS protocol.
- Consider intubating the patient using RSI technique for these situations:
  1. Airway is compromised.
  2. Inadequate ventilation.
  3. SpO_2 could not be maintained above 94% despite using non-rebreathing mask.

Note: If possible, pericardiocentesis should be done before intubation as excessive ventilatory pressures reducing venous return may cause cardiac arrest.

- Establish large bore (14G/16G) IV lines in both cubital fossae. Initial resuscitation fluid of choice is a crystalloid (Hartmann's or normal saline)
- Obtain blood for investigations:
  1. GXM for 6 units of whole blood
  2. FBC, urea/electrolytes/creatinine, and ABG

Indications for chest tube insertion after a trauma

- Pneumothorax, haemothorax, or open chest wound.
- Rib fractures requiring positive pressure ventilation.
- Selected patients with suspected severe lung injury, especially those being transferred by air or ground vehicle.
- Patients undergoing general anaesthesia for treatment of other injuries (eg cranial or extremity), who are suspected of significant lung injury.

Indications for ED thoracotomy in trauma setting

- Blood loss in ED not responsive to rapid crystalloid infusion.
- Witnessed arrest or acute deterioration.
- Penetrating trauma with vital signs or signs of life (pupils respond to light, any spontaneous respirations, any movement to pain or non-agonal cardiac rhythm) in field or ED.
- Penetrating thoracic wounds even without signs of life in field or ED (best with short duration of CPR).

ED thoracotomy not recommended

- Penetrating non-thoracic trauma without vital signs of life in the field.
- Blunt trauma without vital signs or signs of life in the ED.

DIAGNOSIS OF THREE POTENTIALLY LIFE-THREATENING CONDITIONS

- Evidence of chest trauma and hypotension. Consider three treatable causes:
  1. Massive haemothorax

2. Tension pneumothorax
3. Pericardial tamponade

- It is vital to pick up these conditions and manage them within minutes as they can kill in minutes! There is no time for investigations.

TREATMENT FOR SPECIFIC CHEST CONDITIONS

Tension pneumothorax

- **Key diagnostic features**: signs of chest trauma, signs of pneumothorax, hypotension, severe respiratory distress and neck vein distension.
- Immediate **therapy**:
  1. Perform needle thoracotomy: 14G needle, 2nd intercostal space in the midclavicular line.
  2. Followed by tube thoracotomy at 5th intercostal space, between anterior and midaxillary line.
- Key points:
  1. The diagnosis is a **clinical** one and treatment decisions are based on high index of suspicion.
  2. Performing a CXR to confirm diagnosis causes delay and perhaps death.

Note: A simple traumatic pneumothorax should not be ignored as it can progress to a tension pneumothorax.

Open pneumothorax

- **Pathophysiology**: large chest wall defect with equilibration of intrathoracic and atmospheric pressure, producing a 'sucking chest wound'.
- **Management**:
  1. Provide adequate oxygenation and ventilation.
  2. Cover defect with a sterile dressing, taped on 3 sides to produce a 'flutter-valve' effect.
  3. **Do not tape all sides** as this may create a tension pneumothorax.
  4. Then insert chest tube.

Note: Chest tubes should not be inserted through penetrating wounds because they are apt to follow the missile tract into the lung or diaphragm and damage those organs or restart massive bleeding.

Flail chest

- **Definition**: occurs when 2 or more ribs are fractured at two points.
- **Diagnosis** is based on the following features:
  1. Paradoxical movement of chest wall segment (this itself does not cause hypoxia)
  2. Respiratory distress
  3. External evidence of chest trauma
  4. Pain on respiratory effort

Note: The main cause of hypoxaemia in flail chest is due to the underlying pulmonary contusion although pain with restricted chest wall movement and underlying lung injury contribute to patient's hypoxia.

- **Management**:
  1. Ensure adequate oxygenation.
  2. Ensure adequate ventilation.

Note: Patients with isolated flail chest injuries can often be managed without ventilatory support, especially if the chest pain can be adequately relieved.

  3. Provide judicious fluid therapy.

Note: Fluid overloading should be prevented or rapidly corrected in flail chest patients with pulmonary contusion or adult respiratory distress syndrome.

  4. Adequate pain relief administered IV.

- **Indications for early mechanical ventilation in flail chest**:
  1. Shock
  2. ≥3 associated injuries
  3. Severe head injury
  4. Previous pulmonary disease
  5. Fracture of ≥8 ribs
  6. Age >65 years

Note: When a patient requires ventilatory support, it is much safer to apply it 'prophylactically' before actual ventilatory failure develops.

- **Controversial treatment**: splinting the flail segment may worsen ventilation.

Massive haemothorax

- **Defined** as >1,500 ml of blood lost into the chest cavity at initial output.
- Basic steps in **management** include:
  1. Ensure adequate oxygenation (administer 100% oxygen).
  2. Establish 2 large bore IV access and fluid resuscitation.
  3. Blood transfusion and correction of coagulopathy.
  4. Tube thoracocentesis.
  5. Beware of sudden cessation of blood drainage: check for blocked tube.
- **Indications for thoracotomy** (urgent cardiothoracic consult):
  1. Initial blood drainage >1,500 ml.
  2. Ongoing drainage of >500 ml/h for the first hour, 300 ml/h for 2 consecutive hours or 200 ml/h for 3 consecutive hours.
  3. Persistent transfusion requirements.
  4. Large retained pneumothorax especially if associated with continued bleeding.
  5. Continued haemodynamic instability.
  6. Suspicion of oesophageal, cardiac, great vessel or major bronchial injuries.

Note: Think of possible damage to great vessels, hilar structures and heart in penetrating anterior chest wounds medial to nipple line and posterior chest wounds medial to scapula.

Cardiac tamponade

- Diagnosis requires a high index of suspicion. Certain combinations of features point towards this possibility:
  1. Chest trauma and hypotension
  2. Beck's triad (hypotension, muffled heart sounds, distended neck veins)

Note: Beck's triad is seen in only 50% of cases. Neck veins in cardiac tamponade may not be distended until coexistent hypovolaemia is at least partially corrected; a muffled heart sound is the least reliable sign in Beck's triad.

  3. Chest trauma and pulseless electrical activity
  4. Kussmaul's signs (increased neck distension during inspiration and pulsus paradoxus)

- Other supporting evidence that may be present include:
  1. Enlarged cardiac shadow in CXR (rare) or
  2. Small ECG voltages (uncommon) or
  3. Pericardial fluid demonstrated on 2D Echo or FAST, which is definitive
- **Management**:
  1. Ensure adequate oxygenation of patient (give 100% O_2).
  2. Establish large bore IV lines.
  3. Give IV fluid bolus 500 ml stat.
  4. Treat pericardial tamponade by pericardiocentesis.
     a. ECG guided (with ECG lead attached to pericardiocentesis needle)
     b. 2D Echo guided. This can be diagnostic or therapeutic

Note: Aggressive fluid resuscitation helps maintain cardiac output and buys time for patient. **Never** probe blindly with a needle as risk of iatrogenic cardiac injury is high.

Pulmonary contusion

- This refers to an injury resulting in disruption of pulmonary tissue architecture, disruption of alveolar membrane with bleeding and oedema into the alveolar spaces.
- Features of pulmonary contusion usually take time to develop.
- **Causes** include:
  1. Blunt and penetrating trauma
  2. Blast injuries
  3. Compressive injuries
- Possible **clinical signs** are:
  1. Respiratory distress
  2. Decreased breath sounds
  3. Crepitations in the affected lung field
  4. Hypoxaemia
- **Management**:
  1. Administer supplemental oxygen.
  2. Provide ventilatory support, if necessary.
  3. Provide judicious fluid therapy.

Tracheobronchial injuries

- Tracheobronchial injuries are difficult to pick up in a trauma patient. Diagnosis requires a high index of suspicion.
- The possible **aetiology**:
  1. Penetrating injuries
  2. Acceleration-deceleration force
  3. Blast injuries
- **Clinical signs** include:
  1. Haemoptysis
  2. Subcutaneous emphysema
  3. Tension pneumothorax
  4. Persistent pneumothorax despite treatment
- **Management**:
  1. Administer supplemental oxygen.
  2. Provide ventilatory support.
  3. Patient may require more than one chest tube.
  4. Early cardiothoracic consultation.

Blunt cardiac injury (BCI)/myocardial contusion

- **Special considerations**:
  1. Clinically, there are few reliable signs and symptoms that are specific to BCI.
  2. The presence of a sternal fracture does not predict the presence of BCI.
  3. Neither CK-MB analysis nor bedside cardiac troponin T are useful in predicting which patients have or will have complications related to BCI.
  4. An abnormal ECG (ST and T waves changes) is sensitive for BCI.
- **Management**:
  1. Triage patient to critical care area.
  2. Secure ABC, give oxygen.
  3. Perform an ECG.
- **Management decisions**:
  1. If **ECG is normal**, the risk of patient having a BCI that requires treatment, ie a complication, is insignificant, and the **patient may be discharged** (assuming there is no **other** reason to admit).
  2. If **ECG is abnormal** (dysrhythmia, ST segment changes, ischaemic changes, AV block, unexplained sinus tachycardia), the **patient should be admitted** for continuous cardiac monitoring.
  3. If the patient is **haemodynamically unstable**, an **echocardiogram** should be performed.

Note: Nuclear medicine studies add little when compared to Echo and are therefore not useful if an Echo has been performed.

Traumatic aortic disruption

- Most patients with traumatic aortic disruption die on site.
- Those who survive to reach hospital probably have a contained haematoma and will potentially deteriorate rapidly.
- **Telltale signs**:
  1. Blunt or penetrating injuries to the chest or acceleration/deceleration injury
  2. Hypotension despite lack of external sources of bleeding
  3. Massive haemothorax
  4. Weaker or absent peripheral pulses
  5. Principal chest x-ray features
     a. Widened mediastinum
     b. Left-sided pleural effusion
     c. Blunting of left aortic knuckle
- **Management**:
  1. Assess according to ATLS protocol
  2. CT thorax if patient is fit enough for transport
  3. GXM for at least 6 units of whole blood: call Cardiothoracic and General Surgery stat

Rib fractures

- Management is influenced by the level and number of rib involved as well as underlying visceral injuries.

Note: Many clinically significant rib fractures cannot be visualized on CXR. The main purpose of CXR in patients with possible rib fractures is to eliminate associated haemothorax, pneumothorax, lung contusion, and other organ injury.

- **Upper rib (1–3) fractures and scapular fractures**:
  1. Application of large force
  2. Increased trauma risk to head and neck, spinal cord, lungs, great vessels
  3. Mortality up to 35%
- **Middle rib (4–9) fractures**:
  1. Most common: significance increases if multiple. Simple rib fractures without complications can be managed on an outpatient basis.
  2. **Admit** for observation if patient:
     a. Is dyspnoeic
     b. Has pain unrelieved
     c. Is elderly
     d. Has poor preexisting lung function
- **Lower rib (10–12) fractures**: associated with risks of hepatic and splenic injuries.

Note: Prophylactic chest tube insertion should be done for all trauma patients who are to be intubated in the presence of rib fractures. Associated injuries often missed include cardiac contusion, diaphragmatic rupture and oesophageal injuries.

Traumatic diaphragmatic rupture

- **Indicators** of a possible diaphragmatic rupture:
  1. Persistent or progressive respiratory distress
  2. Bowel sounds in the chest
  3. **Chest x-ray** features
     a. Vague and indistinct diaphragmatic shadow
     b. Herniation of abdominal organs into the chest cavity
     c. Displacement of NG tube into chest cavity more commonly on the left
- Diagnosis requires a high index of suspicion.
- All patients should be referred to General Surgery for laparotomy.

Crush injuries to the chest

- **Prognosis** depends on duration of application of the crushing force:
  1. <5 min (transient force applied and prognosis is good)
  2. >5 min (poor prognosis)
- Crush injury to the chest produces **traumatic asphyxia**
  1. Plethora of upper body
  2. Petechiae of upper body
  3. Cerebral oedema
- **Management**:
  1. Ensure oxygenation.
  2. Provide ventilation.
  3. Treat associated injuries.
  4. Admit for observation.

Penetrating injury to the chest

- Important points to **note**:
  1. Do not remove foreign object from wound.
  2. For penetrating injury below the nipple line, always consider intraabdominal injuries.

Subcutaneous emphysema

- **Aetiology**:
  1. Airway injuries
  2. Lung and pleural injuries
  3. Oesophageal or pharnygeal injuries
  4. Blast injuries
- **Signs**:
  1. Crepitus
  2. Swelling of face, neck or tissues involved
- **Management**: subcutaneous emphysema rarely requires treatment. The underlying cause should be managed instead. Assume patients with

subcutaneous emphysema have underlying pneumothorax even not visible on CXR. Hence, patients with subcutaneous emphysema after chest trauma should have a chest tube inserted before being placed on a ventilator.

Oesophageal trauma

- **Indications** of a possible oesophageal trauma:
  1. Subcutaneous emphysema
  2. Mediastinal air in the absence of a pneumothorax
  3. Retropharyngeal air on lateral neck x-ray
  4. Left-sided pleural effusion: drainage tested positive for amylase
  5. Left pneumo or haemothorax without a rib fracture
  6. Severe blow to the lower sternum or epigastrium and patient is in pain or shock out of proportion to the apparent injury
  7. Particulate water in the chest tube after the blood begins to clear
- Patient should be referred to the General Surgeon for further management.

Laryngeal trauma

- Although it is a rare injury, it can present with acute airway obstruction.
- **Diagnosis** is triad of:
  1. Hoarseness
  2. Subcutaneous emphysema
  3. Palpable fracture
- **Management**:
  1. If the patient's airway is totally obstructed or if the patient is in severe respiratory distress, attempt intubation.
  2. If intubation is unsuccessful, an emergency tracheostomy is indicated.
  3. Surgical cricothyroidotomy, although not preferred for this situation, may be life saving if emergency tracheostomy fails.
  4. Contact ENT specialist and anaesthetists early.

References/further reading

1. Robertson C, Redmond AD. *The Management of Major Trauma*. 2nd ed. Oxford: Oxford University Press; 1994.
2. Skinner D, ed. *ABC of Major Trauma*. 2nd ed. London: BMJ Books; 1996.
3. Eastern Association for the Surgery of Trauma (EAST) Practice Parameter Workgroup for Screening of Blunt Cardiac Injury. www.east.org. 1998.
4. Thoracic Trauma. In: Committee on Trauma of the American College of Surgeons. *Advanced Trauma Life Support for Doctors Student Course Manual*. 6th ed. Chicago: American College of Surgeons; 1997:125–141.
5. Wilson RF, Steiger Z. Thoracic trauma chest wall and lung. In: Wilson RF, Walt AJ, eds. *Management of Trauma: Pitfalls and Practice*. 2nd ed. Baltimore: Williams & Wilkins; 1996:314–342.
6. Wilson RF, Stephenson LW. Thoracic Trauma: Heart. In: Wilson RF, Walt AJ, eds. *Management of Trauma: Pitfalls and Practice*. 2nd ed. Baltimore: Williams & Wilkins; 1996:343–360.

98 Trauma and infections, hand

Peng Li Lee

☛ **Special Tips for GPs**

- Preserve an amputated part by wrapping it in a clean piece of gauze soaked with moist saline, and placing the wrapped part in a clean and dry container. Put the container on ice. **Do not** place the amputated part directly on ice.

ACUTE NAIL BED INJURIES

- **Classifications**:
  1. Simple laceration of nail bed and subungual haematoma
  2. Crushing laceration of nail bed
  3. Avulsion laceration of nail bed
  4. Lacerations with associated fractures
  5. Lacerations with loss of skin and pulp
  6. Fingertip amputations
- Nail bed injuries generally do well after primary repair and less so with reconstruction, so the initial repair is vital. Hence with the exception of (1), all other nail bed injuries should be admitted for repair in the OT where finer instruments and loupe magnification are available.
- **X-ray** is required for most fingertip and nail bed injuries. The presence of a distal phalanx fracture adds 2 considerations to the management:
  1. Need for reduction: an unstable displaced fracture may require K-wire fixation.
  2. Risk of infection with open fracture: cover with broad spectrum antibiotics.

SUBUNGUAL HAEMATOMA

- **Classification**: percentage of area beneath the nail in which blood is visualized.
- **Treatment**: trephine with a red hot tip of an unfolded paper clip (Figure 1):
  1. Digital block is not required except for the most nervous patient. The nail plate (which is itself insensate) will burn and evaporate as the heated tip penetrates. The heated paper clip tip is cooled instantly upon encounter with the flush of blood and further penetration and injury to the nail bed is rare. Do not apply pressure but allow the heat to penetrate the nail plate as this avoids ramming the paper clip into the nail bed (risk of osteomyelitis).

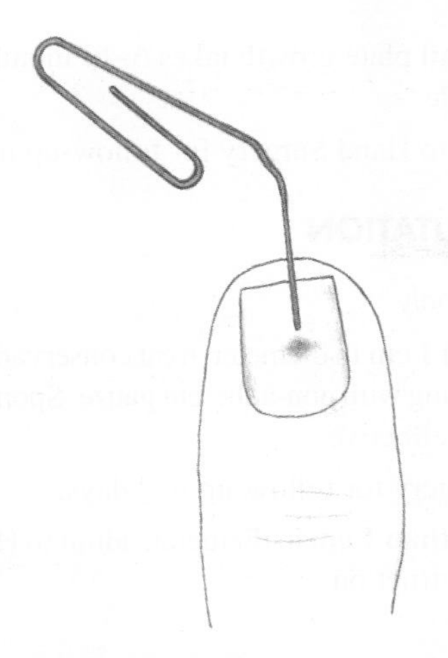

Figure 1: Trephine of subungual haematoma with the red hot tip of an unfolded paper clip

2. Prepare the injured finger with povidone-iodine (not alcohol as it is flammable).
3. Place two holes side by side to facilitate drainage. The haematoma is evacuated with gentle massage followed by soaking in the povidone-iodine.

- **Follow-up** with antibiotic ointment, dressing and protective splint.
- For subungual haematoma greater than **50%**, hand literature supports nail removal, exploration and suturing of nail bed.

SIMPLE LACERATION OF NAIL BED

- **Principles of treatment**: minimal debridement, preservation of as much tissue as possible and splinting with nail plate.

1. Digital block with 1% lignocaine (allow 10 min for full effect).
2. Place a rubber band or penrose tourniquet at the base of the finger.
3. Finger tip is cleansed and draped.
4. The nail plate should be gently elevated with blunt forceps and gently removed with a haemostat using continual pressure.
5. Lacerations are repaired using 6/0 plain catgut or dexon suture.
6. The nail plate is irrigated with normal saline and used as a splint over the repaired nail bed. A non-absorbable suture, eg Prolene, is placed through the nail plate and then through an area just proximal to the nail sulcus as an anchor (sutures to be removed in 3 weeks).
7. If the nail plate is not available, the foil from the suture package may be used to keep the nail fold open.

- Advise patients: nail plate growth takes 6–12 months and nail deformity may be unavoidable.
- **Disposition**: refer to Hand Surgery for follow-up in 2–3 days.

DIGITAL TIP AMPUTATION

With skin/pulp loss only

- For defect **less than 1 cm** in diameter, treat conservatively, with meticulous cleansing and dressing with non-adherent gauze. Spontaneous epithelization is simple and cost effective.
- Refer to Hand Surgery for follow-up in 2 days.
- For defect **greater than 1 cm** in diameter, admit to Hand Surgery for skin-graft or flap reconstruction.

With bone exposed

- Admit to Hand Surgery.
- Preserve the amputated part, which may be used for replantation.
- Set up IV plug on uninjured hand.
- Give IV cefazolin 1 g if there is no contraindication. Take swab for culture before antibiotics (send specimen up with patient to ward for despatch).
- Administer tetanus prophylaxis as indicated.
- The amputated part must be wrapped in clean gauze soaked with moist saline, then placed in a clean and dry container and the container placed on ice. **Do not** place the amputated part itself directly on ice.
- X-ray the amputated part: 2 views (AP and lateral).

FLEXOR TENDON INJURIES

Flexor tendon injuries are frequently seen in ED. The most common mechanism is laceration. The role of the ED physician is to make an accurate diagnosis through a thorough examination and this requires a revision and understanding of the function of the flexor tendons. Beware of subtle signs associated with partial laceration which can result in subsequent long-term disability.

Testing the integrity of flexor digitorum superficialis (FDS) and flexor digitorum profundus (FDP)

- Testing FDS function (Figure 2a). With the adjacent fingers held in full extension (prohibiting FDP motion), efforts at finger flexion produce isolated FDS motion, as indicated by solitary flexion of the PIP joint.
- Testing FDP function (Figure 2b). Isolated DIP flexion can only be accomplished with an intact FDP musculotendinous unit.

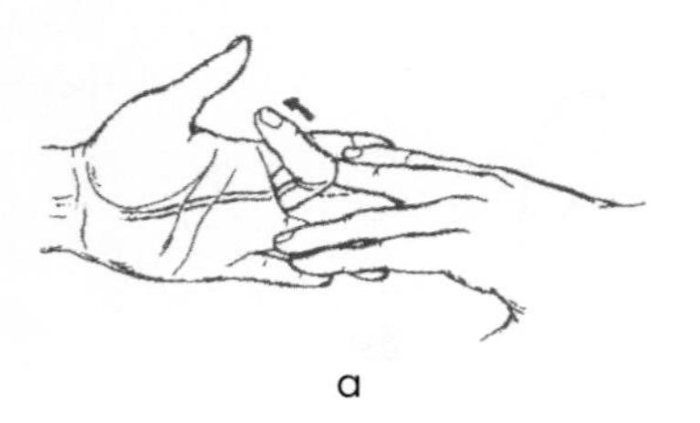
a

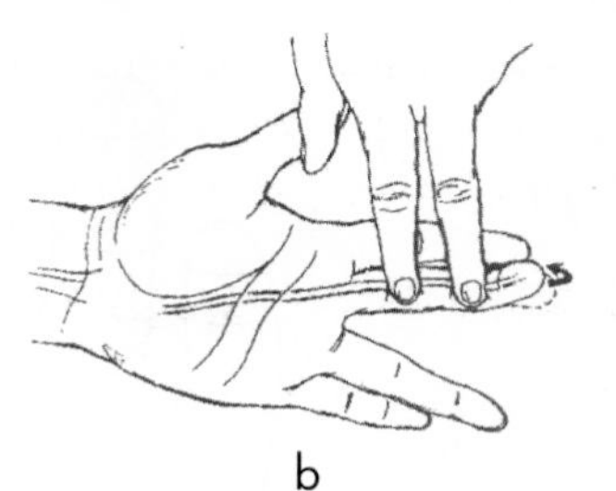
b

Figure 2: Testing the integrity of (a) flexor digitorum superficialis and (b) flexor digitorum profundus functions

Note: Viewing an intact tendon through a lacerated sheath does not mean that the tendon is uninjured. The tendon may have been in a different position when the injury occurred and at the time of examination, the lacerated part of the tendon has moved proximally or distally and out of view. Test and document the integrity of the accompanying digital nerves (use 2-point discrimination of an unfolded paper clip, approximately 5 mm apart).

Pertinent history

- Mechanism of injury: laceration and closed/blunt trauma
- Occupation
- Dominant hand

X-ray

- X-ray the digit for the following reasons:
- Exclude FB in lacerated wound.
- Exclude the avulsion of FDP insertion at the base of the distal phalanx in closed rupture (lateral film).

Implications of zoning

- Timing of repair
  1. Primary repair (within 24 hours) is recommended. If this is delayed to 3 weeks, repair may require a tendon graft.
  2. Zones III, IV and V (Figure 3) mandate urgent surgical repair because of frequent accompanying injuries to adjacent structures.
- Outcome
  1. Zone II historically classified as 'no-man's land' because of the difficulty in surgical approach and the poorer outcome when 2 repaired tendons (FDS and FDP) are expected to glide within a fibrous sheath.
  2. Zone III generally has a favourable outcome after the primary repair.

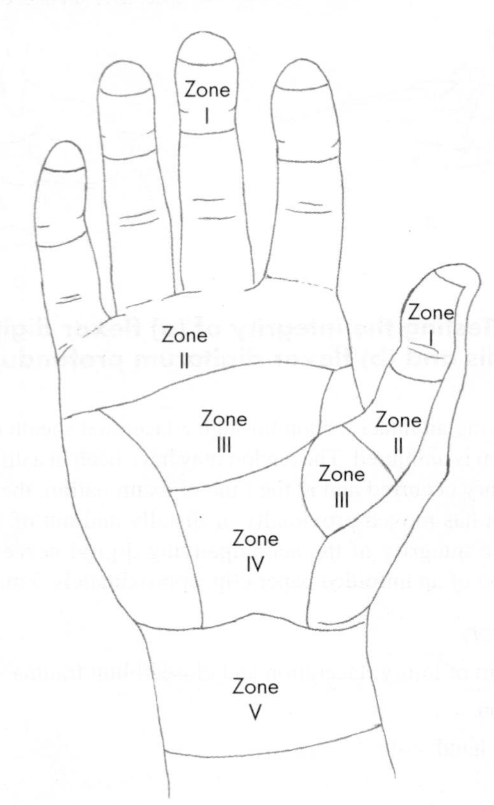

Figure 3: Classification of flexor tendon zones (by Verdan)

Management of flexor tendon injury at ED

- Admit to Hand Surgery for primary repair.
- Tetanus toxoid according to regime.

PARTIAL FLEXOR TENDON LACERATION

- **Diagnosis**: may be difficult.
- **Clue**: more pain on active movement than anticipated.
- **Significance**
  1. delayed rupture
  2. painful and restricting tenosynovitis
- All partial lacerations of tendon will require exploration. Injury involving less than 25% can be treated by trimming the lacerated ends. A laceration of 50% or more requires formal repair.
- **Management in ED**: admit for exploration.

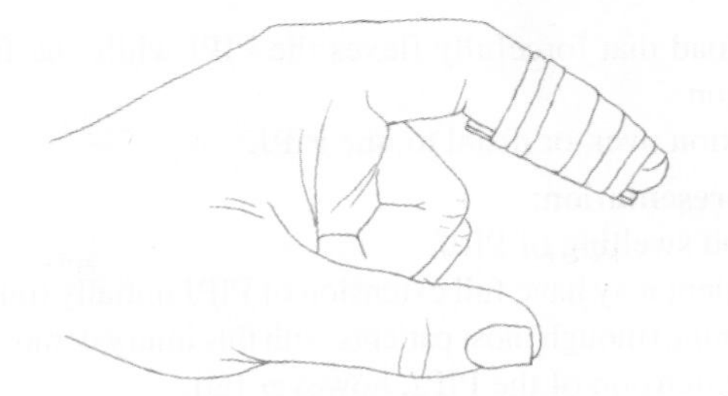

Figure 4: A mallet finger splint

EXTENSOR TENDON INJURY

Mallet finger

- Disruption of the insertion of extensor tendon to terminal phalanx.
- **Mechanism of injury**:
  1. Blunt trauma via acute flexion of the DIPJ by an axial load to the terminal phalanx, eg catching a ball
  2. Laceration, which is less common.
- **Clinical presentation**:
  1. Pain, swelling and tenderness of DIPJ
  2. Inability to extend the DIPJ
  3. Volar subluxation of DIPJ
- **X-ray digit**: look for fracture at the base of distal phalanx.
- **Management** depends on the type of injury
  1. Closed injury without fracture: mallet splint (Figure 4) for 6 weeks. Follow up with Hand Surgery in 5 days.
  2. Tendon avulsion with small bone fragment (<33%): mallet splint. Follow up with Hand Surgery in 5 days.
  3. Tendon avulsion with large bone fragment: admit for surgical repair.
  4. Open injury: admit for surgical repair.

Mallet splint

- Apply volar splint to distal phalanx, keeping the DIPJ in slight hyper-extension while allowing the PIPJ and MCPJ free movement.

BOUTONNIERE DEFORMITY

- Disruption of the central slip of extensor tendon over the PIPJ. The lateral bands, which normally lie dorsal to the axis of rotation and therefore extend the joint, now fall volar to this axis and become paradoxical flexors of the PIPJ.
- **Mechanism of injury**:
  1. Direct blow to the dorsum of PIPJ.

2. Axial load that forcefully flexes the PIPJ while the finger is held in extension.
3. Laceration over, or distal to, the PIPJ.

- **Clinical presentation**:
  1. Pain and swelling of PIPJ.
  2. The patient may have full extension of PIPJ initially (due to lateral slips functioning) though most patients with this injury demonstrate weakness in the extension of the PIPJ, however full.
  3. Boutonniere deformity is often not evident after acute injury but develops in 10–14 days.
  4. Most have associated dislocation that had been reduced prior to arrival in the ED; demonstration of instability is limited by pain.
- **X-ray digit**: typically normal but if the lateral view demonstrates an avulsion fracture of the dorsal base of the middle phalanx, the diagnosis is confirmed.
- **Diagnosis**: requires high index of suspicion for any injury at the PIPJ. Diagnosis is often not apparent at once due to the acute swelling.
- **Management** depends on the type of injury:
  1. Closed injuries: boutonniere splint. Follow up with Hand Surgery in 5 days.
  2. Open injuries: admit for primary repair.

Boutonniere splint

- Apply volar splint over PIPJ, keeping it in full extension, and leaving DIPJ and MCPJ free (Figure 5).

DISRUPTION TO EXTENSORS OVER MCPJ

- This is usually an open injury.
- Important to **exclude** a human tooth bite/punch to teeth (ask specifically as patients often deny this part of history) because
  1. High risk of septic arthritis if a tooth wound is missed.

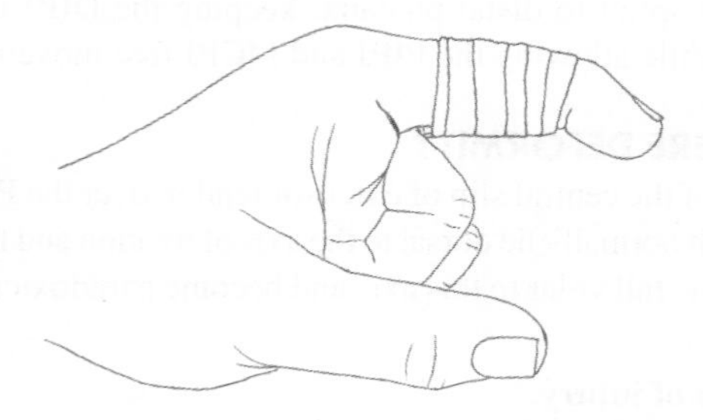

Figure 5: A boutonniere splint

2. Aggressive wound debridement and antibiotics are required.
3. Secondary closure considered versus primary closure.

- **Findings**: extension of MCPJ may still be present because of the sagittal bands at the side of the tendons
- **X-ray** of MCPJ to look for
  1. FB, eg tooth fragment.
  2. Radiolucency within MCPJ
  3. Injury to metacarpal head.
- **Admit** for surgical repair.
- **Start** IV antibiotics and give tetanus prophylaxis as indicated.

ISOLATED THERMAL BURNS OF HAND

Minor burns

- First- and second-degree (superficial and superficial partial thickness)
- Tetanus prophylaxis
- Provide analgesia
- Local therapy:
  1. TG dressing with or without silver sulphadiazine cream (contraindicated in pregnancy and sulfa allergy).
  2. Hand dressed within a clean polythene bag to encourage mobilization.
  3. Elevate hand in arm-sling to reduce swelling.
- Refer to Hand Surgery for follow-up in 1–2 weeks.

Deep dermal burns

- Third- and fourth-degree (deep partial and full thickness)
- Tetanus prophylaxis.
- Circumferential full thickness injury of the limb may induce compression injury distally: important to check neurovascular status. Urgent escharotomy may be required.
- **Disposition**: admit to Hand Surgery for wound care, possibly skin grafting.

Note: (1) Prophylactic systemic antibiotics are not routinely recommended, (2) partial thickness can be differentiated from full thickness injury by the loss of pin prick sensation, and (3) consider non-accidental injury in paediatric age group.

CHEMICAL BURNS OF THE HAND

- The depth of burns is directly related to the length of contact with the offending agent.
- **Document**: chemical involved, length of exposure and treatment initiated on-site, eg washing/antidote.

- **Management**:
  1. Chemical powders should be brushed off.
  2. Irrigate with copious amount of saline/water.
  3. Elevate hand.
- **Hydrofluoric acid burn: a hand emergency!** Refer to *Burns, Minor* for further details.
  1. Very painful.
  2. Causes deep damage until fluoride ion is neutralized with Ca^{2+}.
  3. For superficial injury, topical application with calcium gluconate mixed with sterile KY gel.
  4. For deeper or extensive injury, consider subcutaneous injection of 10% calcium gluconate into the base and around the burn using a 27G needle. Try to avoid performing a digital block as an analgesic manoeuvre since this will certainly remove the pain but will also remove the one parameter to determine the efficacy of therapy with calcium gluconate, ie pain.

ELECTRICAL BURNS OF THE HAND

- **2 elements** to consider:
  1. Flash burn, which causes deep dermal burns.
  2. Passage of current through the body. Possible complications are cardiac dysrhythmias and myoglobinuria with resultant ARF.
- **History**: differentiate low-voltage domestic supply (240 V 50 MHz) from high voltage industrial supply.
- **Examination**:
  1. Search for entrance and exit sites.
  2. May have thermal burns secondary to ignition of clothing.
  3. Assess the limb circulation and the neurovascular status.
- **Management at ED**:
  1. 12-lead ECG and cardiac monitoring for arrhythmia.
  2. Check urea/electrolytes/creatinine, creatine kinase, LDH.
  3. X-ray of the suspected joint dislocation from catatonic contractions of muscles secondary to high electrical voltage.
  4. Treat dermal burns as outlined above.
- **Disposition:** Admit to General Medicine for cardiac monitoring if dysrhythmia or cardiovascular collapse occurs.

HAND INFECTIONS

Paronychia

- Nail fold abscess.
- **Presents with** subungual tissue swelling and redness with or without frank pus.
- Screen for DM.

- **Treatment**:
  1. Early: oral antibiotics, eg cloxacillin (versus *S. aureus*) and warm soaks daily.
  2. Late: oral antibiotics and I&D of abscess under digital block.
- **Drainage methods**: (refer to Figures 6 and 7)
  1. Slide blade into nail sulcus near the point of maximal tenderness.
  2. Remove a longitudinal section of nail if subungual abscess is present.
- **Disposition:** refer to Hand Surgery for follow-up on the next working day for dressing.

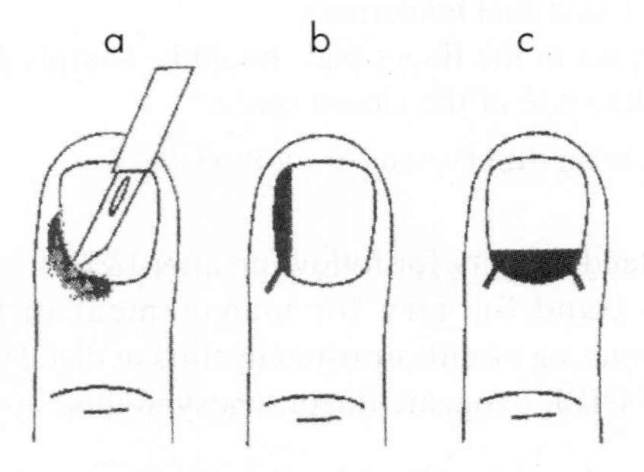

Figure 6: Drainage of paronychia

(a) The eponychial fold is elevated from the nail for a simple paronychium, (b) the lateral nail is removed if pus tracks under it. A small eponychial incision may be necessary, and (c) the proximal nail is removed if pus tracks under it. Two incisions will be needed to remove it.

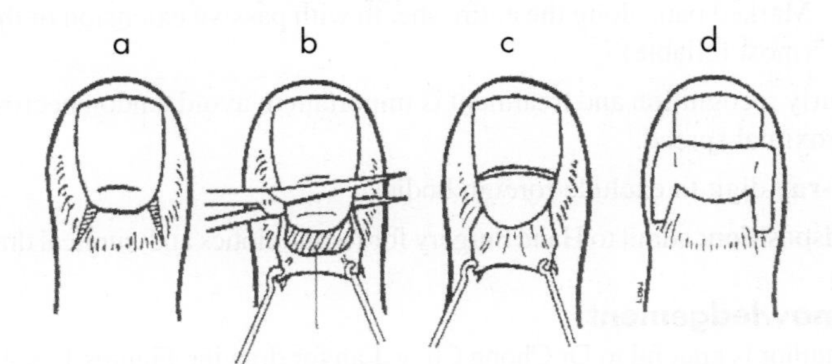

Figure 7: Treatment of a proximal subungual abscess

(a) Expose the edge of the proximal nail plate, (b) elevate and incise the proximal one-third of the plate and clean the nail bed, (c) leave the distal two-thirds to act as a physiologic dressing. Care should be taken not to disrupt the nail matrix, and (d) use a Bismuth impregnated gauze as a wick for approximately 48 hours.

Felon

- Infection of the distal pulp space of a digit.
- Presents with swelling, pain and redness of the finger tip.
- **X-ray**: exclude FB and bony involvement.
- **Treatment**: incision and drainage under digital block.
- **Drainage methods**
  1. High lateral incision (avoid the neurovascular bundle): begin 5 mm distal to skin crease of DIPJ and extend to the end of the nail plate.
  2. Longitudinal palmar incision; the choice of incision is based on finding the point of maximal tenderness.
  3. Fibrous septae in the finger pad should be sharply incised to provide adequate drainage of the closed space.
- **Antibiotics**: cloxacillin (versus *S. aureus*).
- **Disposition**
  1. Refer to Hand Surgery for follow-up after I&D.
  2. Admit to Hand Surgery for management in the presence of complications, eg osteitis **or** osteomyelitis of distal phalanx, pyogenic arthritis of DIPJ, pyogenic flexor tenosynovitis.

Suppurative flexor tenosynovitis

- Infection in the flexor tendon sheath that usually follows a penetrating injury.
- **Clinical features**: Kanavel's 4 cardinal signs
  1. Uniform swelling of the digit
  2. Semiflexed resting position of digit
  3. Tenderness along the entire course of sheath
  4. Marked pain along the entire sheath with passive extension of the digit (most reliable)
- Early recognition and treatment is important to avoid tendon necrosis and proximal spread.
- **X-ray** digit to exclude foreign bodies.
- **Disposition:** admit to Hand Surgery for IV antibiotics and surgical drainage.

Acknowledgement

The author is grateful to Dr Chong Chew Lan for drawing Figures 1, 3, 4 and 5.

References/further reading

1. Uehara DT, ed. The hand in emergency medicine. *Emerg Med Clin N Am*. 1993;11(3):758.
2. Della-Giustina DA, Coppola M, eds. Orthopedic emergencies Part I. *Emerg Med Clin N Am*. 1999;17(14):817.
3. Martin DS, Collins ED. *Manual of Acute Hand Injuries*. St Louis: Mosby; 1998.
4. American Society for Surgery of the Hand. *The Hand: Primary Care of Common Problems*. New York: Churchill Livingston; 1990.

99 Trauma, head

Shirley Ooi

CAVEATS

- Head injury is the leading cause of mortality and morbidity after trauma.
- Although there is usually no specific treatment for primary brain injury, some **secondary brain injury** is **preventable or treatable**.

Note: **Primary brain injury** is the damage produced directly by the original mechanical forces. **Secondary brain injury** occurs after the initial trauma.

- **Hypoxaemia** and **hypotension** are the most frequent systemic insults causing **secondary brain injury**.
- **Do not** assume that **altered mental state** in a head-injured patient is due to alcohol intoxication. It may be caused by hypoglycaemia, hypercarbia, hypotension or other concomitant drug intoxication.
- **Skull fractures** greatly increase the likelihood of underlying brain injury (Table 1).
- A **lucid interval** should warrant special efforts to rule out an acute **extradural haematoma**.
- All patients with major trauma should be assumed to have a head injury and cervical spine fracture until proven otherwise.
- One cannot rely on neurologic assessments until adequate perfusion and oxygenation have been obtained.
- Proper observation of a head-injured patient means repeated careful neurological examination.
- **Do not** attribute **hypotension** in a trauma patient to be due solely to head injury. Other sources of blood loss should be looked into.
- Hypertension and bradycardia (**Cushing's reflex**) signify a rising intracranial pressure.
- Unilateral pupillary dilation or sluggish response to light indicates a developing mass on the side of pupillary dilation. These signs develop in the late stages of rising intracranial pressure.

Table 1: Risk of intracranial haematoma after head injury

		Risk of intracranial haematoma
Orientated	No skull fracture	1 in 6,000
Disorientated	No skull fracture	1 in 120
Orientated	Skull fracture	1 in 30
Disorientated	Skull fracture	1 in 4

- A new focal motor deficit is an important sign that the patient needs immediate, aggressive care.
- **Never sedate the restless head-injured patient** without ordering a head CT scan because it may herald the development of an intracranial haematoma and should be investigated appropriately.

> ☛ **Special Tips for GPs**
> - **Not all** patients with **mild head injury** or **scalp lacerations** need to have **skull x-rays** taken. Refer to criteria given.
> - There must be a reliable caregiver at home before any patient with head injury can be discharged. Remember to follow up with proper discharge instructions.

MANAGEMENT

Skull x-rays

- **Indications for skull x-rays** (SXR): Controversy has surrounded the question of who should have skull x-rays. In most centres, the criteria for ordering skull x-rays are also those for admission regardless of the skull x-ray findings. Hence, **SXRs in general should not be ordered** for those with **mild head injury who are to be admitted for observation** with the **exception** of the following situations:
  1. Large boggy scalp haematoma preventing the accurate palpation of an underlying depressed skull fracture (in which case a head CT scan should be ordered).
  2. Suspected radioopaque foreign body in scalp lacerations (eg cut by broken glass).

  Moreover, about 50% of all intracranial abnormalities resulting from head trauma do not have an associated skull fracture. Hence, the presence of a skull fracture should raise the suspicion of an intracranial lesion, but the absence of a skull fracture does not diminish the need for a head CT scan.

Note: Simple scalp laceration is not a criterion for skull x-ray. The wound should be palpated before T&S to rule out the presence of fracture.

- **What to look for in skull x-rays**
  1. Linear or depressed skull fractures
  2. Midline position of calcified pineal gland (displacement of >3mm to one side suggests large intracranial haematoma present)
  3. Air-fluid levels in sinuses (including sphenoidal sinuses)

Note: A fluid level in sphenoidal sinus detected on a lateral SXR taken with a horizontal beam suggests **basal skull fracture**. **Base of skull fracture** is

not an indication for urgent head CT scan if the GCS is 15 but is an **indication for admission**. Recent studies have found **no evidence** for use of **prophylactic antibiotics** in **basal skull fractures.** This is because occult CSF leakage can continue over months and years and delayed meningitis can sometimes occur many years after the injury. Hence, there is no rational basis for an arbitrary one- or two-week course of antibiotics. Antibiotics should be given only if there is evidence of posttraumatic meningitis, usually due to *Strep pneumoniae.* This is almost universally sensitive to benzyl penicillin.

4. Aerocoele
5. Facial fractures
6. Foreign bodies
7. Diastasis (widening) of sutures

CT scan

- **Indications for emergent head CT scan after head injury**
  1. GCS ≤13 in the absence of alcohol intoxication or skull fracture
  2. GCS ≤14 in the presence of skull fracture
  3. Unilateral dilated pupil in the presence of altered mental state
  4. Depressed skull fracture
  5. Focal neurological deficit
  6. Head injury patient requiring ventilation
  7. Head injury patient requiring general anaesthetic for other forms of surgery

Note: Use of emergent head CT is somewhat controversial. According to ATLS guidelines, all patients even with mild head injury need to have CT scan. However, in hospitals practising a more conservative approach, ordering CT scans for all head-injured patients may not be cost effective and practical. Hence, skull x-rays are usually used as a form of screening tool although its cost effectiveness is also controversial and in general is not recommended.

Resuscitation

The **priorities** in resuscitation are according to ATLS principles, ie:

- Airway and cervical spine control
- Breathing

Note: Causes of **respiratory impairment** include (1) central causes such as drugs and brainstem injury, and (2) peripheral causes such as airway obstruction, aspiration of blood/vomit, chest trauma, adult respiratory distress syndrome and neurogenic pulmonary oedema.

- Circulation
  1. Blood investigations include FBC, urea/electrolytes/creatinine, coagulation profile, GXM ±serum ethanol level.

Note: A blood alcohol level <2 g/l makes it likely that altered consciousness is due to the head injury and not to alcohol consumption. However, a high alcohol level cannot be assumed to be the reason for altered consciousness in the injured patient.

2. Do a bedside glucose level in all head-injured patients with altered conscious level to exclude hypoglycaemia!

- Neurological assessment
- **Indications for intubation in head injury**
  1. Coma (GCS <8).
  2. Rapidly deteriorating GCS of ≥2.
  3. GCS ≤14 in the presence of unilateral dilated pupil.

Note: Although a dilated or fixed pupil in an injured patient is usually due to an intracranial haematoma and/or brain damage, it may also be caused by expanding eye trauma, direct injury to the third cranial nerve, various drugs, intracranial aneurysms, hypoxia, hypotension, seizures and expanding intracranial aneurysms.

4. Clinical respiratory distress, a rate >30/min or <10/min, or an abnormal ventilatory pattern or in general, hypoxaemia not correctable by 100% O_2 by non-rebreather mask.
5. Concomitant maxillofacial injuries.
6. Repeated convulsions.
7. Concurrent severe pulmonary oedema, cardiac or upper abdominal injury.

Note: Hyperventilation should be used in moderation to achieve a PCO_2 between 30–35 mm Hg if there are indications of raised intracranial pressure. In general, the PCO_2 level should be between 35–40 mm Hg. Check **ABG** 10–15 min after hyperventilation.

- **Indications for use of Mannitol in head injury**
  1. Comatose patient with initial normal reactive pupils but then develops pupillary dilation with or without hemiparesis.
  2. Bilateral dilated and non-reactive pupils that are not hypotensive.

     Dosage of Mannitol: 1 g/kg BW, ie [5 × BW(kg)] ml of 20% Mannitol as a rapid infusion over 5 min

     Precautions before use of Mannitol:

     a. Insert urinary catheter
     b. Ensure patient is not hypotensive
     c. Ensure patient does not have chronic renal failure

Note: Hyperventilation and IV Mannitol will buy a grace period of 2 hours at most and no time should be lost in arranging for definitive treatment.

Criteria for referral to neurosurgeon

This may differ according to institutional practice. They include:

- Head injury with deteriorating GCS
- Depressed skull fracture

- Pneumocranium
- Penetrating skull injuries
- Positive head CT scan findings

Criteria for admission of mild head injury

- Loss of consciousness >10 min
- Amnesia
- Posttraumatic seizure
- Clinical signs of base of skull fracture
- Moderate or severe headache or vomiting
- Alcohol intoxication
- Penetrating injury
- Skull fracture
- Significant associated injuries
- No reliable caregiver at home

Head injury instructions

Before discharge, patients should be advised to seek further medical advice in the event of:

- Severe headache
- Frequent vomiting
- Discharge of fluid from nose or ears
- Confusion or inappropriate drowsiness
- Fits

References/further reading

1. Michael DB, Wilson RF. Head injuries. In: Wilson FW, Alexander JW, eds. *Management of Trauma: Pitfalls and Practice*. 2nd ed. Baltimore: Williams &Wilkins; 1996:173–202.
2. Currie DG. *The Management of Head Injuries: A Practical Guide for the Emergency Room.* 2nd ed. Oxford: Oxford University Press, 2000.
3. Head trauma. In: Committee on Trauma of the American College of Surgeons. *Advanced Trauma Life Support for Doctors Student Course Manual*. 2nd ed. Chicago: American College of Surgeons; 1997:181–206.
4. Masters SJ, McClean PM, Arcarese JS. Skull x-ray examination after head trauma. Recommendations by a multidisciplinary panel and validation study. *N Engl J Med*. 1987;316:84–91.
5. Cheung DS, Kharasch M. Evaluation of the patient with closed head trauma: An evidence-based approach. In: Fontanarosa PB, ed. Evidence Based Emergency Medicine Evaluation and Diagnostic Testing. *Emerg Med Clin N Am*, 1999;17(1):9–23

100 Trauma, lower limb

Shirley Ooi

CAVEATS

- Although orthopaedic injuries may look serious, they are often not life- or limb-threatening and are included in Secondary Survey in a multiple trauma patient.
- All **dislocations** are **usually not serious** and only require adequate pain relief as the immediate treatment **except** for the following **3**, which should be reduced as soon as possible:
  1. Knee dislocations (because of popliteal artery compromise)
  2. Ankle dislocations (because of skin necrosis)
  3. Hip dislocations (because of avascular necrosis of the hip)
- For all **joint dislocations** that require manipulation and reduction at the ED, **do not** give **intramuscular (IM) opioids. Give IV opioids** instead. This is because opioids given by the IM route are erratic in their absorption. Hence, when conscious sedation is needed, one is unsure of the dosage to top up for pain relief. This may result in respiratory suppression and hypotension when the full IM dose of opioid is absorbed into the circulation.

> ☛ **Special Tips for GPs**
> - Ankle x-rays are not needed for every case of ankle injury. See section on *Indications for ordering x-rays in ankle injury.*

HIP DISLOCATION

- **Mechanism of injury**
  1. Dashboard injury.

Note: This often results in simultaneous fracture of patella, fracture of femoral shaft and **posterior hip dislocation**.

2. Falls on foot cause **posterior hip dislocation** if the leg is flexed at the hip and adducted, **anterior dislocation** if the hip is widely abducted and **central dislocation** if the femur is in some other part of the abduction or adduction range.
3. Weight falling on person with legs wide apart, knees straight and back bent forward causes **anterior hip dislocation**.
4. Doing a 'split' causes **anterior hip dislocation**.
5. Blow or fall on side causes **central hip dislocation**.

- **Clinical features**
  1. **Posterior hip dislocation**: hip held slightly flexed, adducted and internally rotated, leg appears shortened, femoral head palpable in buttock.
  2. **Anterior hip dislocation**: hip held slightly flexed, abducted and externally rotated. Anterior bulge of dislocated head is seen from side.
  3. **Central hip dislocation**: leg in normal position, tender trochanter and hip and little movement possible.
- **X-ray**: Anteroposterior (AP) view of pelvis and lateral view of the hip involved (Figures 1a, 1b, 1c).

Note: It is important to bear in mind that for **all hip pains**, an **AP view of the pelvis** and the lateral view of the hip involved should be done rather than AP and lateral view of the hip for these 2 reasons:

1. Pubic rami fracture may also present with 'hip pain'. This may be missed if AP hip instead of AP pelvis is done.
2. AP view of the pelvis allows comparison of Shenton's lines on both sides and helps in picking up subtle abnormalities.

- **Complications**
  1. Foot drop from sciatic nerve involvement in **posterior hip dislocation**.
  2. Femoral nerve paralysis and femoral artery compression in **anterior hip dislocation**.

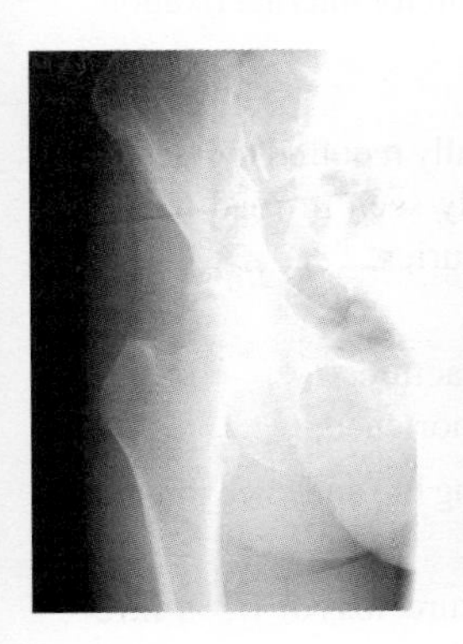

1a: AP view

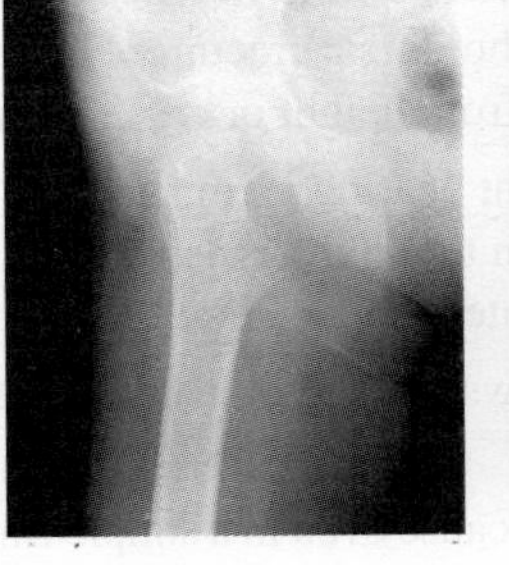

1b: Lateral view

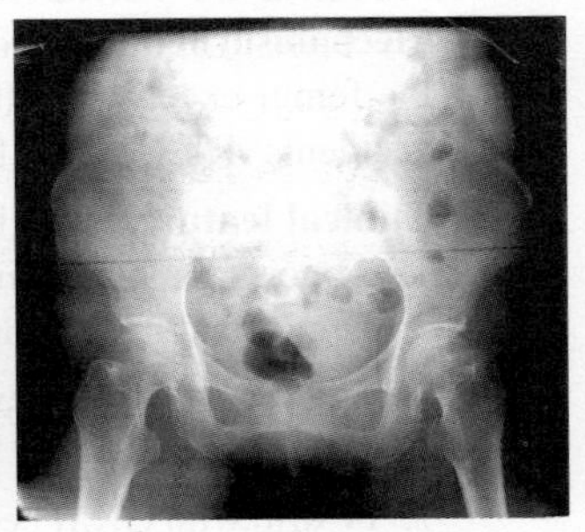

1c: AP view of pelvis

Figure 1: Views of the hip and pelvis

A 60-year-old lady tripped and fell and complained of pain over her right hip with limited range of movement. Figures 1a and b are the AP and lateral views of the right hip. With difficulty, a fracture of the right superior pubic ramus is seen. On repeating an AP pelvic x-ray (Figure 1c), besides the right superior pelvic ramus which is now shown very clearly, an impacted right inferior pubic ramus fracture is seen as well

- **Treatment/disposition**
  1. Pain relief in the form of IV and not IM narcotics **before** x-rays.
  2. Reduction as soon as possible under conscious sedation in the ED.
  3. Check x-ray after reduction and admit for traction.
  4. If unable to reduce, admit for reduction under general anaesthesia.

FRACTURE OF FEMORAL NECK AND TROCHANTERIC FRACTURES

- **Mechanism of injury**: usually from **falls in the elderly**.
- **Clinical features**
  1. Inability to bear weight after a fall, especially in an elderly patient with or without pain in hip.
  2. External rotation and shortening of lower limb.
  3. Tenderness over fracture site in groin.
  4. Pain on attempted movement of hip.
  5. Bruising is a late sign of extracapsular fractures and is absent in acute injuries.
- **X-ray**
  1. AP view of pelvis and lateral view of the involved hip.
  2. Remember to do chest x-ray for an elderly patient before admission
- **Complications**: generally none.
- **Treatment/disposition**: analgesia before x-rays. Admit for internal fixation.

FRACTURE OF FEMORAL SHAFT

- **Mechanism of injury**: **considerable violence** is usually required to fracture the femur except in pathological fractures. Usually seen in road traffic accidents (RTAs), falls from height or crushing injuries.
- **Clinical features**: weight bearing is impossible.
  1. Abnormal mobility in the limb at the level of fracture.
  2. Leg is externally rotated, abducted at hip and shortened.
- **X-ray**: AP and lateral views of femoral shaft (including hip and knee joints).
- **Treatment/disposition**
  1. IV drip with GXM because even in a simple fracture, loss of 1/2–1 litre of blood into tissues with accompanying shock is common.
  2. Give pain relief, eg femoral nerve block, IM or IV narcotics.
  3. Apply Donway's air splint.
  4. Admit for traction or intramedullary nailing.

PATELLAR FRACTURE

- **Mechanism**
  1. By direct violence, eg RTAs with dashboard injury, falls against a hard surface and heavy objects falling across the knee.

2. By indirect violence as a result of a sudden muscular contraction.

- **Clinical features**
  1. Inability to extend knee.
  2. Bruising and abrasion over knee.
  3. Note presence and site of tenderness.
  4. A palpable gap above or beneath the patella.
  5. An obvious proximal displacement of the patella.
- **X-ray**: AP and lateral view of knee.
- **Treatment/disposition**
  1. Give analgesia **before** x-rays.
  2. If undisplaced, apply cylinder backslab and discharge with analgesia, crutches and Trauma Clinic referral.
  3. If displaced, apply cylinder backslab and admit for fixation.

PATELLAR DISLOCATION

- **Mechanism**
  1. Typical history: while running, knee gets stuck and patient falls down. Patient often notices prominent medial bulge from medial femoral condyle (although patella usually dislocates laterally).
  2. Dislocated patella may spontaneously reduce.
- **Clinical features**
  1. Mild knee effusion.
  2. Tenderness on medial aspect of knee.
- **X-ray**: AP, lateral and skyline view. The skyline view is to exclude associated fracture of lateral femoral condyle.
- **Treatment/disposition**
  1. Give analgesia and reduce dislocation.
  2. Apply cylinder backslab for 6 weeks in first dislocation to prevent recurrent dislocation.
  3. If recurrent dislocation, apply pressure bandage for 1–2 weeks.

KNEE DISLOCATION

This is an EMERGENCY!

- **Mechanism of injury**: usually from RTAs, especially from dashboard injury.
- **Clinical features**: swelling, gross deformity, often with marked posterior sag.
- **X-ray**: AP and lateral view of knee.
- **Complications**
  1. Popliteal artery injury: look for pale, cold, pulseless lower limb or paresthesia of lower limb.
  2. Common peroneal nerve palsy.

- **Treatment**
  1. Give IV analgesics.
  2. Reduce dislocation immediately, especially if there is a delay in obtaining X-rays.
  3. Apply cylinder backslab.
  4. Call Vascular Surgeon and Orthopaedic Surgeon and arrange for angiogram.
- **Disposition**: admit all patients.

KNEE HAEMARTHROSIS/EFFUSION

- **Mechanism of injury**: usually from trauma to knee. **Immediate haemarthrosis** is due to:
  1. Torn cruciate ligaments
  2. Torn collateral ligaments
  3. Osteochondral fracture
  4. Peripheral meniscal tear

  Delayed effusion is due to meniscal tear.
- **Clinical features**: Gross swelling from haemarthrosis or effusion.
- **X-ray**:
  1. AP and lateral views of knee. Note fat fluid level in suprapatellar bursa indicating an intraarticular fracture even if a fracture is not seen (Figure 2).
  2. Skyline view is useful in subtle fractures of femoral condyles (especially in lateral dislocation of patella) and patella.

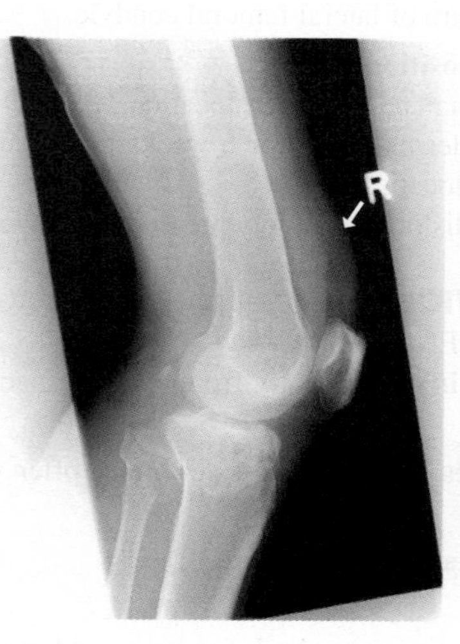

Figure 2: Lateral x-ray of the knee joint

Lateral x-ray of the knee joint shows fractures of tibial plateau, proximal tibia and head of fibula. Note the fat fluid level indicated by arrow showing lipohaemarthrosis.

- **Complications**: beware that patient is not having knee dislocation or concomitant knee fracture.
- **Treatment**:
  1. If knee haemarthrosis is not tense, patient can be discharged with **r**est, **i**ce, **c**ompression (apply crepe bandage) and **e**levation (RICE) treatment.
  2. Give analgesics.
- **Disposition**
  1. Refer to Orthopaedic Clinic within 24–48 hours.
  2. If tense haemarthrosis, patient should be admitted for aspiration.

FRACTURE OF TIBIAL PLATEAU

- **Mechanism of injury**: usually result from severe valgus stress.
- **Clinical features**:
  1. Haemarthrosis
  2. Lateral bruising
  3. Abrasions
  4. Valgus deformity of knee
- **X-ray views**: AP and lateral views of knee.
- **Complications**: note that subtle tibial table fractures may be missed. If patient continues to bear weight on it, the fracture will worsen.
- **Treatment**: give analgesia and apply cylinder backslab.
- **Disposition**: admit for fixation or traction depending on severity of fracture.

FRACTURE OF TIBIA/FIBULA

- **Mechanism of injury**: the tibia is vulnerable to:
  1. Torsional stresses (eg sporting injuries)
  2. Violence transmitted through the feet (eg falls from height, RTAs)
  3. Direct blows (eg RTAs, blows from falling objects)

     Isolated fracture of tibia or fibula may occur from direct violence although relatively uncommon. Indirect violence leads to fracture of both tibia and fibula.
- **Clinical features**:
  1. Pain
  2. Swelling
  3. Deformity
  4. Tenderness
  5. Fracture crepitus over the shin
  6. Very often it is an open fracture because 1/3 of the tibia is subcutaneous
- **X-ray**: AP and lateral views of tibia/fibula (must include knee and ankle joints)
- **Complications**: compartment syndrome in closed fractures and infection in open fractures

- **Treatment/disposition**:
  1. **Closed undisplaced fracture of tibia and fibula**:
     a. Give IM/IV analgesia before x-rays.
     b. Apply above knee backslab.
     c. Repeat x-rays to check final position of fracture.
     d. Admit for observation.
  2. **Closed displaced fracture of tibia and fibula**:
     a. Give IV narcotics before x-rays.
     b. Under conscious sedation with IV midazolam and narcotics, try to reduce the fracture.
     c. Apply above knee backslab.
     d. Repeat x-rays before admission.
  3. **Open fracture of tibia and fibula**:
     a. Give IM/IV analgesics.
     b. Take swab c/s from wound.
     c. Cover wound with dressing.
     d. Check tetanus immunization status.
     e. Give antibiotics (cefazolin).
     f. Apply long leg backslab or temporary splint.
     g. Admit for wound debridement.
  4. **Isolated closed fracture of fibula**:
     a. Give IM analgesics.
     b. Exclude fracture of tibia and injury to ankle joint.
     c. Crepe bandage.
     d. Discharge patient with oral analgesics.
     e. Refer to Orthopaedic Clinic.

Note: Patient can be allowed to bear weight.

ANKLE INJURY

- **Mechanism of injury**: when ankle is very deformed, suspect ankle dislocation. This is an EMERGENCY!

Note: The dislocated ankle must be reduced immediately to prevent skin necrosis.

- **Clinical features**: in every suspected ankle injury, palpate 4 bony points, ie
  1. Medial malleolus
  2. Lateral malleolus
  3. Whole length of fibula and
  4. Base of 5th metatarsal
- **X-ray**: X-rays are unnecessary for every case of sprained ankle.
  Indications for ordering x-rays in ankle injury:
  1. Bone tenderness at the posterior edge (distal 6 cm) or tip of the lateral malleolus.
  2. Bone tenderness at the posterior edge (distal 6 cm) or tip of the medial malleolus.

3. Inability to bear weight both immediately *and* in the ED.
4. In cases where there is sufficient swelling to hinder accurate palpation.
5. In cases where there is clinical instability.
6. In patients >50 years for whom clinical studies indicate a likely incidence of fracture of approximately 30%.
7. For *social reasons*, eg an athlete.

Note: Criteria 1 to 3 are known as the **Ottawa Ankle Rules**.

X-ray views to order are:

1. AP and lateral view of ankle for suspected ankle fracture.
2. Whole fibula if there is tenderness over the fibula higher up to exclude Maissoneuve fracture.
3. Posteroanterior (PA) and lateral view of foot if there is tenderness over the base of 5th metatarsal.

- **Complications**: skin necrosis in delayed reduction of dislocated ankle.
- **Treatment**:
  1. **Sprained ankle**:
     a. Give analgesics at the ED.
     b. Discharge with RICE treatment and analgesics.
     c. Refer to physiotherapist for ankle strapping in a severe sprain.
  2. **Ankle fracture**:
     a. Apply below knee backslab.
     b. Admit for internal fixation except for isolated stable fracture of lateral malleolus below ankle mortise where it can be treated conservatively.
  3. **Ankle dislocation**:
     a. Set up a heparin plug and give IV narcotics before x-rays.

Note: The dislocated ankle must be reduced as soon as possible under conscious sedation with IV midazolam and narcotics, or inhalation of Entonox (N_2O/O_2) to prevent skin necrosis. Hence, if there is a delay in obtaining x-rays for >10–15 min or if there are already signs of circulatory compromise, the ankle should be relocated even before the x-rays are done.

b. Apply short leg backslab after reduction.
c. Do postreduction x-rays.
d. Admit for internal fixation.

FRACTURE OF CALCANEUM

- **Mechanism of injury**: fall from a height on to heels.

Note: Remember to exclude bilateral calcaneal fractures and wedge fracture of spine.

- **Clinical features**:
  1. Heel when viewed from behind may appear wider, shorter, flatter or tilted laterally into valgus.
  2. Tense swelling of heel.
  3. Marked local tenderness.

4. If patient presents later, there will be bruising which may spread to medial side of sole and proximally to calf.

- **X-ray**: AP, lateral and axial views of calcaneum.
- **Treatment/disposition**:
  1. If subtalar joint is not involved:
     a. Apply firm bandaging over wool.
     b. Discharge with crutches, analgesics and advice to elevate limb at home.
  2. If bilateral fractures of calcaneum: admit for rest.
  3. If calcaneum is displaced or crushed:
     a. Apply below knee backslab.
     b. Admit.

FOOT INJURY

Note: Common ones include the following:

- Calcaneal fracture (as mentioned above)
- Tarso-metatarsal dislocations
- Metatarsal fractures
- Phalangeal fractures/dislocations

Tarso-metatarsal (Lisfranc's) dislocations

- **Mechanism of injury**:
  1. Fall on the plantar flexed foot.
  2. Blow to the forefoot as in RTAs.
  3. Blows on the heel when in the kneeling position.
  4. Run-over kerb side accidents.
  5. Forced inversion, eversion or abduction of the forefoot.
- **Clinical features**: swelling and 'drifting' of foot
- **X-ray**: AP and oblique views of foot (Figure 3).

Note: Lisfranc's dislocation is not always readily evident on radiographs and remains the most common misdiagnosed foot fracture.

- **Complications**: dorsalis pedis artery or medial plantar anastomosis may be in jeopardy.
- **Treatment**:
  1. Give analgesics before x-rays.
  2. Apply backslab.
  3. Admit for open reduction and internal fixation (ORIF).

Fracture of metatarsals

- **Mechanisms**: often due to crushing injury.
- **X-ray**: AP and oblique views of foot.
- **Principles of management**:
  1. **If fracture is undisplaced without soft tissue damage**:

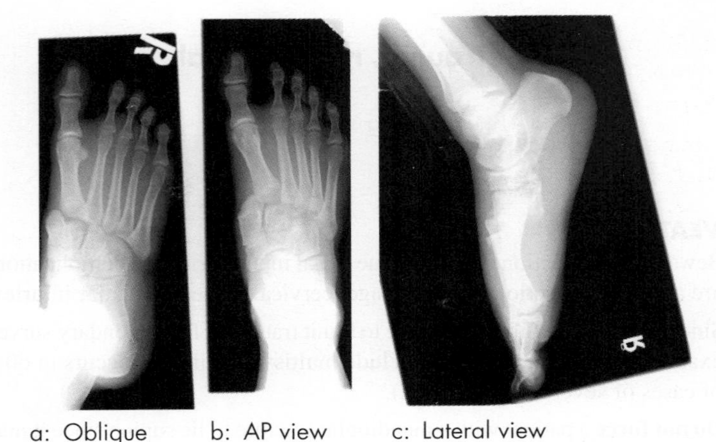

a: Oblique b: AP view c: Lateral view

Figure 3: Views of right foot dislocation

Oblique (Figure 3a) and AP (Figure 3b) x-ray views of the right foot show dislocation of the tarso-metatarsal joints with lateral displacements of all 5 metatarsals (Lisfranc's dislocations). This is further seen on the lateral view of the right foot (Figure 3c).

   a. Give analgesics before x-rays.
   b. Treat symptomatically with crepe bandage or a short backslab extending distally to beyond the toes.
   c. Discharge with non-weight bearing crutches (NWB) and analgesics.
   d. Refer to Orthopaedic Clinic.
2. **If fractures are multiple and undisplaced**, treat conservatively as above.
3. **If fractures are multiple and displaced**:
   a. Admit for operation if fracture is open.
   b. Apply backslab and discharge with analgesics and crutches NWB and early referral to Orthopaedic Clinic for review for ORIF, if fracture is closed.

Phalangeal fracture/dislocations

- **X-ray**: AP and oblique views of foot.
- **Principles of management**:
  1. Attend to soft tissue injuries and nail bed injuries first.
  2. Reduce dislocations using digital blocks or Entonox.
  3. Immobilize fractures and dislocations using adhesive strapping to the adjacent toe.
  4. Discharge with analgesics and referral to Orthopaedic Clinic.
  5. For multiple toe dislocations, admit for reduction.

References/further reading

1. McRae R. *Practical Fracture Treatment*. 2nd ed. Edinburgh: Churchill Livingstone; 1989.

101 Trauma, maxillofacial

Peter Manning • Shirley Ooi

CAVEATS

- Beware the distraction of a grotesque facial injury: principal complications are airway obstruction, haemorrhage, cervical spine and ocular injuries.
- Since many of the injuries are due to blunt trauma, a full secondary survey examination is mandatory to exclude multisystem injury (occurs in 60% of cases of severe facial trauma).
- **Do not force** a patient with a mandibular fracture to lie supine since it may compromise the airway: permit patient to sit up if he/she so feels the need.
- The absence of significant blood loss externally does not preclude internal bleeding sufficient to cause hypovolaemic shock since a supine patient may swallow the blood. Only later, upon vomiting, is the degree of blood loss evident.
- Perform a systematic examination of the face, paying particular attention to the eye examination and status of the bite (occlusion).
- Given that the bones of young children are softer than adults, more force is needed to fracture the paediatric face with a higher incidence of associated intracranial injuries.

☛ Special Tips for GPs

- **Do not force** a patient with a suspected mandibular fracture to lie supine since this may compromise the airway.
- When evaluating a patient with a suspected nasal bone fracture, pay particular attention to looking for a **septal haematoma**. This is a **true ENT emergency** requiring incision and drainage promptly.
- Young children have an increased incidence of frontal bone injury due to its prominence, whereas mid-face injuries are extremely uncommon. Always suspect non-accidental injury if a child presents with a torn frenulum, lip trauma and mid-face bruising.
- The only dental fracture that is a true emergency is the Ellis Class III, identified by bleeding from the pulp.

MANAGEMENT

Broadly speaking, patients can be divided into 2 groups:

- Isolated maxillofacial injury secondary to a relatively small force, eg punch or kick, can be managed in the intermediate or low acuity care area of the department.
- Severe maxillofacial injury secondary to a significant blunt trauma, eg rapid deceleration from a road traffic accident or fall from height, must be managed in the critical care area of the department:
  1. Severe maxillofacial injuries must be managed in the critical care area following the tenets of ATLS.
  2. Establish and **maintain a patent airway** with cervical spine immobilization.
     a. Sit patient up if no spinal injury is suspected **or** if patient feels the need to do so.
     b. Jaw thrust and chin lift.
     c. Tongue traction: (1) fingers, (2) O–silk suture and (3) towel clip.
     d. Endotracheal intubation: awake oral intubation versus rapid sequence intubation versus cricothyroidotomy (refer to *Airway Management/ Rapid Sequence Intubation* for further details).
  3. Administer supplemental oxygen by non-rebreather reservoir mask.
  4. Monitoring: vital signs q 5–10 min, ECG, pulse oximetry.
  5. Establish 1 or 2 peripheral large bore IV lines for volume replacement.
  6. Labs: GXM, FBC, urea/electrolytes/creatinine, coagulation profile.
  7. Facilitate the cessation of ongoing haemorrhage.
     a. Direct pressure
        Pinching nose
        Nasal or throat packing
        Tamponade by Foley catheter
     b. Haemostatic agent tranexamic acid (Cyclokapron®)
        Dosage: 25 mg/kg body weight IV slow bolus over 5–10 min
  8. **X-rays**: the timing of facial x-rays is **not** a priority in multiple injuries. Two radiographic views are:
     a. Occipitomental or OM (Water's) view
     b. Posteroanterior or PA (Caldwell) view
     c. Lateral view
     d. Submentovertical (SMV) or 'jughandle' view
     e. Towne's view

Note: Views a, b, and c above used to be the standard facial views. However, Goh et al (2002) showed that a **single 30-degree OM view** would be **sufficient to screen for maxillofacial trauma**. Hence, if facial fractures are suspected, a single 30° OM view should be ordered only and not facial views.

OM (Water's) view

See Figure 1: good for mid-face, showing orbital rims and floors and blood in maxillary sinus

PA (Caldwell) view

See Figure 2: displays frontal bone and paranasal sinuses. Can sometimes show up the zygomaticofrontal suture diastasis in a tripod fracture better than on OM view.

Lateral view (cross-table or upright)

See Figure 3: facilitates layering of blood in sinuses.

Submentovertical (or 'jughandle') view

See Figure 4: displays zygomatic arch.

Towne's view

See Figure 5: displays mandibular rami and condyles.

Systematic review of OM view using McGrigor's lines

See Figure 6: Trace the 3 lines on the OM view.

- As the lines are drawn, compare the injured with the uninjured side.
- The soft tissue above and below these 3 lines should also be examined.

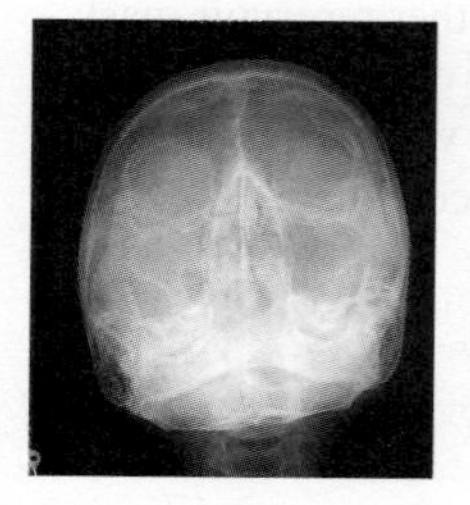

Figure 1: OM (Water's) view

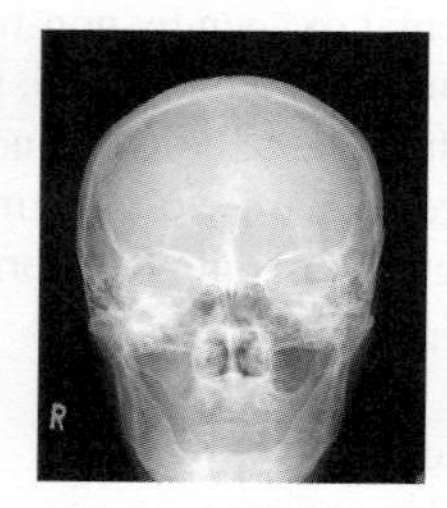

Figure 2: PA (Caldwell) view

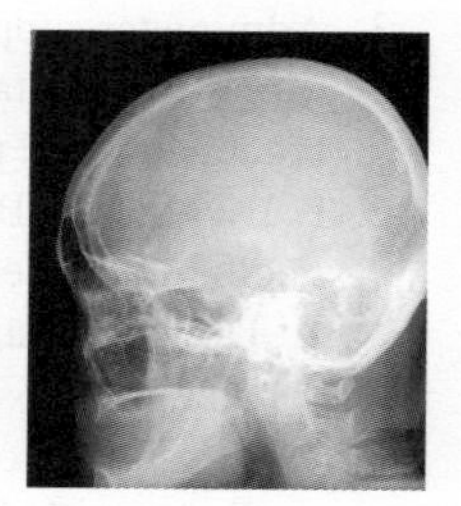

Figure 3: Lateral view

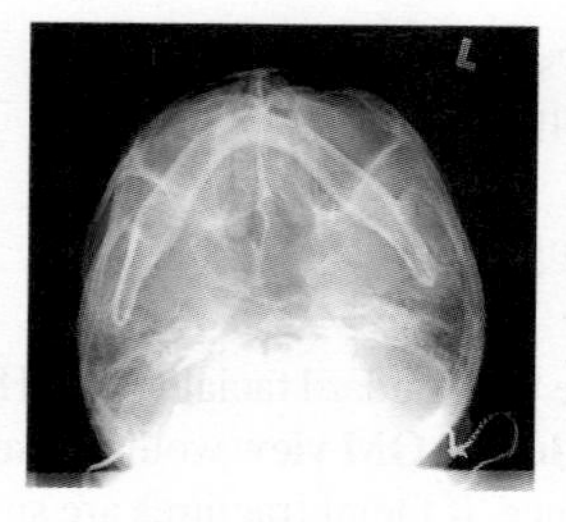

Figure 4: SMV ('jughandle' view)

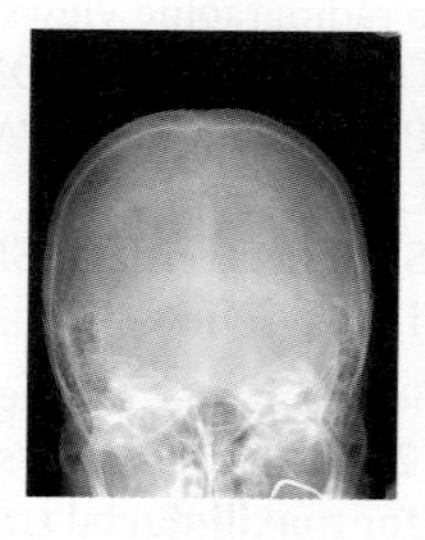

Figure 5: Towne's view

- **Line 1** (Figure 7): start outside the face, tracing through the suture between the frontal and zygomatic bones at the lateral margin of the orbit across the forehead, assessing the superior orbital margin and the frontal sinus to the other side. **Compare injured and uninjured sides**. Look for:
  1. Fractures
  2. Widening of the zygomatic suture
  3. Fluid level in a frontal sinus
- **Line 2** (Figure 8). Start outside the face, trace upwards along the superior border of the zygomatic arch (up the elephant's trunk), crossing the body of the zygoma, to the inferior margin of the orbit, to the contour of nose to the other side of the face. **Compare injured and uninjured sides**. Observe fracture of the zygomatic arch fracture through the inferior rim of the orbit soft tissue shadow in the superior aspect of the maxillary antrum (blow-out fracture).
- **Line 3** (Figure 9). Start outside the face, trace along the inferior margin of the zygomatic arch (under the elephant's trunk), and down the lateral wall of the maxillary antrum to the inferior margin of the antrum, across the maxilla along the line of the teeth to the other side.

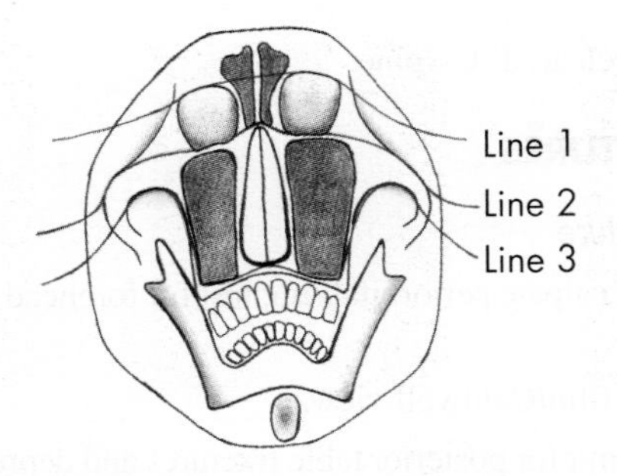

Figure 6: McGrigor's 3 lines

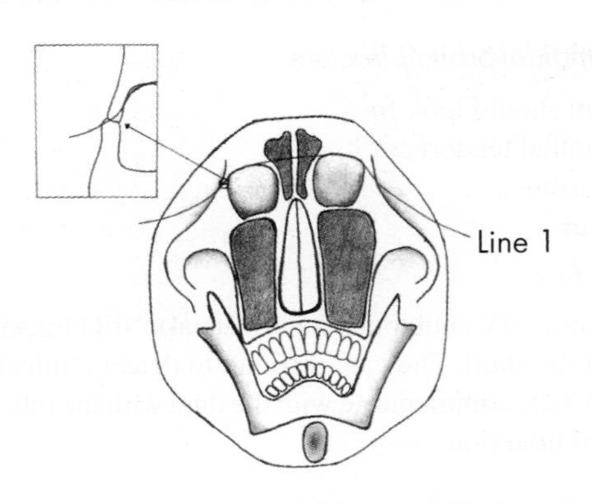

Figure 7: McGrigor's Line 1

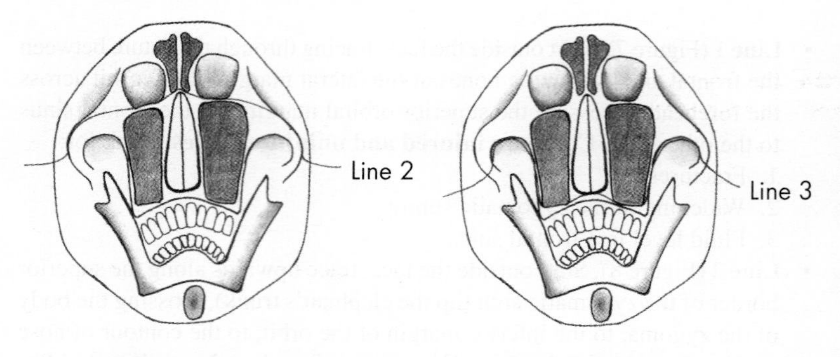

Figure 8: McGrigor's Line 2

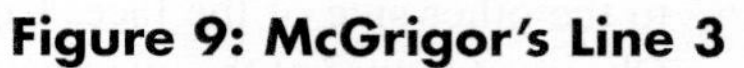

Figure 9: McGrigor's Line 3

Role of computed tomography

- Not a priority in ED management.
- Most valuable for complex facial fractures, especially those involving the frontal sinus, nasoethroid region and the orbits.
- Standard facial x-rays are more useful for 'routine' cases, eg assaults, fall to floor, etc.
- CT requires a 'cleared' C-spine.

SPECIFIC FRACTURES

Frontal bone fracture

- Physical exam: palpate periorbital rim; test for forehead anaesthesia; EOM testing.
- Imaging: skull film/Caldwell view.
- Disposition: admit for posterior table fractures and depressed fractures (IV antibiotics controversial). Both of these fractures are likely to breach the dura with the inherent possibility of intracranial infection.

NEO (naso-ethmoidal-orbital) fracture

- Physical exam should look for:
  1. Medial canthal tenderness
  2. CSF rhinorrhoea
  3. Telecanthus
- Imaging: CT face.
- Disposition: admit (IV antibiotics controversial). NEO fractures may extend to the base of the skull. They are difficult to detect clinically or on x-ray. If present they may communicate with the dura with the inherent possibility of intracranial infection.

'Blow out' orbital fracture

- Result from a direct compression force to the globe (eg from a squash ball). See Figures 10 and 11.

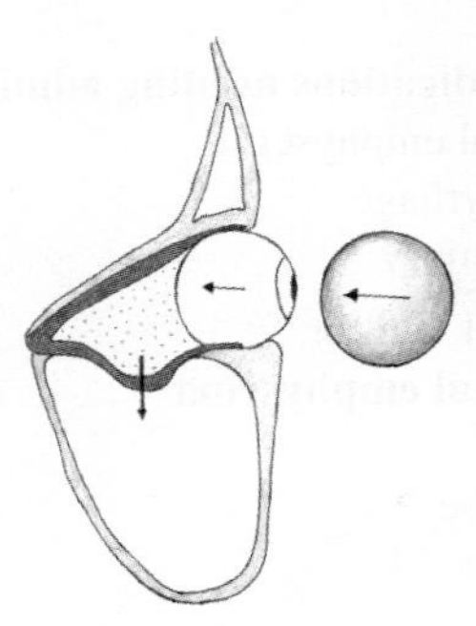

Figure 10: Mechanism of injury causing a blow out fracture of the orbital floor

A frontal impact to the orbit increases intraorbital pressure. The orbit fracture is at the weakest part – the orbital walls – rather than the globe. Alternatively, a blow to the inferior orbital rim causes the orbital floor to buckle and fracture.

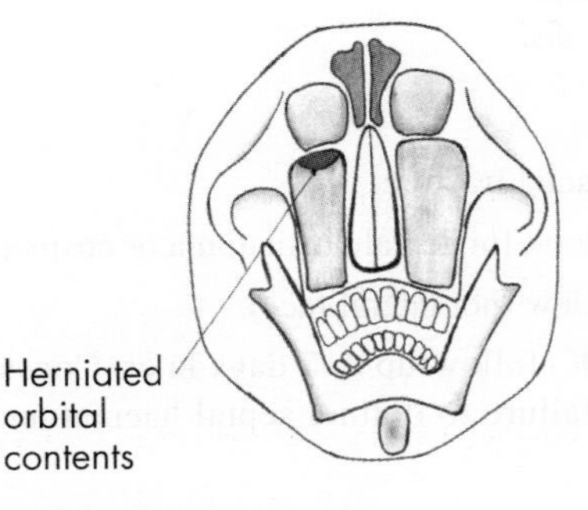

Figure 11: Blow out fracture

The dark shadow represents the 'tear-drop' sign

Note: A blow out fracture of the orbit does not involve the orbital rim. In fact, the finding of an orbital rim fracture should prompt close scrutiny for a 'tripod' fracture of the zygoma.

- Weakest point is inferomedial floor of the orbit (lamina papyracea).
- Herniation of some orbital contents into the maxillary antrum through the floor (**'tear-drop' sign**).
- Physical exam:
  1. Test for infraorbital anaesthesia by tapping for the difference in sensation between the incisors on both sides
  2. Testing of extraocular movements
  3. Visual testing
- Imaging: Water's view.
- Disposition: refer to Plastic Surgery SOC.

Note: Diplopia alone is not an indication for admission.

- **Emergent surgical indications needing admission** are
  1. Compressive orbital emphysema
  2. Retrobulbar haemorrhage
  3. Penetrating globe injury
- **Discharge advice**: look out for
  1. **Compressive orbital emphysema**
     a. Intense eye pain
     b. Proptosis of globe
     c. Ophthalmoplegia
     d. Tense globe
     e. Visual loss

  To prevent compressive orbital emphysema, patients should be advised not to blow their noses.
  2. **Retrobulbar haemorrhage**
     a. In addition to those points in compressive orbital emphysema
     b. Dilating pupil
     c. Pale optic disc

Nasal fracture

- Most common facial fracture.
- Physical exam: look for septal haematoma or cosmetic deformity.
- Imaging: nasal view (not lateral face).
- Disposition: SOC follow-up 4–7 days later. Consult/admit for septal haematoma as failure to drain a septal haematoma will cause septal perforation.

Zygoma: 'tripod' fracture

- Consists of fractures of the floor **and** lateral wall of the orbit, zygomatic arch and lateral wall of the maxillary antrum. See Figure 12.

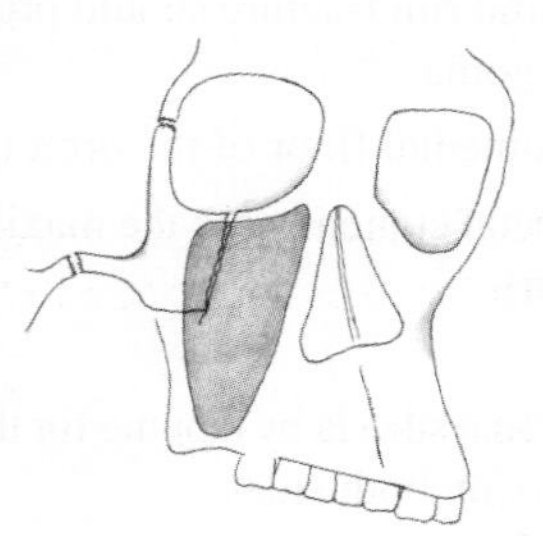

Figure 12: Fracture of the zygomaticomaxillary complex (tripod fracture)

There are fractures through the supporting struts of the malar bone: (1) the zygomatic arch, (2) lateral orbital rim (frontozygomatic suture), (3) inferior orbital rim and orbital floor, and (4) the anterior and lateral walls of the maxillary sinus.

- Physical exam:
  1. Look for lateral subconjunctival haemorrhage
  2. Look for drooping lateral canthus
  3. Test for infraorbital anaesthesia
  4. Examine for open bite
- Imaging: OM (Water's) view.
- Disposition: isolated tripod fracture can be discharged to the Plastic Surgery SOC. Discharge advice should include instructions to return immediately if there is blurring of vision as for blow-out fractures. Patient should be admitted if there is:
  1. Severe diplopia
  2. Trismus
  3. Visual problems

Zygoma: 'arch' fracture

- An isolated arch fracture is common.
- Physical exam: intraoral palpation; worm's eye/bird's eye views.
- Imaging: submental vertex (SMV) view.
- Disposition: SOC follow-up.

LeFort fractures

- Bilateral mid-face injuries.
- High-energy injuries 100× force of gravity. Beware multisystem injury.

Note: Fracture patterns may be mixed, eg LeFort II on one side, and LeFort III on the other side.

- Physical exam: look for mid-face mobility facial lengthening and examine for open bite.
- Imaging: x-rays of OM/PA/lateral views (Table 1). CT best for operative planning.
- Disposition: admit (beware multisystem injury).

Mandibular fractures

- Second most common facial fracture. Patient complains of malocclusion and pain on jaw movement associated with ruptured TM/fracture temporal bone.
- Physical exam:
  1. Assess for intraoral laceration
  2. ROM jaw
  3. Spatula test: place 1 wooden spatula between the teeth and have patient bite gently on it.
  4. Gentle rotation of the blade will produce pain in the presence of a fractured mandible
  5. Dental exam
  6. Test for lower lip anaesthesia

Table 1: Radiographic signs of LeFort fractures

Water's view
Bilateral mid-face fractures are characteristics of all LeFort fractures.
Bilateral maxillary sinus air-fluid levels or opacification are usually present.
LeFort I
Bilateral lateral wall of the maxillary sinus fractures.
Bilateral medial wall of the maxillary sinus fractures (can be difficult to see).
Nasal septum fracture (inferior).
LeFort II (pyramid fracture)
Nasion fracture.
Bilateral inferior orbital rim and orbital floor fractures.
Bilateral fractures of the lateral walls maxillary sinuses.
LeFort III (craniofacial separation)
Nasion fracture.
Bilateral lateral orbital wall fractures (frontozygomatic suture).
Bilateral zygomatic arch fractures.

Source: Table reproduced with permission of the McGraw-Hill Companies, from Schwartz and Reisdorff (2001);[1] p. 361, Table 15–5.

- Imaging: Towne's view, lateral oblique mandible and panorex
- Disposition: admit open fracture for IV antibiotics. Refer closed fracture to outpatient clinic or admit depending on degree of jaw opening.

Tooth fractures

- See Figure 13.
- Fractures of the crown: Ellis classification
- Fractures of the root: <7% dental injuries

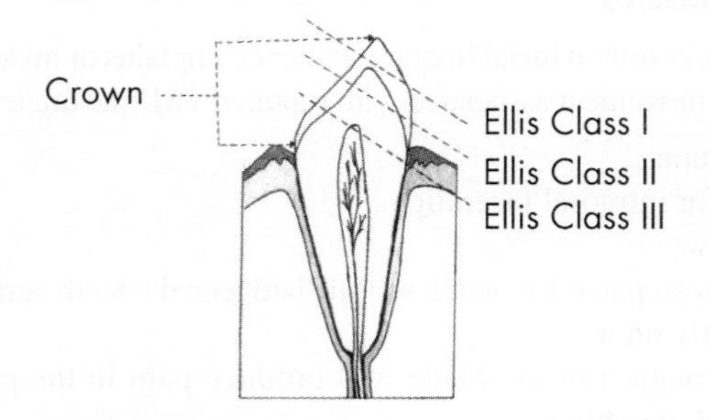

Figure 13: Tooth fractures

Ellis Class I

- Fracture of enamel only: minimal pain.
- Disposition: dentist next day

Ellis Class II

- Fracture of enamel and exposing pinkish or yellow dentin.
- Disposition: stat dental opinion if a child; next day if adult.

Ellis Class III

- Fracture as shown by bleeding or pink blush at the fracture site indicating pulpal exposure. Involves enamel, dentin and pulp exposure.
- Disposition: stat dental opinion. A true dental emergency because the pulp chamber is immediately contaminated. If no dentist is available, a piece of moist cotton can be placed over the exposed pulp and covered with a piece of dry foil or sealed with a temporary root canal sealant.

Acknowledgement

The authors are grateful to Dr Chong Chew Lan for drawing Figures 6, 7, 8, 9, 10, 11, 12 and 13 in this chapter.

References/further reading

1. Schwartz TD, Reisdorff E. *Emergency Radiology*. New York: McGraw-Hill; 2001.
2. Colucciello SA, Sternbach G, Walker SB. The treacherous and complex spectrum of maxillofacial trauma: etiologies, evaluation, and emergency stabilization. *Emerg Med Reports*. 1995;16(7).
3. Raby N, Berman L, deLacey G. *Accident and Emergency Radiology: A Survival Guide*. London: WB Saunders; 1995:36–49.
4. Amsterdam JT. Oral medicine. In Marx JA, Hockberger RS, Walls RM, eds. *Rosen's Emergency Medicine: Concepts and Practice*. 5th ed. St. Louis: Mosby; 2002:901–904.
5. Goh SH, Low BY. Radiologic screening for midfacial fractures: A single 30-deg occipitomental view is enough. *J Trauma*. 2002:52:688–692.

102 Trauma, pelvic

Irwani Ibrahim

CAVEATS

- The common pitfalls in the management of pelvic trauma include:
  1. Failure to consider pelvic fracture in patients with multisystem trauma
  2. Failure to give resuscitation adequately
  3. Failure to recognize associated injuries
- There is more severe blood loss in open pelvic fractures (as opposed to closed) because the tamponading effect of the peritoneum is lost.
- Elderly women often have pelvic fractures with minimal falls because of underlying osteoporosis.
- **Mechanisms of injury**:
  1. Simple falls, avulsions from muscular attachment
  2. Direct blows
  3. Fall from heights, motorcycle accidents, high speed deceleration motor vehicle crashes
- **Associated injuries**: most mortality and morbidity with pelvic fractures occur because of associated trauma involving adjacent blood vessels and nerves and the genitourinary and distal gastrointestinal tract.
- **Cause of death**: main cause of death is uncontrolled bleeding.

> ☛ **Special Tips for GPs**
> - Consider the diagnosis of pubic rami fracture in the elderly with hip pain after a fall.

MANAGEMENT

- ABC as in major trauma management.
- Correct hypovolaemia: at least 2 large bore IV lines should be set up.
- Send blood for FBC, urea/electrolytes/creatinine, coagulation profile and GXM of at least 4–6 units of rapid matched blood.
- Do **physical examination**. **Physical signs** associated with pelvic fracture:
  1. Swelling in suprapubic or groin area
  2. Ecchymosis in external genitalia, medial thigh and flanks
  3. Blood from urethra
  4. Abrasions, contusions of bony prominence
  5. Step-off, instability
  6. Crepitus with bimanual palpation of iliac wings

Note: (1) **Do not** try to **spring** the **pelvis** to assess stability as this is unreliable, unnecessary and may cause additional haemorrhage. (2) Lacerations of perineum, groin or buttock after blunt trauma indicate **open pelvic fracture** unless proven otherwise. (3) Neurological examination should be performed since **sacral plexus injury** can occur.

- **Associated injuries**:
  1. Inspect perineum for open wounds.
  2. Perform rectal examination noting the position of prostate, feeling for bony spicules and looking for blood stains on glove on withdrawing.
  3. Perform vaginal examination for open wounds.
  4. If there is evidence of **urethral injury**, eg blood on meatus, scrotal bruising or high riding prostate, look out for pelvic fracture that can be unstable.
- Do not insert a catheter. Refer to Urologist who may decide to insert a suprapubic catheter.
- Do **x-ray pelvis** to look for disruption of pubic symphysis and asymmetry.
- Give adequate **analgesia**.
- Start **antibiotics** in case of **open fractures**.
- Support unstable pelvic fractures using sandbags.
- Refer to Orthopaedics who may reduce and immobilize the fractures with C-clamp **external fixators**.
- If haemorrhage control fails, consider **angiography** and **embolization**.

References/further reading

1. Committee on Trauma of the American College of Surgeons. *Advanced Trauma Life Support for Doctors Manual*. 6th ed. Chicago: American College of Surgeons; 1997.
2. Wilson RF, Tyburski J, Georgiadis GM. Pelvic fractures. In: Wilson RF, Walt AJ, eds. *Management of Trauma: Pitfalls and Practice*. 2nd ed. Baltimore: William & Wilkins; 1996:578–599.
3. Gillott A, Rhodes M, Lucke J. Utility of routine pelvic x-ray during blunt trauma resuscitation. *J Trauma*. 1988;28(11):1570–1574.
4. Kaneriya PP, Schweitzer ME, Spettell C, et al. The cost-effectiveness of routine pelvic radiography in the evaluation of blunt trauma patients. *Skeletal Radiol*. 1999;28(5):271–273.
5. Mackersie RC, Shackford SR, Garfin SR, et al. Major skeletal injuries in the obtunded blunt trauma patient: A case for routine radiologic survey. *J Trauma*. 1988;28(10):1450–1454.
6. Civil ID, Ross SE, Botehlo G, et al. Routine pelvic radiography in severe blunt trauma: Is it necessary? *Ann Emerg Med*. 1988;17(5):488–490.
7. Koury HI, Peschiera JL, Welling RE. Selective use of pelvic roentgenograms in blunt trauma patients. *J Trauma*. 1993;34(2):236–237.
8. Salvino CK, Esposito TJ, Smith D, et al. Routine pelvic x-ray studies in awake blunt trauma patients: A sensible policy? *J Trauma*. 1992;33(3):413–416.
9. Grant PT. The diagnosis of pelvic fractures by 'springing'. *Arch Emerg Med*. 1990;7(3):178–182.

103 Trauma, pregnancy

Benjamin Leong

CAVEATS

Keep in mind physiological and anatomical changes in pregnancy.

- **Airway considerations (in the primary survey)**
  1. **Intubation may be difficult** with airway oedema present.
  2. There is **increased risk of aspiration** due to reduced lower oesophageal pressure with increased gastric pressure from uterine compression.
- **Breathing/respiratory considerations (in the primary survey)**
  1. **Oxygen consumption increases** by about 15%, resulting in lower oxygen reserve.
  2. **Minute ventilation increases** resulting in physiological hypocarbia. Normocarbia, if detected, may thus actually represent hypoventilation.
  3. **Diaphragmatic splinting** during pregnancy results in reduced functional residual capacity (FRC) and makes pneumothoraces and haemothoraces more life threatening.
  4. **Ventilatory pressures may rise** due to reduced chest wall compliance and diaphragmatic splinting.
  5. As the diaphragm may rise by up to 4 cm, insertion of chest tubes should be **above the 4th intercostal space**.
- **Circulation considerations (in the primary survey)**
  1. **Maternal BP** decreases by 5–15 mm Hg and **heart rate** increases by about 15–20 bpm during the 2nd trimester, but these vital signs should not be dismissed as physiological until adequately evaluated for haemorrhage.
  2. **Maternal blood loss** of up to 35% (about 1.5 litres) may be tolerated before signs of shock are evident.
  3. **Evidence of foetal compromise** may be the 1st sign of maternal haemorrhagic shock as uterine blood flow is diverted to support maternal circulation.
  4. **Untreated hypovolaemic shock** may compromise placental circulation. Maternal shock is associated with up to 80% foetal mortality rate. It may also lead to infarction of the pituitary, which normally increases in size during pregnancy (**Sheehan's syndrome**).
  5. **Supine hypotension syndrome** occurs (usually from the 20th week) when the uterus compresses the inferior vena cava (IVC) and may worsen maternal shock.
  6. **Physiological anaemia** occurs due to maternal blood volume rising by about 50% but with only a 25% corresponding increase in red cell mass.

- **Anatomical considerations (in the secondary survey)**
  1. The **uterus** rises out of the pelvis at **12 weeks**, reaches the umbilicus at **20 weeks**, the xyphisternum at **36 weeks**, and may make assessment of the abdomen more difficult.
  2. The **bony pelvis** is less likely to fracture due to **increased ligamentous laxity**.
  3. The **symphysis pubis** and **sacroiliac joints** may be widened, **mimicking diastasis** on x-ray. Clinical correlation with the mechanism of injury and tenderness is necessary.
  4. IVC compression during pregnancy results in increased pelvic congestion, which may result in torrential **retroperitoneal or pelvic haemorrhage**.

☛ **Special Tips for GPs**

- Prevention is better than cure.
  1. Advise pregnant patients on **proper use of seat belts** in cars: shoulder belts should lie above the uterus and lap belts should lie over the pelvis, below the uterus.
  2. Advise on **proper foot wear** to minimize falls: flat heeled with good grip.
- **Basic measures** that may be performed if the GP is the first responder include:
  1. Proper positioning of the patient (see comments above)
  2. Local bleeding control
  3. Supplemental oxygen (if available)
  4. Early IV fluids (if available)

MANAGEMENT

General principles

- The priorities and ABCs of trauma management do not differ during pregnancy.
- There may be **2** patients to monitor but stabilize the **mother** first.
- **Involve the obstetrician** in addition to the **trauma team early**.
- Manage the patient in a monitored area (high acuity or intermediate acuity care):
  1. Supplemental oxygen.
  2. Monitoring: ECG, pulse oximetry, vital signs q 5–10 min, continuous CTG monitoring for pregnant patients beyond 20 weeks gestation.

- **Patient position**:
  1. If spinal injury is suspected, position the patient with **sandbags** or a **wedge** ('Cardiff wedge') below the right buttock and **manually displace the uterus to the left**.
  2. Otherwise, manage the patient in the **left lateral position**.

Primary survey

- **Clear the airway** as for non-pregnant patients.
- Apply **cricoid pressure** to reduce gastric aspiration in patients with impaired consciousness who have lost their airway protective reflexes.
- Insert a **nasogastric tube** to decompress the stomach.
- **Intubate** if necessary.
- Resuscitate with **IV crystalloids aggressively**. Consider transfusion early. Avoid vasopressors as far as possible, which result in reduced uterine blood flow.
- **Resuscitation in cardiac arrest** should follow guidelines as for non-pregnant patients.
- However, if there is no return of spontaneous circulation after 5 min, **emergency caesarian section** should be considered if the foetus is viable.

Secondary survey

- The secondary survey should **follow the same manner** as in non-pregnant patients.
- The indications for **chest tubes** remain the same. However, do not place the chest tube below the level of the 4th intercostal space.
- In addition, assessment of the uterus and foetus should include:
  1. **Continuous CTG monitoring** for uterine irritability, foetal heart rate decelerations or loss of variability.
  2. **Fundal height and tenderness**
  3. **Foetal movements**
  4. **Vaginal blood**, **amniotic fluid** (vaginal pH >7.5), **cervical effacement** and **impending labour**
- **Injuries and complications unique to pregnancy**:
  1. **Abruptio placentae**
     a. Leading cause of foetal death after blunt trauma
     b. Occurs as a result of sheer stress from blunt trauma or sudden deceleration
     c. Clinical triad of abdominal pain, vaginal bleeding, uterine irritability, but may be occult
     d. Up to 2 litres of maternal blood may accumulate within uterus
     e. Associated with increased risk for DIVC

2. **Uterine rupture**
   a. Uncommon
   b. Usually caused by blunt abdominal trauma
   c. Increased risk among women with history of caesarian section
   d. Clinical features include peritonism, asymmetrical uterus and palpable foetal parts
3. **Preterm labour**
   a. Increased uterine irritability may occur as a result of uterine trauma
   b. Caused by release of arachidonic acid
   c. 90% abort spontaneously
4. **Foetal injury**
   a. Uncommon: the foetus is more likely to suffer compromise from maternal hypoxia or hypovolaemia
   b. May occur either due to penetrating or blunt trauma
5. **Rh sensitization**
   a. Occurs when blood from a Rh positive foetus enters the circulation of a Rh negative mother
   b. Rh immunoglobulin (IM RhoGAM 300 mg) should be considered for all Rh negative mothers who sustain abdominal trauma, in consultation with the obstetrician
6. **Amniotic fluid embolus**
   a. Rare and carries a poor prognosis
   b. May result in cardiovascular collapse, respiratory distress, convulsions or DIVC

Investigations

- FBC, urea/electrolytes/creatinine.
- Coagulation profile.
- GXM (note Rh status of mother).
- Kleihauer test (in Rh negative mothers).
- Necessary **x-rays** and **CT scans** should not be withheld, using lead shields as appropriate, though alternatives such as ultrasound or DPL may be considered.
- The indications for **diagnostic peritoneal lavage** remain the same. However, it should be performed well above the fundus of the uterus, or at least above the umbilicus. As the intestines are displaced superiorly by the uterus, there is an increased risk of bowel perforation in upper abdominal penetrating trauma, and a lower cell count (5,000 cells/mm^3) should be used to define a positive study.
- **Ultrasound** (FAST) is very useful for detecting haemoperitoneum, as well as detecting foetal movement and placental abruption.

Definitive care

- Decisions for definitive treatment for respective injuries should be made between the respective surgeons and the obstetrician.
- **Situations that may require emergent delivery** of the foetus include:
  1. Abruptio placentae
  2. Foetal distress
  3. Maternal cardiac arrest
- Even if no obvious maternal injury has occurred, the patient should have **continuous cardiotocograph monitoring for 4 hours**. Even seemingly trivial injuries may result in placental separation.

Disposition

- Patients with major trauma should be generally admitted to the General Surgical ICU or HD unit.
- Patients may also be admitted to the respective surgical subspecialties depending on the spectrum of injury to the mother (eg isolated traumatic brain injury under neurosurgery or isolated limb fracture under orthopaedics).
- If there has been no obvious significant injury, the patient may be admitted to the labour ward for monitoring.

References/further reading

1. Trauma in women. In: Committee on Trauma of the American College of Surgeons. *Advanced Trauma Life Support for Doctors Manual*. 6th ed. Chicago: American College of Surgeons; 1997:313–323.
2. Wyatt JP, Illingworth RN, Clancy MJ, et al, eds. *Oxford Handbook of Accident and Emergency Medicine*. Oxford: Oxford University Press; 1999:622–623.
3. Scaletta TA, Schaider JJ, eds. *Emergent Management of Trauma*. 2nd ed. New York: McGraw-Hill; 2001:359–368.

104 Trauma, upper limb

Peter Manning • Seet Chong Meng • Shirley Ooi

CAVEATS

- Although orthopaedic injuries look serious, they are often not life or limb threatening and are included in the Secondary Survey in a multiple trauma patient.
- For all joint dislocations that require manipulation and reduction at the ED, do **not** give **IM opioids**. **Give IV opioids** instead. This is because opioids given by the IM route are erratic in absorption. Hence, when conscious sedation is needed, one is unsure of the dosage to top up for pain relief. This may result in respiratory suppression and hypotension when the full IM dose of opioid is absorbed into the circulation.
- For all orthopaedic injuries, always remember to record the neurovascular status before and after manipulation/reduction or application of plaster.

> ☛ **Special Tips for GPs**
> - Remember to give analgesia and splint the fracture or dislocation before referring patient to the ED. Remember that splinting is a form of pain relief.
> - Do not give IM opioids if you are unsure whether patient requires M&R for the fracture or dislocation.

CLAVICULAR FRACTURES

- **Mechanism of injury**:
  1. Most commonly due to a fall on the outstretched hand
  2. May also be due to a direct blow on the shoulder, eg fall on the side
- **Clinical features**:
  1. Tenderness at fracture site
  2. Deformity with local swelling
- **X-ray view**: a single AP view of shoulder is usually adequate.
- **Complications**: rarely, the fracture fragments may endanger the subclavian neurovascular structures.
- **Treatment/disposition**: broad arm sling and review at Orthopaedic Clinic within 5 days.

STERNOCLAVICULAR DISLOCATIONS

- **Mechanism of injury**: usually due to a fall or blow to the front of the shoulder.
  1. Asymmetry of the inner ends of the clavicle
  2. Local tenderness
- **Clinical features**:
  1. Tenderness and swelling over the sternoclavicular joint
  2. Pain with movement of the arm and on lateral compression of the shoulders
  3. With severe injuries, the medial clavicle is displaced relative to the manubrium
  4. Dyspnoea, dysphagia or choking (in patients with posterior dislocations due to compression of mediastinal structures)
- **X-ray view**: AP and oblique views are difficult to interpret; the diagnosis is essentially a clinical one; tomograms or CT may be needed.
- **Complications**: rarely, the dislocation may endanger the great vessels posterior to the clavicle.
- **Treatment/disposition**:
  1. Minor subluxations: broad arm sling/analgesics and review at Orthopaedic Clinic within 3 days.
  2. Gross displacement: admit to Orthopaedics for exploration/reduction under GA.

Note: Life-threatening injuries to adjacent structures occur in up to 25% of posterior dislocations.

ACROMIOCLAVICULAR JOINT INJURIES

- **Mechanism of injury**: usually due to a fall in which the patient lands on the shoulder with the arm adducted or a fall on the outstretched arm.
- **Clinical features**: unusual prominence of the lateral end of the clavicle and local tenderness.
- **X-ray view**: AP view of AC joint (inferior aspects of the acromion and clavicle should form a straight line).

Note: Weight-bearing views add little and only cause the patient pain. They do not change treatment.

- **Treatment/disposition**: broad arm sling and review at Orthopaedic Clinic within 5 days.

SCAPULAR FRACTURES

- **Mechanism of injury**: usually due to significant direct trauma to the posterolateral chest.
- **Clinical features**: local tenderness and swelling and associated injuries (see p. 487).

- **X-ray view**: AP shoulder with or without scapular views.
- **Complications**: scapular fractures are commonly associated with significant intrathoracic injuries such as rib, clavicular and vertebral fractures, injuries to pulmonary vessels and brachial plexus.
- **Treatment/disposition**
  1. Isolated scapular fractures: broad arm sling and analgesics; review at Orthopaedic Clinic within 3 days.
  2. Coexistent intrathoracic injuries: admit under General Surgery for either observation or definitive care of the individual injuries.

SHOULDER DISLOCATIONS

Statistically, 96% are anterior; 3–4% are posterior; 0–1% are inferior (luxatio erecta) dislocations.

Anterior dislocation

- **Mechanism of injury**: usually due to a fall leading to external rotation of the shoulder.
- **Clinical features**
  1. It is typical for the patient to hold the injured arm at the elbow with the other hand
  2. Arm is held in slight abduction
  3. Contour appears 'squared off'
  4. Extremely painful
- **X-ray view**: AP (Figure 1a) and axial (Figure 1b) or Y-scapular views assist in differentiating anterior from posterior dislocations.

Note: X-rays are essential from a medicolegal standpoint to exclude a coexisting fracture **prior to** manipulation and reduction (M&R). There is increasing evidence to suggest that atraumatic recurrent shoulder dislocations **do not need** pre-M&R x-rays. However, this is not widely accepted in orthopaedic circles.

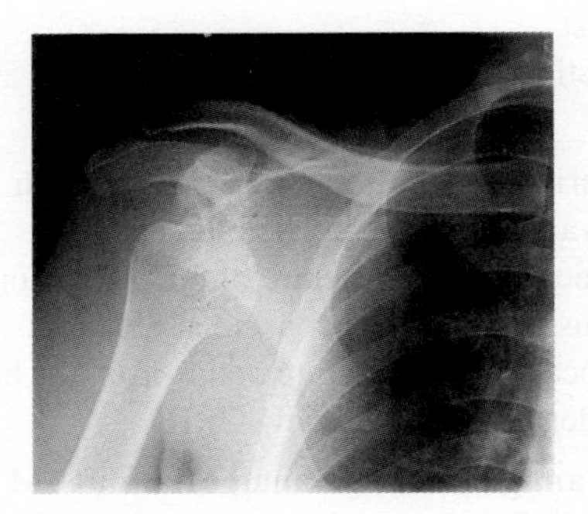

Figure 1a: AP view of shoulder showing anterior shoulder dislocation in the subcoracoid region

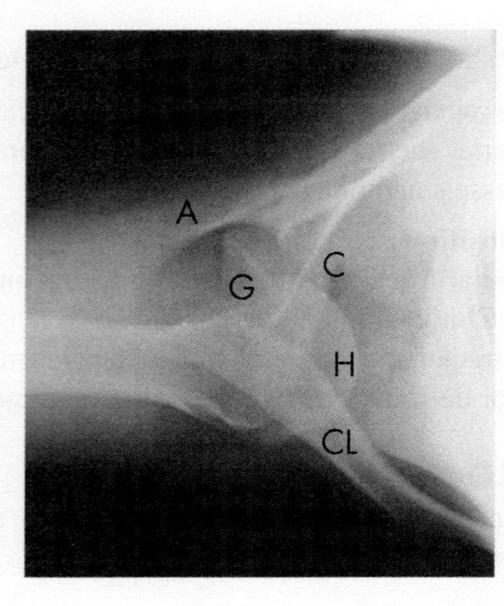

Figure 1b: Axial view of shoulder showing the anatomy of the shoulder

Note the locations of the acromion (A); coracoid (C); glenoid (G); clavicle (CL), head of humerus (H). The acromion and coracoid always point anteriorly. Hence, this x-ray confirms anterior dislocation of the head of humerus.

- **Complications**
  1. Recurrence

Note: Hill-Sachs lesion (compression fracture of the posterolateral aspect of the humeral head) may be seen in patients with previous anterior dislocation.

  2. Avulsion of the greater tuberosity (more common in patients >45 years)
  3. Fractures of anterior glenoid lip
  4. Damage to axillary artery and brachial plexus

Note: Must examine

1. axillary nerve function by checking pin prick sensation over deltoid or 'regimental badge' area
2. pulses at the wrist
3. radial nerve function

- **Treatment**
  1. Isolated anterior dislocation: M&R (for which there are multiple techniques available) under conscious sedation.
  2. Anterior dislocation with fracture of the greater or lesser tuberosities of the humerus: M&R under conscious sedation.
  3. Anterior dislocation with fracture of the proximal humeral shaft: admit for M&R under GA, keep in view ORIF.
- **Sequence of management**: IV analgesia, **not** IM (place IV plug in anticipation of M&R), then x-ray, followed by M&R under conscious sedation.

- **M&R**: traction techniques are preferred and some of the previously popular manipulation techniques are no longer favoured, eg Hippocratic/Kocher's manoeuvres. Traction should be performed in the critical or intermediate care areas where full monitoring can be achieved, with patient under conscious sedation (refer to *Conscious Sedation*).
  1. **Cooper-Milch technique**
     a. Under conscious sedation, place patient in supine position with elbow flexed at 90°.
     b. Extend elbow and very slowly move arm in to full abduction with sustained inline traction while an assistant applies gentle pressure on the medial and inferior aspect of the humeral head.
     c. Following relocation of the head of humerus, which can be almost imperceptible on occasions, adduct the arm gradually.
     d. Apply collar and cuff and order postreduction x-ray.
  2. **Stimson's technique**: a method that employs gravity and which is particularly useful when the ED is very busy.
     a. Administer IV analgesia with the patient lying in the prone position with arm hanging over the side of the trolley with 2.5 kg to 5 kg attached to the arm.
     b. Slowly, over a period of 5 to 30 minutes the gravitational force overcomes the muscle spasm and the shoulder relocates.
     c. Apply collar and cuff and order postreduction x-ray.
  3. **Countertraction technique**: useful as a back-up manoeuvre when either of the above fails.
     a. Under conscious sedation, place patient supine and place a rolled sheet under the axilla of the affected shoulder.
     b. Abduct the affected arm to 45° and apply sustained inline traction while an assistant applies traction in the opposite direction using the rolled sheet.
     c. After relocation, apply collar and cuff and order postreduction x-ray.
     d. **Disposition**: review in Orthopaedic Clinic within 3 days.
  4. **Spasso technique**: although this is not a widely known technique, it has been widely used in our department. We have found it to be one of the easiest methods to use and with high success rates.
     a. Under conscious sedation, bring the affected arm close to the chest wall.
     b. Forward flex the arm at the shoulder and externally rotate it simultaneously. Most of the time even before the shoulder reaches 90° forward flexion, a 'clunk' is heard and the head of the humerus relocates.
     c. Adduct the arm.
     d. Apply collar and cuff and order postreduction x-ray.

Posterior dislocation

- **Mechanism of injury**
  1. Usually due to a fall on the outstretched internally rotated hand or a direct blow to the front of the shoulder.

2. Associated with the violent muscle contractions of convulsions or electrical contact injuries.

- **Clinical features**
  1. The arm is held in internal rotation and adduction.

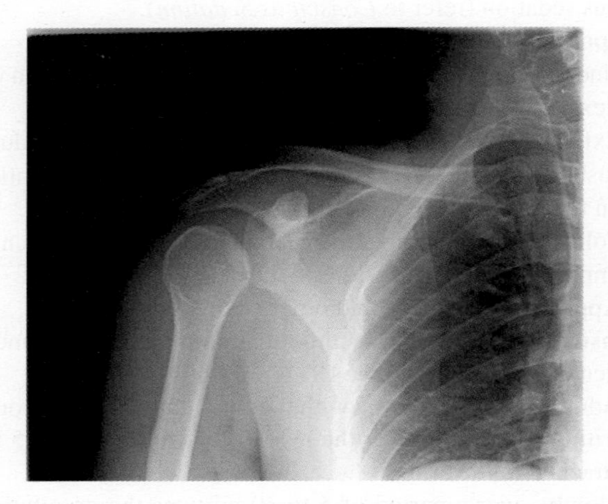

Figure 2a: Posterior dislocation of right shoulder
This view shows the 'light-bulb sign' due to internal rotation of the head of humerus. Note the lack of overlap between head of humerus and glenoid labrum on the AP shoulder view.

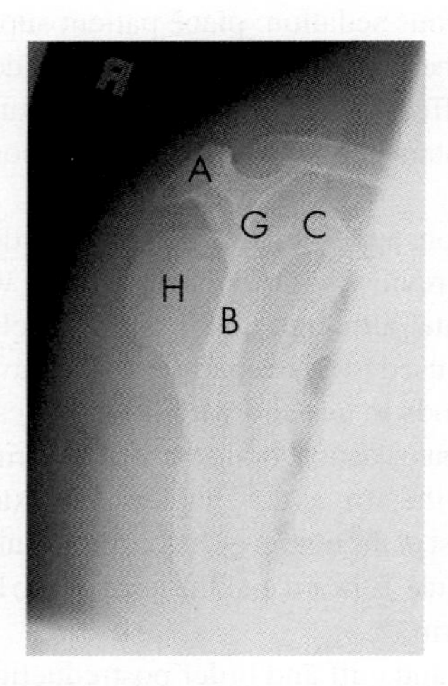

Figure 2b: Y-scapular view
The humeral head (H) is displaced away from the coracoid/chest and is hence a posterior dislocation. The Y is formed by the junction of the scapular blade (B), coracoid (C) and the acromion (A). Normally, the head of humerus should sit at the junction of the Y, which is the glenoid fossa (G).

2. Patient experiences pain and greatly decreased range of movement of the shoulder.

- **X-ray view**: AP (Figure 2a) and Y scapular views (Figure 2b).

Note: It is very easy to miss a posterior shoulder dislocation on the AP view (Figure 2a). Suspect posterior shoulder dislocation if the '**light-bulb sign**' due to internal rotation of the shoulder and the lack of overlap between the head of humerus and the glenoid labrum on AP shoulder view is seen.

- **Complications**: damage to axillary artery and brachial nerve.
- **Treatment**: similar principles as for anterior dislocations.
    1. For isolated posterior dislocation, attempt M&R under IV conscious sedation.
    2. For posterior dislocation with fracture of the tuberosities, attempt M&R under conscious sedation.
    3. For posterior dislocation with fracture of humeral shaft, admit for M&R under GA, keeping in view ORIF.
- **Technique**
    1. Under conditions of IV conscious sedation, apply traction to the arm in a position of 90° abduction.
    2. Sometimes countertraction by an assistant using a rolled sheet under the axilla is required.
    3. Then gently externally rotate the arm.
    4. After relocation in the first time dislocation in the young adult, apply strapping together with collar and cuff.
    5. After relocation in the elderly, apply collar and cuff keeping in view early mobilization.
- **Disposition**: review in Orthopaedic Clinic within 3 days.

Inferior dislocation

- **Mechanism of injury**: usually due to a fall with the arm in an abducted position.
- **Clinical features**
    1. Upper arm abducted with 'hand over head' position.
    2. Loss of rounded contour of shoulder.
- **X-ray view**: AP view is sufficient to make diagnosis.
- **Complications**: damage to axillary artery and brachial nerve.
- **Treatment**: similar principle to other dislocations.
    1. For dislocation with or without fracture of tuberosities, attempt M&R under IV conscious sedation.
    2. For dislocation with fracture of humeral neck, admit for M&R under GA, KIV ORIF.
- **Technique**
    1. Under conditions of IV conscious sedation, apply steady traction to the abducted arm.

2. Sometimes countertraction by an assistant using a rolled sheet placed over the acromion is needed.
3. After relocation, apply collar and cuff.

- **Disposition**: review in Orthopaedic Clinic within 3 days.

PROXIMAL HUMERAL FRACTURES

These fractures may involve the anatomical and surgical necks, either tuberosity, or various combinations.

- **Mechanism of injury**: usually due to a fall on the side, a direct blow to that area, or a fall on the outstretched hand.
- **Clinical features**
  1. Tenderness and swelling over the proximal humerus.
  2. Later, gross bruising gravitating down the arm.
- **X-ray views**: AP and lateral views of the humerus.
- **Complications**
  1. Adhesive capsulitis (frozen shoulder).
  2. Injury to neurovascular structures.
  3. Avascular necrosis humeral head.
- **Treatment**: apply collar and cuff.
- **Disposition**
  1. Severely displaced fractures of the greater tuberosity may require admission for ORIF under GA.
  2. Mildly displaced fractures can be discharged, to be reviewed in Orthopaedic Clinic within 3 days.

HUMERAL SHAFT FRACTURES

- **Mechanism of injury**: usually due to indirect force, such as a fall on the outstretched hand, or a direct blow to the area.
- **Clinical features**
  1. Local tenderness and swelling.
  2. Deformity may be present.
- **X-ray views**: AP and lateral views of the humerus.
- **Complications**: radial nerve palsy (drop wrist) and vascular compromise.
- **Treatment/disposition**
  1. For minimally angulated fracture, apply U slab; more easily done with patient seated on the trolley rather than in supine position, followed by collar and cuff, and review in Orthopaedic Clinic within 3 days.
  2. For severely displaced fractures, perform M&R under IV conscious sedation; apply U slab and collar and cuff, and review in Orthopaedic Clinic within 3 days.
  3. For cases complicated by neurovascular damage, admit to Orthopaedics.

Supracondylar humeral shaft fractures

- **Mechanism of injury**: a fall on the outstretched hand usually occurring in a child.
- **Clinical features**
  1. Tenderness and swelling over the distal humerus and elbow.
  2. Deformity may be present.
  3. The olecranon, and medial and lateral epicondyles preserve their isosceles triangle relationship.
- **X-ray view**: AP and lateral elbow views **(beware lateral condylar fracture: admit for ORIF)**. Look for the 'fat-pad' sign (Figure 3).
- **Complications**
  1. **Brachial artery damage**
     a. Check radial pulse and capillary refill.
     b. Look for pallor and coolness of the extremity, pain, paraesthesia or paralysis of forearm.
  2. Check fingers and thumb for neurological deficit due to radial, ulnar and median nerve involvement.

Note: Document the presence or absence of these features.

- **Treatment/disposition**
  1. If minimal displacement (<10–15°) exists, apply long arm backslab and review in Orthopaedic Clinic in 1–2 days. Give clear written instructions pertaining to signs of developing **compartment syndrome**.

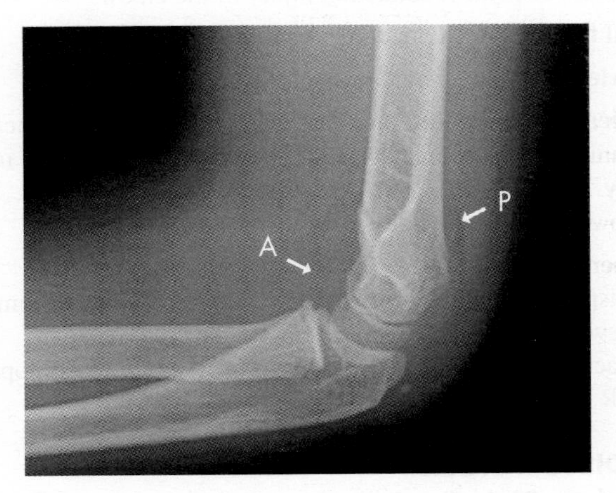

Figure 3: Lateral view of elbow showing anterior (A) and posterior (P) fat-pad sign

A visible anterior fat pad is normal, but the *displacement* of the anterior fat pad as is shown in (A) raises the strong possibility of a fracture. A visible posterior fat pad (P) is always abnormal because the posterior fat pad lies within the olecranon fossa. The 2 commonest causes are a supracondylar fracture of the humerus in a child or a radial head fracture in an adult although any intraarticular fracture can cause a 'fat-pad' sign.

2. If there is considerable swelling in the region of the elbow with a minimally angulated fracture, consider erring on the side of safety and admit a child overnight for observation of the circulation.
3. If displacement >15°, apply long arm backslab and admit for M&R.

MEDIAL EPICONDYLAR FRACTURE OF THE HUMERUS

- **Mechanism of injury**
  1. May be avulsed by the ulnar collateral ligament when the elbow is forcibly abducted.
  2. Avulsion due to sudden contraction of forearm flexor muscles.
  3. Direct trauma.
- **Clinical features**: local swelling and tenderness.
- **X-ray view**: AP and lateral views of the elbow.
- **Complications**: ulnar nerve injury treatment/disposition.
  1. If minimal or no displacement, apply long arm backslab and review in Orthopaedic Clinic within 3 days.
  2. If fracture is more severely displaced, admit for M&R under GA, keeping in view ORIF.

LATERAL CONDYLAR FRACTURE OF THE HUMERUS

Note: This is commonly missed as it could be confused with a supracondylar fracture!

- **Mechanism of injury**: adduction injury of the elbow.
- **Clinical features**: local tenderness and swelling.
- **X-ray view**: AP and lateral views of the elbow.
- **Complications**: no acute complications. The delayed complications are:
  1. Malunion and non-union causing cubitus valgus and tardy ulnar nerve palsy.
  2. Elbow stiffness especially in adults.
- **Treatment/disposition**
  1. Undisplaced or minimally displaced fractures, apply long arm backslab; review in Orthopaedic Clinic within 3 days.
  2. If fracture is displaced >2 mm or rotated, admit to Orthopaedics for M&R under GA, ORIF.

ELBOW DISLOCATIONS

- **Mechanism of injury**: usually due to a fall on the outstretched hand; posterolateral dislocation is the commonest.
- **Clinical features**
  1. Deformity of elbow with tenderness and swelling.
  2. The isosceles triangle relationship between olecranon, and medial and lateral epicondyles is disrupted (cf supracondylar fracture).
- **X-ray view**: AP and lateral views of elbow.

- **Complications**: injury to brachial artery, ulnar nerve or median nerve.
- **Treatment/disposition**: M&R under IV conscious sedation.
  1. With patient supine, apply traction in the line of the limb.
  2. Slight flexion of the elbow may be necessary while maintaining traction.
  3. After relocation, apply long arm backslab.
  4. If no evidence of neurovascular damage exists, review in Orthopaedic Clinic within 3 days.
  5. If even the mildest hint of neurovascular damage exists, admit to Orthopaedics for observation.
  6. Ensure the joint is truly reduced; x-rays can be really tricky.

'PULLED ELBOW' (SUBLUXED RADIAL HEAD)

- **Mechanism of injury**: usually occurs in a child aged 9 months–6 years, due to an abrupt pull on the outstretched hand, ie an axial or distracting force which pulls the annular ligament over the radial head.
- **Clinical features**
  1. The affected arm hangs limply.
  2. Child either complains of pain in the arm or refuses to use the arm.
  3. Local tenderness is evident over the proximal forearm.
  4. Pain is elicited by flexion of the elbow or supination of the forearm.
  5. No swelling or deformity is seen.
- **X-ray view**: not required in the classic scenario; **however**, if there is a history of a fall or a direct blow to the forearm, then order AP and lateral views of the elbow and forearm as clinically indicated.
- **Treatment/disposition**: manipulation without anaesthesia is the norm.
  1. Hold the hand of the affected arm in a 'hand-shaking' position with your other hand behind the elbow with thumb over the head of the radius.
  2. Gently, but firmly, impact the forearm in to the elbow, and forcibly supinate the arm or rapidly alternately pronate and supinate the forearm until an audible or palpable 'pop' is felt. No sling required since child will start to use the arm normally within 5–10 minutes.
  3. Should the above manoeuvre be unsuccessful, the arm should be rested in a sling, when spontaneous reduction usually occurs within 48 hours.
  4. **No referral** to Orthopaedic Clinic is required; simply, the parents and other family members need to be educated as to how to lift a child properly and to not pull the child by the hand or play 'helicopter' with him/her.

Olecranon fracture

- **Mechanism of injury**: usually due to a fall on the elbow, but may also result from a violent contraction of the triceps muscle.
- **Clinical features**: local tenderness and swelling/bruising over the olecranon.
- **X-ray views**: AP and lateral views of the elbow.

- **Treatment/disposition**
  1. If there is minimal or no displacement of the fracture, apply long arm backslab and refer to Orthopaedic Clinic for review within 5 days.
  2. If fracture is displaced, apply long arm backslab and admit for M&R under GA, keeping in view ORIF.

RADIAL HEAD/NECK FRACTURE

- **Mechanism of injury**: due either to a fall on the outstretched hand or to a direct blow on the forearm.
- **Clinical features**: local pain and tenderness, with swelling over the lateral elbow.
- **X-ray views**: AP and lateral views of the elbow.

Note: Occult fractures of the radial neck/head may **only** show a **'positive posterior fat-pad sign'** on the lateral film (Figure 3): always look specifically for this sign!

- **Treatment/disposition**
  1. If the fracture is undisplaced, apply long arm backslab and refer to Orthopaedic Clinic within 5 days.
  2. If the fracture is displaced, apply long arm backslab and admit to Orthopaedics for M&R under GA, keeping in view ORIF.

FOREARM FRACTURES

- **Mechanism of injury**: usually due to direct trauma, but may also result from a fall on the outstretched hand.
- **Clinical features**: tenderness and swelling of the forearm, with deformity if the fracture is displaced.
- **X-ray views**: AP and lateral views of the forearm.

Note: Ensure that the film includes the elbow and wrist so that a Monteggia or a Galeazzi fracture can be excluded. **Never** treat a single forearm bone fracture until you have excluded the above fracture-dislocations.

1. A **Monteggia** fracture-dislocation refers to **a fracture of the ulna** with dislocation of the radial head.

Note: Many legal suits resulted from a missed bowed (greenstick) ulna!

2. A **Galeazzi** fracture-dislocation refers to **a fracture of the radius** with dislocation of the inferior radio-ulnar joint.

- **Complications**: vascular injury or compromise with possible development of compartment syndrome
- **Treatment/disposition**
  1. For fractures with minimal or no displacement, apply long arm backslab and refer to Orthopaedic Clinic within 3 days.
  2. For displaced fractures, attempt M&R under a Bier block. Such attempts can be unsuccessful, whereupon apply long arm backslab and admit to Orthopaedics for ORIF.

COLLES' FRACTURE

- **Mechanism of injury**: usually due to a fall on the outstretched hand.
- **Clinical features**: characteristic 'dinner fork' deformity with local tenderness.
- **X-ray views**: lateral (Figure 4a) and AP (Figure 4b) views of the wrist.
- **Complications**: Malunion; delayed rupture of the extensor pollicis longus; median nerve compression; Sudeck's atrophy.
- **Treatment**
  1. Reduce under Bier's block (refer to *Pain Management*) if fracture is closed and not intraarticular.
  2. Requires monitoring of vital signs and ECG rhythm.
- **Reduction technique**
  1. Apply longitudinal traction to disimpact the fracture.
  2. Then apply flexion and ulnar deviation force to the fragment using finger and thumb or the ball of your thumb.
  3. Following reduction, apply short arm backslab with the forearm in pronation, and ulnar deviation and slight flexion at the wrist.
  4. If re-x-ray shows satisfactory reduction, apply sling and advise the patient to mobilize the shoulder, elbow and fingers of the affected arm.
- **Disposition**
  1. If reduction is satisfactory, refer to Orthopaedic Clinic within 2 days.
  2. If fracture is open or intraarticular, admit to Orthopaedics for M&R under GA or ORIF.

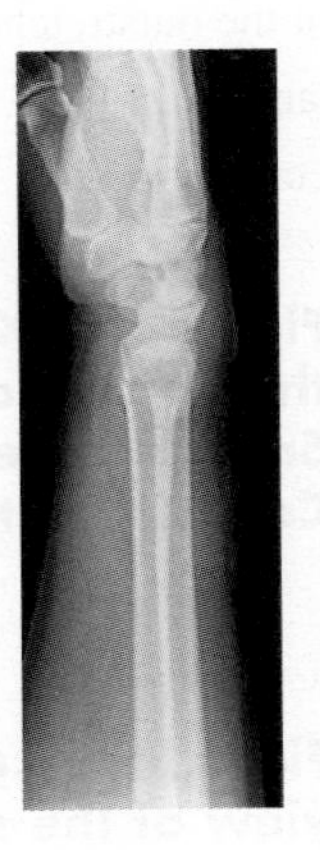

Figure 4a: Lateral view of wrist showing Colles' fracture

Note the posterior displacement of the distal fragment.

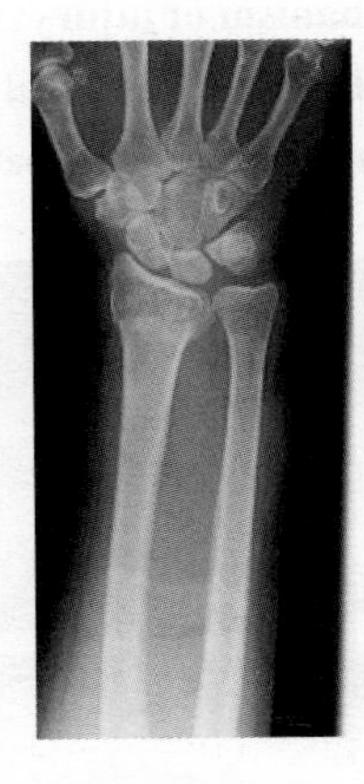

Figure 4b: AP view of wrist showing Colles' fracture

SMITH'S (OR REVERSE COLLES') FRACTURE

- **Mechanism of injury**: usually due to a fall on the back of the hand, with the distal fragment being tilted anteriorly.
- **Clinical features**: local tenderness, swelling, and deformity.
- **X-ray views**: AP (Figure 5a) and lateral views (Figure 5b) of the wrist.
- **Treatment**
  1. Reduce under Bier's block (refer to *Pain Management*) if fracture is closed and not intraarticular.
  2. Requires monitoring of vital signs and ECG rhythms.
- **Reduction technique**
  1. Traction with arm in supination until disimpaction is achieved.
  2. Apply dorsally-directed pressure to fragment.
  3. Apply a short arm volar slab with the forearm in full supination, wrist in dorsiflexion and the elbow in extension first. As this fracture is difficult to hold, a long arm backslab is applied after this with the elbow at 90° flexion.
- **Disposition**
  1. If reduction is satisfactory, refer to Orthopaedic Clinic within 2 days.
  2. If fracture is open or intraarticular, admit to Orthopaedics for M&R under GA or ORIF.

BARTON'S FRACTURE

This is a form of Smith's fracture in which only the anterior portion of the radius is involved.

- **Mechanism of injury**: usually due to a fall on the outstretched hand.
- **Clinical features**: local tenderness, swelling and deformity.
- **X-ray views**: AP and lateral views (Figure 6) of the wrist.

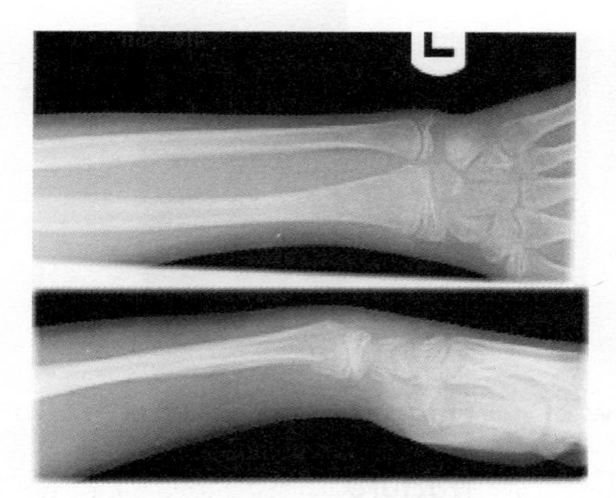

Figure 5a: X-ray of the wrist showing Smith's (reverse Colles') fracture

Figure 5b: Lateral view of the same fracture.

Note the anterior displacement of the fracture fragment.

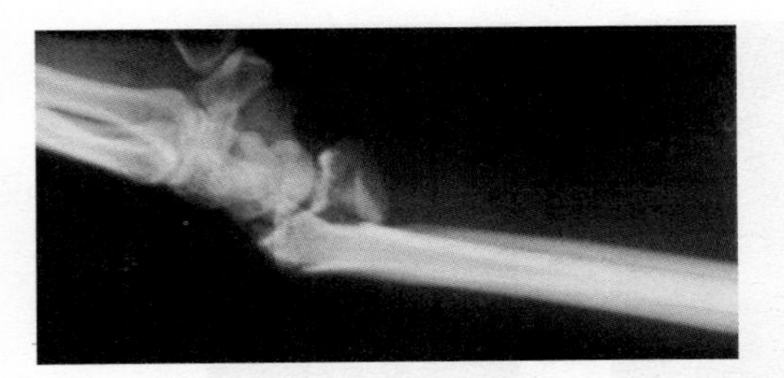

Figure 6: Lateral view of wrist showing Barton's fracture

- **Treatment/disposition**: apply short arm volar slab and admit to Orthopaedics for ORIF.

SCAPHOID (CARPAL NAVICULAR) FRACTURE

- **Mechanism of injury**
  1. Usually due to a fall on the outstretched hand.
  2. Occasionally due to 'kickback' when using a starting handle, pump or compressor.
- **Clinical features**
  1. Pain in the radial border of the wrist.
  2. Tenderness in the anatomical snuffbox and dorsal and ventral aspect of scaphoid.
- **X-ray views**: AP and lateral views of the wrist (Figure 7b), plus, **scaphoid views** (Figure 7a).

Note: Scaphoid views should be ordered in any patient with tenderness around the 'snuffbox' area.

- **Complications**: avascular necrosis/non-union/osteoarthritis/Sudeck's atrophy.
- **Treatment/disposition**
  1. In case of definite scaphoid fracture: apply scaphoid spica splint and review in Orthopaedic Clinic within 5 days.
  2. In cases where there is clinical suspicion of a scaphoid fracture but there is no x-ray substantiation of a fracture, apply scaphoid spica splint and review in Orthopaedic Clinic within 10 to 14 days.

LUNATE DISLOCATION

- **Mechanism of injury**: usually due to a fall on the outstretched hand.
- **Clinical features**: local tenderness and swelling.
- **X-ray views**: AP and lateral views of the wrist (Figure 8).
- **Complications**: median nerve palsy/avascular necrosis/Sudeck's atrophy.
- **Treatment**
  1. Reduction under Bier's block (refer to *Pain Management*).
  2. Requires monitoring of vital signs and ECG rhythm.

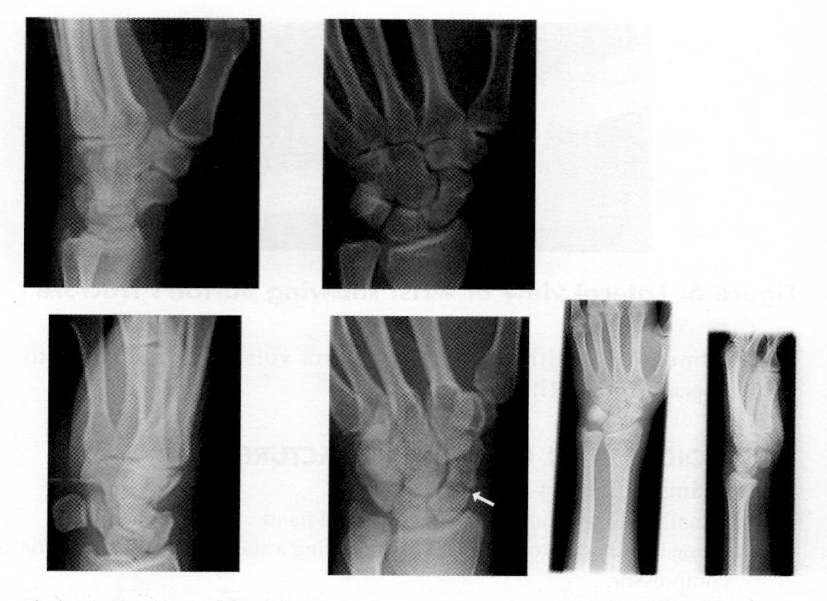

Figure 7a: Scaphoid views

Figure 7b: AP and lateral views of the wrist

Scaphoid views (a) showing fracture at waist of scaphoid indicated by arrow. Note that the fracture is not obvious on the standard AP and lateral views (b) of the wrist.

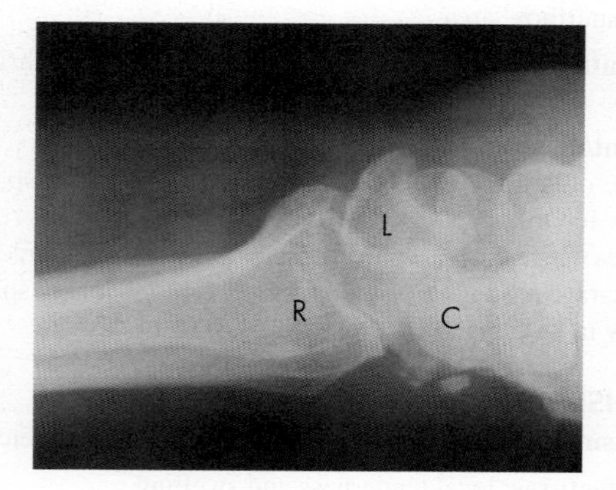

Figure 8: Lateral view of wrist x-ray showing lunate (L) dislocated anteriorly

The concavity of the lunate is empty. The radius (R) and capitate (C) remain in a straight line.

- **Reduction technique**
  1. Apply traction to supinated wrist.
  2. Extend the wrist, maintaining traction.
  3. Apply pressure with the thumb over the lunate.
  4. Flex the wrist as soon as you feel the lunate slip into place.
  5. Apply a short arm back slab in position of moderate flexion of the wrist.
- **Disposition**
  1. With successful reduction, review in Orthopaedic Clinic within 2 days.
  2. If reduction attempts are unsuccessful, apply backslab and admit to Orthopaedics for ORIF.

PERILUNATE DISLOCATION

- **Mechanism of injury/clinical features/x-ray views**: as above.
- Often associated with fracture of the scaphoid bone (Figure 9).
- **Treatment/disposition**: admit to Orthopaedics for ORIF.

METACARPAL FRACTURES

- **Mechanism of injury**: due either to a fall on the outstretched hand or to a direct blow on the hand.
- **Clinical features**: local tenderness, swelling, and deformity.
- **X-ray views**: AP and oblique views of the metacarpal.

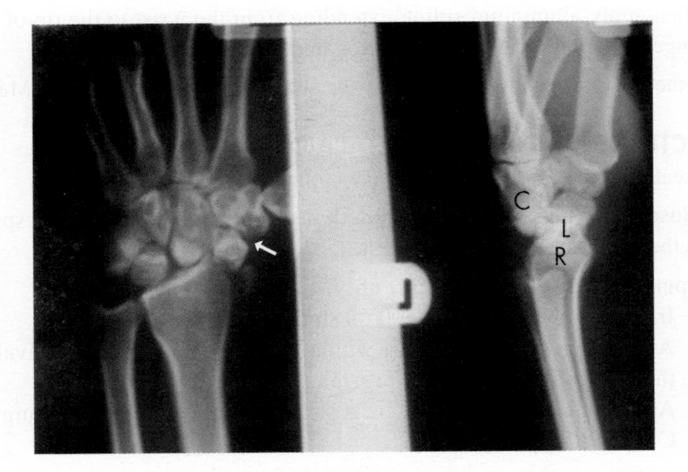

Figure 9: X-ray of the wrist showing a trans scapho-perilunate dislocation

The scaphoid fracture is indicated by an arrow. The whole carpus except the lunate (L) is displaced posteriorly. The concavity of the lunate is empty but the radius (R) and lunate remain in a straight line. The capitate (C) lies posteriorly and out of line.

- **Treatment/disposition**
  1. If the fracture is undisplaced, apply a short arm backslab and review in Orthopaedic Clinic within 2–3 days.
  2. If the fracture is displaced, attempt reduction under Bier's block, followed by application of a backslab. Review in Orthopaedic Clinic within 2–3 days.
  3. If the fracture involves the metacarpal neck, the splint should extend beyond the PIPJ with the MCPJ at 90° flexion. Review in Orthopaedic Clinic within 2–3 days.

BENNETT'S FRACTURE

This is a fracture of the thumb metacarpal, where there is a small medial fragment of bone which may tilt, but which maintains its relationship with the trapezium.

- **X-ray views**: AP and lateral views of the thumb metacarpal.

Note: The vertical fracture line involves the trapezo-metacarpal joint and there is proximal and lateral subluxation of the thumb metacarpal.

- **Treatment/disposition**: Apply scaphoid thumb spica backslab and admit to Hand Surgery for ORIF.

FRACTURES OF THE PROXIMAL AND MIDDLE PHALANGES OF FINGER(S)

- If the fracture is displaced, perform M&R under Entonox or digital block first.
- Then apply aluminium splint, extending from the wrist to the tip of the finger, with the MCPJ at 90° flexion and the IPJs extended.
- If the fracture is undisplaced, apply the aluminium splint without the M&R.

FRACTURES OF TERMINAL PHALANGES

- Treatment of soft tissue injury takes precedence.
- **Closed fractures**: no M&R required; just apply a short aluminium splint to the posterior aspect of the digit.
- **Open fractures (terminal tuft only)**
  1. Irrigate with a minimum 500 ml sterile saline.
  2. Administer IV cefazolin 1 g within 1 hour of the patient's arrival in the ED, before x-ray when possible.
  3. Apply a short aluminium splint posteriorly and review in Hand Surgery Clinic within 3 days.
- **Open fracture (shaft or base)**: administer IV antibiotics as above, apply dressing or aluminium splint and admit to Hand Surgery for ORIF.

References/further reading

1. McRae R. *Practical Fracture Treatment*. 2nd edition. Edinburgh: Churchill Livingstone; 1989.

105 Urolithiasis

JP Travers • Peter Manning

CAVEATS

- Ureteric colic causes patients to roll around rather than lie still.
- Most can be treated with conservative measures, ie increasing fluid intake.
- Give adequate analgesia using NSAIDS or opioid agonists.
- Obstructive uropathy and infection are urological emergencies and mandate admission.
- About 75–80% of stones will pass spontaneously.
- Contributing factors:
  1. Dehydration, high protein and high sodium diet.
  2. Essential hypertension.
  3. Hypercalciuria. Dietary calcium and oxalate does not enhance stone formation.
  4. Men are affected more frequently than women.
- Renal colic-like pain in a patient over 50 years of age, without a past history of kidney problems, might represent an abdominal aortic aneurysm leak or abdominal aortic dissection.

> ☛ **Special Tips for GPs**
> - Most kidney stones can be treated conservatively.
> - Loin to groin pain with haematuria is indicative of kidney stone.
> - Men with pain in the right iliac fossa have appendicitis until proven otherwise.
> - Always consider ectopic pregnancy in women and seek a menstrual history and urinary HCG.
> - Provide adequate analgesia with NSAIDs or opioid narcotics.
> - Renal stones with fever is an urological emergency and should be referred to hospital urgently!

DIFFERENTIAL DIAGNOSIS

See Table 1.

Table 1: Differential diagnosis of renal/ureteric colic
Appendicitis
Salpingitis
Diverticulitis
Pyelonephritis
Ovarian torsion
Prostatitis
Ectopic pregnancy
Bowel obstruction
Carcinoma

Lab tests evaluation

- Do urinalysis for microscopic haematuria. Note that the prevalence of microscopic haematuria in urolithiasis using urine dipstick tests was 95.4%. Thus, in the absence of haematuria with isolated right or left iliac fossa pain, alternative diagnosis to ureteric colic should be considered.
- If possible, do a complete blood count, especially in those with high fever. An elevated white blood cell count associated with fever indicates abscess or infection and is an urological emergency!
- Radiology: KUB and refer to urology clinic for IVU.

Treatment

- Increase fluid intake, which enhances stone dissolution. An adequate fluid intake of 3,000 to 4,000 ml per day is recommended (enough to produce at least 2 quarts of urine in every 24-hour period). Beware in elderly patients who might have a history of congestive heart failure.
- Citrate treatment chelates calcium to form a soluble complex.
- Dietary fibre may have an indirect effect in preventing real stones.
- For intense acute renal colic give prompt analgesia. NSAIDs like diclofenac inhibit prostaglandin-E2 production at the site of the obstruction. Narcotics such as Pethidine® may cause an increase in smooth muscle spasm, making pain worse. Both drugs, however, are relatively contraindicated in pregnancy and in nursing mothers. In pregnancy, stones are more easily passed because of the normal dilation of the ureter. Use allopurinol for uric acid stones.

Disposition

- Refer to urology for admission:
  1. Persistent pain in spite of analgesia
  2. Stone size >8 mm on KUB

3. Patient with known solitary kidney
4. Presence of infection, especially with obstruction

- Refer pregnant patients for early outpatient appointment.

References/further reading

1. Coe FL, Parks JH, Asplin JR. The pathogenesis and treatment of kidney stones. *NEJM*. 1992;327(16):1141–1152.
2. Curhan GC, Willett WC, Rimm EB, et al. A prospective study of dietary calcium and other nutrients and the risk of symptomatic kidney stones. *NEJM*. 1993;328(12): 833–838.
3. Jenkins AD. Upgrading extracorporeal shock wave lithotripsy. *Contemporary Urol*, Oct, 1991;11–12.
4. Lawson RK. Smaller means safer intraureternal electrohydraulic lithotripsy. *Contemporary Urol*, Oct, 1991;51–58.
5. Lingeman JE, et al. Kidney stones: Acute management. *Patient Care*, Aug 15 1990;20–42.
6. Lingeman, JE, et al. Kidney stones: Identifying the causes. *Patient Care*, Sep 30 1990;31–46.
7. O'Brien WM, Rotolo JE, Pahira JJ. New approaches in the treatment of renal calculi. *Am Fam Physician*. Nov 1987;181–194.
8. DeRuiter J. Renal disease, renal stones and UT obstruction. In: McPhee SJ, ed. *Pathophysiology of Disease: An Introduction to Clinical Medicine*. Norwalk, CT: Appleton & Lange; 1995:401–404.
9. Ooi SBS, Kour NW, Mahadev A. Haematuria in the diagnosis of urinary calculi. *Ann Acad Med Singapore*. 1998;27:210–214.

106 Wound care

Irwani Ibrahim • JP Travers • Shirley Ooi

CAVEATS

- **Good history** of events is important to determine possible associated injuries and degree of contamination, eg punch bite, high pressure injection injuries, crush injuries.
- Thorough examination for foreign bodies (FB), tendon function, neurovascular function, contamination and infection is essential.
- Wounds should be explored under **appropriate anaesthesia** for full assessment.
- **Do not** explore neck wounds in the ED, no matter how superficial they may appear.
- Document abnormalities or their **absence**. Photographs may be useful in certain cases, eg assault.
- The following cases should be **x-rayed (AP/lateral)**:
  1. All cases of wounds produced by glass.
  2. Selected cases to exclude open fractures, involvement of joint and exclusion of FB.
- Radioopaque markers (eg paperclip) taped to the wound may help identify the FB in relation to the wound.
- Wound swabs are **not** needed in fresh injuries unless associated with fractures.
- Haemorrhage should be controlled by direct pressure and elevation of the limb: **Do not** use artery forceps or tourniquets.
- **Never** shave an eyebrow.
- **Do not remove** large FBs embedded in the wound.
- **Do not** prescribe antibiotics in patients with normal immune status with little wound contamination.
- Antibiotics **cannot** substitute for good wound debridement.
- Take the opportunity to update the patient's tetanus status.

MANAGEMENT

- If haemorrhage is severe
  1. Secure the airway, breathing and circulation.
  2. Establish large bore IV line(s) and fluid resuscitate.
  3. GXM 2–4 units.
  4. Elevate and compress.

> ☛ **Special Tips for GPs**
> - Refer cases to the ED if unable to achieve a good wound debridement due to time constraint or non-sterile conditions.
> - Beware of innocuous wounds which look 'benign' but may have extensive tissue destruction, eg pressure jet injuries or crush injuries.
> - Beware the so-called 'simple' plantar puncture wound. It is anything but simple (see p. 509).

- **Technique**
  1. Wound cleaning is the most important part of wound care. Wounds should be cleaned with chlorhexidine solution **except** facial wounds (sterile normal saline).
  2. Wounds in hair-bearing areas should have the adjacent hair trimmed with scissors: shaving may predispose the wound to infection through epidermal damage.
  3. Remove all dirt and foreign material that is visible; deep wounds should be irrigated with **at least** 200 ml sterile normal saline.
  4. Local anaesthetic of choice is **1% buffered plain lignocaine**, used for direct infiltration and nerve blocks.
  5. **Explore wounds** when: (a) FB suspected and (b) history suggestive of deep damage with no clinical confirmation.
- **Methods of closure**: if in doubt, suturing is always the best option:
  1. **Steristrips**
     a. These are less painful to apply, and less likely to cause tissue ischaemia.
     b. Saves time.
     c. Suitable for children, flap lacerations in the elderly and skin closure where deep layer sutures have been placed.
     d. Inappropriate over joints
  2. **Tissue glue**
     a. Suitable for small cuts and lacerations in children and most suitable for lacerations which gape <3 mm.
     b. Technique: clean wound and achieve good haemostasis. Appose the wound edges and place the glue along the wound in a continuous line. Hold the edges together for at least 30 seconds to allow the glue to set. Do not place the glue into the wound as it acts as a foreign body.
  3. **Suture technique**
     a. Use 2-layered technique (subcutaneous and skin) in deep wounds to promote better wound healing.

b. Use absorbable sutures, eg Dexon or Vicryl for subcutaneous tissues: Trunk and extremities: 4/0; face: 5/0
c. Use non-absorbable sutures for the skin, eg Prolene or Silk: Scalp: 2/0 Silk; trunk and extremities: 4/0 Prolene; face: 6/0 Prolene
d. In general, one can use one size smaller suture in children and can remove them earlier.

- **Disposition**: consider **admission or referral**
  1. If the wound extends into muscle, is heavily contaminated or there is evidence of sensory or motor damage, or unable to ensure adequate debridement, admit to Orthopaedics.
  2. Admit all wounds with tendon damage. Those with injuries distal to the shoulder should be admitted to Hand Surgery. All others admit to Orthopaedics.
  3. Immunocompromised, eg diabetics, CRF and oncology patients.
  4. Large wounds: exceeding 30–60 minutes of theatre time.
  5. Refer special wounds, eg eyelid lacerations to Plastic Surgery.

WOUNDS NOT SUITABLE FOR PRIMARY CLOSURE

- Bites except face.
- Heavily contaminated wounds.
- Infected wounds.
- Wounds >12 hours old except face.

Wound care

- Wounds should be dressed with a non-adherent dressing, eg Tulle-gras.
- Dressing not necessary for facial and scalp wounds.
- The wound should be kept clean and dry for at least 48 hours after primary closure.
- Suture removal:
  1. Scalp: 7 days
  2. Face: 3–5 days
  3. Limbs: 10–14 days
  4. Trunk: 10 days
- Review contaminated wounds daily; clean wounds can be reviewed at 3–5 days.
- Consider **antibiotics prophylaxis**:
  1. Compound fingertip fractures.
  2. Bite wounds.
  3. Wounds in those at risk, eg valvular heart disease and post-splenectomy.
  4. Penetrating injuries not properly debrided.
  5. Wounds >6 hours old.
  6. Complex intraoral wounds.
  7. Workers at high risk, eg agricultural workers, fishermen.

8. Choice of antibiotics: cloxacillin and penicillin (commonest infecting organisms are *Staphylococcus aureus* and *beta-haemolytic streptococcus*) are cost-effective choices, or Augmentin®.

SPECIAL WOUNDS

Plantar puncture wounds

- Even though the wound looks innocuous, remember that the joints of the foot are not deep, hence joint penetration is a possibility with potential for serious infectious complications. The area from the metatarsal neck to distal toes are at highest risk for infection.
- The **complications** include:
  1. *Staph* and *Strep* soft tissue infections in the majority of patients
  2. Osteomyelitis (90% of osteomyelitis is due to *Pseudomonas aeruginosa)*
- Perform x-ray to exclude foreign body and joint penetration.
- The **management** of puncture wounds is **controversial**. The following are **guidelines** based on different clinical presentations:
  1. **Simple punctures**
     Usually with clean objects such as tacks, needles, small non-rusty exposed nails. If none of the following is seen, ie
     a. Indications of retained FB
     b. Dirty and devitalized wound edges, and
     c. Indurated or excessively tender puncture site skin cleansing and a small application of antibiotic ointment, followed by a Band-Aid should suffice.
     d. Administer tetanus prophylaxis.
  2. **Puncture with retained material**
     a. The puncture is often larger than the above mentioned. The wound edges are contaminated, stellate, or shredded appearing.
     b. Usually due to old nails, exposed bolts and unclean puncturing object that broke during the puncture, or possibly forced sock or shoe fragment into the wound.
     c. After providing anaesthesia, a transverse incision parallel to the wrinkle line of a curled foot is made through the puncture site and any FB is removed.
     d. Thorough irrigation is carried out.
     e. Do not suture the wound. Just apply antibiotic ointment and a Band-Aid.
     f. Administer tentanus prophylaxis.
     g. Use crutches for 2–3 days.
     h. Discharge with antibiotics, eg Augmentin®.
     i. Advise patient to look out for signs of infection.
     j. Review wound early.
  3. **Complicated punctures**
     a. Suspect retained foreign body if puncture site is infected.
     b. Do x-rays to exclude radioopaque foreign body.

c. Give IV broad-spectrum antibiotics, eg Unasyn® or Augmentin®.
d. Administer tetanus prophylaxis.
e. Admit for further management, ie surgical debridement.

Note:

- The use of **prophylactic antibiotics** in uninfected puncture wounds is not supported by clinical studies. They should only be considered in high-risk patients and wounds.
- Extensive coring or debridement of vital tissue, high-pressure irrigation, or deep probing has not been shown to improve outcome.

Flap wounds

- The blood supply of the flap wounds may be compromised, especially distally based flaps.
- Flap wounds are suitable for primary suturing if it occurs in the region of the face or in young patients where quality of the skin is good.
- The skin in the elderly is thin, hence the flap may die if sutured under tension. In this case the wound should be cleaned and apposed with steristrips and reviewed early. The method includes primary excision and grafting, especially if the flap is large.

Scalp wounds

- The scalp has the propensity to bleed to a degree sufficient to require fluid resuscitation. The best way to secure haemostasis of scalp wounds is to remove any gross contaminants and briefly cleanse the wound. Subsequently, use a 2/0 silk suture to take deep bites of all 5 layers of the scalp. This will almost invariably stop the bleeding. It is not necessary to suture or diathermize the bleeding point.
- It is not uncommon for scalp lacerations to be accompanied by large haematomas underlying the wound. These haematomas are potential sources for infection and must be removed prior to closure.
- Do not shave hair. Rather, trim it flush with the scalp. Shaving damages epidermis and hair follicles and may predispose wound to infection. Hair apposition technique (HAT) where hair on both sides of a laceration is apposed with a single twist and held with tissue adhesives is a new technique for treating scalp lacerations.

Eye wounds

- A complete eye examination including visual acuity is mandatory.
- X-ray of the orbits is needed if intraocular FB is suspected, such as when there is history of FB entry but no FB is seen on the surface of the cornea or when there is distortion of the shape of the iris.
- Lid lacerations which cross the lid margins, those through both surfaces of the lid, and those that may have damaged the lacrimal gland or duct

must be referred to Ophthalmology or Plastic Surgery, depending on institutional practice.

Nasal wounds

- Examine for septal haematoma. If present, urgent drainage will be needed.
- Do nasal bone x-ray to exclude fracture to determine the need of prophylactic antibiotics.
- Full thickness laceration will need careful layered suturing. If severe, should be referred to Plastic Surgery.
- The main principle is to **accurately** appose the junction between the skin and the mucosa.

Lip wounds

- It is of **utmost importance** to accurately align the vermillion border if the wound *crosses the junction of the lip and the skin.*
- Through and through wounds should be repaired in layers.

Tongue wounds

- Must check for embedded teeth.
- May consider x-rays to exclude FB.
- Minor wounds need not be repaired.
- Refer large bleeding wounds to Dental Surgery or Plastic Surgery.
- Use absorbable suture with short resorption time, eg catgut 5/0.

Ear wounds

- Give a ring block around the ear to provide anaesthesia.
- Determine if cartilage is involved as suturing is needed before skin closure.
- Always apply pressure (with ribbon gauze) bandage after toilet and suture to prevent subperichondrial haematoma from accumulating. If not, the patient may develop fibrosis and scarring ('cauliflower ear').
- Always give antibiotics and review in 1–2 days.

References/further reading

1. Trott A. *Wounds and Lacerations: Emergency Care and Closure.* St Louis: Mosby Year Book; 1991.
2. Wardrope J. *The Management of Wounds and Burns.* New York: Oxford University Press; 1992.
3. Wedmore IS, Charette J. Emergency department evaluation and treatment of ankle and foot injuries. In: Della-Giustina D, Coppola M, eds. *Emerg Med Clinics N Am.* 2000;18(1):108–109.
4. Ong MEH, Ooi SBS, Saw SM, et al. A randomized controlled trial comparing the hair apposition technique with tissue glue to standard suturing in scalp lacerations (HAT study). *Ann Emerg Med.* 2002;40:19–26.

Specific conditions in Paediatrics

107 Asthma, paediatric

Peng Li Lee

CAVEATS

- Not all wheezers are *asthmatic*.
- Consider the following age-specific differentials in a paediatric wheezer:
  1. **Infancy**: tracheooesophageal fistula, bronchomalacia, bronchopulmonary dysplasia, recurrent aspiration, heart failure, acute bronchiolitis, pneumonia.
  2. **1–5 year old**: acute bronchiolitis, inhaled solid objects, eg peanut (causing a ball-valve obstruction), croup.
  3. **School-age children**: asthma, adenovirus bronchitis.
- Role of **CXR**:
  1. Generally indicated in all first-time wheezers.
  2. Doubt about diagnosis of asthma, eg suspected foreign body inhalation.
  3. Clinical signs suggest pneumonia or pneumothorax.
  4. Response to treatment is abnormally slow or there is clinical deterioration.
  5. Persistent hypoxia or need for ICU care.
- Use of **steroids** in acute exacerbations:
  1. This issue has been very much debated in literature and studies and it involves the benefits of a hastened recovery with steroids versus their potential adverse effects on growth and adrenal function.
  2. General guidelines on the use of steroids:
     a. History of life-threatening asthma.
     b. Patients already on high dose inhaled steroids or low dose oral steroid.
     c. Patients requiring frequent β_2-agonist therapy in this current exacerbation.
  3. Dosage: **1–2 mg/kg/day** (max 40 mg) in 2 divided doses, for a duration of 3–5 days.

MANAGEMENT

See Figure 1 for management of acute asthma.

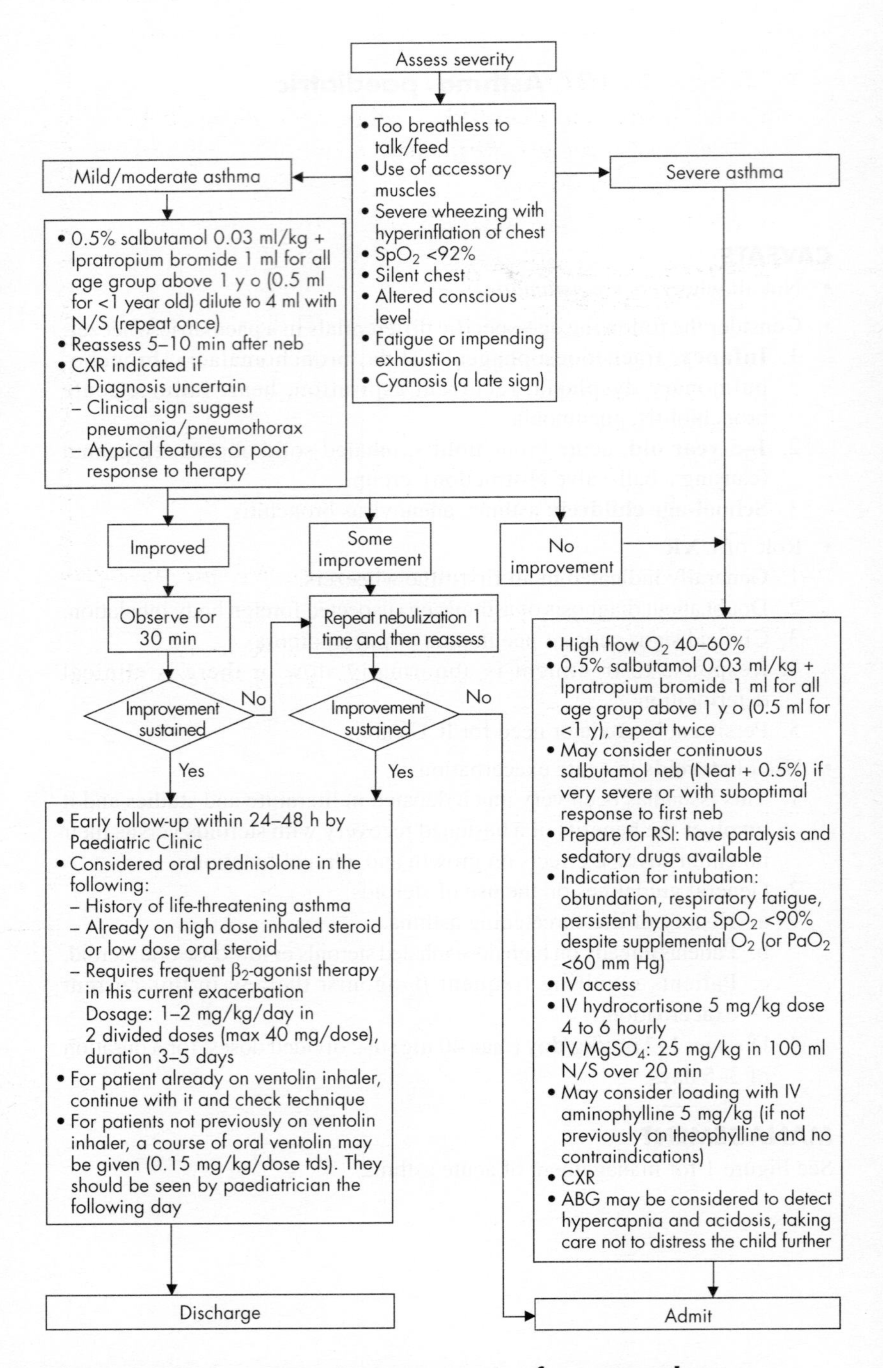

Figure 1: Emergency management of acute asthma

☛ **Special Tips for GPs**

- For all **first-onset paediatric wheezers**, be vigilant in looking for the **differentials** other than asthma, eg exclude foreign body ingestion in a toddler with atypical presentation of 'asthma' such as first onset of sudden wheezing, no preceding or accompanying URTI symptoms, no known history of atopy.
- Not all asthmatics are wheezers. Consider the diagnosis and treatment of asthma in patients who present with persistent cough that is especially worse at night, but who are otherwise well.
- Patients should be referred to hospital for further management if they do not respond after 2 ventolin nebs given in the clinic.

References/further reading

1. Murphy S, Kelly HW, eds. *Pediatric Asthma*. New York: M Dekker; 1999.
2. Hall JB, et al, eds. *Acute Asthma: Assessment and Management*. New York: McGraw-Hill; 2000.

108 Bronchiolitis

Peng Li Lee • Shirley Ooi

CAVEATS

- The term 'bronchiolitis' refers to a viral syndrome in infants (<2 y o) that is characterized by:
  1. Preceding history of common cold symptoms, eg cough, coryza for 2–3 days.
  2. Followed by lower respiratory tract symptoms: dyspnoea, wheezing, difficulty feeding and agitation from airway obstruction.
  3. **Clinical findings** include tachypnoea, nasal flaring, intercostal or subcostal retractions, prolonged expiration with rhonchi and creps, cyanosis.
- **Causative organisms**:
  1. RSV is the most common cause (50–90%)
  2. Parainfluenza, influenza, mumps, adenovirus, echovirus, rhinovirus, *Mycoplasma pneumoniae, Chlamydia trachomatis*

Note: Mycoplasma is the principal agent in school-age children with bronchiolitis.

- **Differential diagnosis**:
  1. Pneumonia
  2. Foreign body
  3. Gastroesophageal reflux
  4. Previously undiagnosed congenital heart disease with heart failure
  5. Previously undiagnosed anatomic abnormalities of airway, eg tracheooesophageal fistula
  6. Early asthma
- Identify **high risk group** for complications of apnoea and acute deterioration, eg:
  1. Premature infants with associated chronic lung disease or bronchopulmonary dysplasia
  2. Congenital heart disease
  3. Cystic fibrosis

MANAGEMENT

Most bronchiolitis cases are self-limiting. Careful monitoring for apnoea and hypoxia and good supportive care remain the cornerstones of management.

- Mandatory **SpO_2** reading: <92% indicate moderate to severe distress.
- Assess **hydration**: poor oral intake from breathlessness and cough-induced vomiting result in dehydration.

> ☛ **Special Tips for GPs**
> - Bronchiolitis is a short-lived, self-limited disease lasting a few days. If the patient is discharged, a follow-up within 24 hours is recommended.
> - Refer all patients with a history of prematurity, congenital heart disease, bronchopulmonary disease, underlying lung disease and compromised immune function for admission.

- Assess severity of **respiratory distress**:
  1. Mild: no retractions
  2. Moderate: intercostal retractions, no cyanosis
  3. Severe: cyanosis, apnoea, hypoxia (<92%), dehydration, severe intercostal retractions
- **CXR** is indicated in ill, atypical signs and difficult respiratory examination in crying infants.
- Indications for hospital **admissions**:
  1. Infants in high risk group (unless symptoms are very mild and parents are confident of managing patients at home).
  2. Young infants <4 months who are at risk of apnoea and rapid progression to more severe disease.
  3. Poor feeding, dehydration, agitation.
  4. Previously seen by several GPs during this current illness with potential worsening of condition especially within 3–4 days of onset of illness.
- Patients for **discharge**:
  1. If they are not in moderate or severe distress, able to feed and are well hydrated.
  2. Parents able to understand and recognize the signs of deterioration: poor feeding, agitation.
  3. Follow-up review in Paediatric Clinic in 1–2 days.

Supportive treatment

- Humidified oxygen therapy.
- Hydration (taking care not to overhydrate as well).

Specific treatment

- **Bronchodilators**:
  1. Often used but efficacy is debatable.
  2. No convincing evidence that they are effective, and in some cases may be associated with detrimental effects (hypoxia from increased V/Q mismatch especially if nebulized without oxygen).

3. In older infants in whom it may be difficult to distinguish bronchiolitis from other forms of virus-induced wheeze, a trial of bronchodilators is reasonable because a proportion of these patients do respond.
4. Generally avoid prescribing for patients who are discharged (alternatively mucolytics, eg bisolvon, may be a better choice).

- **Steroids**: no consistent role in bronchiolitis management in the acute stage.
- **Antibiotics**:
  1. Not indicated routinely unless dual infection is suspected (eg RSV and a bacterial infection) but this is uncommon.
  2. Avoid empiric use of outpatient antibiotics. For patients in whom antibiotics are required, hospital admission should be considered.
- **Ribavirin** is not routinely used but may have a role in selected high risk patients.

References/further reading

1. Everard ML. Acute bronchiolitis and pneumonia in infancy resulting from RSV. In: Taussig LM, Landau LI, LeSouef P, et al, eds. *Pediatric Respiratory Medicine*. St Louis: Mosby; 1998:585–590.
2. Finberg L. Lower respiratory infections. In: Finberg L, Kleinman RE, eds. *Saunders Manual of Pediatric Practice*. 2nd ed. Philadelphia: WB Saunders; 2002:315.
3. Connors K. Bronchiolitis. In: Strange GR, et al. *Pediatric Emergency Medicine: A Comprehensive Study Guide*. New York: McGraw-Hill; 1996:176–180.

109 Febrile fit

Elizabeth Khor • Peter Manning

DEFINITIONS

Diagnostic criteria for febrile fits

- First fit experienced by the child is associated with a temperature of >38° and is usually within the first 24 hours of illness, often as the temperature is rapidly increasing.
- Child is between 6 months and 6 years old.
- No evidence of CNS infection or inflammation.
- No acute systematic metabolic disorder.

Benign febrile fit

- If the fit lasts <15 min.
- The fit does not have significant focal features.
- The fit does not occur in a series with a total duration of >30 min.

Complex febrile fit

- If the febrile fit is longer in duration than a benign febrile fit and with focal features.
- If the fits occur in prolonged series.

CAVEATS

- 4% of normal children between 6 months and 6 years of age will experience a febrile fit.
- Recurrent fits are more likely if a family history exists of febrile fits or if the first febrile fit occurs at >1 year of age.
- Drug history: a Maxolon®-induced oculogyric crisis may mimic a febrile seizure and has a totally different management, ie IM/IV benztropine (Cogentin®).
- Remember to note allergy history prior to the administration of rectal panadol or Voltaren®.
- Note child's posture and temperament:
  1. Opisthotonic posturing in a drowsy child suggests increased intracranial pressure.
  2. An irritable child who is difficult to examine may have meningeal irritation: note that there is a difference between true irritability and the 'crankiness' exhibited by a child who feels unwell.

3. A child with postictal paralysis is more likely to have abnormal neurological signs.

- Remember that **neck stiffness may be absent** in infants or is difficult to elicit in uncooperative children.
- Cyanosis may indicate airway obstruction or aspiration.
- Remember to palpate the **fontanelle** in infants and record the findings.
- Remember to assess for hepatomegaly, which is common in children with sepsis or Reye's syndrome.

> ☛ **Special Tips for GPs**
> - Refer all cases of first febrile fit to the ED.
> - Give antipyretic and do tepid sponging before referring the patient to the ED.

MANAGEMENT

Child actively fitting

- Secure airway.
- Administer supplemental oxygen by mask.
- Administer IV diazepam 0.1–0.25 mg/kg at a rate no faster than 2 mg/minute **or** administer rectal diazepam (Valium®/Stesolid®). This route is more suitable for the GP office:
  1. 5 mg >1 year of age
  2. 2.5 mg for infants

Note: If the fit has exceeded 30 minutes in duration treat as febrile status epilepticus including IV phenytoin infusion in normal saline at 20 mg/kg/body weight at a rate not exceeding 50 mg per minute under ECG monitoring.

- Monitoring: ECG, pulse oximetry.
- Establish peripheral IV line.
- Labs: Stat capillary blood sugar, screen urea/electrolytes/creatinine, ionized calcium and magnesium.
- Measure and record temperature and pulse rate.

Child not fitting

- Measure pulse rate and temperature: if temperature is >38.5°C, administer antipyretics or tepid sponge.
- Administer supplemental oxygen by mask if cyanosis present.
- Consider performing a urinalysis (UC9) to exclude occult UTI.

DISPOSITION

Admission criteria

- First febrile fits since most parents or caregivers are too 'stressed out' to cope at home.
- Suspicion of intracranial or metabolic disease.
- The child has had more than one fit during the current illness.
- Febrile status epilepticus.
- History of recent head injury (within 72 hours).

Discharge criteria

- Hospitalization may not be necessary if **all** the following criteria are met:
  1. Brief (<15 minutes) simple febrile seizure with full recovery and no abnormal neurological signs. This means that when you review the child one hour later, the child behaves normally and can talk, walk or run about the room.
  2. The child is above 2–3 years of age (as it is easier to examine older children, and you are more confident of your clinical signs).
  3. The seizure occurred within the first 24 hours of fever.
  4. You are confident that the cause of the fever is viral in origin (ie you have excluded meningitis, otitis media, pneumonia and that the child is not septic).
  5. The parents are trustworthy, calm and willing to observe the child closely at home, and outpatient follow-up has been arranged within the next 24–48 hours.
  6. You have given clear instructions on how to administer antipyretics and rectal Stesolid (Note: Do not prescribe NSAIDs for more than 48 hours).

  Occasionally, a parent who reports that the patient or siblings have had similar febrile seizures in the past may choose not to admit the child. It is your responsibility that the above six criteria are met before you discharge the patient.

References/further reading

1. Green M, Haggerty RJ, Weitzman M, eds. *Ambulatory Pediatrics*. 5th ed. Philadelphia, PA: WB Saunders; 1999.
2. Barkin RM, Caputo GL, Jaffe DM, et al, eds. *Pediatric Emergency Medicine Concepts and Clinical Practice*. 2nd ed. St. Louis: Mosby; 1997.
3. Reisdorff EJ, Roberts MR, Wiegenstein JG. *Pediatric Emergency Medicine*. Philadelphia, PA: WB Saunders; 1993.

110 Non-accidental injury in paediatrics

Chong Chew Lan

CAVEATS

- **WHO definition**: child abuse or maltreatment constitutes all forms of physical and emotional ill-treatment, sexual abuse, neglect or commercial or other exploitation, resulting in actual or potential harm to the child's health, survival, development or dignity in the context of a relationship of responsibility, trust or power.
- There is a need to consider the culture, attitudes and values prevalent in the society at a given time to diagnose non-accidental injury (NAI). Types of NAI:
  1. Physical abuse
  2. Emotional abuse
  3. Neglect and negligent treatment
  4. Sexual abuse
  5. Exploitation

> ☛ **Special Tips for GPs**
> - Maintain a very high index of suspicion and refer early.
> - Knowledge of the developmental milestones of a child is useful in detecting suspicious history, eg one-month-old infant rolling off the bed and sustaining a skull fracture.

DIAGNOSIS

Diagnosis requires a **high index of suspicion** and is based on a combination of medical findings that are unexplained, implausible and inconsistent with the history obtained, patterns of injury that suggest abuse, and certain characteristics and behaviour of the child and family.

Social indicators of NAI

- **Abused child**
  1. Was unwanted
  2. Was separated from mother soon after birth
  3. Poor bonding with parents
  4. Is a disappointment, whether because of sex or a defect
  5. Is highly irritable and demanding
  6. Is difficult to manage because of illness
  7. Is different from the rest of family

- **Abusive parents**
  1. Were abused or experienced family disruption in their childhood
  2. Lack family support and are unreasonably fearful of caring for their child
  3. Lack parenting skills and/or knowledge of child development, having unrealistic expectations
  4. Have poor impulse control and are generally rigid and authoritarian
  5. Were teen parents
  6. Abuse alcohol and/or other substances
  7. Have physical or mental illness
- **The family**
  1. Has employment and financial stress
  2. Has marital conflict and domestic violence
  3. Experiences crises due to stressful events, eg death in family, recent move, fighting, etc
  4. Loneliness or isolation of mothers when their partners have left or are working away from home; heavy childcare responsibility
  5. Experiences geographic isolation, lack of transportation and lack of social support

Clinical features

- Vague, inconsistent, contradictory, inadequate or implausible story of child's injury.
- Delay in seeking medical attention.
- Inappropriate parent or caregiver response.
- Child is not immunized.
- Failure-to-thrive with or without developmental delay.
- Child with poor hygiene, dental and gum disease and untreated sores.
- Sexual behaviour beyond the child's years and supposed knowledge.
- Multiple injuries of different age.
- Bruises or burns with patterns, eg 3 or 4 oval bruises suggestive of a slap on the face or a grasp around a limb.
- Bruises to padded areas like buttocks, breasts, lower abdomen or medial aspect of both thighs.
- Circular marks around wrists or ankles suggestive of use of physical restraints.
- Injuries to genitalia associated with a vague history.
- Head injuries with vague history.
- Subdural haematoma associated with bilateral retinal haemorrhages in an infant, suggestive of **shaken baby syndrome**.
- Metaphyseal corner fractures, sternal fractures, posterior rib fractures and spiral fractures of long bones in non-ambulatory child.

- Scalds of lower limbs and abdomen with no splash marks or glove and stocking or doughnut pattern, suggestive of immersion burns.
- Cigarette burn marks.
- Sexually transmitted disease in children.
- Need to exclude diseases which may present like NAI, eg osteogenesis imperfecta, haemophilia and idiopathic thrombocytopaenia, Ehlers-Danlos syndrome.

Munchausen Syndrome by Proxy (MSP)

Warning signs:

- Illness is unexplained, prolonged or extremely rare.
- Signs and symptoms have a temporal association with the mother's presence.
- Treatment prescribed is ineffective and not tolerated.
- Other siblings may be similarly affected and there has been NAI or unexplained death of other children.

MANAGEMENT

- When child abuse is suspected, the child should be referred to a paediatric specialist centre according to local protocols.
- **Admission** is recommended. This gives an opportunity for a more thorough history taking and physical examination while the child is in a safe environment. Admission facilitates appropriate investigations and thorough assessment of the child and the family.
- Be firm and polite, and be honest with the parents about the concerns raised by the child's injuries and his/her future well-being.
- If the child's safety is in danger or the parents are uncooperative and insist on discharging the child against medical advice, the medical staff can seek social services or police assistance to authorize the detention of a child in the hospital (gazetted as place of safety).
- Admit the child to the department responsible for treating his presenting medical problem, eg orthopaedic surgery for fracture. These children should then be referred to the paediatrician on-call on the day of admission of the child. The paediatrician and his/her team of doctors will be responsible for the overall management of the child in the hospital and the subsequent follow-up medical care.
- **Alleged child sexual abuse**:
  1. Female victim will be referred to the gynaecologist on call and be seen at the ED as soon as possible. A paediatric surgeon will usually examine the male victim, though evaluation should follow local protocols.
  2. Keep interview and medical examination to a minimum to avoid contamination of evidence and traumatization of the child.

- The police has the primary responsibility in documenting the photographic evidence of all injuries. They should be informed as soon as possible.
- **Keep good notes.**

References/further reading

1. Bechtel K. Identifying the subtle signs of pediatric physical abuse. *Ped Emerg Med Reports*. 2001;6(6):57–67.
2. Singapore Ministry of Health. Responding to Child Abuse and Neglect: Guidelines for the Recognition and Management of Child Abuse and Neglect. Oct 2000;1–31.

111 Trauma, paediatric

Chong Chew Lan

CAVEATS

- Children with multisystem injuries can deteriorate rapidly and develop serious complications.
- The unique anatomical characteristics of children require special consideration in assessment and management.
- The paediatric skeleton is more pliable and therefore internal organ damage is often noted without overlying fractures. For the same reason, the presence of rib fractures in a child suggests high impact injury and multiple, serious organ injuries should be suspected.
- Be aware of the possibility of **non-accidental injury** as a cause of the injuries seen.

> ☛ **Special Tips for GPs**
>
> - Remember the ABCs. Open and maintain airway **with cervical control**. Then give high-flow oxygen if the child is spontaneously breathing. Otherwise, start bag-valve-mask ventilation.
> - If possible, obtain venous access with a 22G canula before the arrival of the ambulance.
> - Call for ambulance as soon as possible.

MANAGEMENT

Airway

- Orotracheal intubation under direct vision with adequate immobilization and protection of cervical spine.
- Preoxygenate before attempting to intubate.
- Use **uncuffed endotracheal tubes (ETT)** for intubation in children. The size of the ETT can be estimated by approximating the diameter of the external nares or the child's little finger. Refer to *Paediatric Drugs and Equipment* for further details.
- **Atropine** (0.1–0.5 mg) should be given prior to intubation to prevent bradycardia during intubation.

- When airway access and control cannot be accomplished by bag-valve-mask or orotracheal intubation, needle cricothyroidotomy is the preferred method. Surgical cricothyroidotomy is rarely, if ever, indicated.

Breathing

- Respiratory rate (RR) in the child decreases with age:
  Infant: 40–60 breaths per minute
  Older child: 20 breaths per minute
- Overzealous ventilation with high tidal volume and airway pressure can result in iatrogenic bronchoalveolar injury. Tidal volume: 7 to 10 ml/kg.
- Pleural decompression is done with tube thoracostomy, as in the adult, at 5th intercostal space, anterior to the midaxillary line. Chest tubes are placed into the thoracic cavity by tunnelling the tube over the rib above the skin incision site.

Circulation

- The increased physiologic reserves of the child allows maintenance of most vital signs in the normal range, even in the presence of severe shock. **The earliest sign of hypovolaemic shock is tachycardia and poor skin perfusion**. A 25% decrease in circulating blood volume is required to manifest the minimal signs of shock:
  1. Tachycardia
  2. Poor skin perfusion
  3. Decrease in pulse pressure
  4. Skin mottling
  5. Cool extremities compared to torso skin
  6. Decreased level of consciousness with dulled response to pain
  7. Decrease in blood pressure
  8. Poor urine output
- Hypotension in the child represents a state of uncompensated shock and indicates severe blood loss of >45% of the circulating blood volume. Tachycardia changing to bradycardia often accompanies this hypotension and is an ominous sign:
  SBP = 70 + (2× age in yrs)
  DBP = 2/3 × SBP

Fluid resuscitation

- Fluid resuscitation in the child is based on the child's weight. The quickest and easiest method of determining the appropriate fluid volume and drug dosages is with the **Broselow resuscitation measuring tape**.
- For **shock**, a **fluid bolus of 20 ml/kg of warmed crystalloid** solution is given. It may be necessary to give a total of 3 boluses of 20 ml/kg of fluid to replace the lost 25% blood volume. **When giving the third bolus of fluid, consider giving 10 ml/kg of type specific blood. Refer stat to a surgeon if there is no improvement after the first bolus of fluid**.

- The **sites** for **venous access** in children, in order of preference, are:
  1. Percutaneous peripheral (2 attempts)
  2. Intraosseous (children ≤6 years of age)
  3. Venous cutdown: saphenous vein at the ankle
  4. Percutaneous placement: femoral vein

  Intraosseous infusion should be discontinued when suitable peripheral access has been established. The preferred site for intraosseous cannulation is the anteromedial surface of the proximal tibia, 2 cm below the tibial tuberosity. This site is unsuitable if it is distal to a fracture site; cannulation can then be performed at the distal femur. Urinary output in adequately resuscitated patients should be 1–2 ml/kg/h.

MANAGEMENT OF SPECIFIC INJURIES

Chest trauma

- Chest injury is a marker for other organ injury since more than two-thirds of children with chest injury also have other organ system injury.
- Rib fractures represent an additional marker for a severe injuring force.
- The specific injuries and their management are identical to those for adults.

Abdominal trauma

- Penetrating abdominal injury dictates the prompt attention of the surgeon.
- Abdominal assessment in children with blunt trauma may be difficult as they are unlikely to cooperate, especially when frightened by the preceding trauma.
- Gastric and urinary decompression may facilitate evaluation.
- Diagnostic aids include:
  1. **Computed tomography (CT)**
     a. Useful in the haemodynamically normal or stabilizing child.
     b. Should be done with double or triple contrast.
     c. Usually requires sedation.
     d. Should not delay further treatment.
     e. Allows for precise identification of injuries.
  2. **Diagnostic peritoneal lavage (DPL)**
     a. Used to detect intraabdominal bleeding in the haemodynamically abnormal child.
     b. Warmed saline solution in volumes of 10 ml/kg (up to 1,000 ml) is run in over 10 min.
     c. Retroperitoneal organ injuries cannot be reliably detected.
     d. Definition of positive lavage is the same for children and adults.
     e. But the presence of blood in the peritoneum does not by itself mandate laparotomy.
     f. Should be performed by the surgeon in the child.

3. **Focused Assessment using Sonography in Trauma (FAST)**
   a. Few studies on the efficacy of ultrasound in the child have been reported.
   b. Selective, non-operative management of children with blunt abdominal injuries is performed in many trauma centres. It has been well demonstrated that bleeding from an injured spleen, liver and kidney is generally self-limiting.
   c. These children should be monitored closely in intensive care with frequent, repeated examination by the surgeon.

Head trauma

- Management is the same as in adults. The GCS is useful. However, the verbal score component must be modified for children. Paediatric verbal score:

Verbal Response	*V score*
1. Appropriate words or social smile, fixes and follows	5
2. Cries, but consolable	4
3. Persistently irritable	3
4. Restless, agitated	2
5. None	1

- As in the adult, hypotension is rarely, if ever, caused by head injury alone, and other causes of hypotension should be excluded. Infants may, albeit infrequently, become hypotensive from blood loss into either the subgaleal or epidural space. This occurs because of open cranial sutures and fontanelle in infants.
- Adequate and rapid restoration of an appropriate circulating blood volume is imperative and hypoxia must be avoided.
- In a young child with open fontanelle and mobile cranial suture lines, signs of an expanding mass may be hidden until rapid decompensation occurs. Therefore, an infant who is not in coma, but who has a bulging fontanelle or suture diastasis, should be treated as having severe head injury.
- Vomiting, seizures and even amnesia are more common in children after head injury. Investigate the child with persistent or worsening vomiting or recurrent seizures with head CT scan.
- **Drugs** frequently used in children with head injury include:
  1. Phenobarbital 2–3 mg/kg
  2. Diazepam 0.25 mg/kg, slow IV bolus
  3. Phenytoin 15–20 mg/kg, administered at 1 mg/kg/min as a loading dose, then 4–7 mg/kg/day for maintenance
  4. Mannitol 0.5–1.0 g/kg (rarely required). This may worsen hypovolaemia and should be withheld early in the resuscitation of the child with head injury

Spinal cord injury

- Spinal cord injury in children is fortunately uncommon.
- Children suffer **s**pinal **c**ord **i**njury **w**ith**o**ut **r**adiographic **a**bnormalities (**SCIWORA**) more commonly than adults. Normal spine radiographs can be found in up to two-thirds of children with spinal cord injury. Therefore, **normal spine x-rays do not exclude significant spinal injury**.
- Spinal cord injury is treated the same way as injuries occurring in adults. For non-penetrating spinal injuries within 8 hours of the injury, methylprednisolone is given at 30 mg/kg within the first 15 min, followed by 5.4 mg/kg per hour for the next 23 hours.

References/further reading

1. Committee on Trauma of the American College of Surgeons. *Advanced Trauma Life Support for Doctors Manual*. 6th ed. Chicago: American College of Surgeons; 1997:201–202.
2. Singapore Ministry of Health. A Guide on Paediatrics. 1997:181.

Miscellaneous useful information

112 Administration of blood products in the ED

Irwani Ibrahim • Peter Manning

CAVEATS

- It should be emphasized that blood and blood products should be administered only when they are clearly indicated and that safer alternatives should be used whenever possible. Replacement therapy should consist only of the component that the patient needs, administered in the smallest volume possible.
- The following **precautions** should be taken:
  1. The first 2 units of whole blood or red cell concentrates may be administered direct from the refrigerator. Warming is necessary when large volumes are given rapidly, ie at rates >50 ml/kg/h. In these cases, blood should only be warmed as it passes through the infusion set.
  2. Blood components must be transfused through standard blood filters designed to retain blood clots and other debris. The exceptions are platelets and cryoprecipitate that should be transfused using the respective infusion sets provided.
  3. In general, blood should **not be transfused** through infusion sets used for other fluids. Some may cause haemolysis (eg **5% dextrose in water**) and others clotting (eg **Hartmann's solution**). Only normal saline may be used for flushing infusion sets for blood transfusions. No medication or intravenous solutions other than normal saline may be added to blood or components.
  4. Flow at high pressure or through small gauge needles may damage red cells. 18/19G needle gives good flow rates.
- During the administration of blood products a close watch is kept on the patient for the earliest signs of transfusion reaction (see below).

BLOOD AND BLOOD PRODUCTS

Whole blood

- In patients with acute blood loss, the restoration of blood volume is more important than red cell replacements. Crystalloids and/or colloids can be used initially in these circumstances, reducing the need for blood transfusion.
- **Indications for whole blood transfusion**:
  1. Acute haemorrhage (despite normal haemoglobin and haematocrit levels)

Note: Following acute blood loss, haemoglobin (Hb) and haematocrit (Hct) may remain normal or nearly normal for an hour or more. Loss of

Table 1: Patient groups at risk from intravascular volume depletion
1. Patients at risk of myocardial ischaemia
2. Coronary artery disease
3. Valvular heart disease
4. Congestive cardiac failure
5. Patients at risk of cerebral ischaemia
6. History of transient ischaemic attacks
7. Previous thrombotic strokes

Table 2: Signs and symptoms requiring blood transfusion in normovolaemic patients at risk
1. Syncope
2. Dyspnoea
3. Postural hypotension
4. Tachycardia
5. Angina
6. Transient ischaemic attack

approximately 20% of blood volume can safely be corrected by crystalloid solutions alone.

2. Blood loss exceeds 25% of the total blood volume.
3. At risk patients (Table 1) developing signs and symptoms (Table 2).

Red blood cells

- **Indications for transfusions of red blood cells**:
  1. Slow continuous blood loss
  2. Acute and chronic leukaemia
  3. Chronic anaemia due to bone marrow failure, uraemia and severe symptomatic iron deficiency or megaloblastic anaemia
- The patient's condition, **not** laboratory test results, is the most important factor in determining transfusion needs.
- Whole blood is **contraindicated in patients with chronic anaemia** because of risk of overload.
- **One unit of red cells** should **raise** the non-bleeding **adult Hb** by about **1 g/dl** and the **Hct** by about **3%**.

Platelets

- **Indications for platelets transfusions**:
  In clinically stable patients with low platelet count, **platelet transfusions are indicated** in:

1. Severely thrombocytopaenic patient in whom life-threatening haemorrhage is occurring or is likely, usually platelet count less than 20×10^9/l.
2. After transfusion of 15 to 20 units of whole blood or red blood cells.

Note: Platelet counts often fall below 80–100 $\times 10^9$/l and platelet transfusions may be indicated for adequate haemostasis underlying major surgery or treatment of severe trauma. The decision to administer platelets should rest on the actual count and not on the replacement formula based on the number of units transfused.

- The emphasis is to treat the patient and not the laboratory result.

Fresh frozen plasma (FFP)

- FFP contains all the clotting factors.
- **Indications**:
  1. Replacement of single factor deficiencies when specific or combined concentrates are not available.
  2. Immediate reversal of warfarin effect in patients at risk of life-threatening haemorrhage.
- In massive transfusion (defined as replacement of a patient's total blood volume within 24 hours), there is no evidence that prophylactic replacement regimes with FFP prevent abnormal bleeding or reduce transfusion requirements. FFP is recommended only in the presence of bleeding and disturbed coagulation.

Cryoprecipitate

Cryoprecipitate is rich in factor VIII, fibrinogen and von Willebrand factor. It is used as a replacement therapy in patients with von Willebrand's syndromes or haemophilia A when viral inactivated factor VIII concentrate is not available.

Factor VIII and factor IX

Viral inactivated factor VIII or factor IX concentrates are used for the treatment of haemophilia A and haemophilia B respectively. See Table 3.

Haemophilia A

Factor VIII (IU) needed = weight (kg) × level desired × 0.5.

Note: 1 vial of factor VIII contains 250 IU.

Haemophilia B

- Factor IX (IU) needed = weight (kg) × level desired.

Note: 1 vial of factor IX contains 500 IU.

- Haemophilia patients with inhibitor should be managed by Haematologist.

Table 3: Factor concentrate level guidelines

Mild bleeding (Level desired 30%)	*Moderate bleeding (Level desired 50%)*	*Severe bleeding (Level desired 75–100%)*
1. Minor or single joint bleeding 2. Muscle bleeding 3. Epistaxis 4. Dental bleeding 5. Haematuria	1. Major or multiple joint bleeding 2. Neck, tongue, pharynx bleeding (without airway compromise) 3. Abdominal bleeding 4. Head trauma without neurological deficit	1. Intracranial bleeding 2. Major operation 3. Major trauma 4. Compartment syndrome 5. Neck, tongue, pharynx bleeding (with airway compromise)

Emergency blood transfusion

- **Emergency blood group 'O' blood** should not be used indiscriminately. It is safer and equally effective in emergencies to make use of crystalloids or colloids first and then matched blood.
- **Group 'O' positive** is used as emergency blood for **Chinese and Malay** patients.
- **Group 'O' negative** is used for **Indian and Caucasian patients** especially females in the reproductive groups.
  The following are categories of blood according to urgency:
  1. **Unmatched emergency blood**, available instantly (no blood group match and no antibody screen).
  2. **Rapid-match blood**, available in 5 to 10 minutes (with blood group match but no antibody screen).
  3. **Full-matched blood**, available in 30 to 45 minutes (with blood group match and antibody screen).
- **Complications of transfusions (immediate reactions)**:
  1. **Haemolytic reaction**: the most serious immediate reaction (0.03% of all transfusions with mortality rate of 10–40%). This reaction most commonly appears before the completion of the first unit of blood.
     a. Patient complains of fever, chills, low back and joint pain, and a sensation of chest tightness. A burning sensation is frequently felt at the IV site. It may also manifest as shock.
     b. **Management** is directed towards the prevention of shock and renal cortical hypoperfusion.
        (1) Terminate the transfusion immediately.
        (2) Vigorous IV fluid therapy and IV frusemide 80–100 mg to maintain a urine output of at least 30 ml/h.
        (3) IV hydrocortisone 200 mg for adult (5 mg/kg for a child).
        (4) Obtain immediate Haematology consultation in ED.

2. **Febrile reaction**: the most common (3–4% of all transfusions) and least serious transfusion reaction.

Note: However, it is impossible clinically, in the early stages, to differentiate the febrile reaction from the more serious immediate haemolytic reaction.

   a. Patient complains of fever, chills and malaise.
   b. **Management**:
      (1) Terminate the transfusion immediately.
      (2) Administer antipyretics.
      (3) IV hydrocortisone 200 mg for adult (5 mg/kg for a child).
      (4) Obtain immediate Haematology consultation in ED.

3. **Allergic reaction**: rare (1% of all transfusions) and occurs before 10 ml of blood has been transfused.
   a. Patient complains of chills and generalized pruritis.
   b. Clinical signs: hypotension, skin flushing, possibly urticaria, angioedema.
   c. **Management**:
      (1) Slow the transfusion rate immediately if only urticaria is present but terminate the tranfusion if fever, angioedema and hypotension develop.
      (2) IV antihistamines.
      (3) IV hydrocortisone 200 mg (5 mg/kg for a child).

Acknowledgement

The authors thank Dr Tien Sim Leng, head of the Singapore General Hospital (SGH) Blood Transfusion Services, for providing Reference 1, the basis for most of the information in this chapter.

References/further reading

1. Singapore General Hospital Blood Transfusion Guidelines. 2nd ed. 1997.
2. Rosen P, Barkin RM, Danzyl DF, et al. *Emergency Medicine: Concepts and Clinical Practice*. 4th ed. St. Louis, MO: Mosby; 1998.

113 Airway management/rapid sequence intubation

Shirley Ooi • Peter Manning

DEFINITION

Rapid sequence intubation (RSI) is the administration of a potent induction agent followed immediately by a rapidly acting neuromuscular blocking agent to induce unconsciousness and motor paralysis for tracheal intubation in patients at risk of gastric aspiration. Assumptions for RSI:

- Patient **unfasted** before intubation and is therefore at **risk for aspiration**.
- Patient **not known or assessed to be difficult to intubate**.
- Administration of the drugs is preceded by a **preoxygenation phase** (refer to second 'P' of RSI for further details) to permit a period of apnoea to occur safely between the administration of the drugs and intubation of trachea **without interposed assisted ventilation**.
- Use of **cricoid pressure or Sellick's manoeuvre** to prevent the aspiration of gastric contents.

INDICATIONS

- The decision to intubate is based on 3 fundamental clinical assessments:
  1. **Is there a failure of airway maintenance or protection?**

Note: Adequacy of airway is confirmed by having the patient speak. Possible inadequate airway includes inability to phonate properly, stridor and altered mental state precluding response to questions. A gag reflex is neither sensitive nor specific as an indicator of loss of airway protective reflexes.

  2. **Is there a failure of ventilation** (eg status asthmaticus) **or oxygenation** (eg severe pulmonary oedema)?
  3. **What is the anticipated clinical course?**
     Patients whose currently acceptable anatomy and physiology can be predicted to deteriorate or work of breathing will be overwhelming with multiple major injuries.
- **If laryngoscopy is unsuccessful,** consider the following:
  1. Is the position of the patient optimal?
  2. Use straight blade if epiglottis is long, floppy or in the way.
  3. Did the person performing Sellick's manoeuvre push the airway out of midline obscuring landmarks?
  4. **BURP** (**B**ackward, **U**pward, **R**ightward, **P**ressure) displacement of larynx.

☛ Special Tips for GPs

- **If the initial or standard bag-valve-mask fails,** ask yourself the following 4 questions:
  1. Do I have the patient in the optimum sniffing position? Caution in the trauma patient.
  2. Have I utilized all of my upper airway adjuncts?
  3. Do I have an optimum mask seal? Eg
     a. Applying KY jelly to a beard
     b. Filling out hollowed cheeks with gauze placed between teeth and cheek mucosa
     c. Reinserting patient's dentures
  4. Have I recruited another person to help optimize BVM technique?

GUIDELINES ON WHEN NOT TO INTUBATE

- If uncomfortable with intubation techniques required and ventilation is adequate.
- If the patient's condition improves during intubation attempts.
- If the respiratory arrest is reversible with a drug (naloxone, flumazenil).
- If the patient has a deformity of the airway or neck (and is stable).
- If the patient has a **do not resuscitate** order.

MANAGEMENT

Remember the **seven Ps of RSI**.

- **Preparation**
  1. Patient must be managed in a resuscitation area.
  2. Monitoring: ECG, pulse oximetry, vital signs q 5 min.
  3. Have sedating agents and paralyzing drugs immediately available (see below).
  4. Prepare airway equipment including stylets, different size blades, oropharyngeal airways or cricothyrotomy tray immediately available.
  5. Have an alternative plan should you fail to intubate.
  6. Have a skilled assistant.
  7. Establish at least 2 peripheral IVs: Hartman's or NS.
  8. Always **anticipate vomiting** in all injured patients. Should a patient vomit, there are 3 manoeuvres to deal with it:
     a. Immediate suction with a large bore Yankauer sucker
     b. Rotate the patient to the lateral position or the 'recovery position'
     c. Put the patient in a Trendelenburg position (if possible)

9. The **assessment of the difficult airway** should be done. Use the '**LEMON Law**' (mnemonic taken from Ref. 1 but details are modified):

L **Look externally** (eg maxillofacial trauma, penetrating neck trauma, blunt neck trauma, and identify difficult ventilation scenarios such as a bearded patient, morbid obesity, extreme cachexia, edentulous mouth with sunken cheeks, abnormal facies).

E **Evaluate** the **'2–3 Rule'** ie at least 2 fingers for mouth opening-interincisor distance or Patil's test (indicates adequate mouth opening), while 3 fingers should fit between the upper border of the thyroid cartilage and the inner border of mentum, ie the thyromental distance (indicates that the larynx is sufficiently low within the neck to permit access by the oral route).

M **Mallampati score** (Figure 1) **and grade of laryngeal view** (Figure 2) for prediction of airway difficulty. Mallampati score (oropharyngeal visualization) correlates with laryngeal visualization.

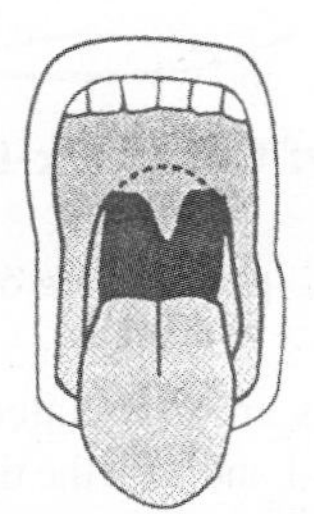

Class I: soft palate, uvula, fauces, pillars visible

No difficulty

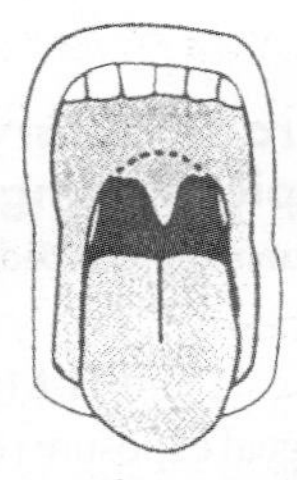

Class II: soft palate, uvula, fauces visible

No difficulty

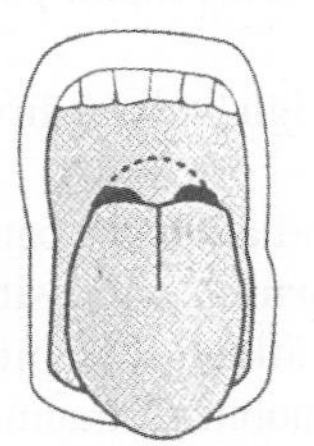

Class III: soft palate, base of uvula visible

Moderate difficulty

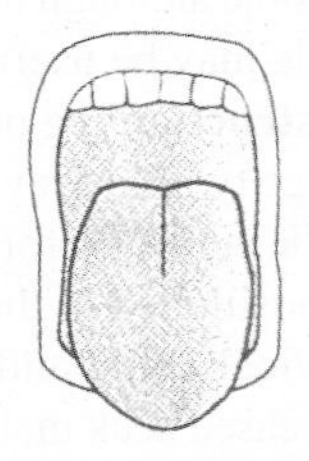

Class IV: hard palate only visible

Severe difficulty

Figure 1 Diagram of Mallampati Score

Source: Diagrams reproduced with permission,[1] p. 34 Figure. 5.1.

Grade 1 is visualization of the entire glottic aperture.

Grade 2 is visualization of just the arytenoids cartilages or the posterior portion of the glottic aperture.

Grade 3 is visualization of only the epiglottis.

Grade 4 is visualization of only the tongue or the tongue and soft palate.

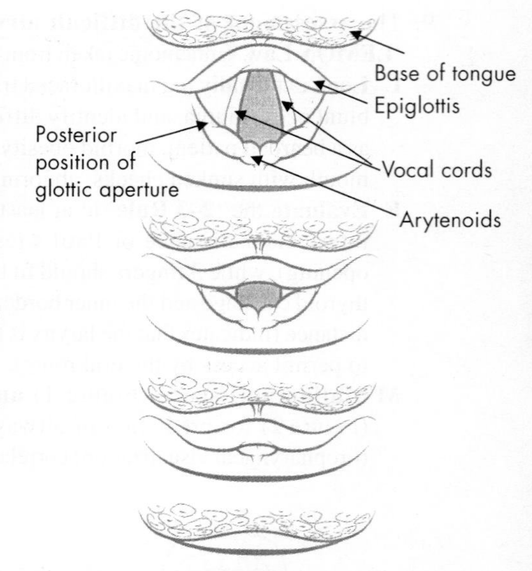

Figure 2: Grade of laryngeal view: Cormack-Lehane laryngoscopic grading system

Source: Diagrams reproduced with permission,[1] p. 53 Figure 6.7.

Classes I and II Mallampati views are associated with superior laryngeal exposure (laryngeal grades 1 and 2) at the time of intubation and low intubation failures. In contrast, Mallampati views classes III and IV are associated with poor laryngeal visualization (laryngeal grades 3 and 4) and with higher intubation failure rates. In the ED, the formal assessment of Mallampati score sitting up is often not possible although the examination of the supine patient with a tongue blade may be useful.

O **Obstruction** (eg presence of foreign body in airway, disruption of integrity of airway)

N **Neck mobility**: for successful ventilation, the patient's neck should be positioned in the '**sniffing morning air position**', ie flexion at cervical spine and extension at atlanto-occipital joint. There is decreased neck mobility in the immobilized trauma patient and those with systemic arthritis.

- **Preoxygenation**
  1. This is the establishment of an oxygen reservoir within the lungs and body tissue to permit several minutes of apnoea to occur without arterial oxygen desaturation. This is essential to the 'no bagging' principle of RSI.
  2. Administration of 100% oxygen with non-rebreathing mask for 5 min replaces the nitrogen of room air in the Functional Residual Capacity

Table 1: Pretreatment drugs for RSI

Lignocaine (1.0–1.5 mg/kg)	For reactive airway disease ('**tight lungs**') or high intracranial pressure (ICP) or '**tight brains**'#
Opioid (fentanyl 2 µg/kg given over 30–60 sec)	When **sympathetic responses** should be blunted (high ICP, aortic dissection, ruptured aortic or berry aneurysm, ischaemic heart disease)*
Atropine (0.02 mg/kg)	To **prevent succinylcholine-induced bradycardia**. For children ≤10 years old and adults with preexisting bradycardia
Defasciculation: non-depolarizing muscle relaxant	For high ICP, penetrating eye injuries

There appears to be little high quality evidence available to show that IV lignocaine suppresses the rises in ICP associated with RSI in HI patients.

* There was no significant difference in the haemodynamic responses to orotracheal intubation by laryngoscopy with or without pretreatment with IV fentanyl.

(FRC) in the lungs with oxygen, allowing several minutes of apnoea time (in healthy 70 kg adult, up to 8 min of apnoea time) before SpO_2 <90%.

3. If patient is unable to be preoxygenated for 5 min before giving paralytic drug, get patient to take 3 to 5 vital capacity breaths in rapid sequence from a 100% oxygen source.

- **Pretreatment**
  1. This is the administration of drugs (Table 1) to mitigate the adverse effects associated with intubation.
  2. It is given 3 min prior to intubation.
- **Paralysis with induction** (see Table 2 for summary of induction agents)
  1. This is the most vital step of the sequence.
  2. Induction agent is given as a rapid push followed immediately by a rapid push of succinylcholine.
- **Protection and positioning**
  1. Sellick's manoeuvre or application of cricoid pressure should be initiated immediately upon the observation that the patient is losing consciousness.
  2. Patient is then positioned for laryngoscopy.

Table 2: Summary of induction agents

Induction agent (Dosage)	*Onset*	*Full recovery*	*Advantages*	*Disadvantages*	*Side effects/caution*	*Special uses*
Thiopentone Elderly: 2.5–3 mg/kg Adult: 3–4 mg/kg Children: 5–6 mg/kg	15–30 sec	3–5 min	Cerebroprotective	Central respiratory depression Hypotension Histamine releasing	Hypotension Asthma Acute intermittent porphyria Variegate porphyria	Head injury with raised ICP
Midazolam 0.1 mg/kg	30–60 sec	0.5–2 h	Amnestic Sedative	Hypotension Suppresses respiration		
Etomidate 0.3 mg/kg (large vein)	15–30 sec	15–30 min	Cerebroprotective Haemodynamic stability		Nausea Vomiting Pain on injection Myoclonic movements Hiccups	Most haemodynamically stable induction agent Head injury Hypotensive patient
Ketamine 2 mg/kg	15–30 sec	15–30 min	Releases catecholamines Analgesic Amnestic	Raises ICP	Raises ICP	Bronchospastic patients Hypotensive patients without head injury Haemodynamic instability due to cardiac tamponade or myocardial disease

- **Placement and proof**
  1. Tube placement within the trachea should be confirmed using end-tidal CO_2 monitoring and aspiration techniques such as the oesophageal detection device.
  2. Cricoid pressure is released after confirmation of correct tube placement and endotracheal tube has been secured.
- **Postintubation management**
  1. Secure endotracheal tube.
  2. Initiate mechanical ventilation.
  3. Do chest x-ray to ensure mainstem intubation has not occurred. However, a more rapid way is to ensure that the proximal end of the cuff is placed 2–3 cm distal to the vocal cords or where the black marking of the ETT is located.
  4. Check BP. See Table 3 for hypotension in the postintubation period.

PRECAUTIONS SHOULD DIFFICULT AIRWAY BE PREDICTED

Do not immediately do a RSI. Consider doing an '**awake oral intubation**'. Sedate patient with IV midazolam 1–2 mg. Spray the pharynx and larynx with liberal amount of lignocaine. Do laryngoscopy and attempt to visualize larynx/vocal cords. Spray liberally on the vocal cords. Intubate if there is fear that patient will deteriorate. If not, get ready for RSI. Further sedation may be needed followed by IV succinylcholine 1.5 mg/kg in an adult.

Table 3: Hypotension in the postintubation period

Cause	*Detection*	*Action*
Tension pneumothorax	Increased peak inspiratory pressure (PIP), difficulty bagging, decreased breath sounds	Immediate thoracostomy
Decreased venous return	Usually seen in patients with high PIPs secondary to high intrathoracic pressure	Fluid bolus, treatment of airway resistance (bronchodilators) Increase expiratory time Try lower tidal volume
Induction agents	Other causes excluded	Fluid bolus, expectant
Cardiogenic	Usually in compromised patient. ECG. Exclude other causes	Fluid bolus (caution), pressors

Source: Table reproduced with permission,[1] p. 13, Box 2.3.

ALTERNATIVE TECHNIQUES IF INTUBATION FAILS

This can be divided into 2 groups of techniques based on the ability for BVM to maintain SpO_2 >90%.

- If **BVM** is **able to maintain SpO_2 >90%**, consider the following airway techniques:
    1. Intubating laryngeal mask airway
    2. Lighted stylets
    3. Retrograde intubation
    4. Cricothyrotomy
- If **BVM** is **unable to maintain SpO_2 >90%**, cricothyrotomy is the procedure of choice.

DRUG THERAPY

Induction agents

Essential for patients who are awake when RSI is being performed to significantly blunt the psychological effects of the procedure and their memory of it. (See Table 2 for summary of induction agents.)

Different intubation scenarios

- **Hypovolaemia** (with low BP): etomidate or ketamine. No drugs if shock is severe. **Avoid** thiopentone and midazolam.
- **Isolated closed head injury** with high ICP, normal or high BP (the desired action is lower cerebral oxygen consumption and cerebral blood flow leading to lower ICP): either thiopentone, etomidate or midazolam. **Avoid** ketamine.
- **Closed head injury** (high ICP) and **hypovolaemia** (with low BP: unresponsive to fluids): etomidate or ketamine. **Avoid** thiopentone and midazolam.
- **Asthma**: either ketamine, etomidate or midazolam. **Avoid** thiopentone.

Paralyzing agents

The optimum drug has a rapid onset of action and short duration. Depolarizing agents are superior to non-depolarizing agents for RSI.

- **Succinylcholine**: the primary agent used in emergency paralysis for airway control. Significant **side effects** include:
    1. Bradycardia (especially in children and those with preexistent bradycardia).
    2. Increased intracranial/intraocular pressures (contraindicated in penetrating globe trauma).
    3. Increased intragastric pressure (may precipitate emesis).
    4. Hyperkalaemia (especially in patients with **chronic** muscle paralysis, eg cerebrovascular accidents and spinal cord injuries).

Note: Increase in plasma potassium after succinylcholine administration is modest (generally <0.5 mmol/l).

5. Hyperkalaemia in chronic renal failure patients before serum potassium known.

Note: There is recent evidence that succinylcholine is generally safe in hyperkalaemia, although the risk undoubtedly rises with increasing potassium levels. The best approach is to avoid succinylcholine use in patients with known, significant hyperkalaemia with serum K^+ >6 mmol/l; rocuronium is a good alternative in such cases. If the K^+ level is not known and morphology on ECG is normal, using succinylcholine is reasonable, even in patients with ESRF. In addition to its consistent, rapid attainment of excellent intubating conditions and its short duration of action, succinylcholine is eliminated independently of renal excretion, a desirable property in ESRF.

6. Fasciculation: aggravated additional musculoskeletal trauma.
7. Rarely, malignant hyperthermia.
   Dosage of succinylcholine: administer 1.0–1.5 mg/kg body weight IV (2 mg/kg in children)

Note: Rocuronium is considered as an alternative to succinylcholine due to its rapid onset of action at 1 min. However, it has a prolonged duration of action unlike succinylcholine.

- **Rocuronium**: a non-depolarizing agent used to prevent succinylcholine-induced muscle fasciculation or to provide a more prolonged paralysis during procedures, eg CT scans.
  Dosage: administer 0.6 mg/kg body weight IV bolus before succinylcholine. Effective duration of action is 20–45 minutes
- **Atracurium (Tracrium®)**: a non-depolarizing agent.
  Dosage: 0.3–0.6 mg/ kg IV bolus. A disadvantage of this drug is substantial histamine release; beware in known asthmatics

SEQUENCE OF EVENTS USING COUNT DOWN MODE

Time (minutes):

−5.00: Preparation

−5.00: Preoxygenation

−3.00: Pretreatment (consider 'LOAD')

0.00: Paralysis with induction

+0.30: Protection

+0.45: Placement and proof

+1.00: Postintubation management

+10.00: CXR to check depth of ETT placement

DISPOSITION

Patients undergoing RSI are candidates for an ICU setting or go straight to the OT following appropriate consultation.

References/further reading

1. Wall RM, Luten RC, Murphy MF, et al. *Manual of Emergency Airway Management*. Philadelphia: Lippincott Williams & Wilkins; 2000.
2. Hals G, Sayre M. The difficult airway: Access, intervention, and stabilization. Part I: Step-by-step techniques for advanced clinical management. *Emerg Med Rep*. 1996;17:23–34.
3. Hals G, Sayre M. The difficult airway: Targeting clinical applications. Part II: Indications and contraindications for intubation and invasive management. *Emerg Med Rep*. 1996;17:35–42.
4. Schow AJ, Lubarsky DA, Olson RP, et al. Can succinylcholine be used safely in hyperkalemic patients? *Anesth Analg*. 2002;95:119–122.
5. Walls RM. Is succinylcholine safe in patients with hyperkalaemia? *J Watch Emerg Med*. 2002;828:3.
6. Butler J. Lignocaine premedication before RSI in head injuries. *Best BETS*.
7. Adachi YU, Satomoto M, Higuchi H, et al. Fentanyl attenuates the hemodynamic response to endotracheal intubation more than the response to laryngoscopy. *Anesth Analg*. 2002;95:233–237.

114 Cardiac dysrhythmias/resuscitation algorithms

Peng Li Lee

ASYSTOLE

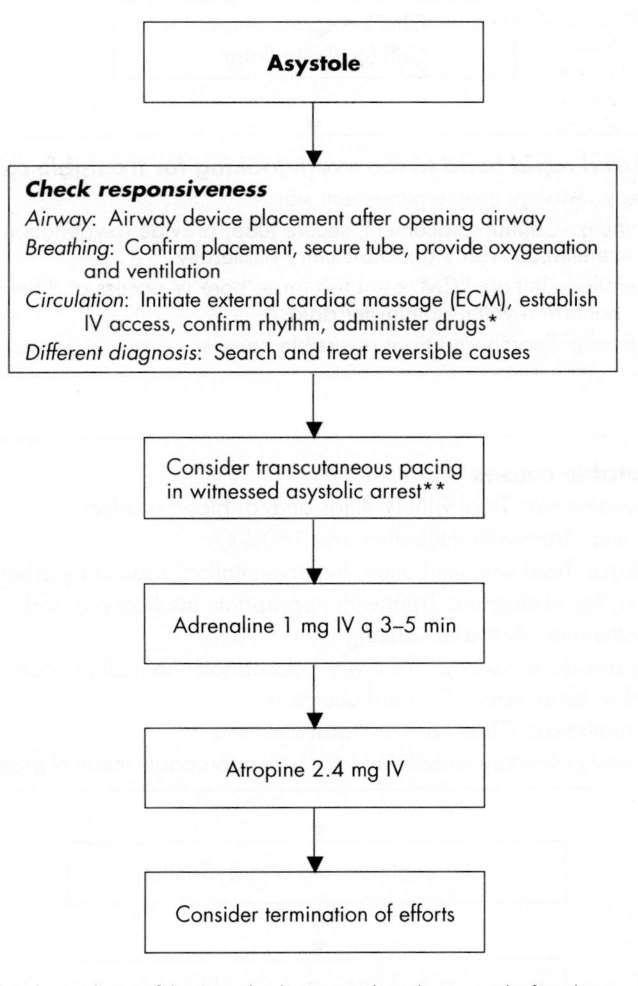

* Peripheral cannulation of the antecubital or external jugular vein is the first choice route.
** Transcutaneous pacing must be initiated at the beginning of the arrest along with drug therapies, otherwise it is not beneficial. Should be reserved for select cases of asystole.

PULSELESS ELECTRICAL ACTIVITY (PEA)

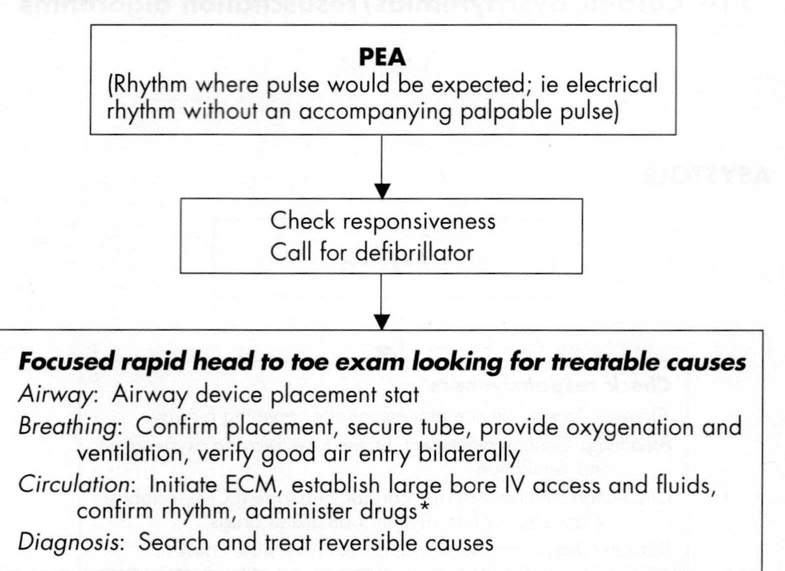

Treatable causes
Hypovolaemia: Treat with IV fluids and/or blood products
Hypoxia: Treat with intubation and 100% O_2
Acidosis: Treat with intubation, hyperventilation, sodium bicarbonate
Hyper/hypokalaemia: Treat with appropriate medical protocol
Hypothermia: Active rewarming
Drug overdose/toxicity: Treat with appropriate medical protocol
Cardiac tamponade: Pericardiocentesis
Pneumothorax: Chest tube or thoracocentesis
AMI and pulmonary embolism: Treat with appropriate medical protocol

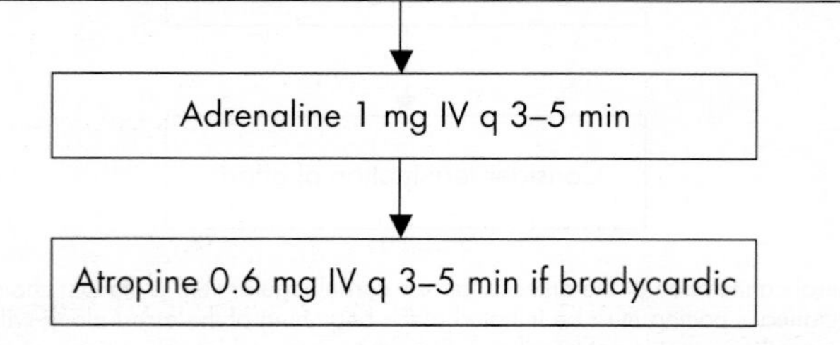

* Peripheral cannulation of the antecubital or external jugular vein is the first choice route.

VF/PULSELESS VT

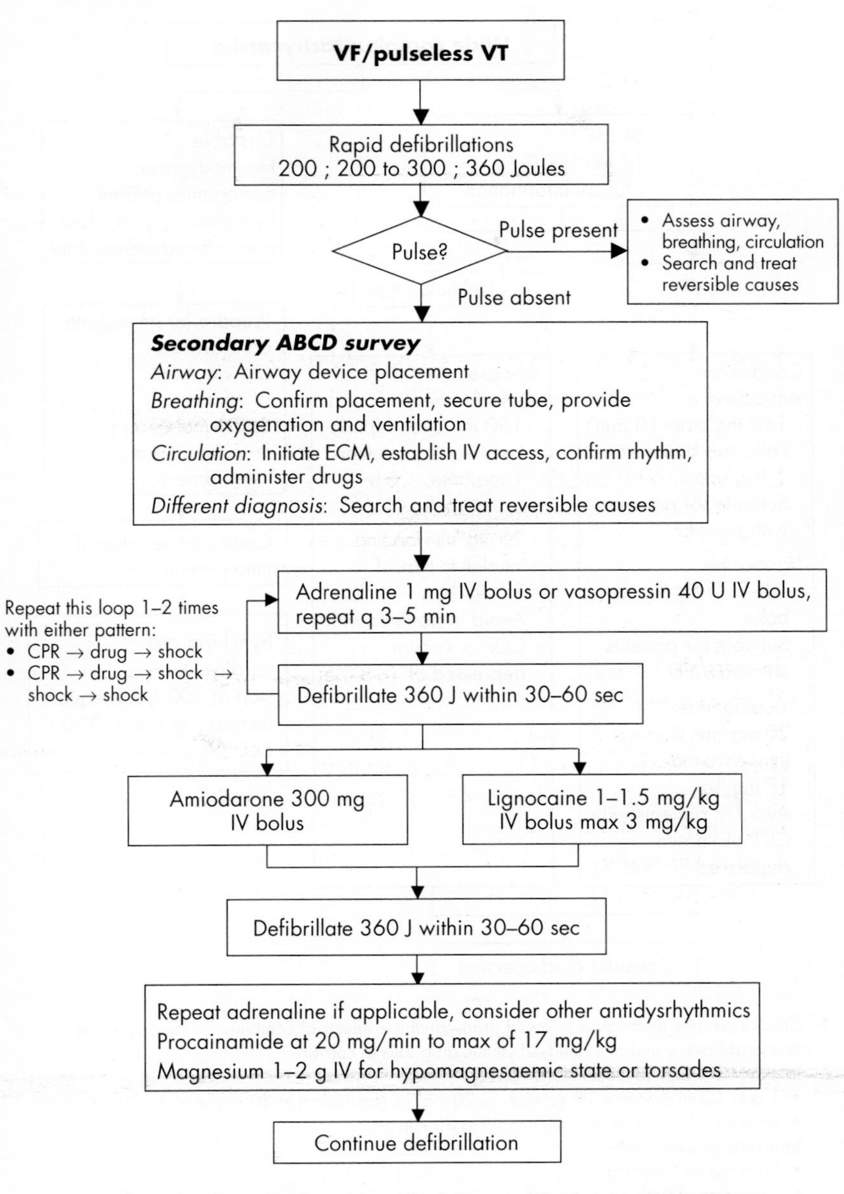

Dilution for procainamide = 1 g in 50 ml dextrose 5% solution ⇒ 20 mg/ml
Loading infusion rate = 1 ml/min (up to 30 min)

WIDE COMPLEX TACHYCARDIA

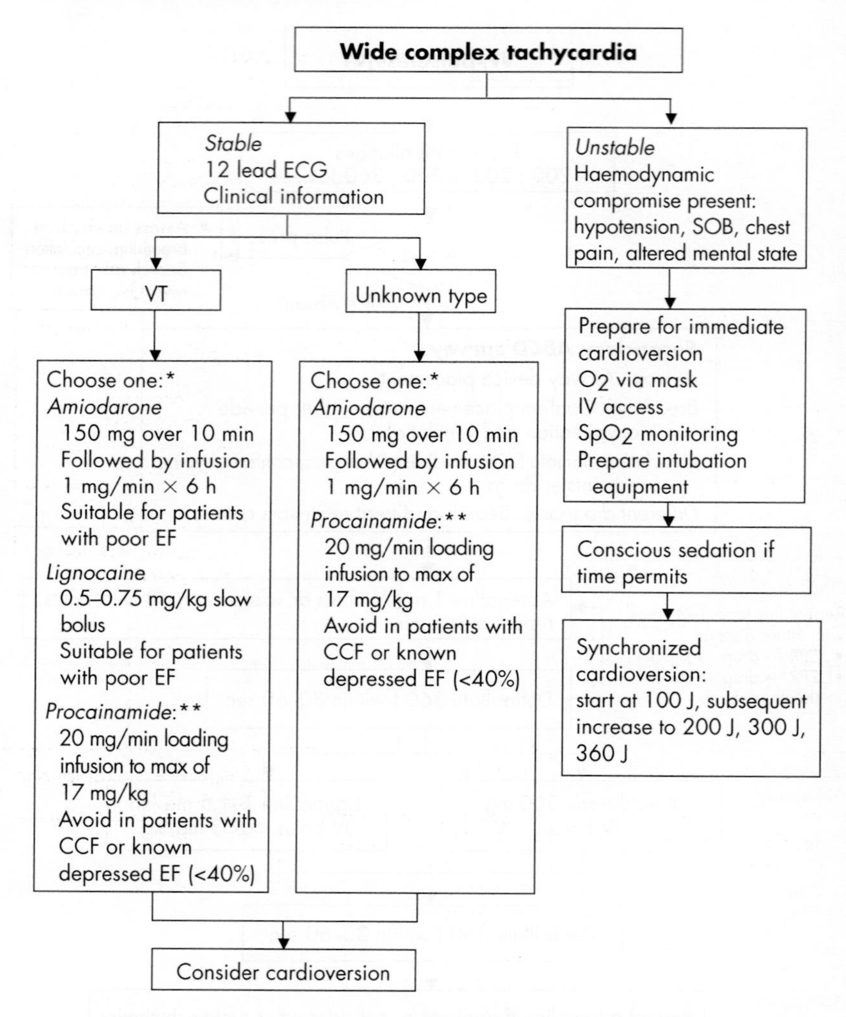

* Choose just one medication to avoid prodysrhythmic effects of combination therapy, move on to cardioversion if one antidysrhythmic drug fails to convert.

** Dilution for procainamide:

- 1 g in 50 ml dextrose 5% solution ⇒ 20 mg/ml (equivalent to 20 mg/min)
- Loading infusion rate at 1 ml/min up to 30 min

Terminate procainamide if

- BP drops ≥15 mm Hg
- Widening of QRS
- Prolonged PR interval

NARROW COMPLEX TACHYCARDIA

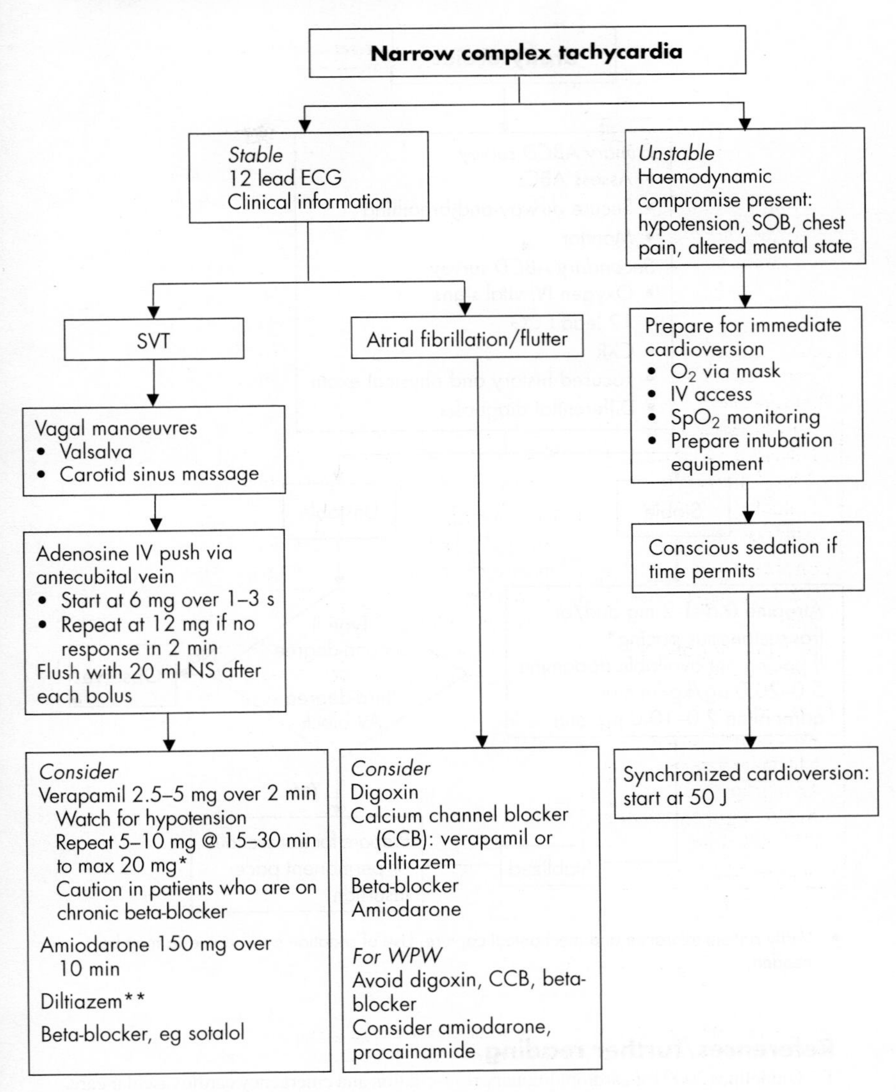

* Suggested method of dilution and administration of *verapamil*
- Dilute verapamil 20 mg in 80 ml normal saline (concentration 0.25 mg/ml)
- Infuse at a rate of 4 ml/min (240 ml/h) to give 1 mg/min
- Maximum dose 20 mg

** Suggested method of dilution and administration of *diltiazem*
- Dilute 50 mg diltiazem in 80 ml normal saline (concentration 0.6 mg/ml)
- Infuse at a rate of 4 ml/min (240 ml/h) to give 2.5 mg/min

BRADYCARDIAS

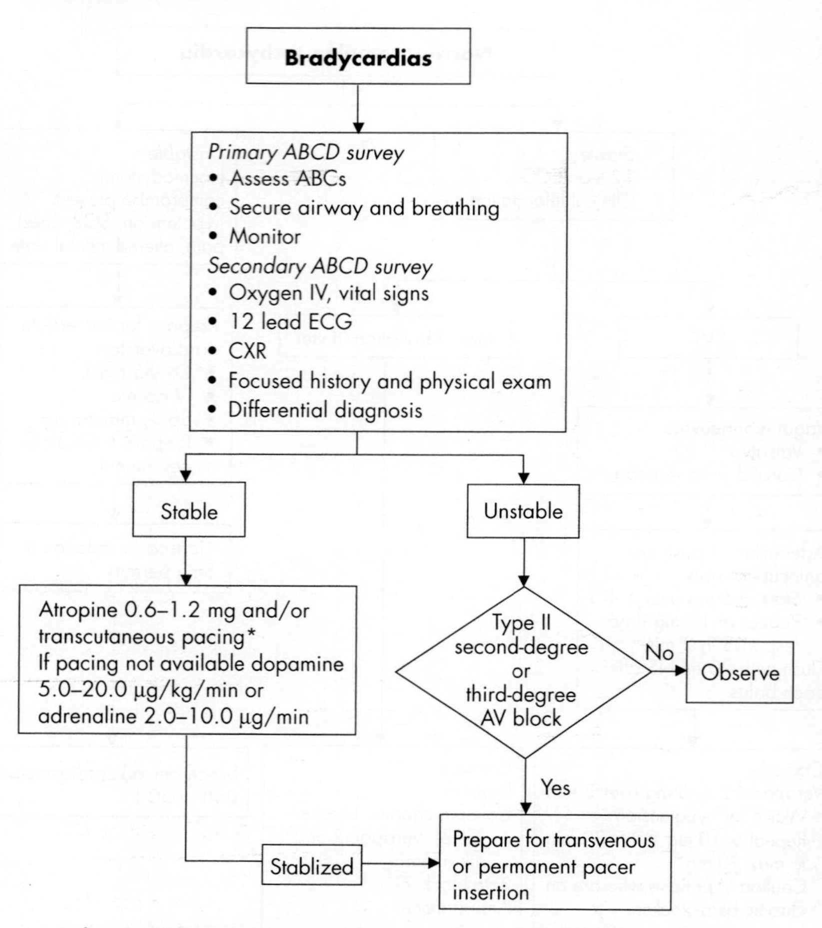

- Verify patient tolerance and mechanical capture. Use of sedation and analgesia may be needed.

References/further reading

1. Guidelines 2000 for cardiopulmonary resuscitation and emergency cardiovascular care. American Heart Association. Supp 1. *Circulation.* 2000;102(8).

115 Cervical spine clearance

Peng Li Lee

CAVEATS

- **X-ray** of the **C-spine** is **not required** if the following criteria are satisfied:
  1. Patient is alert, awake and sober
  2. No complaint of neck pain
  3. No distracting injuries elsewhere in the body or pain during assessment
  4. No cervical spine tenderness on examination
  5. Able to move neck from side to side and flex and extend without pain
  6. No neurological deficits
- In the absence of the above criteria, numerous prospective studies found that no patient had a clinically significant C-spine injury.
- In all other trauma patients, the following should be ordered:
  1. **Plain C-spine x-ray**
     a. AP view
     b. Lateral view or swimmer's view: base of occiput to upper border of T1 should be visualized
     c. Open mouth odontoid view. This may not be possible if a patient will not or cannot cooperate for the open-mouth x-ray. An oblique view of the odontoid process or a foramen magnum view can be done to assess the dens.
  2. **CT scan**: indicated as a supplement to plain x-rays for suspicious areas or inadequately visualized areas.
- **C-collar should be kept on in the following situations**:
  1. When in doubt about the C-spine x-rays findings.
  2. Presence of other acute surgical problems that require the patient to be rushed to the OT before complete workup of the spine is finished.
  3. Comatose, altered mental state and paediatric patients (who are too young to describe their complaints) until after appropriate evaluation by orthopaedic or neurosurgeon.

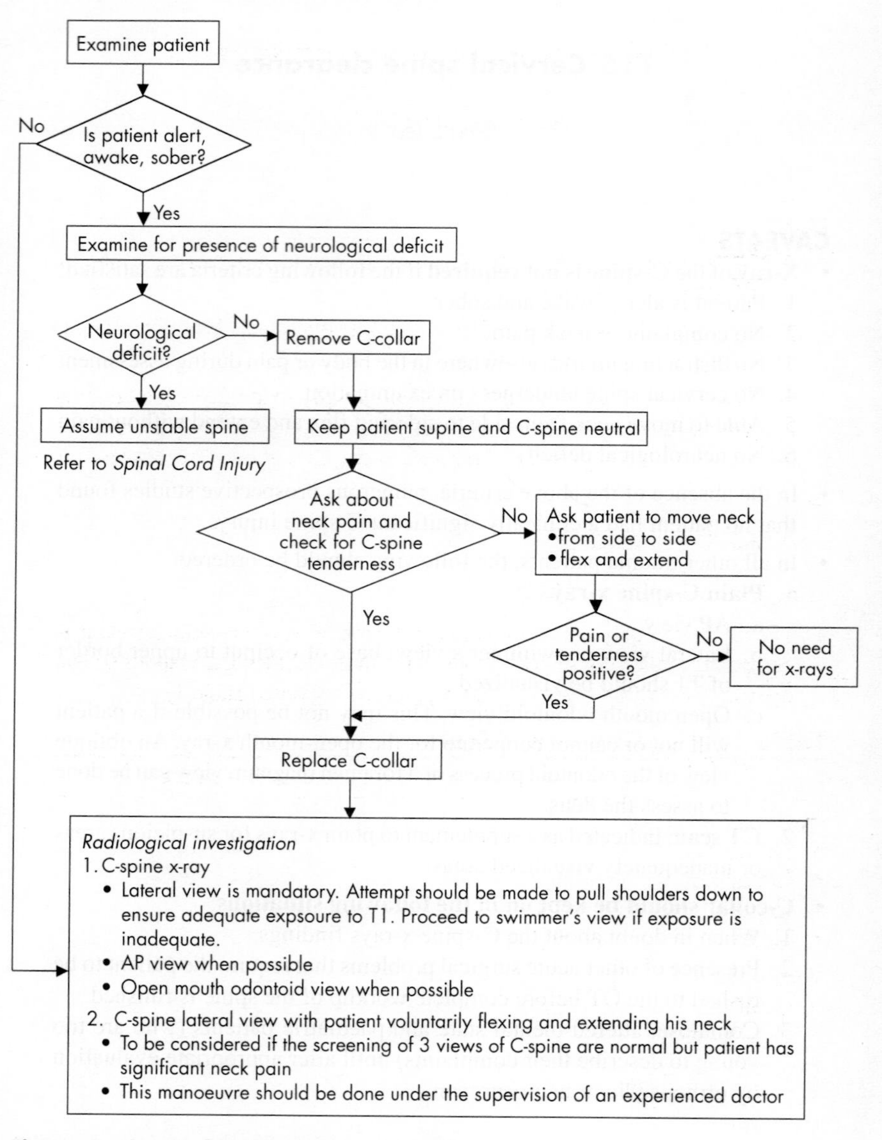

Figure 1: Cervical spine clearance at ED

References/further reading

1. Committee on Trauma of the American College of Surgeons. *Advanced Trauma Life Support for Doctors. Student Course Manual*. 6th ed. Chicago: American College of Surgeons; 1997:215–242.
2. Practice Management Guidelines for Identifying Cervical Spine Injuries following Trauma, by EAST Practice parameter workgroup for cervical spine clearance.

116 Commonly used scoring systems

Chong Chew Lan • Shirley Ooi

USES

- Allows us to quantify the severity of the injury, enabling comparison of injuries between patients.
- This, in turn, allows us to predict and compare outcome. Hence, it is useful in clinical audit and research.
- Trauma scoring is also useful in triage, especially in the field. It augments the clinical judgement of the prehospital personnel, facilitating the transfer of patients to the appropriate facility and the allocation of resources.

PHYSIOLOGIC SCORES

Glasgow Coma Scale (GCS)

- The GCS is widely used to assess a patient's level of consciousness. It is computed as the sum of coded values for three behavioural responses: eye opening, best verbal response and best motor response (Table 1).

Table 1: Glasgow Coma Scale

	Score
Eye opening (E)	
• Spontaneous	4
• To calling	3
• To pain	2
• None	1
Verbal response (V)	
• Oriented	5
• Confused	4
• Inappropriate words	3
• Incomprehensible sounds	2
• None	1
Best motor response (M)	
• Obeys commands	6
• Localizes pain	5
• Withdraws (pain)	4
• Flexion (pain)	3
• Extension (pain)	2
• None (pain)	1
Total GCS points (1 + 2 + 3)	*lowest 3, highest 15*

- The GCS itself can be used to categorize patients:
  1. **Coma**: a patient in **coma** is defined as having **no eye opening (E = 1)**, and **no ability to follow commands (M = 1 to 5)**, and **no word verbalizations (V = 1 to 2)**. This means that all patients with a GCS <8 and most with a GCS = 8 are in coma. Patients with a GCS >8 are not in coma.
  2. **Head injury (HI) severity**: on the basis of the GCS, patients are classified as having:
     a. Severe HI if GCS ≤8.
     b. Moderate HI if GCS = 9 to 13
     c. Mild HI if GCS = 14 to 15
- The GCS can be applied to the paediatric age group. However, the verbal component must be modified for children <4 years old (Table 2).
- GCS has been correlated with mortality and with the Glasgow Outcome Scale, which measures the level of ultimate brain function. It is widely used for prehospital triage and for determining the level of consciousness after hospital admission.

Revised Trauma Score (RTS)

The RTS (Table 3) is based on the GCS, systolic blood pressure (SBP) and respiratory rate (RR). It is widely used in triage. Variables are assigned coded values from 4 (normal) to 0. The coded values of GCS, SBP and RR are weighted and summed to yield the RTS, which takes values from 0 to 7.84. Higher values are associated with better prognoses.

Table 2: Paediatric verbal score

Verbal response	*Score*
Appropriate words or social smile, fixes and follows	5
Cries, but consolable	4
Persistently irritable	3
Restless, agitated	2
None	1

Table 3: Revised Trauma Score

GCS	*SBP*	*RR*	*Coded Value$_c$*
13–15	>89	10–29	4
9–12	76–89	>29	3
6–8	50–75	6–9	2
4–5	1–49	1–5	1
3	0	0	0

RTS = $0.9368\ GCS_c + 0.7326\ SBP_c + 0.2908\ RR_c$ where the subscript c refers to coded value.

ANATOMIC SCORES

Abbreviated Injury Scale (AIS)

The AIS attributes a score between 1 and 6 to each individual injury (Table 4). It has been revised several times since the original 1971 version.

Injury Severity Score (ISS)

- ISS considers the body to comprise 6 regions:
  1. Head/neck
  2. Face
  3. Thorax
  4. Abdomen or pelvic contents
  5. Extremities or pelvic girdle
  6. External structures (skin)
- It is computed as the sum of the squares of the three highest AIS for injuries from different body regions. Possible ISS scores from 1 to 75. Any patient with AIS 6 scores 75 for ISS. The ISS correlates with mortality but has limitations in that it incorporates only the greatest AIS value from each body region, takes into account 3 injuries at most and considers injuries with the same AIS values to be of equal severity regardless of the body region. As a result, some ISS values or interval cohorts contain data on patients with heterogenous injuries, who have substantially different prognoses and are poor bases for prediction of outcome. Nonetheless, it remains the most frequently used summary measure of severity of anatomic injury.

OTHER SCORING SYSTEMS

TRISS methodology is used to quantify the probability of survival (Ps) as a function of injury severity and hence is widely used to compare ‘performances’ (eg one hospital against another). The Ps is calculated by combining ISS with RTS and adding a weighting factor according to the age of the patient. Patients who survive with Ps <0.5 are ‘unexpected survivors’ while patients who die with Ps >0.5 are ‘unexpected deaths’.

References/further reading

1. Wyatt JP, Illingworth RN, Clancy MJ, et al, eds. *Oxford Handbook of Accident and Emergency Medicine*. Oxford: Oxford University Press; 1999:341.
2. Head trauma. In: Committee on Trauma of the American College of Surgeons. *Advanced Trauma Life Support for Doctors. Student Course Manual*. 6th ed. Chicago: American College of Surgeons; 1997:188–190, 304.

Table 4: Abbreviated Injury Scale

Scale	*Attributes of injury*
AIS 1	Minor injury
AIS 2	Moderate injury
AIS 3	Serious injury
AIS 4	Severe injury
AIS 5	Critical injury
AIS 6	Fatal injury

117 Conscious sedation

Peter Manning • Peng Li Lee

DEFINITION

- This term refers to a minimally depressed level of consciousness that retains the patient's protective airway and cardiac reflexes, and the ability to respond appropriately to physical stimulation and/or verbal commands. The agents used to attain this state include sedating agents, with a margin of safety wide enough to render unintended loss of consciousness unlikely, eg midazolam (Dormicum®) and analgesics, eg opioid agonists, which possess sedative side effects and result in respiratory depression.
- An alternative term being coined now is procedural sedation and analgesia or PSA for short.

CAVEATS

- It is assumed that the patient has been assessed for suitability for sedation, which includes the documentation of allergies, current medications and abnormal airway patency.
- In the absence of a senior emergency physician or anaesthetist, consider admitting for general anaesthetic children under the age of 5 years.
- If in doubt regarding your ability to perform conscious sedation in a particular patient, either admit the patient or seek advice from the on-call emergency physician.
- The use of ketamine requires 2 operators. One performs the procedure while the other is responsible for the constant monitoring of the patient's airway and haemodynamic status.

INDICATIONS

- Patients with dislocations of medium and large joints.
- Abscesses for incision and drainage.
- Lacerations in anatomically challenging sites, eg the face in children ≤5 years.

> ☛ **Special Tips for GPs**
>
> - Conscious sedation is not a procedure that you should consider undertaking in the office unless your office set-up includes haemodynamic monitoring capability and **immediate** anaesthesia assistance.

MANAGEMENT

Supportive measures

- Patients must be managed in a monitored area no matter how young and fit they seem or possess a negative past medical history. Idiosyncratic and allergic reactions are difficult to predict.
- Monitoring: ECG, pulse oximetry, vital signs q 5–10 min.
- Supplemental oxygen.
- Have resuscitation equipment immediately available to include:
  1. Oral airways
  2. Bag-valve-mask (BVM) devices
  3. Endotracheal tubes
  4. Defibrillator
  5. Reversal agents naloxone (Narcan®) and flumazenil (Anexate®)

Drug therapy

For dosages of sedating and muscle relaxing agents, see Table 1.

- **Benzodiazepines, eg midazolam (Dormicum®)** have the advantage of being an amnesic agent in addition to being a sedative and muscle relaxant. However, it does not have analgesic properties. Hence it is best used in conjunction with an opioid agonist analgesic.
- **Opiate analgesic/sedating agents, eg morphine, meperidine (Pethidine®), fentanyl (Sublimaze®)**: of these three similar agents, fentanyl has the significant advantage of not producing histamine release (anaphylactoid reaction).
- **Ketamine**: this **dissociative amnesic, sedating agent and weak analgesic** is used primarily in children.

Complications of conscious sedation

- **Respiratory depression** due to midazolam and opioid agonists. Management by:
  1. Oxygen
  2. Bag-valve-mask ventilation
  3. Reversal agents: flumazenil and naloxone (see below)
- **Laryngospasm** due to ketamine. Management by:
  1. Positive pressure ventilation (PPV)
  2. Succinylcholine (IV 1–2 mg/kg or IM 4 mg/kg) if laryngospasm persists after PPV
  3. Airway management with BVM or intubation after paralysis
- **Hypotension** due to midazolam and opioid agonists. Management by:
  1. Trendelenburg position
  2. Normal saline infusion 20 ml/kg
  3. Reversal agents (see use of reversal agents on p. 561)

Table 1: Drug dosages and guidelines

Drug	Dosage		Advantages	Disadvantages/precautions
	Adults	Paediatrics		
Midazolam (Dormicum®, Versed®)	0.1 mg/kg IV in divided doses, alternating with analgesic	Initial dose 0.05 mg/kg IV; then up to a max of 0.1 mg/kg in divided doses, alternating with analgesic	Rapid onset; short duration of action; titratable	Respiratory and CNS depression, especially when used with opioid agonists
Morphine	0.1–0.2 mg/kg IV in divided doses, alternating with sedating agent	0.01–0.04 mg/kg IV in divided doses, alternating with sedating agent	Tried and tested over the years; titratable	Respiratory and CNS depression; also an emetic; slow onset with prolonged action; causes histamine release
Meperidine (Pethidine®)	1.0 mg/kg IV in divided doses, alternating with sedating agent	Same as adult	Shorter duration and less cardiac depression than morphine; titratable	As above for morphine but less emetic; weaker analgesic than morphine
Fentanyl (Sublimaze®)	1–2 μg/kg IV in divided doses, alternating with sedating agent	Initial dose 0.5 μg/kg IV; then up to a max of 2 μg/kg in divided doses, alternating with sedating agent	Rapid onset; short action; rapid recovery; minimal histamine release	Respiratory and CNS depression; chest wall rigidity after large doses
Ketamine	IV use: 1–2 mg/kg	IM use: 3 mg/kg and round up multiples of 5 but ensure final dose is <4 mg/kg. IV use: 1 mg/kg by slow bolus	Does not cause cardiorespiratory depression; is a bronchodilator and is useful in asthmatics	Laryngospasm with large doses (but is uncommon); sialogogue; use comprises a 2-person procedure due to need for constant monitoring; avoid in hypertension, coronary artery disease and CCF
Atropine: adjunct to ketamine	0.6 mg IM or IV up to a dose of 2.4 mg	0.02 mg/kg by IV or IM route (min 0.1mg, max 0.6 mg)	Antisialagogue	

- **Chest wall rigidity** due to fentanyl. Management by:
  1. Naloxone
  2. Succinylcholine (IV 1–2 mg/kg or IM 4 mg/kg) if naloxone fails
  3. Airway management after paralysis
- **Allergic reaction**. Management by:
  1. Adrenaline (1:1,000 SC at 0.01 ml/kg or 1:10,000 IV at 0.05–0.1 ml/kg)
  2. Antihistamine, eg IM or IV diphenhydramine 1 mg/kg
  3. Hydrocortisone (IV 5 mg/kg)

Use of reversal agents

- **Incorrect use**: it is preferable to permit a patient to regain full consciousness naturally without the use of the antidotes naloxone and flumazenil since the half-life of the agents used in conscious sedation is longer than that of the antidotes. Indiscriminate use of the antidotes could therefore be expected to lead to fluctuating levels of consciousness.
- **Correct use**: should the patient become bradypnoeic or even apnoeic during the procedure or become deeply unconscious, then the antidotes naloxone and/or flumazenil should be administered. **Dosages**:

  Naloxone (**Narcan®**): Child 0.01 mg/kg body weight IV q 1 h
Adult 2 mg IV q 1 h

  Flumazenil (**Anexate®**): Child 0.1 mg IV
Adult 0.5 mg IV × 2–5 min apart

Following procedure

- Secure limb or apply dressing to operated part.
- Place patient in recovery position with mild Trendelenburg tilt.
- Continue monitoring till patient is fully awake, can cough (or cry) and moves purposefully.
- Arrange for patient to be escorted home by friend or family.

Disposition

Discharge instructions: For the next 24 hours patient should not:
- Drive a car or ride a motorcycle or pedal cycle.
- Climb to heights.
- Swim.
- Take alcohol or medications that produce drowsiness.

References/further reading

1. Morgan GE, Mikhail MS. *Clinical Anesthesiology*. 2nd ed. Norwalk, CT: Appleton & Lange; 1996.
2. Kandang Kerbau Children's Hospital, Singapore. Paediatric Conscious Sedation Protocol, 1999.

118 Fluid replacement in paediatrics

Peng Li Lee

IV THERAPY FOR PATIENTS NOT IN SHOCK

Total fluid required (ml/24 h)

= Replacement in DS (R) + Maintenance in DS (M)

↓ ↓

$\frac{\%\ \text{dehydration}}{100} \times \text{BW (kg)}$ litres +

Age	ml/kg
Day 1	60
Day 2	90
Day 3	120
Day 4–1 y	150
1–5 y	100
5–10 y	75
>10 y	50

Note: DS (R) is 2.5% dextrose with 0.45% of saline solution
DS (M) is 3.75% dextrose with 0.23% saline solution

Give half the calculated replacement and maintenance volume over the first 8 h.

Example: 3% dehydration in 10 kg, 1 year old child
Replacement volume = (3/100 × 10) litres = 300 ml
Maintenance volume = 10 kg × 100 ml/kg = 1,000 ml
Order at A&E = (300/2) ml D/S (R) followed by (1,000/2) ml D/S (M) over 8 h, ie, at a rate of 81 ml/h infusion

RESUSCITATION FOR SHOCK

- Crystalloids (Hartmann's or NS) = 10–20 ml/kg as quickly as possible over 15 mins to rapidly expand extracellular volume. Repeat as required.

References/further reading

1. Singapore Ministry of Health. A Guide on Paediatrics. 1997:22–23.

119 List of drugs to avoid in G6PD deficiency

Irwani Ibrahim

ANALGESICS

- Acetylsalicylic acid (aspirin)
- Acetophenetidin (Phenacetin®)

SULPHONAMIDES AND SULFONES

- Suphanilamide
- Sulphapyridine
- Sulphadimidine
- Sulphacetamide
- Sulphafurazone
- Dapsone
- Sulphoxone
- Glucosulfone sodium
- Co-trimoxazole

OTHER ANTIBACTERIAL COMPOUNDS

- Nitrofurans: nitrofurantoin, furazolidone, nitrofurazone
- Nalidixic acid
- Chloramphenicol
- *p*-aminosalicylic acid

ANTIMALARIALS

- Primaquine
- Pamaquine
- Chloroquine

CARDIOVASCULAR

- Procainamide
- Quinidine

MISCELLANEOUS

- Vitamin C
- Vitamin K analogues
- Naphthalene (mothballs)
- Probenecid
- Dimercaprol (BAL)
- Methylene blue
- Arsine
- Phenylhydrazine
- Toluidine blue
- Mepacrine

References/further reading

1. Hoffbrand AV, Lewis SM, eds. *Postgraduate Haematology.* 3rd ed. Oxford: Heinemann Professional Publishing Ltd; 1989.
2. Handin RI, Lux SE, Stossel TP, eds. *Blood: Principles and Practice of Hematology.* Philadelphia: Lipincott;1995.
3. Stein JH, ed. *Internal Medicine.* St Louis: Mosby Year Book; 1994.
4. Isselbacher KJ. *Harrison's Principles of Internal Medicine.* 13th ed. New York: McGraw-Hill; 1994.

120 List of drugs to avoid in pregnancy

JP Travers • Lee Sock Koon

CAVEATS

Before prescribing in pregnancy, always consider the benefits of treatment which should outweigh the risks. This list applies to available drugs commonly used in the ED only. Many drugs are known to have adverse effects in pregnancy and only some are safe. In a critical situation the welfare of the mother takes priority over that of the foetus.

Safe	Avoid	Unclear/special precautions	Serious cases only
Antibiotics			
Amoxicillin	Tetracycline	Gentamicin (sensory organ damage)	
Cloxacillin	Co-trimoxazole	Metronidazole (teratogenic in 1st trimester)	
Amoxicillin-clavulanate potassium (Augmentin®)			
Ceftazidime (Fortum®)			
Ceftriaxone (Rocephin®)			
Erythromycin	(not estolate!)		
For pain			
Codeine	Cafergot (caffeine 100 mg ergotamine tartrate 1 mg per tablet)	Hyoscine-N-butylbromide (Buscopan®; safety not established yet)	Ibuprofen
Paracetamol		Pethidine® (not before labour)	Indomethacin (Indocid®)
Fentanyl		Aspirin (avoid in last trimester)	Diclofenac (Voltaren®)
		Bisocodyl (stimulates gravid uterus)	Mefenamic acid (Ponstan®)
		Morphine/pethidine (care in perinatal period)	Naproxen
For vomiting and diarrhoea			
Metoclopramide		Prochlorperazine (Stemetil®; teratogenic in 1st trimester)	
Loperamide		Promethazine (safe in 1st and 2nd trimesters)	

Safe	Avoid	Unclear/special precautions	Serious cases only
		Hyoscine-N-butylbromide (Buscopan®; safety not established yet)	
Epigastric pain/ulcer			
Antacids			Cimetidine/ranitidine (safety not established yet)
Cardiovascular			
Digoxin	ACE inhibitors (captopril, monopril)		Felodipine
Magnesium	Warfarin		Hydralazine (neonatal thrombocytopaenia)
Heparin	Verapamil		GTN/ISDN (safety not established/SP lactation)
Hydrocortisone			Atenolol/propranolol (long use retards foetal growth)
Salbutamol nebulizer			Procainamide (safety not established)
Prednisolone			Amiodarone (not in perinatal period)
			Frusemide (Lasix®)
			Adenosine
			Adrenaline
			Aminophylline (care in perinatal period)
			Theophylline (care in perinatal period)
Neurological and antiepileptics			
	Midazolam		Phenytoin phenobarbitone (teratogenic)
	Sodium valproate		Diazepam
	Lignocaine		Largactil
			Haloperidol
Immunizations			
Antitetanus toxoid (killed vaccines)	MMR, smallpox (live attenuated)		

References/further reading

1. Singapore Ministry of Health. Standard Drugs. 1998.
2. The British Medical Association Guide to Medicine and Drugs, 1999.

121 Needlestick/body fluid exposure

Peter Manning

DEFINITION

This type of contamination usually refers to an incident in which a patient, health care worker (HCW) or member of the public is contaminated with potentially infected body fluids.

CAVEATS

- In hospital, injuries happen during two-handed recapping, or transferring a needle from one person to another during injections, venepuncture or IV cannulation. Approximately one-third of injuries occur distant from the time and place of patient care, eg skin puncture from an uncapped needle in a garbage bag.
- HCWs have seroconverted following both parenteral and **non-parenteral exposures**.
- The risk of contracting hepatitis is much greater than that of HIV.
- Typically, HIV infection in HCWs occurs secondary to accidental inoculation of blood from an HIV-positive source patient.
- A person who tests negative for anti-HIV may nonetheless harbour the virus, and seroconversion may be delayed or absent following inoculation with the virus.

> ☛ **Special Tips for GPs**
>
> - **Postexposure antiretroviral chemoprophylaxis** is now the standard of care and should be implemented immediately after a known HIV-positive exposure (see later section).

MANAGEMENT

- **Patient care considerations**:
  1. **Percutaneous exposure**: attempt to express inoculated site and wash thoroughly under running water. Then disinfect with Chlorhexidine or Povidone iodine and apply a dressing if deemed necessary.
  2. **Mucous membrane exposure**: irrigate the affected area immediately with copious amounts of water.

3. **Non-intact skin exposure**: wash the area with soap and water or an antiseptic hand wash. Then disinfect with Chlorhexidine or Povidone iodine.

Note: For all contacts follow your institutional policy and procedures.

- **Blood/body fluid from an identified source patient**:
  1. Send blood of exposed HCW for HbsAg, anti-HBS, and anti-HIV
  2. Send blood of source patient (only after consent given) for HbsAg and anti-HIV
     a. **Identified source patient is HBV surface antigen (HbsAg) negative**
        (1) HCW with natural immunity to HBV: no further action required
        (2) HCW who has completed HBV immunization: no further action required
        (3) HCW who has not completed HBV immunization: start/complete HBV immunization
        (4) HCW who is HBV surface antigen (HbsAg) positive: no further action required
     b. **Identified patient is HBV surface antigen (HbsAg) positive**
        (1) HCW with natural immunity: no further action required
        (2) HCW who has completed HBV immunization: booster dose of hepatitis B vaccine
        (3) HCW who has not completed HBV immunization: hepatitis B specific HIG within 72 hours and start/complete HBV immunization
        (4) HCW who is HBV surface antigen positive: no further action required
     c. **Identified source patient is HIV antibody negative**
        (1) Determine hepatitis B status of the patient
     d. **Identified source patient is HIV antibody positive**
        (1) HCW is HIV antibody positive: no further action required
        (2) HCW is HIV antibody negative: implement postexposure prophylaxis immediately (see later section) and refer HCW to follow-up according to institutional practice
        (3) Determine hepatitis B virus status of source patient and proceed as previously described

- **Blood/body fluid from unidentified patient**
  1. HCW who has natural immunity to HBV: no further action required
  2. HCW who has completed HBV immunization: booster dose of hepatitis B vaccine
  3. HCW who has not completed HBV immunization: administer hepatitis B specific HIG within 72 hours and start/complete hepatitis B immunization

- **Post-exposure prophylaxis**: if a HCW is exposed to blood or body fluid of HIV positive source patient, consider postexposure retroviral chemoprophylaxis that may reduce the risk of seroconversion (based on animal and human studies). Studies have shown that prophylaxis administered within 24 hours of exposure reduces the transmission of HIV.
  1. Administer prophylaxis immediately: **do not wait** for follow-up appointment in 3 days or so
  2. Prescribe zidovudine (AZT, ZDV, retrovir)
     Dosage: 200 mg PO td × 3 days
  3. If source patient HIV status is unknown but belongs to a high risk group:
     a. obtain blood specimen as above
     b. refer for prompt follow-up, ie <48 hours

References/further reading

1. Centres for Disease Control and Prevention. Public Health Service guidelines for the management of health-care worker exposures to HIV and recommendations for postexposure prophylaxis. *MMWR Morb Mortal Wkly Rep.* 1998;47(RR-7):1–33.
2. Singapore National University Hospital. Infection Control Manual. 2000.

122 Paediatric drugs and equipment

Chong Chew Lan

FORMULAE FOR ESTIMATION OF NORMAL VALUES

- **Weight (kg)** is estimated by:
  1. [2 × age (yr)] + 9 for age <9 years
  2. 3 × age (yr) for age >9 years
- **Surface area (m^2)** is the square root of [Ht (cm) × BW (kg)/3600].
- **Lowest systolic BP in**:
  1. Neonate ~ 60 mm Hg
  2. Infant ~ 70 mm Hg
  3. Thereafter = [70 + (2 × age in yr)] mm Hg

Age (years)	*Heart rate (hr in bpm)*	*Respiratory rate*
<1	110–160	30–40
2–5	95–140	20–30
5–12	80–120	15–20
>12	60–100	12–16

Note: If <5 years: HR >180, consider sinus tachycardia
If >5 years: HR >160, consider sinus tachycardia
All ages: HR >220, consider supraventricular tachycardia
Paediatric estimated **total blood volume** (ml) = **80 × BW** (kg)

EQUIPMENT

- **Paediatric ETT size (mm)** is estimated by **4 + age (yr)/4** (from age 2 years).
- **Paediatric ETT length (cm) from mouth** is estimated by **12 + age (yr)/2.** Add 3 cm for distance from nose (from age 2 years). Alternatively, **(ETT size × 3) cm at mouth** can be used.
  1. **Cardioversion for atrial dysrhythmia**: 1 Joule/kg
  2. **Cardioversion for ventricular dysrhythmia**: 2–4 Joules/kg

Age	*Newborn*	*1 month*	*3 months*	*6 months*	*1 year*
ETT size	3 mm	3 mm	3.5 mm	4 mm	4 mm
ETT length (oral)	9 cm	10 cm	10.5 cm	11 cm	12 cm
Chest tube	8 F	8 F	10 F	10 F	10 F
Urine catheter	5 F	5 F	8 F	8 F	8 F

DRUGS

Resuscitation

Drug	*Concentration*	*Dosage (in mg/kg)*	*Dosage in (ml/kg)*
Adrenaline (IV/IO)	1:10,000	0.01 (up to 0.1 mg/kg/dose if no response)	0.1 (up to 1ml/kg/dose if no response)
Adrenaline (via ETT)	1:1,000	0.1	0.1
Atropine	0.6 mg/ml	0.02	0.03
Bicarbonate	4.2%	1–2 mmol/kg	1–2 ml/kg
Lignocaine	10 mg/ml (1%)	1	0.1
Dextrose	25%	0.5	2
Volume expansion	Crystalloid/colloid		10 repeat 2–3 times if needed

Antifungals

Drug type	*Dosage*	*Remarks*
Nystatin Oral	Neonates: 100,000 U 8 h Child: 500,000 U 6–8 h	
Amphotericin B IV	0.5–1.0 mg/kg/day over 6 h	Test dose: 0.1 mg/kg. Protect from light
Fluconazole Oral and IV	3–6 mg/kg/day 12–24 h	Not recommended for infants

Antivirals

Drug type	*Dosage*
Acyclovir (Zovirax)	
Oral	*Varicella in normal children* 20 mg/kg/dose (max 800 mg) qds × 5 days *HSV in normal children* >2 years: 200 mg 5×/day × 5 days <2 years: 100 mg 5×/day × 5 days
IV	*Varicella or zoster in the immunocompromised/pneumonia/encephalitis* <1 year: IV 10 mg/kg/dose 8 h >1 year: IV 500 mg/m²/dose 8 h Duration: 7 days or until no new lesions have appeared for 48 hours *HSV Encephalitis* IV 10 mg/kg/dose 8 h × 14–21 days (neonates 21 days) *Neonatal HSV infections* IV 10–20 mg/kg/dose 8 h × 14–21 days

Antibiotics

Drug type	*Dosage*	*Remarks*
Ampicillin		Rubella-like rash common with many viral infections, which may not equate to ampicillin allergy
Oral	50–100 mg/kg/day 6 h 100–200 mg/kg/day 6 h (severe)	
IV	200–400 mg/kg/day 4 h (meningitis)	
Amoxicillin		
Oral	50 mg/kg/day 8 h	
Amoxicillin + clavulanic acid (Augmentin®)		
Oral	50 mg/kg/day 12 h (up to 90 mg/kg/day)	
IV	50 mg/kg/dose 8 h	
Amoxicillin + sulbactam (Unasyn®)		
Oral	50 mg/kg/day 12 h	
IV	100–200 mg/kg/day 6 h	
Penicillin V		
Oral	50 mg/kg/day 6 h (treatment) 250 mg bd (rheumatic fever prophylaxis)	
Crystalline Penicillin		
IV	100,000–400,000 U/kg/day 6 h	
Cloxacillin		
Oral	50 mg/kg/day 6 h	
IV	50–200 mg/kg/day 6 h	
Cephalexin (Keflex®)		First-generation cephalosporin
Oral	50 mg/kg/day 6–8 h	
Cefuroxime (Zinacef®, Zinnat®)		Second-generation cephalosporin Good activity against *H. influenzae*
IV	50–100 mg/kg/day 6 h	
Oral	15 mg/kg/dose 12 h	
Ceftazidime (Fortum®)		Third-generation cephalosporin Good for Pseudomonas. Adjust dosing interval in renal failure
IV	100 mg/kg/day 8 h 150 mg/kg/day for meningitis	
Ceftriaxone (Rocephin®)		Third-generation cephalosporin
IV	50 mg/kg/day 12–24 h 100 mg/kg/day 12 h for meningitis	
Erythromycin		
Oral	30–50 mg/kg/day 6 h (bd for EES)	
Clarithromycin		
Oral	15 mg/kg/day bd	
Gentamicin		Can be given at 8, 12 or 24 hourly intervals as long as total dose per day remains the same. Nephrotoxic and ototoxic
IV	(<1/52 old) 2.5 mg/kg/dose 12 h (1/52–1/12 old) 2.5 mg/kg/dose 8 h (>1/12 old) 2 mg/kg/dose 8 h	
Metronidazole		
Oral	30 mg/kg/day 8 h	
Trimethoprim		Not to be used in G6PD deficiency or 2 months of age. 6 mg bactrim contains 1 mg of trimethoprim
Oral	4 mg/kg/dose 12 h	
Nalidixic acid		
Oral	50 mg/kg/day 6 h	
Nitrofurantoin		
Oral	5 mg/kg/day 6 h	

Analgesics/antipyretics/antiinflammatory

Drug type	*Dosage*	*Remarks*
Paracetamol		
Oral	10 mg/kg/dose 6 h	Not to be used <2–3 months old
Ibuprofen		
Oral	20 mg/kg/day 6 h (antipyretic) 20–50 mg/kg/day 4–6 h (antiinflammatory)	Not to be used <1 year old
Diclofenac (Voltaren®)		
Oral/Rectal	0.5–3 mg/kg/day bd (max. 50 mg per dose)	Not recommended <1 year
Pethidine®		
IV/IM	0.5–2 mg/kg/dose (max. dose 75 mg)	
Morphine		
IV	0.1 mg/kg/dose (max. 15 mg) 0.01–0.04 mg/kg/h infusion in NS	
Oral	0.2–0.4 mg/kg/dose 4 h	

Sedatives

Drug type	*Dosage*	*Remarks*
Chloral hydrate		
Oral	30–50 mg/kg/day 6–8 h or stat	Contraindicated in hepatic or renal failure
Midazolam (Dormicum®)		
IV/IM	0.1–0.2 mg/kg/dose (up to 0.5 mg/kg/dose)	
Diazepam (Valium®)		
IV/IM	0.1–0.25 mg/kg/dose (≤0.6 mg/kg in 8 h) 0.2–0.5 mg/kg/day bd or tds	
Oral	<10 kg: 2.5 mg 12 h	
Rectal	>10 kg: 5.0 mg 12 h	
Cardiac cocktail		Given for sedation 30 min before procedure
Promethazine		
IV/IM	0.5 mg/kg/dose	
Pethidine®		
IV/IM	1 mg/kg/dose	
Chlorpromazine (Largactil®)		
IV/IM	0.5 mg/kg/dose	
Conscious sedation		
Ketamine		
IV	1–2 mg/kg/dose	
IM	3–6 mg/kg/dose	
Atropine		
IV/IM	0.02 mg/kg/dose (min. 0.1 mg, max 0.6 mg)	
± Midazolam		
IV/IM	0.1–0.2 mg/kg/dose	

Asthma drugs

Drug type	*Dosage*	*Remarks*
Aminophylline		
IV	5 mg/kg/dose in 1/2 h (loading) 15–20 mg/kg/day over 24 h (max. 500 mg/day)	Omit loading in patients already on theophylline
Hydrocortisone		
IV	4–5 mg/kg/dose 4–6 h	
Prednisolone		
Oral	1–2 mg/kg/day, usually OM × 5 days	
Salbutamol		
Oral	0.1 mg/kg/dose tds/qds 0.03 ml/kg/dose	
Nebulized	0.2–0.3 puff/kg/dose, ie	Continuously q 1/2 hourly q 6 hourly (1 puff = 100 mg)
MDI	2–6 puff 4 h/PRN	
Beclotide®		
MDI	2–6 puff bd	
Ipratropium bromide (Atrovent®)		
Nebulized	0.3–1 ml 4–6 h	
Theophylline (Neulin®)		
Oral	15–20 mg/kg/day 6 h (for SR formulation bd)	

Respiratory drugs

Drug type	*Dosage*	*Remarks*
Dexamethasone		
Oral	For croup: 0.2 mg/kg 12 h × 3 doses	
Adrenaline		
Nebulized	For croup: 0.5 ml/kg/dose (1:1,000) max. 5 ml	
Acetycylsteine (fluimucil)		
Oral	<1 yr: 1/2 satchet bd 1–2 yr: 1/2 satchet tds 2–6 yr: 1 satchet tds 6–10 yr: 2 satchets bd >10 yr: 2 satchets tds	
Bisolvon		
Oral	0.1 mg/kg/dose tds	
Chlorpheniramine		
Oral	0.1 mg/kg/dose tds to qds	
Promethazine		
Oral	<6/12: not recommended 6–12 months: 0.125–0.25 mg/kg/dose bd >12–24 months: 0.125–0.25mg/kg/dose tds	Antihistamine, antitussive and antiemetic
Loratadine		
Oral	0.2 mg/kg daily (max. 10 mg daily)	

Antiemetic

Drug type	*Dosage*	*Remarks*
Metoclopramide (Maxolon®)		
IV/IM Oral	0.1 mg/kg/dose bd or tds	Can cause extrapyramidal reactions usually of the dystonic type
Prochlorperazine (Stemetil®)		
IM	0.2 mg/kg/day qds	May cause oculogyric crisis
Oral	0.4 mg/kg/day tds or qds	
Ondansetron (Zofran®)		
IV Oral	0.2 mg/kg/dose 8 h	Max. per dose: 10 mg

Antidiarrhoea

Drug type	*Dosage*
Lacteol Fort®/Smecta®	
Oral	<1 yr: 1 satchet/day 8–12 h 1–2 yr: 1–2 satchet/day 8–12 h >2 yr: 2–3 satchet 8–12 h
Kaopectate	
Oral	<1 yr: 5 ml tds 2–3 yr: 10 ml tds >3 yr: 15 ml tds

Antispasmodic

Drug type	*Dosage*	*Remarks*
Hyosine-N-butylbromide (Buscopan®)		
Oral IM	0.5 mg/kg/dose tds (max. 40 mg)	Might cause functional ileus in younger children
Propantheline		
Oral	1.5 mg/kg/dose tds	
Infacol wind drops (Simethicone®)		
Oral	<2 yr: 0.2 ml per dose max. × 2 >2 yr: 0.4 ml per dose	
Trimebutine maleate (Debridat®)		
Oral	1 ml/kg/day bd–tds or 24 mg/5kg/day	72 mg/15 ml

Laxatives

Drug type	*Dosage*
Glycerin	
Suppository	Neonate: 1/4–1/2 stat Infant: 1 stat
Lactulose	
Oral	0.5 ml/kg/dose 12–24 h 1 ml/kg/dose hourly till bowel cleared, then 6–8 hourly for hepatic coma
Liquid paraffin	
Oral	1 ml/kg daily (max. 45 ml/day)

Antacids and antiulcerants

Drug type	*Dosage*
Cimetidine	
IV	20–40 mg/kg/day 4–6 h (max. 200 mg)
Oral	
Ranitidine	
IV	1 mg/kg/day 6–8 h
Oral	2 mg/kg/dose (max. 150 mg) 12 h
MMT	
Oral	1–5 yr: 2.5 ml qds 6–12 yr: 5 ml qds
Mylanta	
Oral	0.25 ml/kg/dose 4–6 h
Omeprazole (Losec®)	
IV	2 mg/kg stat (max. 80 mg) then 1 mg/kg/dose 12 h (max. 40 mg)
Oral	0.4–0.8 mg/kg/day

Muscle relaxants

Drug type	*Dosage*	*Remarks*
Succinylcholine		
IV	1–2 mg/kg/dose	Duration of action: 10 min
Atracurium		
IV	0.5 mg/kg bolus	Useful in patients with renal dysfunction
Pancuronium		
IV	0.05–0.1 mg/kg/dose 1–2 h	
Vecuronium		
IV	0.1 mg/kg/dose 1–2 h	

References/further reading

1. Singapore Ministry of Health. *A Guide On Paediatrics*. 1997:126–157.
2. Shann F. *Drug Doses*. 10th ed. Collective Pty Ltd; 1998:1–69.

123 Pain management

Shirley Ooi • Peng Li Lee • Chong Chew Lan

ANALGESIA/SEDATION FOR SHORT PROCEDURES

Joint dislocation, incision and drainage of abscesses, removal of foreign body

First choice	*Second choice*
IV **fentanyl** 2–3 µg/kg to a total of 150 µg, given as small serial doses alternating with small serial doses of IV **midazolam** 0.1–0.2 mg/kg to a total not to exceed 10 mg	IV **meperidine (Pethidine®)** 25–50 mg slow bolus and IV **midazolam** 0.1–0.2 mg/kg

1. The options given are used as adjuncts to local anaesthetics whenever appropriate.
2. Consider adjunct with **Entonox** through self-administered valve system if fear of respiratory suppression (eg elderly, respiratory problems) exist.

Emergency cardioversion

First choice
IV **midazolam** 0.1 mg/kg

Paediatric patient with forearm fracture, joint dislocation, laceration in anatomically challenging sites, eg face

First choice	*Second choice*
IM **ketamine** 2.4 mg/kg and atropine 0.02 mg/kg, or IV **ketamine** 1 mg/kg and atropine 0.02 mg/kg, or IV **fentanyl** 0.5–3 µg/kg and **midazolam** 0.05-0.1 mg/kg	Oral **midazolam** 0.4 mg/kg

1. Refer to *Conscious Sedation*.
2. Local anaesthetics are preferably buffered (1% lignocaine 9 ml to 1 ml 8.4% sodium bicarbonate) to minimize pain on infiltration.

ANALGESIA/SEDATION FOR SEVERE PAIN OF LONGER DURATION

Orthopaedic fractures

First choice	*Second choice*
IV **Pethidine®** 25–50 mg slow bolus	IV **morphine** 3–5 mg initially, repeat every 10 min if necessary.

1. Proper splintage is a form of pain relief.
2. IV metoclopramide 10 mg can be given as an antiemetic if required.

Special cases of fractures

- **Humeral shaft/tibial shaft/radius** and **ulna shaft fractures** before application of plaster

First choice	*Second choice*
Entonox	IV **fentanyl** 2–3 μg/kg slow bolus, and IV **midazolam** 0.1–0.2 mg/kg

1. Allows gross manipulation of fracture prior to plaster application.

- **Femoral shaft fracture**

First choice	*Second choice*
Femoral nerve block (see p. 592)	IV **Pethidine®** 25–50 mg

1. Allows application of traction splint.
2. Femoral nerve block useful if sedation is not indicated, eg concomitant head injury.

- **Forearm/wrist fracture** for manipulation and reduction

First choice
Bier's block with 20 ml 0.5% lignocaine (see p. 581 for details)

1. Allows accurate manipulation and reduction of fracture

- **Palm**

First choice	*Second choice*
Ulnar, median or radial nerve blocks depending on site on involvement	**Bier's block**

1. Do not use Bier's block in children below 8 years old.
2. For Bier's block, **minimum** time between injection and first deflation of cuff should be **20 min**. For children and the elderly this interval should be 30 min.

- **Fingers**

First choice	*Second choice*
Metacarpal block with 1% lignocaine (see p. 585 for details)	**Digital nerve block** (see pp. 584–585) with 1% lignocaine

- **Foot**

First choice
Ankle block

- **Orthopaedic fractures** in the presence of **head injury**

First choice	*Second choice*
IV **tramadol** 50–100 mg	IV or IM **ketorolac** 30–60 mg

1. Tramadol has fewer sedative effects than Pethidine®/morphine.

Non-traumatic neck/back pain

First choice	*Second choice*
IM **NSAIDs**, eg **diclofenac** 75 mg and IV **diazepam** 10 mg (in the presence of muscle spasm)	IM **Pethidine®** 50–75 mg or IV **Pethidine®** 25–50 mg slow bolus

1. Discharge with:
   a. Oral analgesics.
   b. Anarex®/Beserol® two tablets tds or diazepam 2.5–5 mg tds/qds
   c. Soft cervical collar for cervical strain but not for tension myalgia
   d. Heat treatment
   e. Referral for physiotherapy

Abdominal pain

- **Acute abdomen**

First choice	*Second choice*
IV **Pethidine®** 25 mg slow bolus	IV **morphine** 2–5 mg slow bolus

- **Renal/ureteric colic**

First choice	*Second choice*
IM **NSAIDs**, eg **diclofenac** 50–75 mg	IM **Pethidine®** 50–75 mg

- **Abdominal colic** from gastroenteritis

First choice
IM or IV hyoscine-N-butylbromide (**Buscopan**®) 40 mg

Chest pain

- **Ischaemic chest pain**
  1. Angina

First choice
GTN: SL, patch or IV

  2. Myocardial infarction

First choice	Second choice
SL **GTN** and IV **morphine sulphate** 2–5 mg, repeat every 10 min IV metoclopramide 10 mg as antiemetic if needed	If pain is unrelieved after 2–3 doses of IV morphine, and especially if patient is hypertensive or in heart failure, consider I/V **GTN infusion** starting at 5–15 μg/min with dose doubled every 5 mins 1. As tolerated or 2. Until BP/pulse changes or 3. Until pain relief is obtained Alternatively, Entonox as adjunct

a. Refer to *Coronary Syndromes, Acute*.
b. **Caution**: GTN is contraindicated in right ventricular infarct, hypovolaemia or pericardial tamponade.

- **Non-ischaemic chest pain**: pericarditis

First choice	Second choice
IV **dexamethasone** 15 mg	**NSAIDs**

Facial pain

- **Trigeminal neuralgia**

First choice	Second choice
Carbamazepine 100–200 mg bd PO. Increase dosage gradually until pain free or side effects occur (drowsiness, dizziness, unsteadiness)	**Baclofen**® 10 mg tds PO

1. Do FBC before starting carbamazepine
2. Combination of carbamazepine or phenytoin with Baclofen® may be tried

- **Postherpetic neuralgia**

First choice	*Second choice*
Prednisolone 60 mg/day PO × one week, then 30 mg/day × one week, then 15 mg/day × one week	**Amitryptyline** 25 mg–75 mg ON and **fluphenazine** 1–3 mg ON PO once postherpetic neuralgia is established

1. Prednisolone during the acute phase of trigeminal herpes will prevent postherpetic neuralgia

- **Temporal arteritis**

First choice
Prednisolone 30–60 mg/day or 1 mg/kg/day PO

Headaches

- **Migraine**

First choice	*Second choice*
IM or oral NSAIDs, eg IM **diclofenac** 75 mg, or **naproxen** 550 mg PO IV **metoclopramide** 10 mg	SC **sumatriptan** 6 mg Repeat a 2nd dose of 6 mg at least 1 h after 1st dose if symptoms recur; total dose = 12 mg/24 h, or Oral **sumatriptan** 100 mg. If no response, do not give 2nd dose during the same attack. **Ergotamine tartrate** 1–2 mg PO, repeat half-hour later 1. Dosage: ≤4–6 mg/24 h. 2. Dosage: ≤10–12 mg/wk

1. **Sumatriptan** is **contraindicated** in
   a. Uncontrolled hypertension
   b. IHD
   c. Myocardial infarction
   d. Prinzmetal angina
2. Do not give sumatriptan with ergotamine
3. **Ergotamine** is **contraindicated** in
   a. Severe hypertension
   b. Peripheral vascular disease
   c. IHD
   d. Impaired hepatic and renal function
   e. Pregnancy

- **Tension headache**

First choice	Second choice
Paracetamol 1g PO	I/M or oral **NSAIDs**, or oral narcotic type of analgesics, eg codeine, codeine with paracetamol (Panadeine®, Viocodin®)

BIER'S BLOCK (IV REGIONAL ANAESTHESIA)

- **Indications**: M&R of forearm fractures, eg Colles' fracture
- **Contraindications**
  1. Uncooperative
  2. Known hypersensitivity
  3. Paediatric: age <8 years or weight <25 kg
  4. Epilepsy
  5. Severe hypertension, obesity (risk of leakage under tourniquet)
  6. Severe peripheral vascular disease
  7. When pulse needs to be monitored as a guide to reduction, eg M&R of severe supracondylar fracture
  8. Sickle cell disease
- **Preparation**
  1. Medical history
  2. Examination: note baseline BP, CVS and respiratory system
  3. Baseline investigation: ECG for patients >60 years old
  4. Inform patient of procedure, no formal consent required
- **Technique**
  1. Patient placed on monitors: BP, SpO_2, cardiac monitor
  2. Resuscitation equipment ready
  3. IV cannula on each hand
  4. Elevate the affected arm above heart level × 3 min to exsanguinate limb before inflating the tourniquet
  5. **Tourniquet up on affected limb**: **50–100 mm Hg above SBP** (about 250–300 mm Hg for adults)
  6. Check that tourniquet is not leaking and confirm the disappearance of radial pulse before injecting a local anaesthetic (LA) such as **lignocaine**
  7. Note time of LA injection
  8. Blanching of skin is expected and is indicative of the success of anaesthesia
- **Dilution and dosage**
  1. Dilution of LA
     a. dilute **10 ml of 1% lignocaine with 10 ml of normal saline**
     b. 20 ml of 0.5% solution contains 100 mg lignocaine, ie **1 ml = 5 mg**

2. Dosage: **0.4 ml/kg (= 2 mg/kg)** of 0.5% lignocaine solution
3. Suggested dosage schedule

Adult	20 ml
Elderly	15 ml
Child >10 y	10–15 ml
Child <10 y	8 ml

Weight (kg)	ml
25	10
30	12
35	14

   a. **Toxic** dose of lignocaine: **3 mg/kg**
   b. **Tip**: If anaesthesia is incomplete after 20 ml of 0.5% lignocaine, inject 10–15 ml NS to flush more lignocaine peripherally
   c. **Onset**: 3 min

Note: Prilocaine is the drug of choice as it has proven track record of efficacy and safety. However, lignocaine is widely used locally.

- **Deflation**: **Do not deflate** cuff if injection time is **<20 min** as this will result in a high concentration entering the circulation. Lignocaine fixes to tissues after 20 min and cuff release usually produces no adverse effects.
- **Complications**
  1. Lignocaine allergy
  2. Lignocaine toxicity due to inadvertent systemic bolus injection
     a. Early: circumoral numbness, light headedness, tinnitus, slurred speech
     b. Late: unconsciousness, seizures, bradydysrhythmias, hypotension, respiratory arrest
- **Discharge**:
  1. After observation for 2 h
  2. Check limb circulation

SUPRAORBITAL AND SUPRATROCHLEAR NERVE BLOCK (FOREHEAD BLOCK)

- **Anatomy**:
  1. The supraorbital nerve divides into 2 branches and leaves the orbit through 2 notches in the superior orbital margin, about 2.5 cm from the midline. It supplies the sensation to most of the forehead and the frontal region of the scalp.
  2. The supratrochlear nerve emerges from the upper medial corner of the orbit and provides the sensory supply to the medial part of the forehead.
- **Dosage**: 1% lignocaine 3–5 ml with or without adrenaline
- **Technique** (Figure 1):
  1. Insert the needle in the midline between the eyebrows and direct it laterally.
  2. Inject the lignocaine subcutaneously from the point of insertion along the upper margin of the eyebrow.
  3. If the wound extends into the lateral part of the forehead, SC infiltration of lignocaine may be needed lateral to the eyebrow to block the zygomaticotemporal and auriculotemporal nerves.

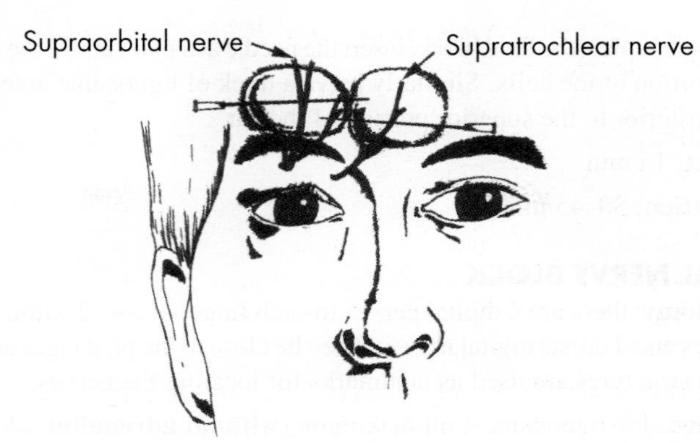

Figure 1: Supraorbital and supratrochlear nerve blocks

- **Onset**: 5 min
- **Duration**: 30–45 min

AURICULAR BLOCK

- **Anatomy**:
  1. The auricle derives its sensory supply from branches of the auriculotemporal, greater auricular and lesser occipital nerves. The vagus nerve supplies sensory nerves to the meatus as well.
  2. The auriculotemporal nerve lies anterior to the pinna while both the greater auricular and lesser occipital nerves lies posteriorly.
- **Dosage**: 1% lignocaine 8–12 ml without adrenaline
- **Technique** (Figure 2):
  1. Insert the needle just beneath the lobule and direct it behind the ear, parallel and just superficial to the bone. Inject lignocaine along this track.
  2. Without reinserting the needle, redirect the needle anterior to the lobule and tragus. Leave a similar trace of lignocaine while withdrawing the needle.

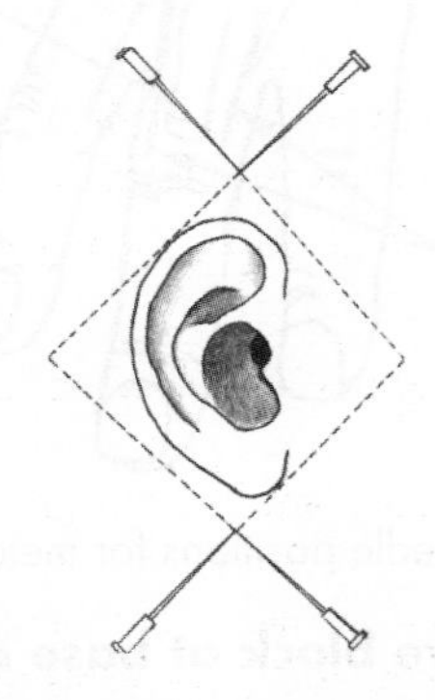

Figure 2: Field anaesthesia of the ear

3. To complete the field block, insert the needle at a point above the superior portion of the helix. Similarly leave a track of lignocaine anterior and posterior to the superior portion of the ear.

- **Onset**: 15 min
- **Duration**: 30–45 min

DIGITAL NERVE BLOCK

- **Anatomy**: there are 4 digital nerves to each finger or toe: 2 palmar digital nerves and 2 dorsal digital nerves. They lie close to the phalanges and these bony structures are used as landmarks for locating the nerves.
- **Dosage**: 1% lignocaine 4 ml maximum (**without adrenaline** added)
- **Technique** (Figures 3 and 4)
  1. **Web space approach**:
     a. Needle (eg 27G) is introduced in the web space just distal to the metacarpal-phalangeal joint and advanced adjacent to the phalanx and directed towards the volar surface of the digit: 1 ml of lignocaine is deposited near the palmar nerve.
     b. The needle is then withdrawn and (without leaving the original puncture site) advanced towards the dorso-lateral aspect of the phalanx until it touches the bone: 0.5 ml of lignocaine is deposited near the dorsal nerve.
     c. The procedure is repeated on the opposite side of the digit.

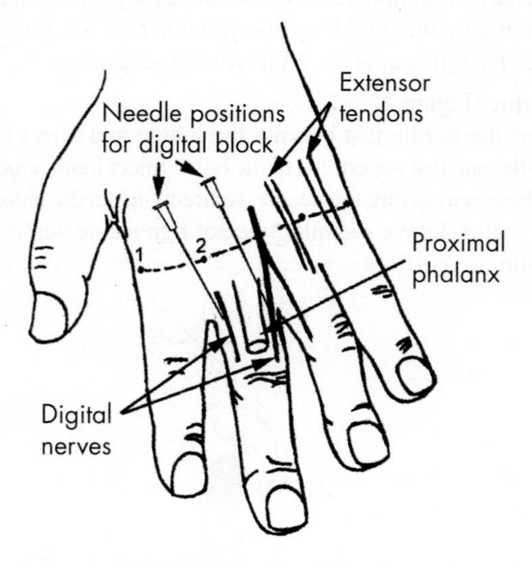

Figure 3: Digital nerve block at base of the finger and at metacarpal level

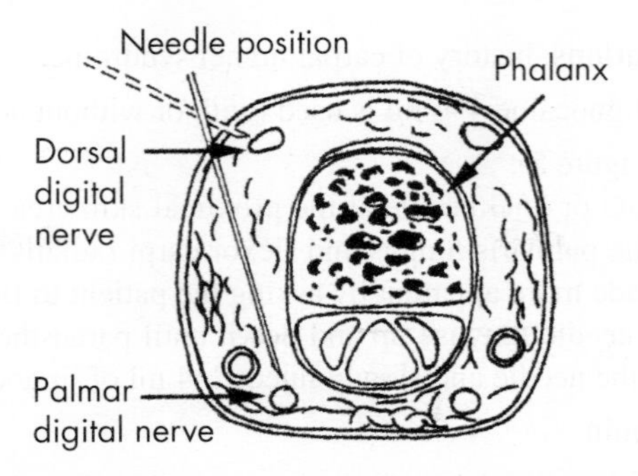

Figure 4: Cross-section of finger/toe

2. The basic procedure for digital block described above may be used for the thumb and the great toe. For the **thumb**, the injections are **near** the **midpoint** as the neurovascular bundle runs in the midline of the thumb.
3. **For 2nd to 5th toes**: a single midline dorsal needlestick can be used to anaesthetize both sides of the toes.
4. **Metacarpal approach**:
   a. Digital nerves can be blocked where they run in the interspaces between the metacarpals.
   b. Insert a needle in the palm through the distal palmar crease, between the flexor tendons of adjacent fingers. Inject 3–4 ml of plain 1% lignocaine. These will anaesthetize the adjacent sites of these 2 fingers. Alternatively, inject 3–4 ml of 1% lignocaine through the distal palmar crease at the midpoint of the base of the finger. This single injection will anaesthetize the finger involved.
   c. Alternatively, a dorsal approach that is less painful can be attempted. Insert a needle to the dorsum of the hand between the relevant metacarpal heads on a level with the distal palmar crease. Place your hand (the operator's) against the patient's palm and advance the needle till you feel the palmar skin is taut. Aspirate, withdraw while injecting till you exit via the dorsal skin. Repeat the procedure on the other side of the relevant metacarpal to anaesthetize the finger involved.

- **Onset**: 5 min
- **Duration**: 45–60 min

WRIST BLOCK

- **Indications**: minor surgery to areas of the hand innervated by the median, ulnar and radial nerve.

Median nerve

- **Anatomy**: at the level of the proximal palmar crease, the median nerve lies superficially between the palmaris longus and flexor carpi radialis (or medial to flexor carpi radialis if the palmaris longus is absent).

- **Contraindications**: history of carpal tunnel syndrome.
- **Dosage**: 1% lignocaine 4–6 ml is used (with or without adrenaline).
- **Technique** (Figure 5):
  1. Insert a 23G or 25G needle at the proximal skin crease of the wrist, between the palmaris longus and flexor carpi radialis (the 2 tendons may be made more apparent by asking the patient to flex the wrist).
  2. Move the needle fanwise up and down until paraesthesia is elicited: withdraw the needle and slowly inject 2–4 ml of lignocaine.
- **Onset**: 5–10 min
- **Duration**: 1.5 h

Ulnar nerve

- **Anatomy**:
  1. Ulnar nerve divides into a dorsal and a palmar branch about 5 cm proximal to wrist.
  2. At the wrist, the palmar branch lies between the flexor carpi ulnaris and the ulnar artery.
- **Dosage**: 1% lignocaine 7–10 ml (with or without adrenaline).

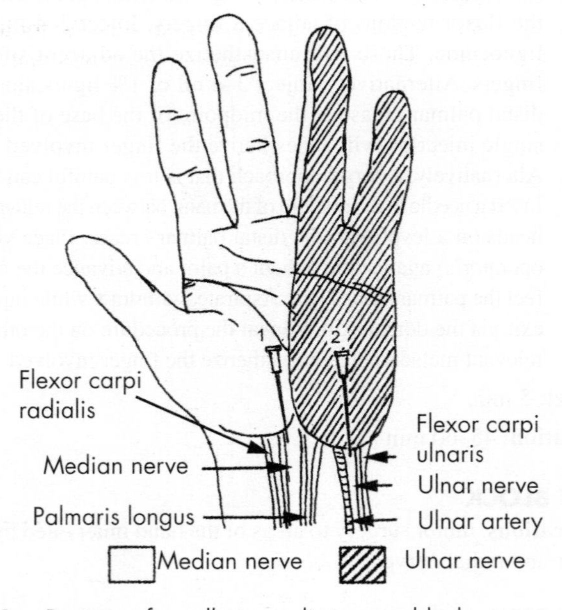

Figure 5: Wrist block showing median and ulnar nerve blocks

- **Technique** (Figure 5):
  1. **Palmar branch**: insert a 23–25G needle between the flexor carpi ulnaris and the ulnar artery at the same level with the ulnar styloid process. If paraesthesia is elicited, withdraw the needle and inject 2–4 ml of 1% lignocaine.
  2. **Dorsal branch**: 5 ml of 1% lignocaine is injected subcutaneously from the tendon of flexor carpi ulnaris around the ulnar aspect of the wrist.
- **Onset**: 5–10 min (faster onset of dorsal branch blockade)
- **Duration**: 1.5 h

Radial nerve

- **Anatomy**: at the level of the wrist the radial nerve gives off superficial branches which lie subcutaneously on the extensor aspect.
- **Dosage**: 1% lignocaine 5 ml (with or without adrenaline).
- **Technique** (Figure 6): subcutaneous infiltration starting from the radial styloid to the ulnar styloid at the level of the wrist.
- **Onset**: 2 min
- **Duration**: 1 h

NERVE BLOCKS AT THE ANKLE

- Lignocaine blocks at the ankle are particularly useful for anaesthetizing the sole of the foot, where local infiltration is very painful and unsatisfactory.

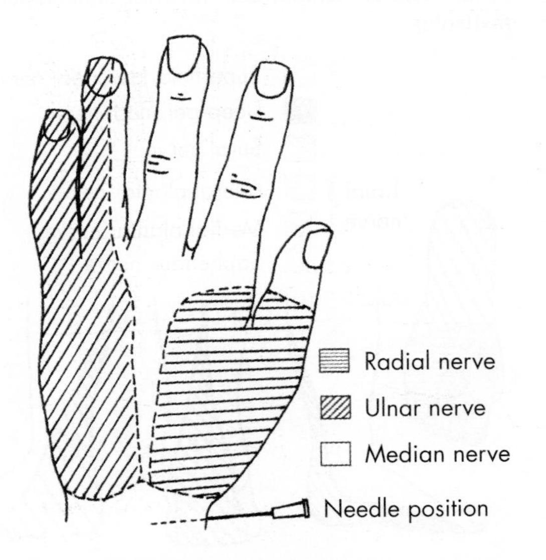

Figure 6: Radial nerve block

- **Anatomy**:
  1. Sensation in the ankle and foot is supplied by 5 main nerves (Figure 7):
     a. **Saphenous nerve** (medial side of the ankle)
     b. **Superficial peroneal nerve** (front of ankle and dorsum of foot)
     c. **Deep peroneal nerve** (lateral side of great toes and medial side of second toe)
     d. **Sural nerve** (heel and lateral side of hind foot)
     e. **Tibial nerve** (which forms the medial and lateral plantar nerves, supplying the anterior half of the sole)
  2. There is significant overlap between the areas supplied by the different nerves, especially on the sole of the foot. It is often necessary to block more than one nerve.
- **Dosage**: 1% lignocaine (with or without adrenaline) 5 ml or 0.5% bupivacaine. Do not use adrenaline in patients with peripheral vascular disease.
- **Technique**:
  1. **Saphenous nerve**: infiltrate LA subcutaneously around the great saphenous vein, anterior to and just above the medial malleolus. Aspirate carefully because of the risk of IV injection.
  2. **Superficial peroneal nerve**: infiltrate LA subcutaneously above the ankle joint from the anterior border of the tibia to the lateral malleolus.
  3. **Deep peroneal nerve**: insert the needle above the ankle joint between the tendons of tibialis anterior and the extensor hallicis longus. Inject 5 ml of LA.
  4. **Sural nerve (Figure 8)**: lie the patient prone. Insert the needle lateral to the Achilles tendon and infiltrate subcutaneously to the lateral malleolus.

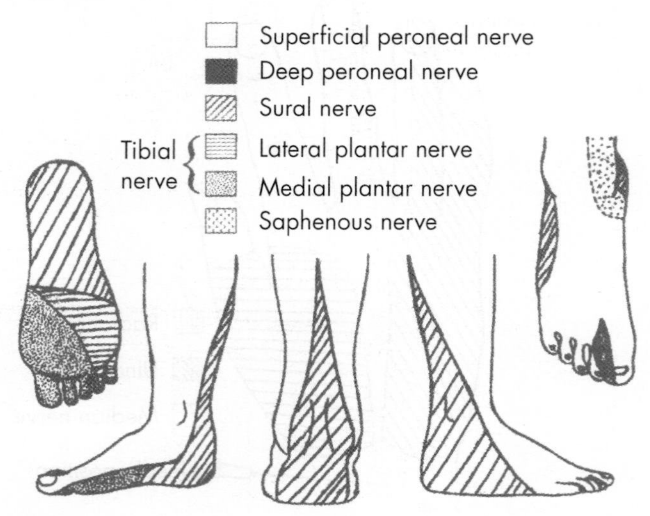

Figure 7: Sensory supply of the foot and ankle

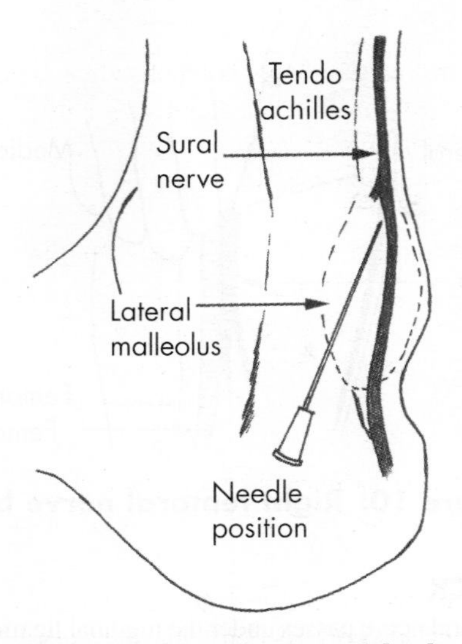

Figure 8: Sural nerve block

5. **Tibial nerve (Figure 9)**: lie the patient prone. Palpate the posterior tibial artery. Insert the needle medial to the Achilles tendon and level with the upper border of the medial malleolus, so the needle tip is just lateral to the artery. Withdraw slightly if paraesthesia occurs. Aspirate. Inject 5–10 ml LA.

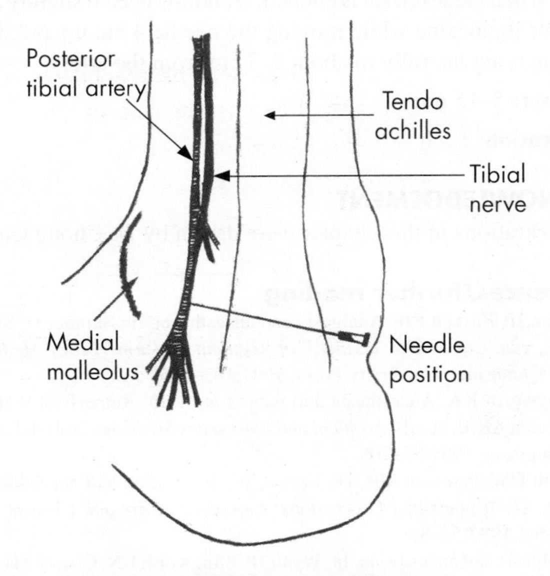

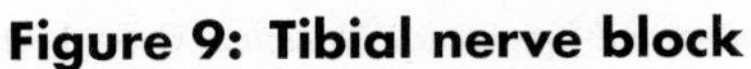

Figure 9: Tibial nerve block

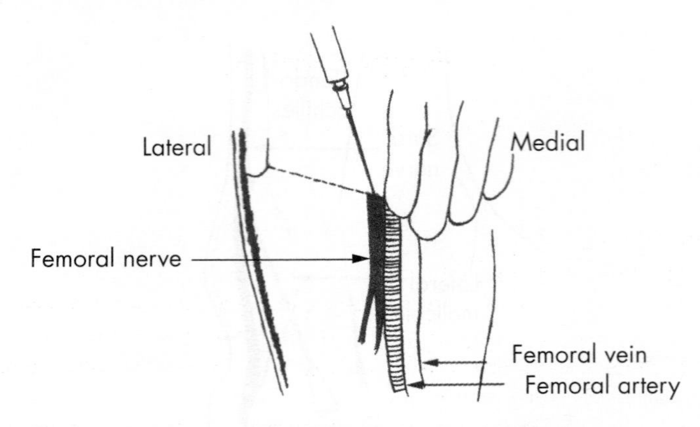

Figure 10: Right femoral nerve block

FEMORAL BLOCK

- **Anatomy**: femoral nerve passes under the inguinal ligament to enter the thigh and lies lateral to the femoral artery (mnemonic: VAN: vein lies most medial).
- **Dosage**: 1% lignocaine 10–15 ml.
- **Technique** (Figure 10):
  1. Use a 21–23G needle at least 4 cm long.
  2. Palpate for femoral artery.
  3. Insert needle perpendicular to skin and just lateral to the artery as it emerges under the inguinal ligament.
  4. When paraesthesia is elicited, withdraw needle slightly and inject 10 ml of lignocaine while moving the needle 4 cm up and down, gradually moving laterally to about 2–3 cm from the artery.
- **Onset:** 5–15 min
- **Duration**: 1.5 h

ACKNOWLEDGEMENT

All illustrations in this chapter were drawn by Dr Chong Chew Lan.

References/further reading

1. Nolan JP, Baskett PJF. Analgesia and anaesthesia. In: Skinner D, Swain A, Peyton R, et al, eds. *Cambridge Textbook of Accident and Emergency Medicine*. Cambridge, NY: Cambridge University Press; 1997:183–205.
2. Illingworth KA. Anaesthesia and pain control. In: Rutherford WH, Illingworth RN, Marsden AK, et al, eds. *Accident and Emergency Medicine*. 2nd ed. Edinburgh: Churchill Livingstone;1989:83–106.
3. Smith DW, Peterson MR, De Berard SC. Infiltration and nerve block anesthesia. In: Trott AT. *Wounds and Lacerations: Emergency Care and Closure*. 2nd ed. St Louis: Mosby; 1997:53–89.
4. Analgesia and anaesthesia. In: Wyatt JP, Illingworth RN, Clancy MJ, et al., eds. *Oxford Handbook of Accident and Emergency Medicine*. Oxford: Oxford University Press; 1999:282–324.

124 Simple statistics

JP Travers • Shirley Ooi

DESIGN ISSUES

- **Random allocation/sampling**
  1. In random allocation/sampling, each individual has a known chance (usually equal) of being allocated a treatment/being selected.
  2. For random sampling, use either random number tables or a computer-generated sampling plan.
  3. For random allocation, use a block-randomization design for balanced allocation.
  4. Both random sampling and allocation deal with possible **bias** at treatment allocation.
- **Bias**: this is the error related to the ways the targeted and sampled populations differ. It is also called the **measurement/systematic error** and it threatens the validity of a study. Examples of bias include:
  1. Volunteer bias: subjects may have a vested interest to enter trial.
  2. Selection bias: subject selection may affect outcome (choose from 1 group type only).
  3. Response bias: placebo effect and desire to please doctor!
  4. Assessment bias: assessor should not be investigator (blind) or subject (double blind).
- **Confounder**: a variable more likely to be present in one group of subjects than another that is related to the outcome of interest and thus potentially confuses or 'confounds' the results, eg age or gender in a study on treatment of IHD.
- **Blinding/masking**: this is a technique to increase objectivity and decrease subjectivity of assessing the efficacy of a treatment. Types of blinding:
  1. **Single blind**: only the patient is unaware of whether he is in the treatment or control group.
  2. **Double blind**: both patient and investigator are unaware.
  3. **Triple blind**: patient, investigator and assessor are unaware.

  However, the current trend is to report on who were blinded rather than use terms like single, double or triple blind.
- **Sample size**: Sample size increases with
  1. Bigger power

Note: **Power** is the ability of test statistics to detect a specified alternative hypothesis or difference of a specified size when the alternative hypothesis is true. More loosely, it is the ability of a study to detect an actual effect or difference.

2. Smaller effect size

DATA ISSUES

Data types

- **Quantitative/numerical data** for which the differences between the numbers have meaning on a numerical scale.
  1. **Continuous scale** has values on a continuum, eg age.
  2. **Discrete scale** has values equal to integers, eg number of fractures.
- **Qualitative (categorical) data**
  1. **Nominal scales** have no ranking order (eg gender).
  2. **Ordinal scales**: there is an inherent order or ranking among the categories (eg Stage I and IV of disease).

Summarizing data

- **Measures of the middle (central tendency)**: the decision on which measure of central tendency is to be used depends on 2 factors: (1) scale of measurement (ordinal or numerical) and (2) shape of the distribution of measurements.
  1. **Mean** (arithmetic): the sum of the observations divided by the number of observations, ie 2, 5, 8, 3, 4 is 22/5 = 4.4 (used if the variable is normally distributed). This is used for numerical data and for symmetric (not skewed) distributions.
  2. **Median** is the central value of the distribution (used if the variable is skewed), ie half of the observations are smaller and half are larger. For 1, 3, 4, 5, 7, the median and mean are both 4 but for 1, 3, 4, 7, 8, 12, 13, 20, 30 the median is 8 but the mean is 10.88. It is also equal to the 50th percentile. This is used for ordinal data or for numerical data whose distribution is skewed.
  3. **Mode** is the value that occurs most frequently. For example, the mode for 2, 2, 2, 3, 3, 4, 5 is 2. Mode is used primarily for bimodal distribution.
- **Measures of spread (dispersion)**
  1. **Range** is the difference between the largest observation and the smallest observation. This is used with numerical data when the purpose is to emphasize extreme values.
  2. **Degrees of freedom:** total number of observations (n) made – 1 or ($n - 1$).
  3. **Variance**: the sum of the deviations from the mean for all observations (n) made in a sample group will always be 0 (ie +2 mm Hg, +1 mm Hg, 0 mm Hg, −1 mm Hg, −2 mm Hg = 0 mm Hg). Therefore we have to square this sum to produce a +ve value (this gets rid of the minus sign, +4, +2, 0, +2, +4). If we divide this sum by the degrees of freedom ($n - 1$), we obtain the variance (12/5 = 2.4). So if the deviations from the mean are large and the number of observations (n) is small, then the variance will be large! The **variance is a numerical**

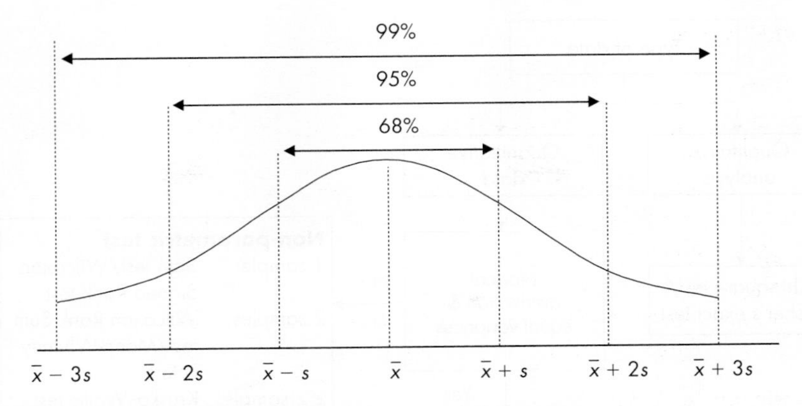

Figure 1: A bell-shaped or normal distribution
95% of the observations lie between $\bar{x} - 2s$ and, $\bar{x} + 2s$ where $\bar{x}$ is the mean of the observations.

unit only and not descriptive, ie 2.4 and not 2.4 mm Hg. To change it back to descriptive, we use the standard deviation.

4. **Standard deviation(s)** is a measure of the spread of data about their mean (Figure 1). This is used with symmetric (not skewed) numerical data. It is this square root of the variance and it is a way of reverting to descriptive terms.

$$s = \sqrt{\frac{\Sigma(x - \bar{x})^2}{n - 1}}$$

where $\bar{x}$ = mean
n = number of observations
s^2 = variance

5. **Standard error** provides an estimate of how far the calculated true value of the mean of the sample population is from the unknown value of the mean of the parent population. The larger the sample size, the closer the sample mean to the parent population mean and the smaller the standard error. Therefore the sample is more representative of the parent.
6. **Percentile** is a number that indicates the percentage of distribution less than or equal to that number. This is used, in the following 2 situations:
   a. When the median is used, ie with ordinal data or with skewed numerical data.
   b. When the mean is used but the objective is to compare individual observations with a set of norm.

HYPOTHESIS TESTING

- **Null hypothesis**: this hypothesis or states that there is no difference or no effect between the groups under study.

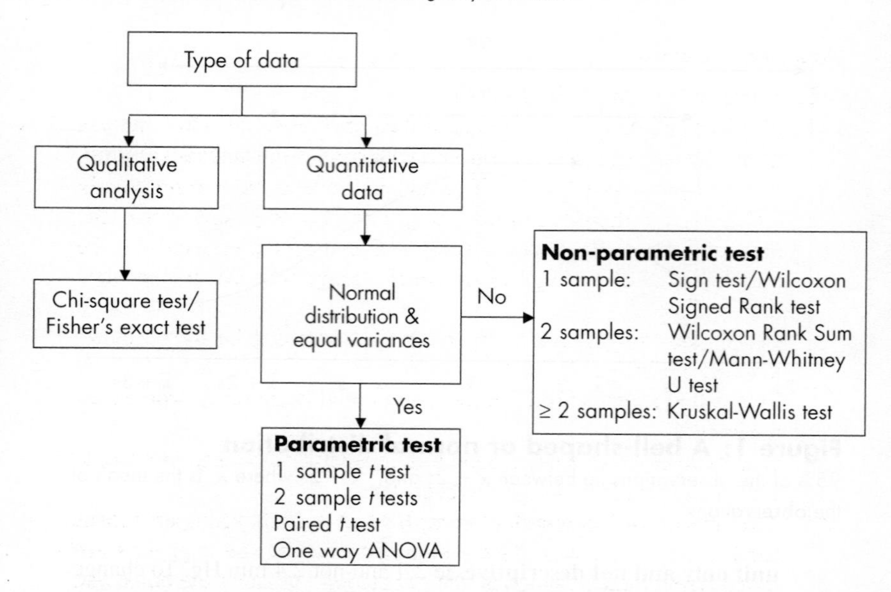

Figure 2: How to decide on types of statistical tests to use

- **Alternative hypothesis**: this is the opposite to the null hypothesis. It is the conclusion when the null hypothesis is rejected.
- **Type I error**: this is the error that results if a true null hypothesis is rejected or if a difference is concluded when there is no difference.
- **Type II error**: this is the error that results if a false null hypothesis is not rejected or if a difference is not detected when there is a difference.
- **Probability** p: This is the number of times an outcome occurs in the total number of trials. p is the probability that the difference obtained between 2 groups is due to chance (usually taken as significant if less than 5% [$p<0.05$] or less than 1 in 20).
- **95% confidence interval** states that you are 95% confident that the unknown parameter such as the mean or proportion is contained within the interval.

TEST TYPES

Figure 2 summarizes the decision-making on statistical test usage.

Qualitative data

For evaluating categorical versus categorical variables (whether there is any association between 2 categorical variables), use **Chi-square** test. If the Chi-square test assumptions are not satisfied (usually if the sampling size is small), use **Fisher's exact** test.

Quantitative data

- **Parametric tests or student's *t* test**
  1. Ideal for comparing two groups of data in 'before and after' studies (**paired *t* test**) or between two groups with **similar normal distribution.** A *t* test is used to determine if the mean of one group is significantly different from the mean of another group. The larger the *t* value, the more significant the difference, ie $t = 7.8$ at $p < 0.05$ means that the probability of obtaining a *t* value of this magnitude due to chance is less than 5%.
  2. **One-tailed *t* test** is used if a treatment is assumed to be always better than the control.
  3. **Two-tailed *t* test** is used if a treatment could be better or worse than the control.
  4. **One-sample *t* test** is used to determine whether the mean of a single variable differs from a specified constant.
  5. **Two-sample or independent-sample *t* test is** used to compare means for 2 groups of cases. The assumption is that the 2 groups are independent random samples, the population variances are equal and the observations are normally distributed in each population.
  6. **Paired-samples *t* test** compares the means of 2 variables for a single group. The assumption is that the difference to the 2 paired variables follows a normal distribution.
  7. **Analysis of variance (ANOVA)**
     a. **One-way ANOVA** produces a one-way analysis of variance for a quantitative dependent variable by a single (independent) variable. The assumptions are that the observations are normally distributed in each population, all the population variances are equal and all the groups are independent random samples.
     b. If used for 3 or more group comparisons, ANOVA will only show **if there is a difference between the groups** but will not identify where the difference(s) is/are. If a difference is found, then a post-hoc test (usually Bonferroni correction) is used to identify where the differences are between the groups.

- **Non-parametric tests such as Mann-Whitney U test or Wilcoxon Rank Sum test** is used when normality assumptions are not satisfied.

- **Correlation analysis** is used to establish if there is a linear relationship between 2 quantitative or ordinal variables, eg rising exam score versus IQ. If normality assumptions are satisfied for the 2 variables, use Pearson correlation. Otherwise use Spearman correlation.

- **Regression analysis** is used to quantify a linear relationship between a continuous outcome variable and a continuous/qualitative independent variable (eg comparing increasing age versus rise in serum cholesterol; this is a **simple linear regression. Muliple linear regression** is used when more than one continuous/qualitative independent variables are being used (gender, race, cholesterol levels)

STATISTICS USED IN DIAGNOSTIC TESTS

	Definition	*Based on Figure 3*
Sensitivity	Population of people with a target disorder in whom a test result is positive, ie **PID** = **P**ositive (test) **i**n **D**isease	$\frac{a}{a+c}$
Specificity	Proportion of people without target disorder in whom a test result is negative, ie **NIH** = **N**egative **i**n **H**ealth	$\frac{d}{b+d}$
Positive predictive value (PPV)/ Predictive value of a positive test	The proportion of time that a patient with a positive diagnostic test result has the disease being investigated	$\frac{a}{a+b}$
Negative predictive value (NPV)/ Predictive value of a negative test	The proportion of time that a patient with a negative diagnostic test result does not have the disease being investigated	$\frac{d}{c+d}$
Likelihood ratio of a positive test [L.R.(+)]	The relative likelihood that a positive test would be expected in a patient with (as opposed to one without) a disorder of interest	$= \frac{a/(a+c)}{b/(b+d)}$ $= \frac{\text{sensitivity}}{1-\text{specificity}}$
Likelihood ratio of a negative test [L.R. (−)]	The relative likelihood that a negative test would be expected in a patient with (as opposed to one without) a disorder of interest	$= \frac{c/(a+c)}{d/(b+d)}$ $= \frac{1-\text{sensitivity}}{\text{specificity}}$

Test	*Disease*	
	Present	*Absent*
+ve	True positive (a)	False positive (b)
−ve	False negative (c)	True negative (d)

Figure 3: Probable outcomes of test results

CONCEPTS USED IN THERAPY ARTICLES

	Definitions	*Formula*
Control risk (Rc)	Risk of the event among control patients	
Treatment risk (Rt)	Risk of the event among treated patients	
Relative Risk Reduction (RRR)	% risk lost	$\frac{Rc - Rt}{Rc}$
Relative Risk (RR)	% risk remaining	$\frac{Rt}{Rc}$
Absolute Risk Reduction (ARR)	Absolute risk lost	$Rc - Rt$
Number need to treat (NNT)	The number of patients who need to be treated over a specific period of time to prevent one bad outcome	$\frac{1}{ARR}$

References/further reading

1. Bland M. An *Introduction to Medical Statistics*. Oxford: Oxford Medical Publications, Oxford University Press; 1993.
2. Byrne D. *Publishing Your Medical Research Paper*. Baltimore: Williams & Wilkins; 1998.
3. Dawson-Saunders B, Trapp RG. *Basic and Clinical Biostatistics*. 2nd ed. Norwalk, CT: Appleton & Lange; 1994.
4. Guyatt, G, Rennie D, eds. *Users' Guide to the Medical Literature*: *A Manual for Evidence-based Clinical Practice*. USA: AMA Press; 2002.
5. Chan YH. Randomised controlled trials (RCTs): Essentials. *Singapore Med J*. 2003;44(2):60–63.
6. Chan YH. Randomised controlled trials (RCTs): Sample size – The magic number? *Singapore Med J*. 2003;44(2):172–174.
7. Chan YH. Biostatistics 101: Data presentation. *Singapore Med J*. 2003;44(6):280–285.
8. Chan YH. Biostatistics 102: Quantitative data: Parametric and non-parametric tests. *Singapore Med J*. 2003:44(8):391–396.

125 Tetanus immunization schedule

Suresh Pillai

TETANUS PRONE WOUNDS

- Wounds with delay of ≥6 hours before seeking medical treatment
- Penetrating wounds
- Contaminated wounds
- Septic wounds
- Presence of devitalized tissue
- Denervated and/or ischaemic tissue
- Burns
- Crush wounds
- Open fractures

Table 1: Anti-tetanus toxoid immunization schedule

		Clean wound	*Tetanus prone wound*
Complete course ATT booster[a]	<5 y <5 y	Nil	Nil
Complete course ATT booster	5–10 y 5–10 y	Nil	ATT
Complete course ATT booster	>10 y >10 y	ATT	ATT
Incomplete course or unknown status		ATT + full ATT course[b]	ATT + full ATT course + HTIG[c]

a. ATT 0.5 ml tetanus toxoid IM

b. Full ATT course 0.5 ml ATT IM stat, 6 weeks, 6 months

c. HTIG Human tetanus immune globulin 250 IU at different site from ATT

References/further reading

1. Tetanus immunization. In: Committee on Trauma of the American College of Surgeons. *Advanced Trauma Life Support for Doctors Manual*. 6th ed. Chicago: American College of Surgeons; 1997:385–389.

126 Useful formulae

Chong Chew Lan

Many clinical problems may be deciphered with the aid of 'mathematical equations'. When appropriately applied, these can help in the formulation of differential diagnosis, interpretation of laboratory data and clinical management. The following are useful formulae for daily practice.

- **Calculated serum osmolality in mmol/l = (2 × Na + urea + glucose)**
  1. Need to be >350 mOsm/kg H_2O for diagnosis of hyperosmolar non-ketotic coma. **Normal range is 286 ± 4 mOsm/kg H_2O.**
  2. Calculated serum osmolality can also be used to calculate the **osmolal gap.**
  3. **Osmolal gap =** measured serum osmolality – calculated serum osmolality.
  4. The '**normal**' osmolal gap is arbitrarily set at **10 mOsm/kg H_2O**. In the ED setting, an elevated osmolal gap usually represents the presence of ethanol or other toxic alcohols such as methanol, ethylene glycol, isopropyl alcohol, proteins or lipids.

- **AG (anion gap) = Na (mmol/l) – [chloride (mmol/l) + bicarbonate (mmol/l)]**

  The **normal range is 7 ± 4 mEq/l**. The reference range for the AG has shifted 'downwards'. Historically, the 'normal' AG has been 12 ± 4. The newer 'normal' range is 7 ± 4, which reflects the current methods for measuring Na^+, Cl^- and HCO_3^-. This downward shift in the normal AG value is primarily due to an upward shift in the chloride value that has accompanied changes in laboratory assessment methods. AG is useful in the evaluation of patients with metabolic acidosis. See Table 1 (p. 162) and Table 2 (p. 163) respectively for causes of high and normal AG.

- **Acid base disorders**: for more details, refer to *Acid Base Emergencies*.
  1. The diagnosis of acid base disorders can be complicated and the recognition of mixed **acid base disorders** (Figure 1) often proves elusive. Unless the clinician knows what degree of compensation is expected of a disorder, he/she may not recognize the existence of an overlapping second disorder.
  2. Rules of compensation in acid base disorders (PCO_2 in mm Hg; HCO_3^- in mmol/L):

Primary disturbance	Normal compensatory response
Metabolic acidosis	$PCO_2 = (1.5 \times HCO_3^-) + 8 \pm 2$
Metabolic alkalosis	$PCO_2 = [(0.6 \times HCO_3^- - 24)] + 40)$
Acute respiratory acidosis	$\Delta HCO_3^- = (0.1 \times \Delta PCO_2)$
Acute respiratory alkalosis	$\Delta HCO_3^- = (0.2 \times \Delta PCO_2)$
Chronic respiratory acidosis/alkalosis	$\Delta HCO_3^- = (0.4 \times \Delta PCO_2)$

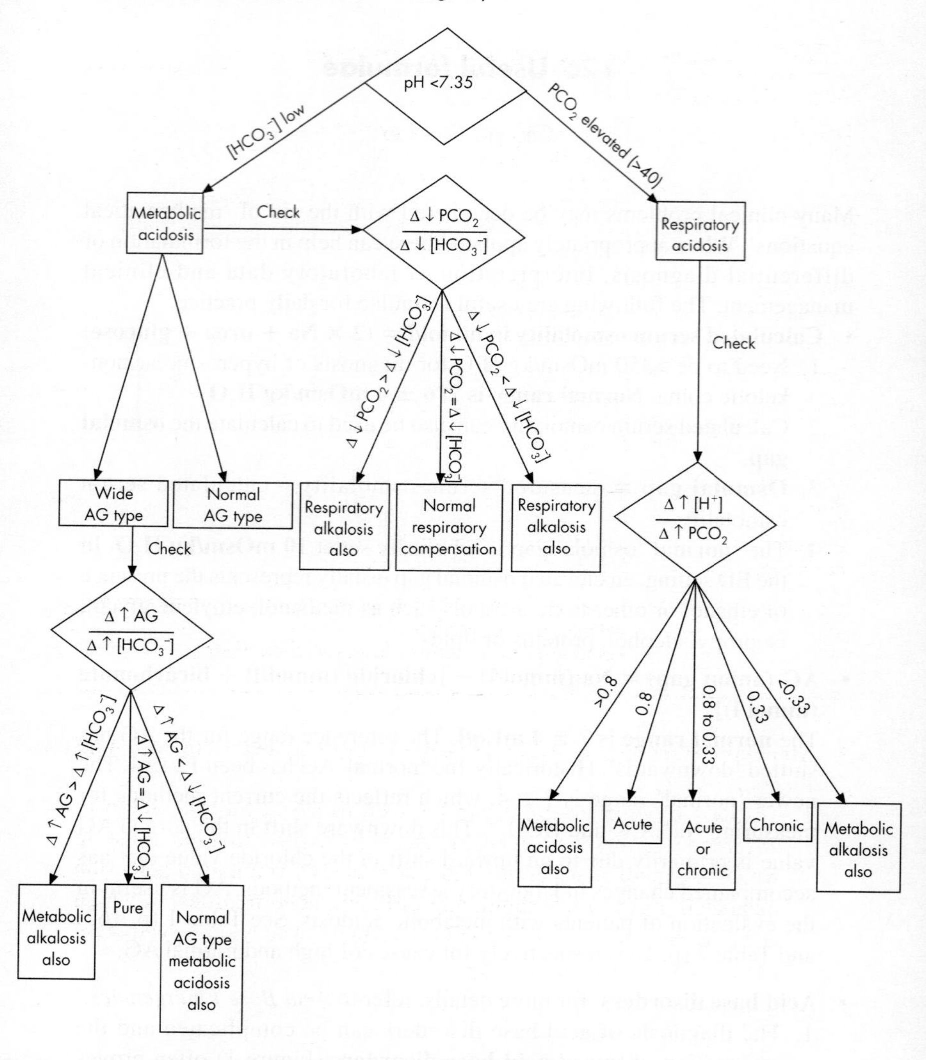

Figure 1: Algorithm for determination of type of acidosis and mixed acid base disturbances when pH indicates acidaemia

Figure reproduced with permission of the McGraw-Hill Companies, from Tintinalli JE, Kelen GD, Stapczynski JS, et al, eds. *Emergency Medicine: A Comprehensive Study Guide*. New York: McGraw-Hill; 2000:133, Fig. 21–2A.

- **Bicarbonate deficit (mEq) = 0.5 × wt (kg) × (desired − measured) bicarbonate**

  In the absence of superimposed respiratory acid base disorder, a serum bicarbonate level of 15 mEq/l can be used to calculate the bicarbonate deficit. One-half of the bicarbonate deficit is replaced immediately and the rest is infused over the next 4 to 6 hours.

Table 1: Causes of prolonged QT interval

Acquired long QT syndrome	
Drugs	• Class 1A, 1C and III antidysrhythmics (eg quinidine, procainamide, disopyramide, sotalol and amiodarone) • Psychotropic agents (eg tricyclic antidepressants, phenothiazines, tetracyclic agents and haloperidol) • Others: organophosphates, erythromycin, pentamidine, astemizole, terfenadine
Electrolyte abnormalities	• Hypokalaemia • Hypomagnesaemia • Hypocalcaemia
Cardiac abnormalities	• Myocardial ischaemia • Myocarditis • Complete AV block • Sinus node dysfunction
Intracranial disease	• SAH
Altered nutritional state	• Liquid protein modified fast diet • Starvation (anorexia nervosa)
Congenital	• Jervell and Lange-Nielsen syndrome (autosomal recessive with congenital deafness) • Romano-Ward syndrome (autosomal dominant) • Sporadic type

- **Alveolar-arterial (A-a) oxygen gradient**: for more details, refer to *Acid Base Emergencies*.
  1. The A-a oxygen gradient can be used to assist the physician in differentiating between hypoxia caused by hypoventilation alone, in which A-a gradient is normal, and that caused by ventilation-perfusion mismatch, right to left shunt, and diffusion abnormalities, in which A-a gradient is abnormal. For ABG taken in room air at sea level (partial pressures expressed in mm Hg),

     $$\text{A-a gradient} = \left[(760 - 47) \times FiO_2 - \frac{PaCO_2}{0.8}\right] - PaO_2$$

     where FiO_2 is expressed in decimal
  2. To account for age-dependent variations,

     $$\text{normal A-a gradient} < \frac{\text{age}}{4} + 4$$

  3. The A-a gradient can assist the emergency physician in determining the causes of hypoxia but literature remains unclear as to how to interpret a normal A-a gradient in the setting of a suspected pulmonary embolus.
- **QT interval**
  1. Useful rule of thumb: The QT interval should be less than one-half the R-R interval. More precisely,

     $$\textbf{corrected QT interval (QTc)} = \frac{\mathbf{QT}}{\sqrt{\mathbf{RR}}}$$

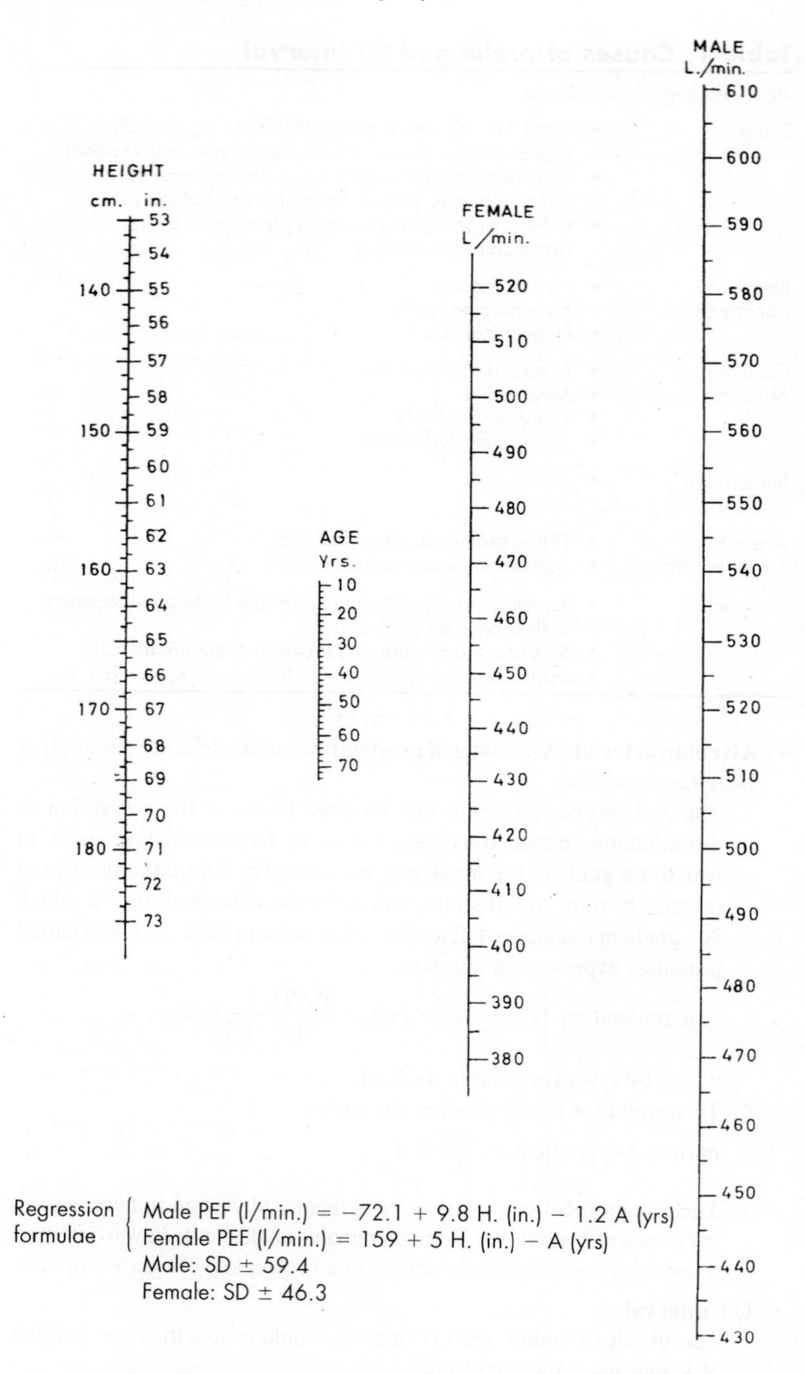

Figure 2: PEFR nomogram for adult Chinese in Singapore (Use height and age)

2. Normal QTc = 0.42 sec.
3. See Table 1 for causes of prolonged QT interval

- **Diagnostic tools for the evaluation of azotemia**
  1. **Fractional excretion of sodium**

$$FE_{Na} = \frac{\text{Urine (Na)/Plasma (Na)} \times 100}{\text{Urine (Cr)/Plasma (Cr)}}$$

  2. **Renal failure index (RFI)**: $RFI = \frac{Urine_{Na} \times Plasma_{Cr}}{Urine_{Cr}}$

  3. **Urine findings in prerenal azotemia and acute tubular necrosis**

Diagnostic tool	**Prerenal azotemia**	**ATN**
Urine osmolality U_{osmo} (mOsm/kg)	>500	<350
Urine sodium U_{Na} (mEq/l)	<20	>40
Urine/Plasma creatinine (U/P Cr)	>40	<20
Renal Failure Index (RFI)	<1	>1
Fractional excretion of sodium FE_{Na^+}	<1%	>1%
BUN/Cr ratio (mg/dL)	>20	≤10

- **Peak flow** (Figure 2)
  Peak flow for men (l/min) = **[3.95 − (0.0151 × age)] × ht** (cm)
  Peak flow for women (l/min) = **[2.93 − (0.0072 × age)] × ht** (cm)

- **Conversion factor between different units**
  kPa = 0.133 × mm Hg; **mm Hg** = 7.5 × kPa
  °F = (9/5°C) + 32; °C = 5/9(°F − 32)
  serum creatinine, mg/dL = mmol/l × 88.4
  serum urea, mg/dL = mmol/l × 2.8
  serum glucose, mg/dL = mmol/l × 18

References/further reading

1. Hope RA, Longmore JM, McManus SK, et al. *Oxford Handbook of Clinical Medicine*. 4th ed. Oxford: Oxford University Press; 1998:630–633.
2. Marino PL. *The ICU Book*. 2nd ed. Baltimore: Williams & Wilkins; 1998:340–342.
3. Nacouzi V. Fluids, electrolytes and acid-base disorders. In: Cline DH, Ma OJ, Tintinalli JE, et al, eds. *Emergency Medicine: A Comprehensive Study Guide* Companion Handbook. 5th ed. New York: McGraw-Hill; 2000:46–52.
4. James JH, Bosker G. Mathematical formulas, equations, and diagnostic aids in emergency medicine: Practical and systematic approaches to solving complex clinical problems. *Emerg Med Rep*. 1995;16(26):255–266.
5. David DN, Kelen GD. Acid-base disorder. In: Tintinalli JE, Kelen GD, Stapczynski JS, et al, eds. *Emergency Medicine: A Comprehensive Study Guide*. 5th ed. New York: McGraw-Hill; 2000:128–140.

127 Views of x-rays to order

Shirley Ooi

SKULL VIEWS

X-ray views	Indications	Remarks
Standard views		
1. Anteroposterior (AP)	Suspected vault fracture	Refer to *Trauma, Head* for indications of ordering skull XR
2. Lateral (right or left according to side of injury)	Suspected vault fracture Fluid in the sphenoidal sinus in base of skull fracture	
Additional views		
1. Towne's	Suspected occiput fracture	Can only be taken if cervical spine injury has been excluded.
2. Tangential	To evaluate suspected depressed skull fracture	

FACIAL VIEWS

Refer to *Trauma, Maxillofacial* for illustrations of the x-rays.

X-ray views	Indications	Remarks
1. 30-degree occipitomental (OM) view	Suspected maxilla, zygomatic complex and orbital floor fracture	This single view is enough as a radiologic screening for midface fractures. Refer to p. 469 for further explanation. Need to exclude cervical spine injury first
2. Submentovertical ('jug handle') view	Suspected zygomatic arch fracture	Need to exclude cervical spine injury first
3. Nasal bone (lateral view)	Suspected nasal bone fracture	This x-ray may not be necessary as management is based on clinical evaluation of deformity
4. Orthopantomogram (OPG) view	To visualize the whole of mandible for suspected fracture	If OPG view is not available, at the ED, 3 plain films, ie a PA and 2 oblique views of the mandible can be done instead

CERVICAL SPINE X-RAYS

- This is one of the 3 standard x-rays done in a multiple trauma victim.

Note: Following trauma, there is **no need** for **cervical spine x-ray** in any patient who meets **all** the criteria on p. 553.

- An important neck injury may still be present despite normal plain cervical spine x-rays. Clinical history and examination must always take precedence over apparently normal x-rays.

X-ray views	*Remarks*
1. Lateral (to include top of T_1 vertebral body)	In a multiple trauma patient a lateral cervical spine x-ray is the only view required in the initial phase.
Swimmer's view	Done if the C_7/T_1 junction is not visualized on lateral cervical spine x-ray. Sensitivity of lateral view alone ±swimmer's view is 85%. **Note**: If x-ray is done to exclude **FB**, the request should be '**x-ray neck (soft tissue lateral)**'.
2. Anteroposterior	Sensitivity of lateral, AP and open-mouth views combined is 92%.
3. Open mouth AP	To show the C_1-C_2 articulation.

ABDOMEN AND PELVIS VIEWS

X-ray views	*Indications*	*Remarks*
Standard views		
1. Supine AXR	To identify 'free' air/ pneumoperitoneum To indentify air/fluid interfaces To identify ectopic calcifications	**Note: The erect CXR is a fundamental part of the examination of an acute abdomen as it is the most sensitive x-ray for detecting a small pneumoperitoneum**. 1.0 ml of free air can be demonstrated
Additional views		
2. Erect AXR	Air-fluid levels	**Note**: Air-fluid levels are not pathognomonic of intestinal obstruction. Causes of air-fluid levels on erect AXR: 1. Ileus 2. Intestinal obstruction 3. Gastroenteritis
3. Left lateral decubitus	To visualize air-fluid levels or pneumoperitoneum in patients who are unable to sit upright or stand	

CHEST VIEWS

X-ray views	*Indications*	*Remarks*
Standard views		
1. PA or AP CXR		**PA CXR** should be obtained whenever possible as it enables a more accurate diagnosis of heart size and mediastinal width. **AP films** can be done supine or sitting. **Note**: Pneumothorax and pleural effusions are difficult to see on supine or upright portable CXR. In general CXR should be done in **full inspiration** Only **exception** is when a small pneumothorax or diagnosis of inhaled foreign body ('gas trapping') is suspected when an **expiratory film** is requested instead.
Specialized views		
2. Lateral CXR	Useful to confirm and localize: 1. Intrapulmonary opacities 2. Hilar abnormalities (adenopathy, masses, increased vascularity) 3. Cardiomegaly, heart chamber enlargement and aortic abnormalities 4. Small pleural effusions	Rarely useful in an emergency situation. **Note**: Retrosternal and retrocardiac regions are better seen on the lateral than on PA CXR.
3. Oblique CXR	Rib fractures	
4. Lateral decubitus CXR	Small pleural effusion and to differentiate from pleural thickening	PA CXR taken with patient lying on his or her side (usually abnormal side down)
5. Sternal view	Suspected fractured sternum	

THORACIC AND LUMBAR SPINE VIEWS

X-ray views	*Indications*
Standard views	
1. Lateral 2. Anteroposterior	Suspected malignancy with possible metastases to the spine History of significant trauma to spine Fever and tenderness suggesting osteomyelitis Acute, unexplained neurological deficit

UPPER LIMB VIEWS

Refer to *Trauma, Upper Limb* for x-ray examples.

X-ray views	Indications	Remarks
Shoulder		
1. AP	Standard view to evaluate shoulder pathology	
2. Axial view		Equivalent to looking up into patient's armpit. Disadvantages: 1. Abducting the injured arm may be painful 2. Pain may make it difficult to obtain a technically optimal film. 3. The head of the humerus sits on the glenoid. Orientation is easy; the fingers (the acromion and coracoid processes) always point anteriorly.
3. Y-scapular view		For patient who cannot abduct arm. Anterior is on the side of the rib cage.
4. Lateral transthoracic view	Only useful for assessing humeral fractures and not dislocation	
Humerus		
1. AP	Standard view for humeral injuries	
2. Lateral	Standard view for humeral injuries	
Elbow		
1. AP	Standard view for elbow injuries	**Note**: In normal patients, the posterior fat-pad is never visible as it is within the olecranon fossa, but the anterior fat-pad may be seen closely applied to the humerus. Whenever a posterior **fat-pad sign** or 'sail sign' is present, but no obvious fracture, look carefully for a radial head fracture in adult or supracondylar fracture of humerus, especially in children.
2. Lateral	Standard view for elbow injuries	

UPPER LIMB VIEWS (*continued*)

X-ray views	*Indications*	*Remarks*
3. Oblique	Only for subtle injuries of radial head and distal humerus	
Radius and ulna		
1. AP 2. Lateral	Standard view for forearm injuries	
Wrist		
1. AP 2. Lateral	Standard view for wrist/ distal forearm	
3. Scaphoid views	When scaphoid fracture suspected	These include PA and AP oblique with wrist in ulnar deviation besides the above 2 standard views.
Hand		
1. PA 2. PA oblique 3. Lateral	Standard views for hand injuries To visualize foreign bodies	**Note**: The standard radiograph projections of the whole hand are required to evaluate the base of the proximal phalanges and metacarpals.
Digits		
1. PA 2. Lateral	Standard views for injury to the digits	**Note**: When injury is confined to the distal end of a single digit, radiography should be limited to that digit.

LOWER LIMB VIEWS

X-ray views	*Indications*	*Remarks*
Hips		Do not order AP and lateral x-ray of hip. Instead order x-ray pelvis AP and lateral of hip. AP view of pelvis:
1. AP pelvis 2. Lateral view of that symptomatic joint	Standard view for hip injury	• Allows assessment and comparison of pelvic rami on both sides • A pubic ramus fracture can mimic signs and symptoms of a neck of femur fracture and may be missed on an AP view of hip.
Femur (Shaft) 1. AP 2. Lateral	Standard view for femoral shaft injuries	
Knee 1. AP 2. Lateral	Standard view for knee injuries	**Note**: A fat-fluid level within the suprapatellar bursa should be regarded as indicating an intraarticular fracture.
3. Skyline view	Special view; use in subtle fractures of: 1. femoral condyles (especially in lateral dislocation of patella) 2. patella	
Tibia/Fibula 1. AP 2. Lateral	Standard view for tibia/fibula injuries	
Ankle 1. AP 2. Lateral	Standard view for ankle injuries	
3. Axial view of calcaneum	Special view for calcaneal injuries (in addition to AP and lateral views of ankle)	
Foot 1. AP 2. Oblique	Standard view of foot injuries	

Index

Page numbers in **bold** print refer to main entries

Q